AF789572

Handbook of Experimental Pharmacology

Volume 84

Editorial Board

G.V.R. Born, London
P. Cuatrecasas, Research Triangle Park, NC
H. Herken, Berlin
A. Schwartz, Cincinnati, OH

Antituberculosis Drugs

Contributors

K. Bartmann · H. Iwainsky · H. H. Kleeberg · P. Mišoň
H. A. Offe · H. Otten · D. Tettenborn · L. Trnka

Editor
K. Bartmann

Springer-Verlag
Berlin Heidelberg New York
London Paris Tokyo

Professor Dr. med. KARL BARTMANN
Julius-Lucas-Weg 67
D-5600 Wuppertal 1

With 68 Figures

ISBN-13: 978-3-642-72875-4 e-ISBN-13: 978-3-642-72873-0
DOI: 10.1007/978-3-642-72873-0

Library of Congress Cataloging-in-Publication Data. Antituberculosis drugs. (Handbook of experimental pharmacology; v. 84) Includes bibliographies and index. 1. Antitubercular agents. 2. Tuberculosis – Chemotherapy. I. Bartmann, K. (Karl) II. Series. [DNLM: 1. Antitubercular Agents. W1 HA51L v. 84/QV 268 A633]
QP905.H3 vol. 84 615'.1 s 87-20782 [RC311.3.C45] [616.9'95061]
ISBN-13: 978-3-642-72875-4 (U.S.)

This work is subject to copyright. All rights are reserved, whether the whole or part of the material is concerned, specifically the rights of translation, reprinting, re-use of illustrations, recitation, broadcasting, reproduction on microfilms or in other ways, and storage in data banks. Duplication of this publication or parts thereof is only permitted under the provisions of the German Copyright Law of September 9, 1965, in its version of June 24, 1985, and a copyright fee must always be paid. Violations fall under the prosecution act of the German Copyright Law.

© Springer-Verlag Berlin Heidelberg 1988
Softcover reprint of the hardcover 1st edition 1988

The use of registered names, trademarks, etc. in this publication does not imply, even in the absence of a specific statement, that such names are exempt from the relevant protective laws and regulations and therefore free for general use.

Product liability: The publisher can give no guarantee for information about drug dosage and application thereof contained in this book. In every individual case the respective user must check its accuracy by consulting other pharmaceutical literature.

2122/3130-543210

List of Contributors

K. BARTMANN, Julius-Lucas-Weg 67, D-5600 Wuppertal 1

H. IWAINSKY, Forschungsinstitut für Lungenkrankheiten und Tuberkulose, Karower Str. 11, GDR-1115 Berlin-Buch

H. H. KLEEBERG, Tuberculosis Research Institute, Private Bag X 385, Pretoria 0001, South Africa

P. MIŠOŇ, Research Institute for Technical Development, Kobateky 1400, Prag 4, Czechoslovakia

H. A. OFFE, Charlottenburger Str. 19/C 512, D-3400 Göttingen-Geismar

H. OTTEN, Institut für Chemotherapie, Bayer AG, Postfach 91709, D-5600 Wuppertal 1

D. TETTENBORN, Bayer AG, Forschung und Entwicklung Medizin, Aprather Weg, Postfach, D-5600 Wuppertal 1

L. TRNKA, Research Institute for Tuberculosis and Respiratory Diseases, 18071 Praha 8 – Bulovka, Czechoslovakia

Preface

This volume deals specifically with those antituberculosis drugs which passed the preclinical phase and have been or are used in the treatment of tuberculosis and other mycobacterial diseases (except leprosy) in at least some parts of the world. Despite this restriction, there are 14 such drugs, and as a result this volume has reached rather large proportions. To prevent it from becoming even larger and more unwidely, most derivatives of antituberculotics have been omitted, especially where it is claimed that they provide only better bioavailibility or tolerability. Only in the chapter on the chemotherapy of diseases due to so-called atypical mycobacteria is the clinical use of the drugs described to a certain extent. In addition to antituberculotics, also discussed are antimicrobials which have been found to be effective against these mycobacteria.

The sequence in which the drugs are described is historical, reflecting not the time of discovery but rather the first clinical application. This order was selected for reasons which are now no longer relevant.

In this volume less emphasis is placed on detection, biological or synthetic production of antituberculotics, and structure-activity relationships. In contrast, emphasis is put on the degree, type, and mechanism of antimycobacterial activity, pharmacokinetics, and biotransformation in animals and man, on experimental pharmacodynamics, and on the toxicity of antituberculotics used therapeutically. Thus, all the information which is today designated "preclinical data" is dealt with in extenso. Also described in detail is how, slowly and over many years, experimental chemotherapy of tuberculosis has become increasingly adapted to clinical problems as models have been elaborated which are more and more representative and offer a more reliable basis for predictions. Animal experiments have played an indispensable role in this research and have saved numerous human lives.

With respect to the rationale of and the results obtained during the development of therapeutic regimens, the reader may profit from referring in the subject index to the entries "treatment of infected animals – combined; intermittent; in phases; preventive."

During the time covered by this volume (about 1945–1985), the classification of microorganisms has been refined, and consequently names have been changed to a considerable extent. When it proved impossible to reliably transpose old classifications and nomenclature into the current systems, the author's nomenclature is used.

Gaps in the information about the toxicology and/or biotransformation and pharmacokinetics of some of the antituberculotics, especially the older ones, should not be a cause of concern. We have followed the principle that all available data must be reported, but in the early days preclinical investigations were not as sophisticated as they are today and produced relatively little data. On the other hand, drugs like the tetracyclines, which have a very limited use in tuberculosis but widespread application against infections caused by rapidly growing bacteria, have undergone numerous tests and a great deal of data is available which must all be taken into account. For these types of drugs the reader can also consult other volumes of the *Handbook of Experimental Pharmacology:* volume 62 on aminoglycoside antibiotics, volume 67 on beta-lactam-antibiotics, and volume 78 on tetracyclines.

Tuberculosis is one of the few infectious diseases which require combined chemotherapy. Combinations of drugs are discussed in the section on the last mentioned single drug in the combination. For instance, combinations of isoniazid with *p*-aminosalicylic acid or streptomycin are dealt with in the section on isoniazid, but combinations of isoniazid with ethambutol or rifampicin in the sections on the latter drugs.

Abbreviations have generally been used for the antituberculotics. A list of these abbreviations is given on p. XXIV.

A severe barrier to obtaining comprehensive information is the multiplicity of languages used for scientific communication. The contributors have tried to take into consideration relevant publications in English, German, French, other Romance languages such as Italian, Spanish, and Rumanian, and in several Slavic languages such as Czech, Polish, and Russian. Because of their different mother tongues, the authors have been able to help each other in covering many languages, as the lists of references show.

It has taken a long time to complete this book. At times it was unclear whether we would ever be successful. Handbook-writing has, for most authors, become an almost unmanageable task as all are burdened with too many duties, mostly of a nonscientific nature. The editor wishes to express his sincere and warm thanks to the contributors, who not only finished their papers but, despite all difficulties, also updated them to the level of knowledge in 1985–1986.

Contributors and editor offer, many thanks to Professor Dr. HANS HERKEN for being our ever patient and encouraging representative of the Editorial Board over the many years as the authors struggled with their manuscripts.

The editor gratefully acknowledges a grant from Bayer AG for the translation of a considerable part of the book into English.

K. BARTMANN

Contents

CHAPTER 5

Experimental Pharmacology and Toxicology of Antituberculosis Drugs

List of Abbreviations for Antituberculotics and Some of Their Derivatives

Drug	*Abbreviation*
Capreomycin	CM
Cycloserine	CS
Ethambutol	EMB
Ethionamide	ETH
Isoniazid	INH
Kanamycin	KM
Morphazinamide	MZA
Oxytetracycline	OTC
Para-aminosalicylic acid	PAS
Protionamide	PTH
Pyrazinamide	PZA
Rifampicin	RMP
Streptomycin	SM
Terizidone	TZ
Tetracycline	TC
Thiocarlide	DATC
Thiosemicarbazone (Thioacetazone, Thiacetazone)	TSC
Viomycin	VM

CHAPTER 1

Historical Introduction and Chemical Characteristics of Antituberculosis Drugs

H. A. OFFE

A. p-Aminosalicylic Acid (PAS)

In 1940 BERNHEIM observed that virulent *Mycobacterium tuberculosis* cultures are stimulated in their respiration under the influence of small quantities of benzoic and salicylic acids without these acids themselves being oxidized. Subsequently LEHMANN (1946a, b) established that this stimulation is reversed at higher concentrations of salicylic acid. He therefore looked among the many salicylic acid derivatives for antimetabolites that, like the pair sulphanilamide-p-aminobenzoic acid, would be capable of competitively displacing salicylic acid from the reaction site. In 2-hydroxy-4-aminobenzoic acid, as described by SEIDEL in 1901 and by SEIDEL and BITTNER in 1902, Lehmann found a substance (PAS) that fulfilled his expectations and called it β_m-aminosalicylic acid. He also found that other hydroxyaminobenzoic acids did not have this inhibitory effect, and that the substance acts specifically only against *Mycobacterium tuberculosis* strains. Lehmann described not his fundamental microbiological metabolic experiments but also the animal-experimental and clinical studies he performed with PAS.

Industrially, PAS can be readily obtained in a variety of ways. The principal method for its manufacture (CIBA 1889) is the KOLBE-SCHMITT synthesis from m-aminophenol and carbon dioxide. However, on storage PAS decomposes unless special protective measures are taken, reverting to the starting materials. The m-aminophenol has no tuberculostatic activity and is less well tolerated.

The structural formula of PAS is as follows:

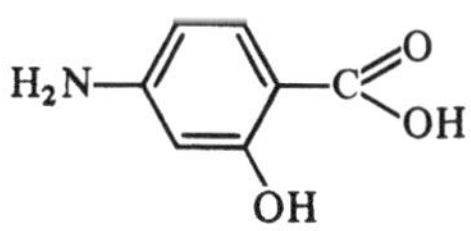

Its empirical formula is $C_7H_7NO_3$ (molecular weight 153.13). The acid crystallizes from alcohol-ether mixtures in colorless needles with a completely uncharacteristic melting point, since heating promotes the release of carbon dioxide. Melting points between 147 °C and 240 °C have been reported (BEILSTEIN 1973).

In water PAS is less well soluble than its salts, the hydrochloride and the sodium salt. 100 g of a saturated aqueous solution contains, at 15 °C, 0.185 g of PAS, this figure rising to 0.193 g at 37 °C. 100 g of a saturated alcoholic solution contains 4.5 g of PAS at room temperature, while a corresponding ethereal solution contains 1.2 g of PAS. PAS is more soluble in urine than in pure water.

The p-aminosalicylic acid hydrochloride, $C_7H_7NO_3 \cdot HCl$, has a melting point of 220 °C–229 °C and is readily soluble in water. The solution is strongly acidic and is more resistant to decarboxylation than PAS itself.

The sodium salt of p-aminosalicylic acid, $C_7H_6NO_3Na \cdot 2H_2O$ (molecular weight 211.1), is very soluble in water (1 g/2 ml). A 1% solution is practically neutral; it resists decarboxylation up to 100 °C but is not sterilizable by heat.

PAS reacts with iron(III) chloride to give a deep violet color. PAS can be detected in the urine with Ehrlich's reagent; it forms a yellowish-red precipitate. The concentrations of PAS and of its derivatives can be determined microbiologically by the vertical diffusion test. Many photometric and spectrophotometric methods of PAS analysis have been described, e.g., by CHARNEY and KUNA (1951). For a summary of these methods see OTTEN et al. (1975).

The taste of free PAS is described as sharp to bitter. For further data on its characteristics, impurities, and stability see HAIZMANN (1953).

References

Beilstein (1973) Handbuch der Organischen Chemie, 4. Aufl. Beilstein Institut für Literatur der Organischen Chemie (Hrsg). Springer, Berlin Heidelberg New York 3. Ergänzungswerk, Bd 14, 2. Teil, Syst Nr 1911, p 1436

Bernheim F (1940) The effect of salicylate on the oxygen uptake of the tubercle bacillus. Science 92:204; also 1941 J Bact 41:387–395

Charney J, Kuna M (1951) The spectrophotometric determination of para-aminosalicylic acid and its acetyl derivative in human urine. Am Rev Tuberc 64:577–578

Ciba (1889) DRP 50 835. Friedländer 2:139

Haizmann R (1953) Die Behandlung der Tuberkulose mit Para-Amino-Salicyl-Säure. Zentralbl Tbk forsch 62:1–208

Lehmann J (1946a) Chemotherapy of tuberculosis. The bacteriostatic action of p-aminosalicylic acid and closely related substances upon the tubercle bacillus, together with animal experiments and clinical trials. Sv Läkartidn 43:2029–2041

Lehmann J (1946b) p-Aminosalicylic acid in the treatment of tuberculosis. Lancet I: 15–16

Otten H, Plempel M, Siegenthaler W (1975) Antibiotika-Fibel, 4. Aufl. Thieme, Stuttgart, p 620

Seidel H (1901) Über Derivate der Nitrophtalsäuren. Ber dtsch Chem Ges 34:4351–4353

Seidel H, Bittner JC (1902) Darstellung der β_m-Aminosalicylsäure. Monatsh Chemie 23:431–433

B. Streptomycin (SM) – Dihydrostreptomycin (DHSM)

The inability of penicillin culture broths to act on gram-negative and tubercle bacilli led WAKSMAN to look among the soil fungi that he had long been working on (Actinomyces and Streptomyces species) for strains that did not have this deficiency (cf. BRUNNER 1962; HOFFMANN 1972). Besides several species whose metabolites did indeed inhibit gram-negative bacteria but were also toxic to mammals, Schatz and co-workers (SCHATZ et al. 1944) found in *Streptomyces griseus* a fungus whose culture filtrates had a relatively low toxicity and acted not only against some gram-negatives but also against mycobacteria. The active substance was named streptomycin after a fungus that Waksman had isolated and described as *Actinomyces griseus* as early as 1919 and which had since been renamed *Streptomyces griseus*.

Salts of streptomycin were then obtained in the pure form by adsorption, elution and precipitation techniques, and put to successful clinical use in the treatment of tuberculosis already in 1944.

In addition to SM, a number of related substances are found in the fermentation media of *Streptomyces griseus* or other fungal species (see HOFFMANN 1972 for review): streptomycin B, mannosidostreptomycin, dihydrostreptomycin, dihydrostreptomycin B, reticulin = hydroxystreptomycin, mannosidohydroxystreptomycin, and demethylstreptomycin. Apart from dihydrostreptomycin, none of these have acquired any therapeutic significance. The dihydro derivative was used for some time, but is no longer recommended.

Elucidation of the structure of SM revealed that SM is a strongly basic glycoside (an aminoglycoside) as a result of its guanido groups (Gu) and one amino group. Its empirical formula is $C_{21}H_{39}N_7O_{12}$ and its molecular weight 581.58.

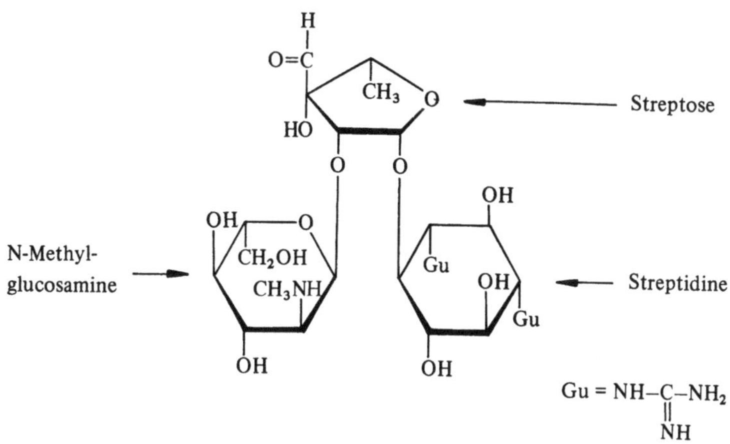

Within the glycoside inositol substituted with two guanido groups – streptidine – is connected via 5-desoxy-3-aldehydo-l-lyxose, or streptose, with N-methyl-2-l-glucosamine. The formation of numerous derivatives with carbonyl reagents and the reaction with fuchsin sulphurous acid suggests the presence of an aldehyde group (in the streptose constituent) in SM. Against this is the fact that the IR and NMR spectra of SM sulphate fail to show the bands characteristic of a C=O group. From this ARONSON et al. (1964) concluded that an intramolecular reaction occurs between the $-NCH_3$ and the aldehyde group, so that a carbinolamine structure must also be borne in mind as a possibility. Moreover, this could be in equilibrium with a cyclic imonium salt. Equilibria between the three structures is also possible.

Free SM is a colorless substance that dissolves in water with a strong basic reaction and decomposes soon after being isolated. Its solubility in organic solvents is low. The methylamino group and the two guanido groups give rise to the formation of virtually neutral salts with three equivalents of acid. A detailed summary of salts with inorganic and organic acids, and of double salts, e.g., with $CaCl_2$ and complex compounds, will be found in HOFFMANN (1972).

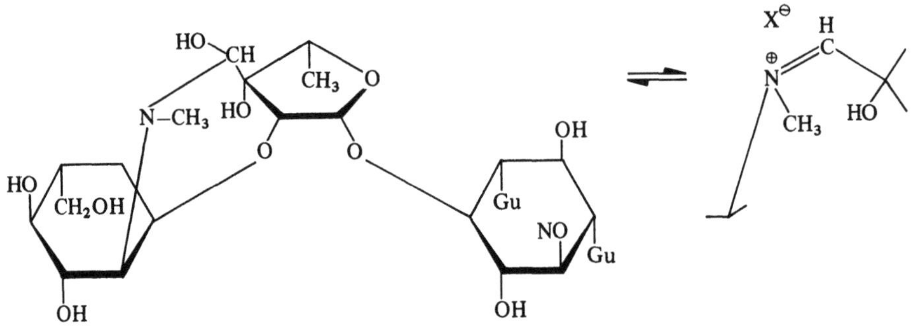

Carbinolamine Cycl. imonium salt

Of the salts, the sulphate is used most commonly for therapeutic purposes. SM sulphate [$(C_{21}H_{39}N_7O_{12})_2 \cdot 3\,H_2SO_4$; molecular weight 1457.42] is a solid, colorless substance with good stability (unlike the free base) when dry, although so far it has only been obtained in an amorphous state. It contains 79.8% of SM. SM sulphate is readily soluble in water at room temperature (more than 2%). The specific rotation $[\alpha]_D^{25}$ of an aqueous solution (c=1) is -79 °. It is stable for a prolonged period over a wide range of pH (3–8). For further data on its stability, especially at higher temperatures, see OTTEN et al. (1975) and HOFFMANN (1972).

In attempts to titrate SM in the presence of methyl orange (helianthine) as indicator, the poorly soluble SM helianthate is precipitated out.

SM was only successfully synthesized 30 years after the isolation of the natural product (UMEZAWA et al. 1974a, b). The presence of 15 optical asymmetric centres was a particular difficulty. Although the laborious total synthesis is of considerable scientific interest, it has no relevance for easier accessibility of SM. The three characteristic degradation products of SM, N-methylglucosamine (KUEHL et al. 1947), streptose (DYER et al. 1965) and streptidine (WOLFRAM et al. 1950) were synthesized at a substantially earlier stage.

SM can be determined microbiologically and by chemical methods. A microbiological method due to SABATH et al. (1971) makes use of a slight modification of the standard agar diffusion method. The characteristic reaction of SM (in contrast to dihydro-SM) on treatment with strong alkali leads to the formation of maltol, whose violet color reaction with iron(III) chloride constitutes the basis for colorimetric SM determinations (SCHENCK and SPIELMAN 1945). The absorption of maltol itself (274 nm in 0.1 N HCl, 317 nm in 0.1 N NaOH) can likewise be used for analytical determination of SM (BOXER et al. 1947).

DHSM has a CH_2OH-group in the streptose-moiety instead of the CHO-group of SM.

References

Aronson J, Meyer WL, Brock TD (1964) A molecular model for chemical and biological differences between streptomycin and dihydrostreptomycin. Nature (Lond) 202:555–557

Boxer GE, Jelinek VC, Leghorn PM (1947) The colorimetric determination of streptomycin in clinical preparations, urine and broth. J Biol Chem 169:153–165
Brunner R (1962) Die Antibiotica, Band 1, 2. Teil, 1–2. Carl, Nürnberg
Dyer JR, McGonigal WE, Rice KC (1965) Streptomycin. II. Streptose. J Am Chem Soc 87:654–655
Hoffmann H (1972) In: Erhart G, Ruschig H (Hrsg) Arzneimittel, 2. Aufl, Bd 4, Teil 1. Verlag Chemie, Weinheim, pp 314–315
Kuehl FA, Flynn EH, Holly FW, Mozingo R, Folkers K (1947) Streptomycin antibiotics XV. N-methyl-glucosamin. J Am Chem Soc 69:3032–3035
Otten A, Plempel M, Siegenthaler H (1975) Antibiotika-Fibel, 4. Aufl. Thieme, Stuttgart, p 390
Sabath LD, Casey JI, Ruch PA, Stumpf LE, Finland M (1971) Rapid microassay of gentamycin, kanamycin, neomycin, streptomycin, and vancomycin in serum or plasma. J Lab Clin Med 78:457–463
Schatz A, Bugie E, Waksman SA (1944) Streptomycin, a substance exhibiting antibiotic activity against gram-positive and gram-negative bacteria. Proc Soc Exp Biol Med 55:66–69
Schenck JR, Spielman MA (1945) The formation of maltol by the degradation of streptomycin. J Am Chem Soc 67:2276–2277
Umezawa S, Takahashi Y, Usui T, Tsuchiya T (1974a) Total synthesis of streptomycin. J Antibiot 27:997–999
Abstr 14th Interscience Conf on Antimicrob Agents and Chemother, Session 33. San Francisco
Umezawa S, Takahashi Y, Usui T, Tsuchiya T (1974b) Total synthesis of streptomycin
Wolfram ML, Olin SM, Polgiase WJ (1950) A synthesis of streptidine. J Am Chem Soc 72:1724–1729

C. Thiosemicarbazone (TSC) [Thioacetazone, Thiacetazone, p-Acetaminobenzaldehyde]

After investigations on sulphonamides had revealed that thiazole and thiodiazole derivatives such as (I) (Domagk and Hegler 1942) exert a certain influence on mycobacteria, work on this class of substances gathered further impetus.

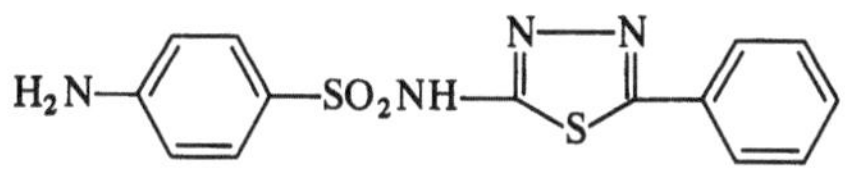

I

It was found (Domagk et al. 1946) that one of the preliminary products (III) used for the synthesis of phenylamino-thiodiazole (II), possessed a much greater tuberculostatic activity. In experiments at modifying this benzaldehyde-thiosemicarbazone (III) (Behnisch et al. 1948, 1950), it was found that replacement of the sulphur by oxygen or the =NH-group attenuated the effect and, moreover, that

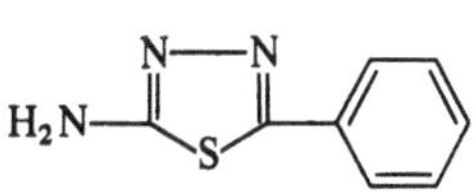

II

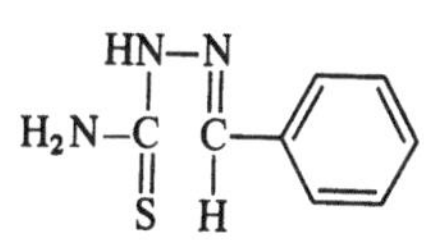

III

thiosemicarbazones of aliphatic aldehydes and ketones were of no interest in this context. In contrast to this, the use of aromatic aldehydes, especially p-substituted, and of some heterocyclic aldehydes yielded products that exerted an influence on mycobacteria not only in vitro but also in vivo (Domagk 1948) and subsequently in clinical practice as well (HEILMEYER 1949). Out of these compounds p-acetaminobenzaldehyde-thiosemicarbazone = acetylamino-benzaldehyde-thiosemicarbazone = amithiozone = thiacetazone = Tibione = TB I/698 = Conteben = TSC was selected for therapeutic application in 1946.

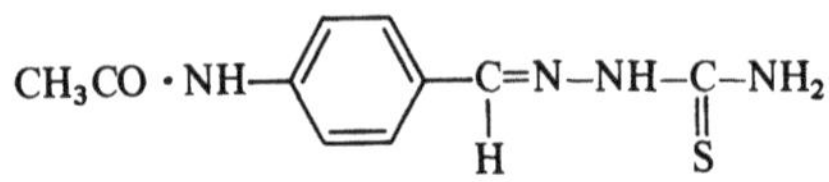

TSC

TSC has the empirical formula $C_{10}H_{12}N_4OS$ (molecular weight 236.29). In its manufacture it is precipitated from the aqueous-alcoholic solution in the form of yellow crystals that melt with decomposition at 233 °C.

The compound is moderately soluble in water: 88 µg/ml at 20 °C and 172 µg/ml at 37 °C (BEHNISCH et al. 1950). It is substantially more soluble in the blood serum and urine (BEHNISCH et al. 1950), as also in aqueous solutions at pH > 7.5. Its solubility in 50% sulphuric acid is 10%. 5% solutions for intracavernous injection can be made up with 50% aqueous antipyrine solution (POLSTER 1950). TSC is moderately to poorly soluble in most organic solvents; 40 mg/ml dissolves in methylacetamide and 10 mg/ml in propylene glycol.

Some 60%–70% of people find the taste of TSC bitter (KUHN and ZILLIKEN 1950). This perception of taste goes hand in hand with that for monophenylthiourea and is seemingly genetically determined. The correlation between intolerance and the bitter taste perception was studied by KNÜCHEL (1950).

TSC forms complexes with heavy metal salts. The grey-green copper complexes have been described, among others, by CARL and MARQUARDT (1950).

TSC can be determined biologically by the serial dilution test; many chemical methods have also been described, most of them based on removal of the acetyl group, subsequent diazotization, and coupling. Among other compounds, methyl (WILDE 1950), ethyl (WERNITZ 1950), phenyl (WOLLENBERG 1950), and aminoethyl (HEILMEYER and HEILMEYER 1950) derivatives of α-naphthylamine have been used for coupling with the diazonium compound. The dyes formed are subjected to colorimetry either directly or after extraction with amyl alcohol.

References

Behnisch R, Mietzsch F, Schmidt H (1948) Neue schwefelhaltige Chemotherapeutica. Angewandte Chemie 60:113–115

Behnisch R, Mietzsch F, Schmidt H (1950) Chemical studies on thiosemicarbazones with particular reference to antituberculous activity. Am Rev Tuberc 61:1–7

Carl E, Marquardt P (1950) Kupferkomplexbildung und tuberkulostatische Chemotherapeutica. Z Naturforsch 4b:280–283

Domagk G, Hegler C (1942) Chemotherapie der bakteriellen Infektionen. Hirzel, Leipzig, p 136–137

Domagk G, Behnisch R, Mietzsch F, Schmidt H (1946) Über eine neue, gegen Tuberkelbazillen in vitro wirksame Verbindungsklasse. Naturwissenschaften 33:315

Domagk G (1948) Die experimentellen Grundlagen einer Chemotherapie der Tuberkulose. Beitr Klin Tuberk 101:367–394

Heilmeyer L (1949) Die Chemotherapie der Tuberkulose. Dtsch Med Wochenschr 74:161–167

Heilmeyer J, Heilmeyer L (1950) Quantitative Bestimmung kleiner Mengen von Benzaldehydthiosemicarbazon und dessen Derivaten (TBI/698) in Körperflüssigkeiten. Arch Exp Path Pharmakol 210:424–430
Knüchel W (1950) Beziehung zwischen Geschmack und Verträglichkeit von Conteben. Neue Med Welt 1:1487
Kuhn R, Zilliken F (1950) Über den Geschmack von p-Acetaminobenzaldehyd-thiosemicarbazon. Naturwissenschaften 37:167
Polster W (1950) Zur Lösung von Conteben in Wasser für intravenöse Injektionen. Tbk Arzt 4:594–595
Short EI (1961) The detection of thiacetazone in urine. Tubercle (Lond) 42:524–528
Wernitz W (1950) Eine photometrische Nachweismethode des TBI/698 im Harn. Klin Wochenschr 28:200–201
Wilde W (1950) Nachweis von TBI/698 in Körpersäften und Sekreten. Med Monatsschr 4:106–107
Wollenberg O (1950) Über die kolorimetrische Bestimmung von Thiosemicarbazonen im Harn. Dtsch Med Wochenschr 75:899–902

D. Pyrazinamide (PZA)

CHORINE's observation (1945) that nicotinamide (I) has an effect on the growth of mycobacteria led not only to one of the ways by which isoniazid is obtained (cf. p. 8) but also gave rise to the discovery of the antituberculotic activity (YEAGER et al. 1952) of the very similar pyrazine-2-carboxylic acid amide (II).

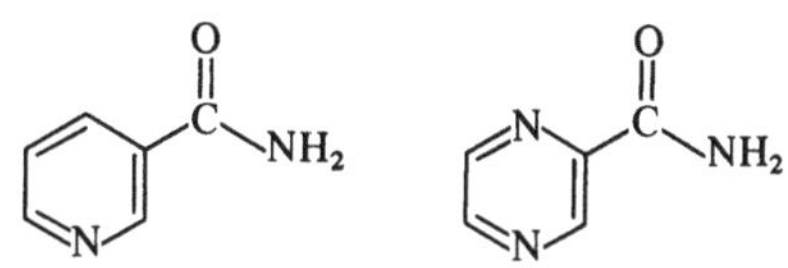

I II

The activity of PZA was reported by the working groups at Lederle Laboratories (KUSHNER et al. 1952) and at Merck Laboratories in the USA (SOLOTOROVSKY et al. 1952).

Like PAS (1901) and INH (1912), PZA had already been known for some time (DALMER and WALTER 1936; HALL and SPOERRI 1940) and was manufactured, among other things, as an intermediate for the synthesis of 2-aminopyrazine which was being investigated as an antibacterial agent. However, PZA itself was evidently not studied for antibacterial activity.

PZA has the empirical formula $C_5H_5N_3O$ (molecular weight 123.1) and melts at 188 °C–189 °C. At room temperature it dissolves to the extent of 1.5% in water, forming a stable solution; it is poorly soluble in organic solvents.

With sodium nitroprusside (sodium nitropentacyanoferrate) PZA gives rise to an orange color, even in low concentrations, this color being detectable in the urine of people treated with PZA (RAO et al. 1956; KRAUS et al. 1961). The color can be measured photometrically (λ_{max} = 495 nm) in samples containing more than 10 µg/ml (STOTTMEIER et al. 1969). PZA has been determined microbiologically in the vertical diffusion test by STOTTMEIER et al.

Morphazinamide ($C_{10}H_{14}N_4O_2$, molecular weight 222.2) is a further development of PZA. It is obtained from PZA with morpholine and formaldehyde by the Mannich reaction. In the body PZA is formed by hydrolysis, the reverse of this reaction.

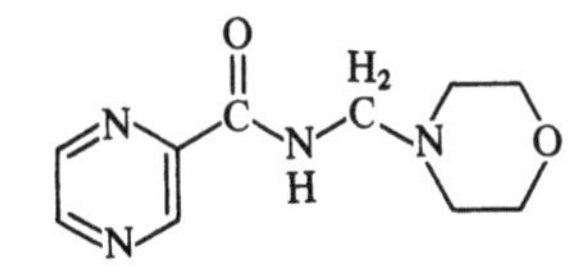

References

Chorine V (1945) Action de l'amide nicotinique sur les bacilles du genre Mycobacterium. C R Acad Sci (Paris) 220:150–151
Dalmer O, Walter E (1936) Verfahren zur Herstellung von Derivaten der Pyrazinmonocarbonsäure. DRP 632:257
Ellard GA (1969) Absorption, metabolism and excretion of pyrazinamide in man. Tubercle (Lond) 50:144–158
Felder E, Tiepolo K (1962) Verfahren zur Herstellung von Pyrazincarbonsäure-aminomethylamiden. DAS 1129:492
Hall SA, Spoerri PE (1940) Syntheses in the pyrazine series. II. Preparation and properties of aminopyrazine. J Am Chem Soc 62:664–665
Kraus P, Krausová E, Šimáně Z (1961) A paper strip test for detection of cycloserine and pyrazinamide in urine. Tubercle (Lond) 42:521–523
Kushner S, Dalalian H, Sanjurjo JL, Bach FL Jr, Safir SR, Smith VK Jr, Williams JH (1952) Experimental chemotherapy of tuberculosis. II. The synthesis of pyrazinamides and related compounds. J Am Chem Soc 74:3617–3621
Rao KVN, Eidus CVJ, Tripathy SP (1965) A simple test for the detection of pyrazinamide and cycloserine in urine. Tubercle (Lond) 46:199–205
Solotorovsky M, Gregory FJ, Ironsin EJ, Bugie EJ, O'Neill RC, Pfister K (1952) Pyrazinoic acid amide an agent active against experimental murine tuberculosis. Proc Soc Exp Biol Med 79:563–565
Stottmeier KD, Beam RE, Kubica GP (1969) The absorption and excretion of pyrazinamide (PZA) in rabbits and tuberculous patients. Trans 27th Pulm Dis Res Conf VAAF:16
Yeager RL, Munroe WGC, Dessau FL (1952) Pyrazinamide (Aldinamide) in the treatment of pulmonary tuberculosis. Am Rev Tuberc 65:523–534

E. Isoniazid (INH)

Isonicotinic acid hydrazide (isonicotinoylhydrazine, pyridine-4-carboxylic acid hydrazide, isoniazid, INH) was first prepared by MEYER and MALLY (1912) at the German Charles University in Prague from ethyl isonicotinate and hydrazine hydrate. For 38 years no one saw any reason to study INH for its suitability as an antituberculotic, especially since GARDNER (1951), while studying the chemically very similar product obtained from the reaction of hydroxylamine with ethyl isonicotinate, had failed to observe any tuberculostatic activity.

The effect of nicotinic acid amide discovered by CHORINE (1945) led H. FOX to start a search for antituberculotic agents among pyridine derivatives. After many other pyridine derivatives it was the turn of the thiosemicarbazone of pyridine-4-aldehyde (BEHNISCH et al. 1948; LEVADITI et al. 1951, 1952; FOX 1951), to be tested. In contrast to the methods used by earlier investigators, the requisite pyridine-4-aldehyde was prepared via isonicotinic acid ester (I), isonicotinoylhydrazine (II), and benzenesulphonylisonicotinoylhydrazine (III) and immediately reacted with thiosemicarbazide (IV) to thiosemicarbazone (V).

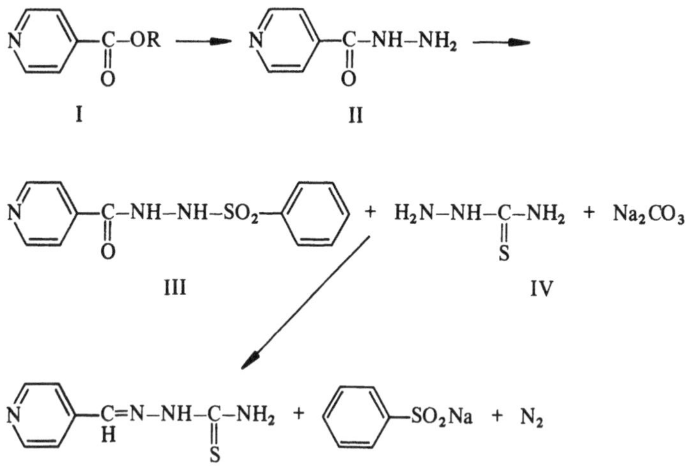

V

Investigation of all the products of this reaction sequence revealed that I and III were inactive, while V had an activity comparable to that of TSC (cf. p. 5). According to GRUNBERG and SCHNITZER (1952), on the other hand, in animal experiments the intermediate product II, INH, surpassed all known agents in its activity.

OFFE et al. (1952a, b) started from very different preconditions. Comparison of TSC (VI) with phthalic hydrazide derivatives (VII) by BUU-HOI et al. (1949) suggested a systematic modification of structure VIII common to VI and VII (OFFE et al. 1952a, b). DOMAGK (1951) found the benzalhydrazone VIII (R_1=H, R_2=phenyl, R_3=pyridyl) to be highly active. The isonicotinic acid hydrazide upon which this hydrazone is based, the 526th preparation, proved to be best of the entire series investigated (OFFE et al. 1952a–c).

In 1952 the companies to which the two working groups belonged, namely F. Hoffmann La Roche u. Co. AG in Basle and Farbenfabriken Bayer AG in Leverkusen, issued a joint statement that "after combined consideration of the relevant

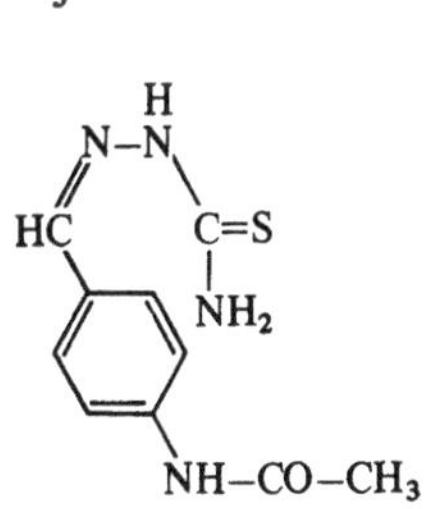

VI

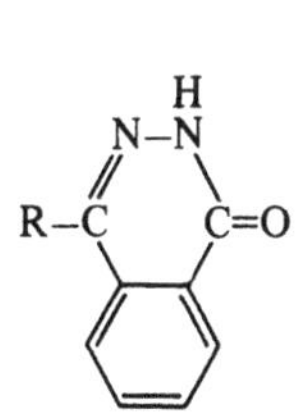

VII

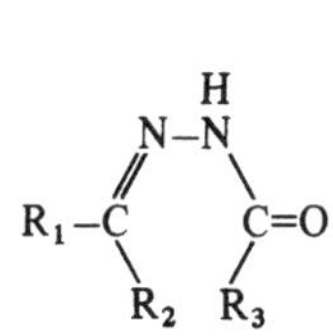

VIII

findings, within the framework of completely independent research in the sphere of tuberculosis, they had both found the hydrazide of isonicotinic acid to be antituberculotic. The two companies had independently of each other started clinical tests on isonicotinic acid hydrazide in 1951".

At the same time as the two above-mentioned groups, BERNSTEIN et al. (1952), at the Squibb Institute for Medical Research, discovered that INH was an antituberculotic agent. The latter company did not give out any information about their method of producing INH.

INH has the empirical formula $C_6H_7N_3O$ (molecular weight 137.15). Its solubility in water is 13% at 22 °C and 25% at 37 °C. It is 20% soluble in boiling methanol and ethanol and only about 2.5% soluble in methanol and ethanol at 20 °C. INH is poorly soluble in organic solvents immiscible with water. It reacts easily with acetone, with the formation of a soluble hydrazone. A very detailed review of the chemical, physico-chemical, and physical properties of isoniazid was published by KRÜGER-THIEMER in 1956.

Isoniazid can be determined by microbiological and chemical methods. The microbiological techniques are particularly suitable for quantitative assays in tissues. There is a very wide variety of chemical detection and determination methods, some of which are also used for metabolite determinations. A detailed summary has been given by OTTEN et al. (1975). Techniques used in the last years are polarography (SUSHKIN and GUZEEVA 1978) and gaschromatography (FRÁTER-SCHRÖDER and ZBINDEN 1976) or gaschromatography combined with mass spectrometry (LAUTERBURG et al. 1981).

INH forms complexes with many heavy metal salts. It reduces ammoniacal silver salt solutions yielding silvered mirrors. It reacts easily with aldehydes and ketones to give hydrazones, as is also the case with physiological and food constituents such as glucose, pyruvic acid, and oxalacetic acid. These reaction products are encountered as typical metabolites of INH, as well as acetylisonicotinoylhydrazine (acetyl INH), diisonicotinoylhydrazine, N-isonicotinoyl-glycine (isonicotinuric acid), and isonicotinic acid.

Attempts have been made to modify INH chemically to obtain isoniazid derivatives with improved pharmacokinetic, toxicological, and antituberculotic properties, especially for combatting the INH-resistant mycobacteria. Reviews by KRÜGER-THIEMER (1956), OFFE (1956), and BERNSTEIN et al. (1953a, b) show that although some derivatives do approach INH in activity and exhibit one advantage or another, on the whole isoniazid is superior to them all in activity.

References

Behnisch R, Mietzsch F, Schmidt H (1948) Verfahren zur Herstellung von Thiosemicarbazonen. DBP 927:505

Bernstein J, Lott WA, Steinberg BA, Yale HL (1952) Chemotherapy of experimental tuberculosis. V. Isonicotinic acid hydrazide (Nydrazid) and related compounds. Am Rev Tuberc 65:357–364

Bernstein J, Jambor WP, Lott WA, Pansy F, Steinberg BA, Yale HL (1953a) Chemotherapy of experimental tuberculosis. IV. Derivatives of isoniazid. Am Rev Tuberc 67:354–365

Bernstein J, Jambor WP, Lott WA, Pansy F, Steinberg BA, Yale HL (1953b) Chemotherapy of experimental tuberculosis. VII. Heterocyclic acid hydrazides and derivatives. Am Rev Tuberc 67:366–375
Buu-Hoi NP, Dechamps G, Hoán N, Le Bihan H, Ratsimamanga AR, Binon F (1949) Dérivés de la phtalazine d'intérêt biologique. Comptes Rendues de l'Academie de Sciences 228:2037–2039 [cited from Ann Inst Pasteur 72:580 (1946)]
Chorine V (1945) Action de l'amide nicotinique sur les bacilles du genre Mycobacterium. C R Acad Sci (Paris) 220:150–151
Domagk G (1951) O. V. Bollinger-Vorlesung München, 13. Dez. 1951
Domagk G, Offe HA, Siefken W (1952) Weiterentwicklung der Chemotherapie der Tuberkulose. Beitr Klin Tuberk 107:325–337
Fox HH (1951) Synthetic tuberculostatics show promise. Chem Eng News 29:3963–3964
Fox HH, Gibas JT (1952) Synthetic tuberculostats. IV. Pyridine carboxylic acid hydrazides and benzoic acid hydrazides. J Org Chem 17:1653–1660
Fratér-Schröder M, Zbinden G (1976) A gaschromatographic assay for the determination of isoniazid N-acetylation; observation in rats with induced constant urine flow. EXPEAM 32:767
Gardner TS, Wenis E, Smith FA (1951) The synthesis of compounds for the chemotherapy of tuberculosis. II. Hydroxamic acid derivatives. J Am Chem Soc 73:5455–5456
Grunberg E, Schnitzer RJ (1952) Studies on the activity of hydrazine derivatives of isonicotinic acid in the experimental tuberculosis of mice. Quart Bull Sea View Hosp 13:3–11
F. Hoffmann La Roche + Co. AG und Farbenfabriken Bayer AG (1952) Experientia 8:364
Jouin JP, Buu Hoi NP (1946) De l'activité des représentants de quelques séries chimiques sur la pousse du bacille de Koch. Ann Inst Pasteur 72:580–606 (see p 590)
Krüger-Thiemer E (1956) Chemie des Isoniazids. J Ber Borstel 3:192–424
Krüger-Thiemer E (1958) Biochemie des Isoniazids. J Ber Borstel 4:299–509
Lauterburg BH, Smith CV, Mitchell JR (1981) Determination of isoniazid and its hydrazino metabolites, acetylisoniazid, acetylhydrazine, and diacetylhydrazine in human plasma by gaschromatography-mass spectrometry. J Chromatogr 224:431–438
Levaditi C, Girard R, Vaisman A, Ray A (1951) Comparison entre le GHOG de Girard et le TB I de Domagk du point de vue de leur activité antituberculeuse chez la souris. C R Soc Biol (Paris) 145:60–65
Levaditi C, Girard R, Vaisman A, Ray A (1952) Activité antituberculeuse de la γ-pyridinealdéhydethiosemicarbazone (G 527), isomere du G 469. Ann Inst Pasteur 82:102–104
Meyer H, Mally J (1912) Über Hydrazinderivate der Pyridincarbonsäuren. Monatsh Chemie 33:393–414
Offe HA, Siefken W, Domagk G (1952a) Neoteben, ein neues hochwirksames Tuberculostaticum und die Beziehungen zwischen Konstitution und tuberculostatischer Wirksamkeit bei Hydrazinderivaten. Naturwissenschaften 39:118 119
Offe HA, Siefken W, Domagk G (1952b) Hydrazinderivate und ihre Wirksamkeit gegenüber Mycobacterium tuberculosis. Z Naturforsch 7b:446–462
Offe HA, Siefken W, Domagk G (1952c) Hydrazinderivate aus Pyridincarbonsäuren mit Carbonylverbindungen und ihre Wirksamkeit gegenüber Mycobacterium tuberculosis. Z Naturforsch 7b:462–468
Offe HA (1956) Konstitution und tuberkulostatische Wirksamkeit in der Neotebenreihe. Medizin und Chemie 5:130–141
Otten H, Plempel M, Siegenthaler W (1975) Antibiotika-Fibel, 4. Aufl. Thieme, Stuttgart, p 599–601
Sushkin AG, Guzeeva SA (1978) Polarographic determination of isoniazid in the urine. Prob Tuberk 56, issue 7:76–79

F. Tetracyclines

We shall consider here only the two tetracyclines used in the treatment of tuberculosis, namely oxytetracycline (Terramycin) = OTC and tetracycline = TC.

I. Oxytetracycline (Terramycin, OTC)

Oxytetracycline (OTC) is the result of systematic screening of soil samples collected all over the world for antibiotic-producing microorganisms. It was discovered and isolated in the Biochemical Research Laboratories of Chas. Pfizer and Co. Inc. (KANE et al. 1950/51). OTC is produced by *Streptomyces rimosus*. In the initial isolation, a culture filtrate of the microorganism was extracted with n-butanol and transferred into dilute acid to give a crude concentrate. Chromatography on Florisil yielded a high potency fraction which was purified further by extracting into butanol and re-extracting into dilute acid. Pure crystalline OTC dihydrate was obtained by dissolving the crude material in dilute acid adjusting to neutrality with alkali and repeating this procedure (REGNA and SOLOMONS 1950/51).

The empirical formula of the free base is $C_{22}H_{24}O_9N_2$ and the molecular weight 460.4. The basic structure of tetracyclines is formed by 1,4,4a,5,5a,6,11,12a-octahydronaphthacene with the two chromophoric regions A and BCD (see Fig. 1). The characteristic substituents are given in Table 1.

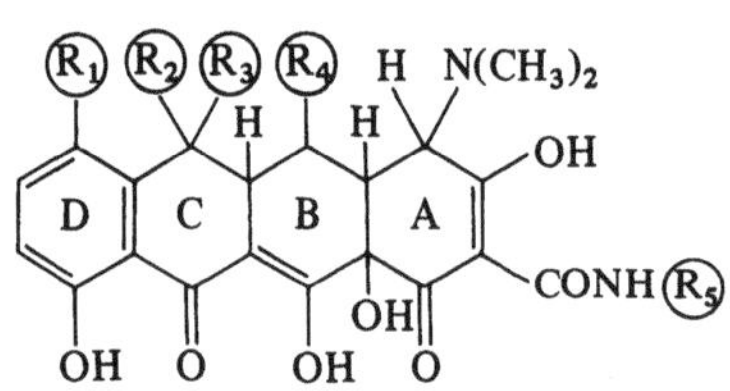

Fig. 1. The basic structure of tetracyclines

Table 1. Substituents of OTC and TC

	R_1	R_2	R_3	R_4	R_5
OTC	H	CH_3	OH	OH	H
TC	H	CH_3	OH	H	H

The tetracyclines are yellow, crystalline, odorless, photosensitive, amphoteric compounds with a bitter taste. Titration of OTC hydrochloride in aqueous solutions gave pK values of 3.5, 7.6, and 9.2. The anhydrous substance melts with decomposition at 181 °C–182 °C. The crystals of OTC dihydrate have the following refractive indices: $\alpha = 1.634$, $\beta = 1.646$, $\gamma = >1.70$. OTC is optically active. The $[\alpha]_D^{25}$ for c = 1% in methanol is +26.5 ° (REGNA and SOLOMONS 1950/51). The tetracyclines have typical UV-absorption spectra. In 0.1 *M* phosphate buffer of

Table 2. Solubilities of OTC in various solvents (mg/dl) at 25 °C (REGNA and SOLOMONS 1950)

Solvent	Free base	Hydro-chloride	Sodium salt
Water, pH 1.2	314		
pH 5.0	0.5		
pH 7.0	1.1		
pH 9.0	386		
Ethanol	120	120	80
Methanol	200	300	15
Acetone	70	25	20
Butanol	1.9	33	110
Dioxan	90	53	80
Acetic acid	–	3000	–

pH 4.5 OTC dihydrate has an $E_{1\,cm}^{1\%}$ of 240 at 249 nm, 322 at 276 nm, and 301 at 353 nm. The spectrum is pH-dependent. In methanol OTC hydrochloride has an $E_{1\,cm}^{1\%}$ of 331 at 265 nm and 283 at 366 nm. In the infrared characteristic absorption bands are found between 650 cm^{-1} and 3600 cm^{-1}. In aqueous solutions OTC fluoresces yellow in the pH range of 5–10.

The solubilities of the base, the hydrochloride, and the sodium salt in various solvents are listed in Table 2. The solubility in water is strongly pH-dependent, with a minimum between pH 3 and 7 and with maxima at pH 1.2 and 8–9 (Table 2). In the dry crystalline state OTC and its hydrochloride do not exhibit any demonstrable loss of biological potency after prolonged storage. When stored at 50 °C for 4 months the hydrochloride loses less than 5% of its activity. OTC can be heated to 100 °C for 4 days without any loss of activity. The stability of the aqueous solutions depends on the pH; it is greatest at pH 1.0 to 2.5, remaining intact for at least 30 days under these conditions at both 5 °C and 25 °C. The same applies to solutions with a pH between 3.0 and 9.0 at 5 °C.

In accordance with their amphoteric character, the tetracyclines form complexes with metal cations and inorganic and organic anions as well as with neutral substances (e.g., urea, caffeine, polyvinylpyrrolidine) and biopolymers such as serum albumin, lipoproteins, globulins, and RNA. The first method of determination was a microbiological one – turbidimetric assay with Klebsiella pneumoniae (KERSEY 1950). Chemical methods are based on fluorescence of the tetracyclines, which is intensified by chelate formation with metal cations (CASWELL and HUTCHISON 1971; MANI and FOLTRAN 1971). With nickel sulphate OTC and TC form 1:1 complexes which can be determined complexometrically (ŠŤÁHLAVSKÁ et al. 1972). The concentration of tetracyclines can be determined by high-performance liquid chromatography, though this does necessitate certain preparatory measures (PRYDE and GILBERT 1979).

II. Tetracycline (TC)

Following the clarification of the chemical structure of chlortetracycline (aureomycin), tetracycline was obtained in the course of a catalytic hydrogenation of aureomycin (BOOTHE et al. 1953; CONOVER et al. 1953). Soon thereafter MINIERI et al. (1953/54) described its isolation from the culture filtrate of *Streptomyces viridifaciens*.

Its empirical formula is $C_{22}H_{24}N_2O_8$ and its molecular weight 444.4. The structure is given in Fig. 1 and Table 1. The anhydrous base melts with decomposition at 170 °C to 175 °C. It crystallizes in orthorhombic needles with refractive indices $\alpha = 1.57$, $\beta = 1.64$ and $\gamma = 1.75$. The substance is optically active ($[\alpha]_D^{25} = -239°$ for c = 1% in methanol). The pK values are 3.30, 7.68, and 9.69. The UV spectrum maxima are at 220, 268, and 355 nm for solutions in 0.1 N HCl.

Table 3. Solubility of TC in various solvents (mg/dl) at 28 ± 4 °C (FRANK and RIEDL 1962)

Solvent	Free base	Hydrochloride
Water	170	1090
Ethanol	>2000	790
Methanol	>2000	>2000
Acetone	1740	75
Dioxan	1460	770
Ethyl acetate	1730	75

The dry substance remains stable for months even at room temperature. The solubilities of TC and TC·HCl in various solvents are listed in Table 3. The stability of TC is greater than that of OTC in neutral solution but somewhat lower in alkaline solution.

Complex formation and the detection methods are the same as for OTC.

References

Boothe JH, Morton II J, Petisi JP, Wilkinson RG, Williams JH (1953) Tetracycline. J Am Chem Soc 75:4621

Boothe JH, Morton II J, Petisi JP, Wilkinson RG, Williams JH (1953/54) Chemistry of tetracycline. Antibiotics Annual, pp 46–48

Caswell AH, Hutchison JD (1971) Selectivity of cation chelation to tetracyclines: evidence for special conformation of calcium chelate. Biochem Biophys Res Commun 43:625–630

Conover LH, Moreland WT, English AR, Stephens CR, Pilgrim FJ (1953) Terramycin. XI. Tetracycline. J Am Chem Soc 75:4622–4623

Dürckheimer W (1975) Tetracycline: Chemie, Biochemie und Struktur-Wirkungsbeziehungen. Angew Chem 87:751–764

Frank A, Riedl K (1962) Tetracycline. Chemie und Eigenschaften. In: Brunner R, Machek G (Hrsg) Die Antibiotika Bd I, Teil 2. Hans Carl, Nürnberg, pp 314–375

Kane JH, Finlay AC, Sobin BA (1950/51) Antimicrobial agents from natural sources. Ann NY Acad Sci 53:226–228

Kersey RC (1950) A turbidimetric assay for terramycin. J Am Pharm Assoc Scientific Ed XXXIX:252–253

Mani J-C, Foltran G (1971) Fluorescence des chélates des tétracyclines. Bull Soc Chim Fr: 4141–4146
Minieri PP, Firman MC, Mistretta AG, Abbey A, Bricker CE, Rigler NE, Sokol H (1953/54) A new broad spectrum antibiotic product of the tetracycline group. Antibiotics Annual: 81–87
Pryde A, Gilbert MT (1979) Applications of high performance liquid chromatography. Chapman and Hall, London New York
Regna PP, Solomons IA (1950) The chemical and physical properties of terramycin. Ann NY Acad Sci 53:229–237
Šťáhlavská A, Tawakkol MS, Slánský V, Fršlinková M (1972) Komplexometrische Gehaltsbestimmung einiger Tetracyclin-Antibiotica und von Chloramphenicol. Pharmazie 27:456–457

G. Viomycin (VM)

Viomycin, an antibiotic very similar to capreomycin (see p. 25), was isolated by BARTZ et al. (1951) from *Streptomyces floridae* and in the same year by FINLAY et al. (1951) from *Streptomyces puniceus*. It was later isolated as vinactin A from *Streptomyces vinaceus* by MAYER et al. (1954) and found to be identical with tuberactinomycin B from *Streptomyces griseoverticillatus* var. *tuberacticus* by IZUMI et al. (1972) and NODA et al. (1972). The tuberactinomycins A, N, and O produced by the latter organism are very similar to VM and SM.

Viomycin ($C_{25}H_{43}N_{13}O_{10}$, molecular weight 685), a pale yellowish powder, is a strong base that forms salts, among them a sulphate, pantothenate, picrate, reineckate, pantothenate-sulphate, and a hydrochloride-hydrobromide. The sulphate (decomposition point 280 °C) is soluble in water (7.8 mg/ml), forming a weakly acidic solution that remains stable over a few days. $[\alpha]_D^{25} = -32$ ° (c of the sulphate in water = 1). Its solubility in organic solvents is low. A characteristic feature of VM, as of CM, is the UV-absorption: at 268 nm ($\varepsilon = 24\,000$) in acidic and neutral media and at 282.5 nm in alkaline media. The Sakaguchi, biuret, and ninhydrin tests are all positive and the maltol, Molisch and Benedict tests negative. VM can be determined spectrophotometrically in Seignette's salt solution in the presence of copper sulphate (532 nm).

On vigorous acid hydrolysis VM yields two l-serines (Ser), one l-α,β-diaminopropionic acid (Dapr), one l-β-lysine (β-lys), and one viomycidin (Vd), as well as one urea and a little carbon dioxide and ammonia. After hydrogenation of VM, capreomycidine is isolated in the course of hydrolysis in place of Vd (cf. p. 25–26).

The amino acid sequence in the cyclic peptide now seems to be confirmed. Whereas initially (BYCROFT et al. 1971) the sequence assumed for CM:

β-Lys-Dapr-Chromophore-Dapr-Ala-Capreomycidine (ring bracket from Dapr to Capreomycidine)

was extrapolated as follows to the VM molecule:

β-Lys-Dapr-Chromophore-Ser-Ser-Vd, (ring bracket from Dapr to Vd) the sequence:

β-Lys-Dapr-Ser-Ser-Chromophore-Vd

is now regarded as correct (BYCROFT 1972). It may be that there is an analogous sequence for CM. A ureidodehydroserine residue is regarded as the chromophore and source of the urea in hydrolysis, the following structure thus emerging for VM:

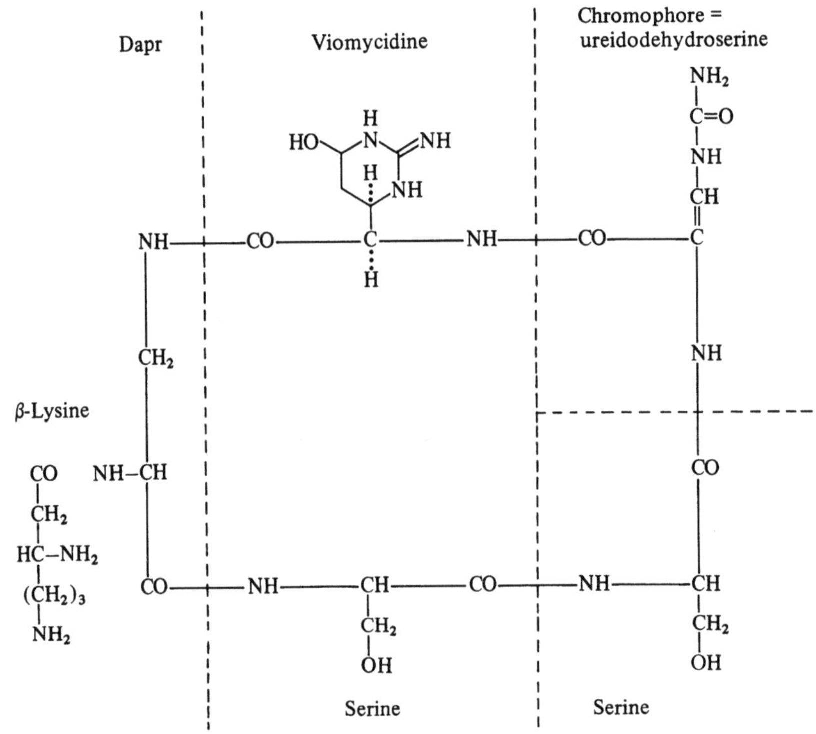

A review of the methods for the determination of VM has been published by OTTEN et al. (1975). Spectroscopically, VM is characterized by strong UV-absorption at 268 nm ($\varepsilon = 24000$) in neutral and acid media, this absorption shifting to 285 nm ($\varepsilon = 15000$) in 0.1 N sodium hydroxide (BYCROFT et al. 1971). When investigated spectrophotometrically in Fehling's solution, VM exhibits absorption at 532 nm (OTTEN loco cit.).

References

Bartz QR, Ehrlich J, Mold JD, Penner MA, Smith RM (1951) Viomycin, a new tuberculostatic antibiotic. Am Rev Tuberc 63:4–6

Bycroft BW, Cameron D, Croft LR, Hassanali-Walji A, Johnson AW, Webb T (1971) The total structure of viomycin, a tuberculostatic peptide antibiotic. Experientia 27:501–503

Bycroft BW (1972) The crystal structure of viomycin, a tuberculostatic antibiotic. J C S Chem Comm: 660–661
Finlay AC, Hobby GL, Hochstein F, Lees TM, Lenert TF, Means JA, P'An SY, Regna PP, Routien JB, Sobin BA, Tate KB, Kane JH (1951) Viomycin, a new antibiotic active against mycobacteria. Am Rev Tuberc 63:1–3
Izumi R, Noda T, Ando T, Take T, Nagata A (1972) Studies on tuberactinomycin III. Isolation and characterization of two minor components tuberactinomycin B and tuberactinomycin O. J Antibiot 25:201–207
Mayer RL, Eisman PS, Konopka EH (1954) Antituberculosis activity of vinactane. Experientia 10:335–336
Noda T, Take T, Nagata A, Wakamiya T, Shiba T (1972) Chemical studies on tuberactinomycin III. The chemical structure of viomycin (tuberactinomycin B). J Antibiot 25:427–428
Otten H, Plempel M, Siegenthaler W (1975) Antibiotika-Fibel. 4. Aufl. Thieme, Stuttgart, p 657

H. Cycloserine (CS)

In 1952 Kurosawa isolated from Streptomyces "K 300", under the name of orientomycin, an antibiotic that later (1956/57) proved to be identical with one obtained in 1955 from *Streptomyces lavendulae* (Shull and Sardinas 1955), *Streptomyces orchidaceus* (Hidy et al. 1955; Harned et al. 1955), and *Streptomyces garyphalus* (Kuehl et al. 1955). After the structural had been clarified it was recognized as a cyclic derivative of serinehydroxamic acid and was given the generic name cycloserine (CS).

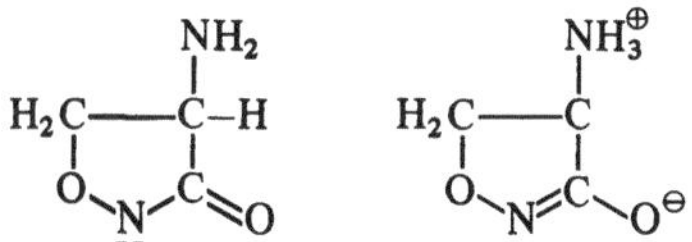

Cycloserine

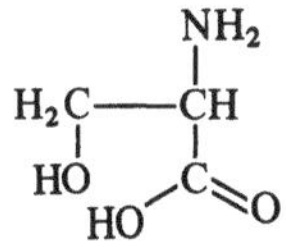

Serine

Its chemical designations include D-4-aminoisoxalidine-3-one and D-4-aminoisoxalidinone. Apart from being obtained by fermentation, the compound can also be synthesized (Folkers et al. 1955; Plattner et al. 1957). As a substance with an asymmetric centre, it occurs in the D- and L-forms. Only the D-form, which also occurs as a natural product, is referred to as cycloserine.

CS has the empirical formula $C_3H_6N_2O_2$ (molecular weight 102.09) and forms colorless crystals said to melt between 152 °C and 156 °C. The substance is readily soluble in water. Its specific rotation (see Freerksen et al. 1959 for a review) of $[\alpha]_D^{25} = 116$ ° (c=1.17 in water) and $[\alpha]_{5461}^{25} = +137 \pm 2$ ° (c=5 in 2 N HCl) depends to some extent on concentration and the pH. As an amphoteric substance, CS forms both a hydrochloride and salts with metals. It has a UV absorption maximum at 219 nm–226 nm. Its isoelectric point is at pH 6.0. In acidic and neutral solutions CS is relatively easily hydrolyzed, as is also the case in solutions that contain proteins (FREERKSEN et al. 1959). CS is largely stable in alkaline media (FUST et al. 1958). Sterile solutions should not be prepared by thermal treatment but by sterile filtration. Apart from methanol, CS is poorly soluble in organic solvents. It can be concentrated from dilute solutions by cation exchangers.

CS can be determined both microbiologically and chemically. A detailed review of the methods has been given by IWAINSKY et al. (1970). The blue color given with alkaline sodium nitroprusside after subsequent treatment with acetic acid (RAO et al. 1965) offers a suitable method for qualitative detection, spots containing 1.6 µg thus being discernible on paper (FREERKSEN et al. 1959, p 319). According to JONES (1957), the sodium nitroprusside method can also be used for spectrophotometry (FREERKSEN 1959, p 321). CS gives a brownish-yellow color with ninhydrin.

By reaction of CS with terephthalaldehyde an azomethin is formed, the Terizidone:

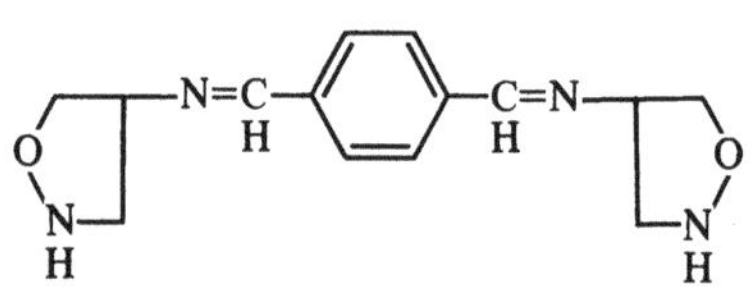

It has the empirical formula $C_{14}H_{14}N_4O_4$ (molecular weight 302.25). The antibacterial activity and the side reactions are similar to CS (BIANCHI et al. 1965).

References

Bianchi S, Felder E, Tiepolo U (1965) Terizidone. Una nuova base di Schiff della D-cicloserina. Il Farmaco (Ed Pr) 20:366–371

Eidus L (1968) Kontrollmethoden zum Nachweis der Tuberkulostatica zweiter Ordnung im Urin. Beitr Klin Tuberk 137:196–203

Folkers K, Stammer CH, Wilson AN, Holly FW (1955) Synthesis of D-4-amino-3-isoxazolidone. J Am Chem Soc 77:2346–2347

Freerksen E, Krüger-Thiemer E, Rosenfeld M (1959) Cycloserin (D-4-amino-isoxazolidin-3-on). Antibiot Chemother 6:303–396

Fust B (1958) D-Cycloserin. Die Medizinische 12:470–478

Harned RL, Hidy PH, Kropp la Baw EK (1955) Cycloserine. I. A preliminary report. Antibiot Chemother 5:204–205

Hidy PH, Hodge EH, Young VV, Harned RL, Brewer GA, Philipps WF, Runge WR, Stavely HE, Pohland A, Boas H, Sullivan HR (1955) Structure and reaction of cycloserine. J Am Chem Soc 77:2345–2346

Iwainsky H, Grunert M, Reutgen H, Sehrt I (1970) Nachweis und Bestimmung antituberkulös wirksamer Verbindungen. Pharmazie 25:505–513

Jones LR (1956) Colorimetric determination of cycloserine, a new antibiotic. Analyt Chem 28:39–41

Kuehl FA, Wolf FJ, Trenner NR, Peck RL, Howe E, Hunnewell BD, Downing G, Newstead E, Folkers K (1955) D-4-amino-3-isooxazolidone, a new antibiotic. J Am Chem Soc 77:2344–2345

Kurosawa H (1952) Studies on the antibiotic substances from actinomyces. XXIII. The isolation of an antibiotic produced by a strain of streptomyces "K 30". J Antibiot Ser B 5:682–688

Plattner PA, Boller A, Frick H, Fuerst A, Hegedues B, Kirschensteiner H, Majnoni St, Schlaepfer R, Spiegelberg H (1957) Synthesen des 4-amino-3-isoxalidinons (Cycloserin) und einiger Analoga. Helv Chim Acta 40:1531–1552
Rao KVN, Eidus L, Jacob CV, Tripathy SP (1965) A simple test for the detection of pyrazinamide and cycloserine in urine. Tubercle 46:199–205
Shull GM, Sardinas JL (1955) Pa-94, an antibiotic identical with D-4-amino-3-isoxalidinone. Antibiot Chemother 5:398–399

I. Thioamides: Ethionamide (ETH) – Protionamide (PTH)

The antituberculotic effect of nicotinamide (I) (CHORINE 1945) and INH (OFFE et al. 1952; BERNSTEIN et al. 1952; Fox et al. 1952) suggested that a closer investigation of the various pyridinecarboxylic acid derivatives might prove useful. Whereas pyridine-2-carboxylic acid (picolinic acid) failed to yield any derivatives with appreciable activity apart from the hydrazide, and in the case of pyridine-3-carboxylic acid (nicotinic acid), (I) proved to have the peak activity, modification at the carboxyl group and alkylation of pyridine-4-carboxylic acid (isonicotinic acid) did lead to some interesting new products.

Table 1. Antituberculotic activity of various pyridine-carboxylic acid amides. The activity is indicated as (+) to (+++) or (−)

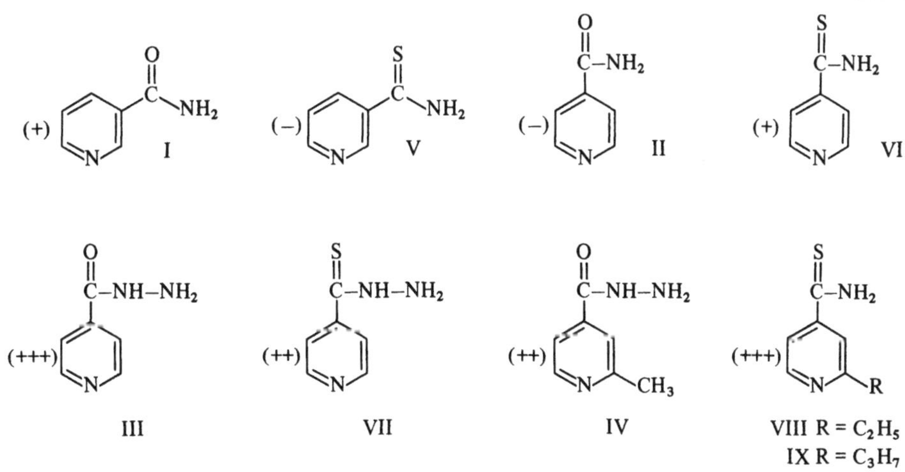

The incorporation of sulphur in the acid amide group of (I) resulted in the inactive thioamide V. Similarly, thio-INH (VII) was less active (KÖNIG et al. 1954), than INH (III). Alkyl substitution of isoniazid (III) in position 2 to give IV reduced the effect if the substituents contained more than one carbon atom (EFIMOVSKY and RUMPF 1954; ISLER et al. 1955). On the other hand, exchanging the oxygen for sulphur in the $CONH_2$-group of the basically inactive isonicotinamide (II) to give isonicotinic acid thioamide (VI) gave rise to marked activity

(Gardner et al. 1954; Meltzer et al. 1955). Substance (VI) is too toxic to be used in therapy. Substitution in position 2 of compound (VI) by alkyl groups (VIII, IX) reduced the toxicity and gave rise to the therapeutically usable compounds 2-ethylthioisonicotinamide (= ethionamide, ETH, Aetina, VIII) and 2-n-propylthioisonicotinamide (protionamide, PTH, IX) (Grumbach et al. 1956).

Ethionamide (ETH) is obtained in yellow crystals with a melting point of 166 °C. Its empirical formula is $C_8H_{10}N_2S$ and its molecular weight 166 (Libermann et al. 1956). Protionamide (PTH) likewise forms yellow crystals and has a melting point of 142 °C. Its empirical formula is $C_9H_{12}N_2S$ and its molecular weight 180. Both ETH and PTH are stable in the dry state and both are poorly soluble in water. Dimethyl sulphoxide dissolves them to the extent of about 40%, while their solubility in alcohol and dimethylformamide is considerable. Both thioamides are not very resistant to acids and alkalis. Oxygen and oxidizing agents result in the formation of the thioamide-S-oxides, which have been observed as metabolites and have also been found to exhibit antituberculotic activity.

In vitro, i.e., under the various conditions in liquid nutrient media, ETH and its sulphoxide are partially inactivated (Grunert et al. 1968); ETH remains unaffected by blood and gastric juice after 24 h whereas under the same conditions ETH sulphoxide is degraded in blood. The stability findings relating to ETH may as a rule be extrapolated to PTH. A synopsis by Bieder et al. (1966) provides information on the ETH metabolites excreted with the urine: as a result of S-oxidation, N-methylation, desulphurization, and deamination, the following are formed during the metabolism of ETH: ETH sulphoxide, 2-ethylisonicotinamide, 2-ethylisonicotinic acid, and the N-methyl compounds 1-methyl-2-ethyl-4-thiocarbamoylpyridinium, 1-methyl-2-ethyl-4-carbamoyl-6-oxodihydropyridine, 1-methyl-2-ethyl-4-thiocarbamoyl-6-oxodihydropyridine, 1-methyl-2-ethyl-4-S-oxothiocarbamoyl-6-oxodihydropyridine, 1-methyl-2-ethyl-4-carbamoylpyridinium. The three 6-oxo derivatives exhibit blue fluorescence on UV irradiation.

Besides its microbiological determination in the vertical diffusion test, ETH can be determined by chemical methods that are also applicable to PTH (Pütter 1964, 1972; Harnanansingh and Eidus 1970). Use is made here of the absorption of the yellow sulphoxide at 400 nm after extraction of the test samples with ether or chloroform. The absorption of ETH can be checked by the same principle (Eidus and Harnanansingh 1968) or by making use of the blue-fluorescing metabolite if its presence is accentuated with potassium ferricyanide (Eidus 1968). A polarographic method has been described by Tikhonov et al. (1976).

References

Bernstein J, Lott WA, Steinberg BA, Yale HL (1952) Chemotherapy of experimental tuberculosis. V. Isonicotinic acid hydrazide (Nydrazid) and related compounds. Am Rev Tuberc 65:357–364

Bieder A, Brunel P, Mazeau L (1966) Identification de trois nouveau métabolites de l'éthionamide: chromatographie, spectrophotometrie, polarographie. Ann Pharm Fr 24:493–500

Chorine V (1945) Action de l'amide nicotinique sur les bacilles du genre Mycobacterium. C R Acad Sci (Paris) 220:150–152

Efimovsky O, Rumpf P (1954) Recherches sur l'acide méthyl-2-pyridine-carboxylique-4. Bull Soc Chim Fr 1954:648–649
Eidus L (1968) Kontrollmethoden zum Nachweis der Tuberkulostatica zweiter Ordnung im Urin. Beitr Klin Tuberk 137:196–203
Eidus L, Harnanansingh AMT (1968) A urine test for control of ingestion of ethionamide. Am Rev Resp Dis 98:315–316
Fox HH, Gibas JT (1952) Synthetic tuberculostats. IV. Pyridine carboxylic acid hydrazides and benzoic azid hydrazides. J Org Chem 17:1653–1660
Gardner TS, Wenis E, Lee J (1954) The synthesis of compounds for the chemotherapy of tuberculosis. IV. The amide function. J Org Chem 19:753–757
Grumbach F, Rist N, Libermann D, Moyeux M, Cals S, Clavel S (1956) Activité antituberculeuse expérimentale de certains thioamides isonicotiniques substitués sur le noyau. C R Acad Sci 242:2187–2189
Grunert M, Werner E, Iwainsky H, Eule H (1968) Veränderungen des Äthionamides und seines Sulfoxydes in vitro. Beitr Klin Tuberk 138:68–82
Harnanansingh AMT, Eidus L (1970) Micro method for the determination of ethionamide in serum. Int J Clin Pharmacol 3:128–131
Isler O, Gutmann H, Straub O, Fust B, Boehni E, Studer A (1955) Chemotherapie der experimentellen Tuberkulose. II. Kernsubstituierte Isonicotinsäurehydrazide. Helv Chim Acta 38:1033–1046
König HB, Siefken W, Offe HA (1954) Schwefelhaltige Derivate von Pyridincarbonsäuren und davon abgeleitete Verbindungen. Chem Ber 87:825–834
Libermann D, Moyeux M, Rist N, Grumbach F (1956) Sur la préparation de nouveaux thioamides pyridiniques actifs dans la tuberculose expérimentale. C R Acad Sci (Paris) 242:2409–2412
Meltzer RJ, Lewis AD, King JA (1955) Antituberculous substances. IV. Thioamides. J Am Chem Soc 77:4062–4066
Offe HA, Siefken W, Domagk G (1952) Neoteben, ein neues hochwirksames Tuberculostaticum und die Beziehungen zwischen Konstitution und tuberculostatischer Wirksamkeit von Hydrazinderivaten. Naturwissenschaften 39:118–119
Pütter J (1964) Photometrische Bestimmung des 2-Äthyl-isothionicotinylamid in Organen und Körperflüssigkeiten. Arzneim Forsch 14:1198–1203
Pütter J (1972) Bestimmung von Prothionamid und Äthionamid sowie den entsprechenden Sulfoxiden im Blutplasma. Arzneim Forsch 22:1027–1031
Tikhonov VA, Grigalyunas AP, Guzeeva SA (1976) Polarographic investigation of the blood ethionamide and prothionamide concentration in patients with tuberculosis of the lungs. Prob Tuberk 54, issue 5:75–78

J. Kanamycin (KM)

In the course of systematic screening of Streptomyces species for their ability to inhibit both gram-negative and gram-positive bacteria and, in addition, for the absence of toxicity giving rise to delayed damage, a mixture of three basic antibiotics fulfilling these requirements was isolated from Streptomyces K2J, a newly isolated soil fungus (UMEZAWA et al. 1957; TAKEUCHI et al. 1957). The hitherto unknown fungus was given the name *Streptomyces kanamyceticus* and the antibiotics were called Kanamycin A, B, and C. Of these three, under specific fermentation conditions Kanamycin A makes up the greatest part of the mixture and, because of its lower toxicity, embodies the therapeutically useful principle.

By intensive acid hydrolysis KM is degraded to three fragments, whose closer examination (CRON et al. 1958) revealed that KM A had an aminoglycoside structure.

Kanamycin A (KM) is concentrated from the culture broths by exchange resins and is purified via salt formation. It cannot be extracted from aqueous solutions with ethyl acetate (UMEZAWA et al. 1957). However, it can be extracted from the aqueous solution at pH 7–9 into solvents immiscible with water if stearic acid, dichlorophenol, or the like has been added (MEIDA et al. 1957).

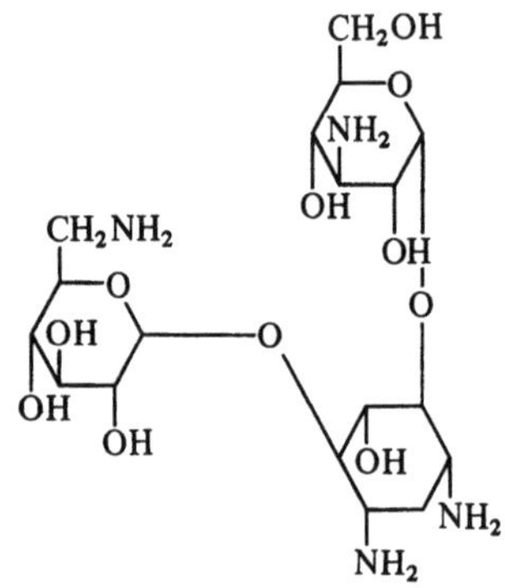

The free KM base ($C_{18}H_{36}N_4O_{11}$: molecular weight 484.50) is not used. It is soluble in water, but not in organic solvents. Many kanamycin salts are prepared in the crystalline state, some of which are used. After dissolution in 0.1 N sulphuric acid, the optical rotation of KM is $[\alpha]_D^{24} = +146°$ (c=1) (CRON et al. 1958). KM sulphate ($C_{18}H_{36}N_4O_{11} \cdot H_2SO_4$; molecular weight 582.58) decomposes at temperatures of around 250 °C. It crystallizes as the monohydrate (molecular weight 600.58) and the water of hydration is difficult to remove. In water the rotation of its plane of polarization is $\alpha_D^{23} = +121°$ (c=1) (MEIDA et al. 1957). It is readily soluble in water (360 mg/ml) but not easily soluble in 50% methanol (5 mg/ml). The pH of the aqueous solution (10 mg/ml) is 7.8. The pH-dependence of the solubility ranges from 770 mg/ml at pH 3 to 200 mg/ml at pH 8 (GRANATEK et al. 1960). Other water-miscible solvents, such as alcohol and tetrahydrofuran, cause KM sulphate to crystallize out from the aqueous solution.

Crystalline KM hydrochloride can be obtained from KM sulphate. The reineckate (salt of $[(NH_3)_2Cr(SCN)_4]H$) is suitable for isolation purposes. The picrate, helianthate, and flavianate are precipitated out of aqueous solutions as poorly soluble salts. Salts with sulphurous acid, higher alkyl sulphuric acids, C-substituted hydroxymethanesulphonic acids, citric acid, 3-phenylsalicylic acid, and glucuronic acid are described for special uses [see HOFFMANN (1972) for a summary].

For a substance of this constitution the stability of KM and its salts is unusually good. In the dry state KM and its salts are resistant to decomposition for a long time (GRANATEK et al. 1960). In aqueous solution, especially at pH 6–8, KM remains stable for many months. After boiling in 5% aqueous ammonia for 1 h, 90% of the activity is preserved. The sulphate can be heated in water for an hour with only 5% loss of activity. By contrast, the molecule is destroyed by boiling for 15 min in 4 N hydrochloric acid.

KM dissolved in pyridine gives a positive ninhydrin reaction. The Molisch test (red) and the Elson-Morgan test are positive, while the Sakaguchi test, the maltol test, and reactions with reducing sugars are negative. If KM is heated to 100 °C for 100 min with 40% sulphuric acid, a substance with the UV spectrum of furfurol (275 nm–280 nm) is obtained.

UMEZAWA et al. (1968a) succeeded in the complete synthesis of KM A and also (UMEZAWA et al. 1968b) of KM C. The complete syntheses play no part in the accessibility of the kanamycins, although partial-synthetic modifications of the kanamycins are relevant; amongst these an aminohydroxybutyric acid derivative of kanamycin A, amikacin (=BB-K8) has become of interest for infections due to gramnegative pathogens.

Chemical, physical, microbiological, and enzymatic methods are available for the detection and determination of KM (for a review see OTTEN et al. 1975). For simple determination in 3 h, possibly in the presence of penicillin and cephalosporin antibiotics, use is made of a method based on the inhibition of the pH increase in urea solutions such as is caused by Proteus mirabilis (NOONE et al. 1971). In addition, KM can be detected by high-performance liquid chromatography (PRYDE and GILBERT 1979).

References

Cron UJ, Fardig OB, Johnson DL, Palermiti FM, Schmitz H, Hooper IR (1958) The chemistry of kanamycin. Ann NY Acad Sci 76:27–30

Granatek AP, Duda S, Buckwalter FH (1960) Pharmaceutical properties and stability of kanamycin. Antibiot Chemother 10:148–156

Hoffmann H (1972) Antibiotika. Kanamycin. In: Ehrhart G, Ruschig H (Hrsg) Arzneimittel, Bd 4, Teil 1. Verlag Chemie, Weinheim, pp 354–358

Meida K, Ueda M, Yagishita K, Kawaji S, Kondo S, Murase M, Takeuchi T, Okami Y, Umezawa H (1957) Studies on kanamycin. J Antibiot Jpn Ser A 10:228–231

Noone P, Pattison IR, Samson D (1971) A simple rapid method for assay of aminoglycoside antibiotics. Lancet II:16

Otten H, Plempel M, Siegenthaler W (1975) Antibiotika-Fibel. 4. Aufl. Thieme, Stuttgart, p 408

Pryde A, Gilbert MT (1979) Application of high performance liquid chromatography. Chapman and Hall, London New York

Takeuchi T, Hikiji T, Nitta K, Yamazaki S, Abe S, Takayama H, Umezawa H (1957) Biological studies on kanamycin. J Antibiot Jpn Ser A 10:107–114

Umezawa H, Ueda M, Maeda K, Yagishita K, Kondo S, Okami Y, Utahara R, Osato Y, Nitta K, Takeuchi T (1957) Production and isolation of a new antibiotic, kanamycin. J Antibiot Jpn Ser A 10:181–188

Umezawa S, Tatsuta K, Koto S (1968a) The total synthesis of kanamycin A. J Antibiot Jpn 21:367–369

Umezawa S, Koto S, Tatsuta K, Tsumura T (1968b) The total synthesis of kanamycin C. J Antibiot Jpn 21:162–163

K. Thiocarlide (DATC)

After the thiocarbazones (I) had been successfully modified, it seemed a good idea to try further variations of these thiocarboxylic acid amides with the aim of discovering more effective antituberculotic agents. These endeavours led on the one hand to the thioamides (II), such as ETH and PTH (see the relevant sections), and on the other hand to the derivatives (III) with two aromatic or heterocyclic rings (HUEBNER et al. 1953).

I 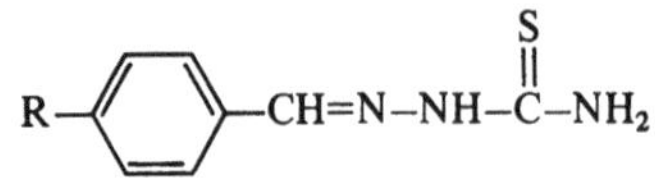

II 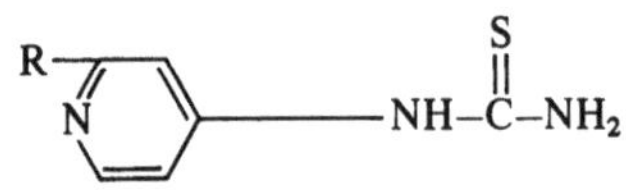

III 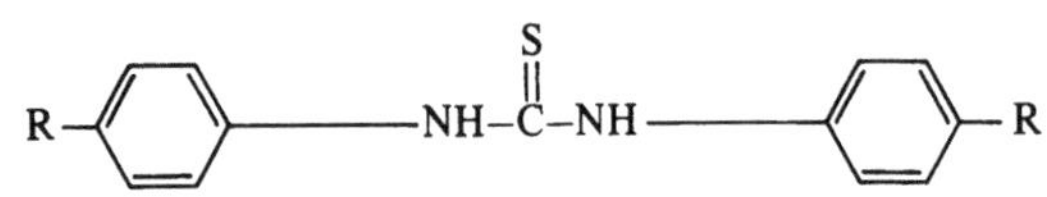

Many of these compounds display antimycobacterial activity, a fact that prompted their study for the treatment of leprosy and tuberculosis. Although some of them are used outside Germany for both these indications, only thiocarlide (DATC) [III,R = $(CH_3)_2CH$-CH_2-CH_2-O-) is still used in the Federal Republic of Germany.[1]

Thiocarlide, 4,4′-diisoamyloxy-N,N′-diphenylthiourea, 4,4′-diisoamyloxythiocarbanilide, DATC, is obtained inter alia from the corresponding amyloxyaniline with that type of mustard oil, which in turn is obtained from this amyloxyaniline.

DATC crystallizes from alcohol in colorless plates (BUU-HOI and XUONG 1953). Its melting point is given as 148 °C–149 °C, although it depends very much on the rate of the heating. The empirical formula is $C_{23}H_{32}N_2O_2S$ and the molecular weight 400.5. Like other thioamides, DATC is very poorly soluble in water.

For comprehensive variations of the diphenylthiourea upon which DATC is based and for their antituberculotic characteristics see WINKELMANN's review (1972).

For a method of detecting DATC see MEISSNER (1965) and BLOEDNER(1965).

References

Buu-Hoi NP, Xuong ND (1953) Sur les composés tuberculostatiques du groupe de la thiourée et leur méchanisme d'action. C R Acad Sci 237:498–500

Bloedner CD (1965) Bakteriologische Blutspiegeluntersuchungen bei Mono-Medikation von Isoxyl. Beitr Klin Tuberk 130:245–254

Huebner CF, Marsh JL, Mizzoni RH, Mull RP, Schroeder DC, Troxell HA, Scholz CR (1953) A new class of antituberculous drugs. J Am Chem Soc 75:2274–2275

Meissner G (1965) Resorption und Ausscheidung von Isoxyl im Serum sowie im Lungengewebe. X Congresso Argentinico de Tisiologia y Pneumologia, Mar des Planta, 28 Nov–2 Dec 1965

Winkelmann E (1972) Mittel gegen mycobakterielle Erkrankungen (Tuberkulose, Lepra). In: Ehrhart G, Ruschig H (Hrsg) Arzneimittel, Bd 4, Teil 1. Verlag Chemie, Weinheim, pp 167–170

[1] In 1986 no more on the market.

L. Capreomycin (CM)

In 1960 HERR et al. isolated an antibiotic from the fermentation liquid of *Streptomyces capreolus* that chiefly inhibited the growth of mycobacteria. This was capreomycin (CM).

CM reacts with 2 moles of sulphuric acid to form a sulphate with a CM content of around 77%. The sulphate is a colorless crystallizate that readily dissolves in water and in formamide, less readily in dimethyl sulphoxide and in propylene glycol, and poorly in the usual organic solvents such as methanol, ethanol, acetone, chloroform, benzene, and aliphatic hydrocarbons.

Chromatographically, the mixture known as CM can be resolved into four very similar substances (HERR et al. 1966) designated as CM IA, CM IB, CM IIA, and CM IIB. The mixing ratios of these four are given by HERR et al. (1966) as about 25:67:3:6 and by BYCROFT et al. (1971) as about 30:60:3.3:6.6. The principal component (CM IB), making up approximately two-thirds of the mixture, has been most thoroughly studied (BYCROFT et al. 1971).

Clarification of the structure (BYCROFT et al. 1971) revealed that the four CM, viomycin (cf. p. 15; 16), and the tuberactinomycins (not used for therapeutic purposes) are members of a family of closely related antibiotics. This relationship explains the parallel resistance of CM and VM.

CM IB has four basic groups (pK_a 6.2, 8.2, 10.1, and 13.3) and, with 2 moles of sulphuric acid, forms a sulphate having the empirical formula $C_{25}H_{44}N_{14}O_7 \cdot 2H_2SO_4$ (molecular weight 850.79) and giving the ninhydrin and biuret reactions. The Sakaguchi, Fehling, Molisch, and $FeCl_3$ tests are negative. It is not attacked by proteolytic enzymes (HERR et al. 1966). After complete acid hydrolysis (HERR et al. 1966; BYCROFT et al. 1971) α,β-diaminopropionic acid (Dapr), alanine (Ala), β-lysine (β-Lys), and capreomycidine (Cap) are formed, in molar ratios of 2:1:1:1; as well as urea, carbon dioxide, and traces of glycine. Cap, an unusual amino acid related to viomycidine (BYCROFT et al. 1968), is α-(2-iminohexahydro-4-pyrimidyl) glycine. It has been successfully synthesized,

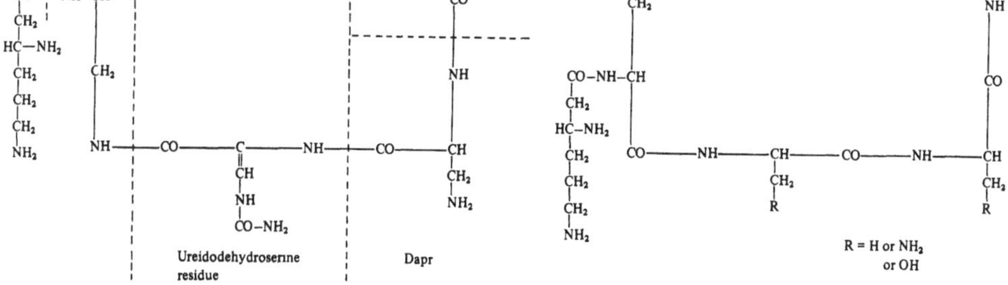

A B

structurally linked with viomycidine, and sterically assigned (BYCROFT et al. 1968).

CM IA differs from the main component CM IB by virtue of the fact that it contains serine in place of the alanine (BYCROFT et al. 1971).

CM IIA and CM IIB correspond in their ring skeleton to CM IA and CM IB but differ from the latter by the absence of the β-Lys side chain (BYCROFT et al. 1971). CM IIA and CM IIB may possibly be artefacts. The bioactivity of CM IA and CM IB is some 2.5 times that of CM IIA and CM IIB.

One of the features shared by CM and viomycin is ultraviolet absorption at 268 nm in water and at 285 nm in 0.1 N sodium hydroxide, which is due to a dehydroserine residue condensed with urea.

CM is thought to have structure A, though in view of its relationship with viomycin structure B cannot be ruled out.

According to VOIGT and MAA BARED (1970), capreomycin can be determined colorimetrically by heating its solution in sulphuric acid with an acetic acid diacetylmonoxime solution. The absorption maximum of the yellow color produced is 475 nm.

References

Bycroft BW, Cameron D, Croft LR, Johnson AW (1968) Synthesis and stereochemistry of capreomycidine [α-(2-imino-hexahydro-4-pyrimidyl)-glycine]. Chem Commun: 1301–1302

Bycroft BW, Cameron D, Croft LR, Hassanali-Walji A, Johnson AW, Webb T (1971) Total structure of capreomycin I B, a tuberculostatic peptide antibiotic. Nature 231:301–302

Herr EB Jr, Haney ME, Pittenger GE, Higgens CE (1960) Isolation and characterization of a new peptide antibiotic. Proc Indiana Acad Sci 69:134

Herr EB Jr, Haney ME, Pittenger GE (1961) Capreomycin: a new peptide antibiotic. 14oth Meeting Am Chem Soc, Abstract no 49c

Herr EB Jr, Redstone MO (1966) Chemical and physical characterization of capreomycin. Ann NY Acad Sci 135:940–946

Voigt R, Maa Bared AG (1970) Zur chemischen Bestimmung von Capreomycin. Pharmazie 25:471–472

M. Ethambutol (EMB)

Because of the marked antituberculotic activity observed, aliphatic polyamines and substituted ethylenediamines were prepared for investigation in a series of experiments. Among these compounds N,N′-diisopropyl-, disec.-butyl-(I)-, and di-tert.-butylethylene diamine were found to more or less correspond in activity to SM. On the basis of the comparisons in these extensive investigations (SHEPHERD and WILKINSON 1962) between the copper-complexing capacity and constitution it was decided to introduce additional hydroxyl groups into two of the alkyl groups.

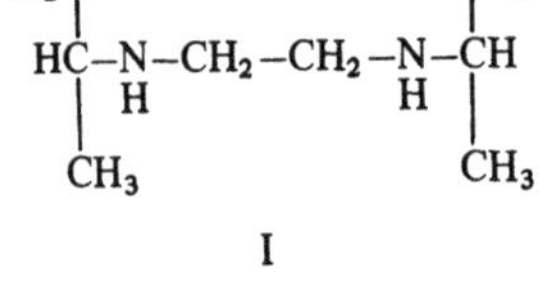

I

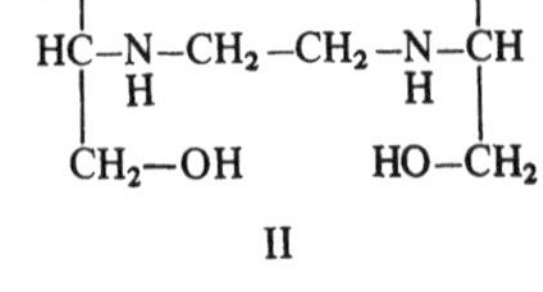

II

The compound found to have the best properties in the experimental series was a bis-hydroxy derivative of I, which gives a specific type of chelate, namely N,N′-bis-(1-hydroxy-sec.-butyl)ethylenediamine (II).

Owing to the presence of two asymmetric centres in the molecule, a (−)-form, a (±)-form, and a meso-form of II can occur in addition to the (+)-isomer. Study of all these forms (WILKINSON et al. 1961) revealed that the (+)-form is the most active. Originally known as (+)-2,2-(ethylenediimino)-di-1-butanol (WILKINSON et al. 1962), it is mentioned in the literature as D-N,N′-bis-(hydroxymethyl-propyl)ethylenediamine. The generic name of this most active of the isomers is ethambutol (EMB).

The ED_{50} in mg/kg/day after oral administration of the meso-form to the mouse is 500, while that of the (±)-form is 90 and that of the pure (+)-isomer 45; the (−)-form is inactive in vivo.

The base obtained from (+)-2-amino-1-butanol by heating with an ethylene halide is separated from the less soluble meso-form (m.p. 135.8–136.5 °C) and has a melting point between 87.5 °C–88.8 °C. Its dihydrochloride melts at 198.5 °C–200.3 °C. The racemate melts at 75 °C–76 °C and its dihydrochloride at 179 °C–180 °C.

(+)-2,2-(Ethylenediimino)-di-1-butanol (=EMB), empirical formula $C_{10}H_{24}N_2O_2 \cdot 2\,HCl$, has an optical rotation of $[\alpha]_D^{25} = +13.7°$ at c=2 in water, the corresponding value for its dihydrochloride under the same conditions being $[\alpha]_D^{25} = +7.6°$. After dissolution and crystallization from hot alcohol the dihydrochloride precipitates out in the form of colorless crystals with a melting point of 201.8 °C–202.6 °C (molecular weight 277.2).

The free base is reported as being readily soluble in chloroform, while the hydrochloride is readily soluble in water. The aqueous solution is thermostable and can be kept for a long time without decomposition.

In a thin-layer chromatogram (n-propanol, ammonia, water), EMB can be visualized as a blue spot by a mixture of 10% aqueous solutions of sodium nitroprusside, sodium carbonate, and acetaldehyde (1:1:1) (REUTGEN and GRUNERT 1969). For spectrophotometric determination in pharmaceutical products and in urine, the formation of a copper complex with Folin's reagent and measurement of the absorption at 265 nm or 610 nm have been recommended (REUTGEN and GRUNERT 1969). A further method that can be used for the determination of EMB is spectrophotometry of the bromthymol blue-EMB complex at 405 nm (STRAUSS and ERHARDT 1970).

References

Reutgen H, Grunert M (1969) Nachweis und Bestimmung von Ethambutol auf chemischem Wege. Pharmazie 24:148–152

Shepherd RG, Wilkinson RG (1962) Antituberculous agents. II. N,N′-Diisopropylethylenediamine and analogs. J Med Pharm Chem 5:823–835

Strauss I, Erhardt F (1970) Ethambutol absorption, excretion and dosage in patients with renal tuberculosis. Chemother 15:148–157

Wilkinson RG, Shepherd RG, Thomas JP, Baughn C (1961) Stereospecificity in a new type of synthetic antituberculous agent. J Am Chem Soc 83:2212–2213

Wilkinson RG, Cantrall MB, Shepherd RG (1962) Antituberculous agents. III. (+)-2,2-(Ethylenediimino)-di-1-butanol and some analogs. J Med Pharm Chem 5:835–845

N. Rifampicin (RMP)

Study of the metabolic products of *Streptomyces mediterranei* (SENSI et al. 1959), the rifamycins, and those of *Streptomyces spectabilis* (SIMINOFF et al. 1957), the streptovaricins, *Streptomyces tolypophorus* (KISHI et al. 1969), the tolypomycins, and *Streptomyces hygroscopicus* var. *geldanus* var. *nova* (DE BOER et al. 1970), the geldanamycins, led to the discovery of a group of compounds with an unusual structure not previously encountered in nature. Synthetic compounds of this kind, with an aliphatic chain looped like a handle over an aromatic system, had already been described by LÜTTRINGHAUS and GRALHEER in 1942 as ansa compounds (like I; ansa = Latin for handle).

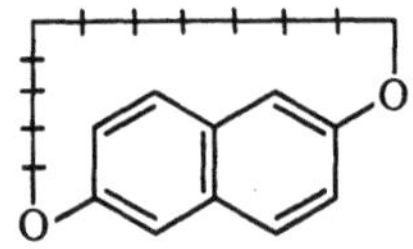

I

Accordingly, the new group of antibiotics obtained from Streptomycetes became known as the ansamycins.

Although the streptovaricins do have a certain activity against *Mycobacterium tuberculosis* (RHULAND et al. 1957), among the ansamycins the rifamycins are the most important for the treatment of tuberculosis.

Rifamycin B in particular, isolated as the largest fraction from the mixture of seven rifamycins under special culture conditions (addition of diethylbarbituric acid to the culture medium), became the starting point for further modifications.

Rifamycin B is oxidized to rifamycin O, which has also been observed as a constituent of the fermentation mixture. From rifamycin O rifamycin S is formed by hydrolysis, and then by reduction rifamycin SV, its formyl derivative yields with 1-amino-4-methylpiperazine the partially synthetic 3-(4-methyl-1-piperazinyliminomethyl)rifamicin SV (MAGGI et al. 1966). Because of its therapeutic importance, this last compound was given the generic name of rifampicin. Other names are rifaldazine, rifampin, RMP, and R/AMP.

Rifampicin is one of many semisynthetic rifamycin derivatives characterized, like the natural products of this group, by a certain degree of biological activity. In contrast to the derivatives with a hydrogen in place of the azomethine side chain, the special significance of rifampicin lies in the fact that it is orally absorbed and that, in comparison with other derivatives, in which the said hydrogen has been substituted, it has a particularly strong antituberculotic activity.

The empirical formula of RMP is $C_{43}H_{58}N_4O_{12}$, which corresponds to a molecular weight of 822.97. Whereas most of the ansamycins are yellow to green, RMP crystallizes in reddish-orange plates with a melting point of 183 °C–188 °C (decomp.). It is not very soluble in water. As a piperazine derivative, it dissolves better in acidic solutions ($pH < 6$) than at higher pH (> 6). However, it should be noted that in stronger acids ($pH < 2.3$) hydrolysis of the azomethine bond occurs, with the formation of formylrifamycin SV and aminomethylpiperazine. In alkaline media the hydroquinone group is sensitive to atmospheric oxygen. The solution can be protected from its partial oxidation to rifampicinquinone by the ad-

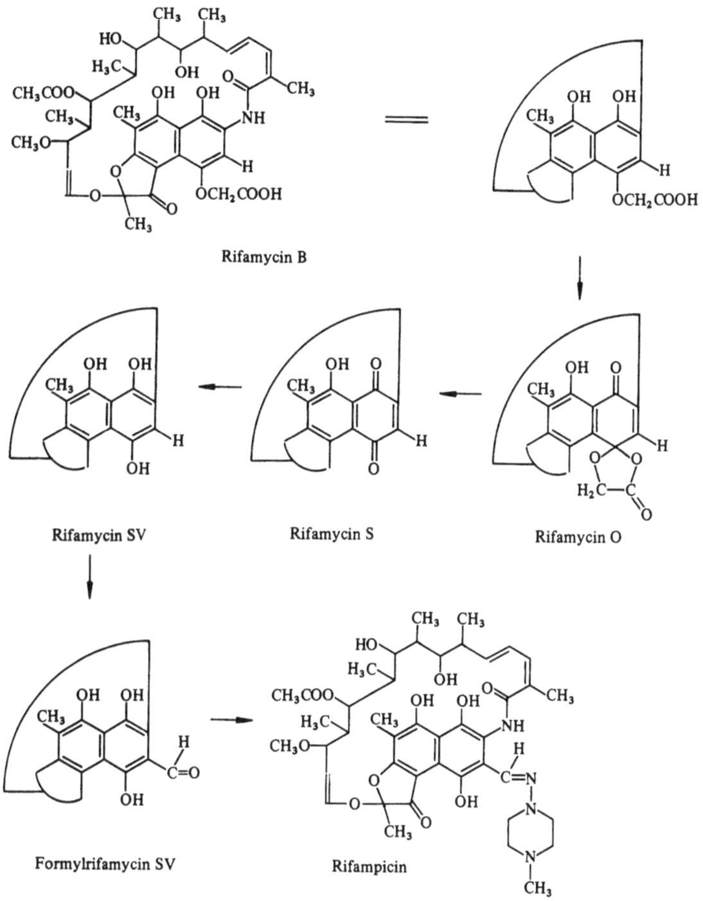

dition of ascorbic acid. The in-vitro and in-vivo activity of rifampicinquinone is the same as that of RMP. Similarly, the activity of the deacetylated derivative on *Mycobacterium tuberculosis* in vitro cannot be distinguished from that of RMP. RMP is better soluble in organic solvents – with the exception of aliphatic hydrocarbons, carbon tetrachloride, and cold acetone – than in water. Dimethyl sulphoxide is recommended for the preparation of a stock solution for dilution with water.

RMP can be detected in the urine, inter alia, by a pink to red color it gives with iron(III) nitrate in nitric acid solution. The sensitivity limit is 3 µg/ml (EIDUS and HARNANANSINGH 1969). The color can be extracted with a mixture of chloroform and ether. Spectrophotometric analysis of RMP and its deacetylated derivative can be carried out by measuring the absorption maxima at 333 nm and 472 nm (EIDUS et al. 1969). NMR, IR, and UV spectra of RMP are given in MAGGI et al. (1966). For the microbiological detection of RMP see ARIOLI et al. (1967) and BINDA et al. (1971). For further analytical methods see OTTEN et al. (1975).

References

Arioli V, Pallanza R, Furesz S, Carniti G (1967) Rifampicin, a new rifamycin. I. Bacteriological studies. Arzneim Forsch 17:523–529
Binda G, Domenichini E, Gottardi A, Orlandi B, Ortelli E, Pacini B, Fowst G (1971) Rifampicin, a general review. Arzneim Forsch 21:1908–1969
De Boer C, Meulman PA, Wnuk RJ, Peterson DH (1970) Geldanamycin, a new antibiotic. J Antibiot 23:442–447
Eidus L, Ling GM, Harnanansingh AMT (1969) Laboratory investigation of rifampin. Int J Clin Pharmacol 2:296–299
Eidus L, Harnanansingh AMT (1969) Simple procedures for checking rifampin in urine. Am Rev Resp Dis 100:738–739
Kishi T, Asai M, Muroi M, Harada S, Mizuta E, Terao E, Miki T, Mizuno K (1969) Tolypomycin. I. Structure of tolypomycinone. Tetrahedron Letters No 2:91–95
Lüttringhaus A, Gralheer H (1942) Über eine neue Art atropisomerer Verbindungen. Liebigs Ann Chem 550:67–98
Maggi N, Pasqualucci CR, Ballotta R, Sensi P (1966) Rifampicin: a new orally active rifamycin. Chemotherapia 11:285–292
Otten H, Plempel M, Siegenthaler W (1975) Antibiotika-Fibel 4. Aufl. Thieme, Stuttgart, p 532
Rhuland LE, Stern KF, Reames HR (1957) Streptovaricin. III. *In vivo* studies in the tuberculous mouse. Am Rev Tuberc Pulm Dis 75:588–593
Sensi P, Margalith P, Timbal MT (1959) Rifomycin, a new antibiotic. Preliminary report. Il Farmaco Ed Sci 14:146–147
Siminoff P, Smith RM, Sikolski WT, Savage GM (1957) Streptovaricin. Am Rev Tuberc Pulm Dis 75:576–587

CHAPTER 2

Experimental Evaluation of Efficacy

L. TRNKA, P. MIŠOŇ, K. BARTMANN, and H. OTTEN

A. Introduction

L. TRNKA and P. MIŠOŇ

Experiments offer the possibility of varying several conditions and thus of assessing the importance of particular technical details. Studies of the therapeutic efficacy of antituberculotics involve three variables: the tuberculous disease, the drug, and the pathogen.

Tuberculosis is largely a chronic disease characterized by a complex pathogenesis determined by the struggle between the microbe and the host. In consequence specific lesions evolve in the organs in which tubercle bacilli survive as facultatively intracellular parasites, as growing, proliferating or dormant, persisting bacilli.

The antituberculotic drugs – chemotherapeutics or antibiotics – interact as a third partner with the host and the bacillus. The therapeutic efficacy of antituberculotics is due to their direct antibacterial effect: reversible or irreversible damage to the vitality of the bacilli. The outcome depends, however, on the intensity and the duration of contact between the drug and the bacillus. This contact is modified by biotransformation of the drug. On the other hand, the drug may influence various functional or morphological systems of the host organism.

Of the many possible experimental conditions only those are meaningful that contribute to the concepts of chemotherapy in man. The success achieved during the last 20 years in the chemotherapy of tuberculosis is the result of well-designed experimental research.

The conditions are simplest for the in-vitro tests. The complex situation in a live host is replaced by cultivation of the tubercle bacilli in artificial media, which facilitates a direct study of the influence of drugs.

Experiments in vitro allow, in contrast to experiments in animals, an investigation of many strains, study of the speed and pattern with which resistance to the various compounds develops, study of cross-resistance with already known antituberculotics, and studies into the effect of combinations with other drugs and of the mode of action.

Most questions of this type can be dealt with by certain variants of the culture techniques. From the results conclusions are then drawn about the events in the lesions, though they will be correct only if the tubercule bacilli behave under the metabolic conditions in vitro as they behave in the microenvironment of the tuberculous lesions. Some authors have in fact observed certain differences in the metabolism between tubercle bacilli grown in vitro and in vivo. It must be pointed out that animal experiments – like in vitro tests – do not allow an absolutely reliable prediction of the clinical value of a given antituberculotic, but they can supply valuable information on special aspects, from which indications can be derived about the therapeutic value in man. In-vitro tests remain indispensable at the first level of evaluation in the search for antituberculotics.

Animal experiments constitute the second level. They are closer to clinical trials, because the part played by the host comes into play, but in contrast to clinical trials the conditions can be chosen largely at will. This holds true for the selection of the animal species and breed, the type and severity of the infection, the rating of the course of the disease, and its modification by treatment with many morphological, microbiological, and other techniques on groups of statistically significant size.

The treatment begins either immediately with the infection as a prophylactic measure or after the development of the disease to a certain extent, as prevention of further spread or as therapy of already established lesions. The course of the infection in treated and untreated animals can be compared either longitudinally or by cross-sections at the beginning and end of the treatment, or on the basis of survival rates during and after therapy.

Prophylactic and therapeutic animal experiments make it possible to compare the efficacy of various antituberculotic agents and their combinations within a relatively favorable period. If the experimental conditions are adequately chosen, differences in pharmacokinetics taken into account, and the results critically interpreted, animal experiments provide valuable information for the planning and design of clinical studies.

The macro-organism can be replaced by cell cultures for the study of some aspects, in particular for studies of the effect of antituberculotics on phagocytosed, intracellularly located tubercle bacilli. However, this technique too has some drawbacks, which must be borne in mind in an evaluation of the data.

The various types of experiments – in-vitro tests, animal experiments, and cell cultures – are designated as models because the various experimental components can be modified to evaluate their importance for the test outcome and their relevance for the treatment of human tuberculosis.

The systematic investigation of antituberculotics includes as a last step the controlled clinical study, which – in tuberculosis – is time-consuming, technically demanding, and expensive. Such studies can be carried out only in a limited number. Their design depends to a large extent on the information derived from the experimental models. They must be reserved for particular clinically important aspects. It is clear, therefore, that experimental models have played and still play an eminent role in the development of antituberculotic chemotherapy.

One of the principal tasks of experiments is the screening of substances for antimycobacterial activity. This is done mainly in the laboratories of the pharmaceutical industry. Many thousands of synthetic compounds and natural products have been tested in vitro during the last 40 years, and many of them have also been tried in tuberculous animals, on infected tissue cultures, or on infected eggs. Positive results provide the basis for further research. Sometimes they are wrongly taken or presented as definite proof of clinical effectiveness.

The second principal task of experimental models is the development of basic principles to guide a rational application of antituberculotics in man. Within this framework hypotheses are tested for the optimization of drug regimens from the aspects of efficacy, duration of treatment, type of drug application, prevention of bacterial resistance, etc. Many of the proved principles of present-day clinical chemotherapy have been derived from laboratory research results.

Countless papers have been published on these two tasks of experimental chemotherapy and for their sensible evaluation it is necessary to appreciate the possibilities and the limitations of the methods used. In Part B of this chapter the methodological aspects of practical relevance to experimental models will therefore first be discussed, to prevent misinterpretations and to explain differing results. Part C, then, will deal with the various antituberculotic drugs.

B. Methods. Their Limitations, Advantages, and Disadvantages

L. TRNKA and P. MIŠOŇ

I. In-Vitro Tests

1. Determination of Minimal Inhibitory Concentrations (MIC)

The standard technique for an evaluation of the antimycobacterial activity of a compound is the determination of its minimal inhibitory concentration (MIC), which is usually defined as the lowest of a series of graded concentrations that prevents the growth of bacilli in or on culture media under specified conditions.

In this type of investigation the following solid media have mainly been used: egg media according to Löwenstein-Jensen or ATS, substrate of Hohn etc., agar media as devised by Middlebrook (7 H 9, 7 H 10), or Tarshis' blood agar. Growth is easily recorded by estimating or counting the numbers of colonies developing after incubation for a certain period of time.

Fluid media are cheaper and easier to prepare. Among those used are Kirchner-Herrmann, Šula, Dubos-Davis, and the completely synthetic media of Proskauer and Beck or Sauton. Tween 80, a component of the Dubos medium, antagonizes the activity of some substances. The proportion of the inoculum that is able to grow at a certain concentration is much more difficult to estimate in fluid media than on solid media.

Some antituberculotics are partly inactivated by binding to ingredients of the medium or by the elevated temperature needed for the coagulation of the egg media. This results in an increased MIC. Proteins are the major causes of inactivation (HEJNÝ and MELICHAR 1965). Because the MIC depends to such an extent on the culture conditions, a satisfactory estimate of the antimycobacterial potency of a given substance can be obtained only by using different culture techniques. The substance must be distributed evenly throughout the medium in a biologically active state. This presents no difficulties with the water-soluble substances. If the solubility in water is insufficient, various organic solvents can be used, which in the concentrations used must be free of their own inhibitory activity. This applies particularly to dioxan (MEISSNER 1965). Changes of the pH of the medium by the substance under test should also be considered. Growth usually means growth as apparent to the naked eye. The endpoint is either absence of any visible colonies or a defined small proportion of the inoculum. The concentrations in the medium are usually reported in weight per unit volume or – for ill-defined substances – in units per volume. Sometimes the concentrations are also given in volume percent, as molarities, or simply in terms of the dilution factor. The test strains are certain reference strains of M. tuberculosis and their substrains resistant to the known antituberculotics, like the strain H37 Rv or H37 Rv-SM-R; in addition, bovine, avian, and strains of so-called atypical mycobacteria, and finally a number of "wild" strains, i.e., ones freshly isolated from patients supposedly never treated with antituberculotics. The number of colony-forming units in the inoculum must be standardized, because the MIC varies with the size of the inoculum. Larger inocula lead to higher MIC's. One reason is the

Table 1. Antimycobacterial activity of capreomycin in vitro (TRNKA et al. 1966)

Medium Concentrations (μg/ml)	Löwenstein-Jensen					Proskauer-Beck				
	4	8	16	32	MIC	0.5	1	2	4	MIC
Strains										
H 37 Rv	+	+	o	o	16	+	+	o	o	2
H 37 Rv-SM-R	+	o	o	o	8	+	+	o	o	2
H 37 Rv-PAS-R	+	o	o	o	8	+	+	o	o	2
"1314" poly R	+	+	+	o	32	+	+	+	o	4

+ = growth; o = no growth.

larger number of resistant mutants in larger inocula. These mutants selectively survive and constitute the starting point for the development of a homogenous resistant population. The selection of resistant strains is much easier if large inocula are used. Data on MIC's can be interpreted only if the number of colony-forming units in the inoculum is counted or at least estimated. Since during incubation the antituberculotics are inactivated by binding or decomposition, the MIC's of most antituberculosis drugs depend on the time of the incubation. This point is important for the standardization of the methods, but also in the case of slowly growing cultures which need longer incubation periods than those prescribed by the standard techniques. The influence of the incubation time on the MIC on egg medium was studied by BARTMANN et al. (1966). Whereas with some drugs, e.g., INH, the endpoint was reached after 3 weeks, with other drugs the MIC continued to increase up to the end of the investigation (10 weeks).

Table 1 presents as an example the determination of the MIC's for capreomycin on solid Löwenstein-Jensen and in fully synthetic fluid Proskauer-Beck media. The tubes with and those without growth could be clearly differentiated. The MIC was easy to determine.

Sensitivity tests as a guide for the treatment of patients are carried out worldwide by three standard techniques (KREBS 1975; BARTMANN 1980): the absolute minimal concentration method, taking "no growth" as the endpoint (Deutsches Zentralkomitee zur Bekämpfung der Tuberkulose), the proportion method, in which a defined proportion of the inoculum is taken as the endpoint (CANETTI et al. 1963; 1969), and the determination of the resistance ratio between the MIC of the strain in question and the MIC of a reference strain (Laboratory Subcommittee of the BMRC). The basic methodological aspects have been discussed by CANETTI (1965), CANETTI et al. (1969), GÁLVEZ-BRANDON and BARTMANN (1969), KREBS (1975) and BARTMANN (1980). At present, the technique most widely used is the proportion method.

Apart from these standard procedures, diffusion tests have been used (SCHMIEDEL 1958; FINK and SCHRÖDER 1973). In the last few years rapid tests have been tried, making use, e.g., of isotopes (REUTGEN 1973; KUNZE et al. 1977; SNIDER et al. 1981) or of continuous optical-density recording (HUSSELS et al. 1981). However, whatever technique is used for the determination of the MIC,

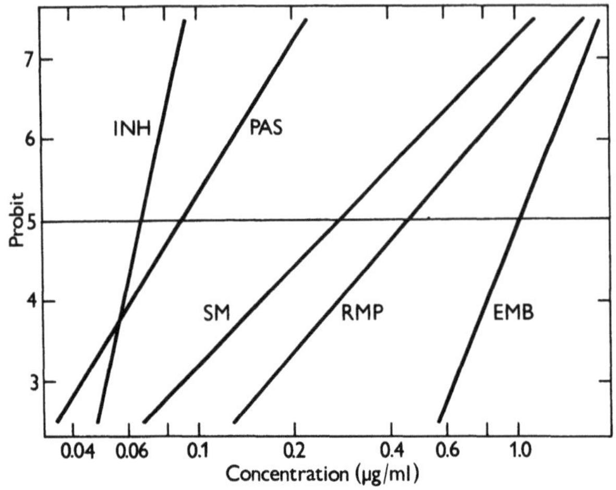

Fig. 1. Dose-effect regression lines for isoniazid (*INH*), streptomycin (*SM*), rifampicin (*RMP*), p-aminosalicylic acid (*PAS*), and ethambutol (*EMB*) in vitro (solid Dubos media with Tween and albumin). TRNKA et al. (1974)

interlaboratory comparisons are possible only to a limited extent, because despite every effort many technical details cannot be sufficiently standardized.

More detailed information on the inhibitory activity of antituberculotics than is given by the all-or-none MIC technique can be obtained by establishing the proportion of the inoculum that grows at various partly inhibitory concentrations. From data of this kind regression lines of the inhibitory activity versus drug concentration can be calculated, as shown in Fig. 1. Both the position of the line with respect to the X-axis, (i.e., concentration) and its slope characterize the antimycobacterial activity.

2. Cross-Resistance

Cross-resistance means that a given strain resistant to a certain substance also exhibits resistance to another substance, to which it was not exposed. Cross-resistance can therefore be detected simply by comparing MIC's. Cross-resistance is found mainly between substances of similar structure and/or similar mode of action. A distinction must be drawn between one-way cross-resistance (e.g., ETH-resistant strains are also resistant against CM, but not vice versa) and two-way cross-resistance (e.g., many ETH-resistant strains are resistant against TSC, and TSC-resistant strains are also resistant against ETH). Table 2 gives an overview of the cross-resistance between antituberculotics now in clinical use. It has been compiled from the literature and personal experience. Cross-resistance is designated as "partial" if not all the bacilli of a given strain display cross-resistance, but only a certain fraction of them.

Detection of cross-resistance may restrict the practical importance of a new drug right from the beginning.

Table 2. Cross-resistance in vitro between antituberculotics used in clinical practice. (After TRNKA et al. 1966)

Ethionamide	⇄	Thiosemicarbazones
Ethionamide	→	Capreomycin[a]
Ethionamide	⇄	Thiocarlide[a]
Thiocarlide	⇄	Thiosemicarbazones
Streptomycin	→	Kanamycin[a]
Viomycin	→	Kanamycin[a]
Viomycin	⇄	Capreomycin[a]
Capreomycin	←	Kanamycin[a]

[a] Partial cross-resistance.
→ = one-way cross-resistance.
⇄ = two-way cross-resistance.

3. Type of Action

The "type of action" denotes the manner in which the vitality of the microbes is influenced by a given substance. If growth is inhibited without irreversible damage to the bacilli, the action ceases at the end of the exposure and the type of action is said to be bacteriostatic. If the growth inhibition is accompanied by an irreversible damage (which continues after the exposure has ended), the type of action is said to be bactericidal. To some extent this differentiation is an oversimplification, because (in contrast to disinfectants) nearly all "bactericidal" drugs kill the bacilli only if these are in a state of active metabolism and not in the resting state; and on the other hand, the "bacteriostatic" drugs may lead to death of the bacilli if applied for a long time. Nevertheless, the above dichotomous differentiation is of great clinical importance, since the duration of treatment can be shortened the more the drug combination applied acts bactericidally (see Part C).

For the determination of the type of action the bacteria have to be cultured in fluid medium that allows submerse and fairly homogenous growth. The dynamics of multiplication and death can then be followed in time by turbidimetric, biochemical, or quantitative culture techniques. For an exact measurement of the proportion of the inoculum that has remained viable after drug action for a certain time it is necessary to separate the drug and the microbes at the end of the selected period. This is often done by dilution down to concentrations which per se are non-inhibitory, possibly in association with measures ensuring physical or chemical inactivation of the drug. Another separation technique is culture of the bacilli in permeable plastic bags which are first placed in the drug-containing medium and at the end of the exposure taken out and washed to remove the drug. Filtration through membrane filters has also been used for the removal of drugs (ZEBROWSKI 1966; DICKINSON 1969; STOTTMEIER et al. 1969).

By experiments of this kind the killing kinetics can be determined, as well as the lag phase of the surviving bacilli before the resumption of multiplication. This lag phase is of special importance for the design of intermittent treatment regimens (DICKINSON 1969; DICKINSON and MITCHISON 1970; MITCHISON and DICKINSON 1971).

Detailed studies on the role of the concentration and time of exposure in the induction of the lag phase have shown that the growth-inhibiting action of INH depends within broad limits on the time-concentration product. For bactericidal effects, however, longer exposures to higher concentrations are required (ARMSTRONG 1960; BARCLAY and WINBERG 1964; ARMSTRONG 1965). The effects of RMP and SM depend predominantly on the drug concentration, that of EMB more on the duration of the exposure (BEGGS et al. 1968; BEGGS and JENNE 1970; BEGGS and WILLIAMS 1971). These experiments do not provide any direct guidelines for the development of regimens in human chemotherapy, but they do give some ideas for designing experimental in-vivo conditions.

II. Animal Experiments

A comprehensive review on this subject has been written by WAGNER (1964). Whereas in vitro the *antimycobacterial* activity of a given substance is tested, what is checked in the animal is its *therapeutic* activity. Therapeutic activity means efficacy, even if the macroorganism has modified the growth conditions of the bacilli and the drug concentrations that reach the bacilli.

After infection the tubercle bacilli multiply, spread through the body, and give rise to lesions of various types in which the exposure to drugs is modified. After its administration the drug is distributed into the various compartments of the body, metabolized, and excreted. From the enteral or parenteral depot the drug is first transported into the circulation, where it is partly bound to the proteins and other fluid or cellular blood components as well as to components of the inner vascular walls. Only the free (unbound) fraction [1] is distributed into the extracellular spaces, where the substance is again partly bound. The free fraction reaches the site of the infection, but also the organs and tissues in which it is metabolized and eliminated. If the blood supply to the lesions is poor the drug's concentration curve in the lesions may be quite different from that in the blood. Transport only by diffusion results in longer invasion and elimination times and thereby transforms the blood-concentration curve more or less into a plateau at a relatively low level. In most cases the concentration in the lesions cannot be measured directly. As a reference value the concentration in the plasma water may be used, because it is equal to the concentration in the interstitial water after diffusion equilibrium has been reached. The courses of the blood- or plasma water-concentrations with time, often called blood-level curves, are the consequence of two opposite processes: invasion and elimination. Normally, the rate of the two processes is proportional to the actual concentration, i.e., the curves can be described by exponential functions. After repeated dosage the shape of the blood level curve is determined not only by the doses applied but also by the dosage interval. There are many other factors which also influence the blood level, such as the content of body water, age, sometimes sex, physiopathological condition of the patient, and so on.

As has been summarized by BARTMANN (1974), it can be assumed that with the bacteriostatics a concentration equivalent to the MIC in vitro is sufficient.

[1] Except the relatively small proportion of the drug which is bound to serum proteins and exudes with them during inflammation through the altered walls of the vessels.

With the bactericidal drugs, however, the concentration should be as high as is needed for the maximal killing effect, provided that the necessary dosage does not give rise to any untoward reactions. With the bacteriostatic drugs the concentration in the lesions that corresponds to the MIC should not fall below this level during the dosage interval. With bactericidal drugs this may happen, because the multiplication of the surviving organisms begins only after a lag phase, which in the case of the tubercle bacillus takes one or more days.

Since the pathological features of tuberculosis in animals are similar more or less to that in man, it is important to select an animal model best suited to answer the particular questions. In most cases a generalized infection is produced, which, if untreated, ends in death. In an acute course of the infection the tubercle bacilli multiply constantly and death ensues within a few weeks, without any major variations in the survival times. In a subacute or chronic course the number of the bacilli in the organs becomes stabilized after initial multiplication and the survival times are more irregular. As acute infections are more uniform, they are preferable for answering many, mainly basic, questions.

The methods and the criteria of evaluation depend on the speed of the course of the disease. In an acute tuberculosis mortality data can be used. In a chronic form of the disease what one needs is criteria that characterize the dynamics. Among these, the counting of culturable bacilli in the organs has proved especially useful. In some animal species this laborious technique can be replaced by counting the specific lesions in the organs or on their surface. Another, less specific, method is the determination of the organ weights or the specific weight of the lungs. Histological techniques have been used. Their results can be scored for a statistical evaluation. In larger animals X-rays of the lungs are informative. The data too can be scored. By their bacteriostatic or their bactericidal activity antituberculotics inhibit the multiplication of the tubercle bacilli. The number of bacilli that can be recovered from the organs by culture decreases. If the treatment lasts long enough, a state may be reached in which bacilli no longer can be demonstrated by the usual microbiological techniques. Some authors have spoken of "sterilization of the organs" in this context, but in most cases this is not adequate because relapses occur if one waits for several months after the end of the therapy or if one subsequently treats the animals with cortisone in doses that reduce their immunocompetence (GRUMBACH et al. 1970).

It has been shown by several investigators that sensitive bacteria can also resist the action of antituberculotics if they go over into a morphological or metabolic state that enables them to survive in the presence of active concentrations. Microbiological demonstration of these so-called persisters may be difficult, because their culture may be hampered and their staining properties (acid fastness) may be lost, e.g., if they transform into spheroplasts. It is not certain whether such a stage is reached only by virtue of the host or whether the additional action of certain antituberculotics, like CS, is required. What is certain, however, is that the persisters can switch over to proliferation if the conditions are favorable, and this can have important consequences and end in a manifest relapse of the disease.

If the proliferation of the tubercle bacilli is inhibited by chemotherapy, the specific lesions heal and the death rate becomes reduced. The morphology of the specific lesions shows large differences between the various animal species, and

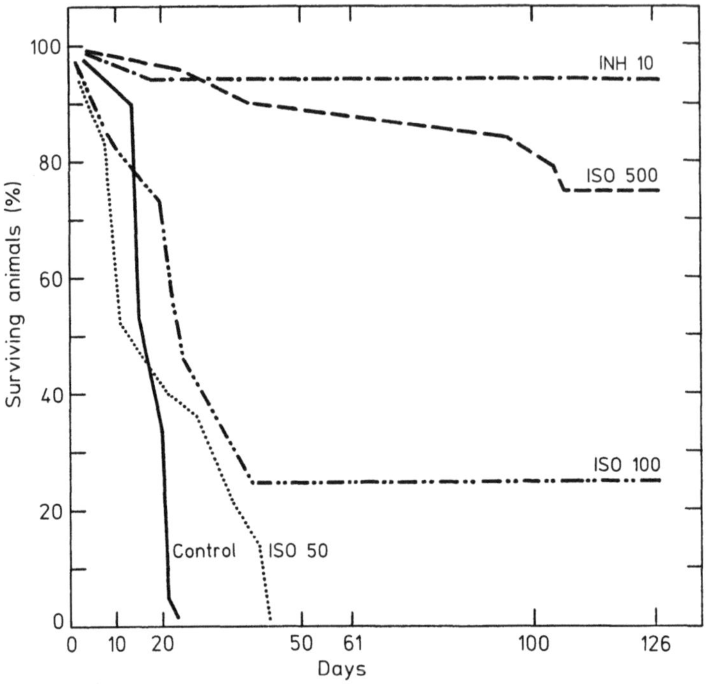

Fig. 2. Mortality of tuberculous mice under continuous treatment with isoniazid (*INH*, 10 mg/kg) or Isoxyl-DATC (*ISO*-50, 100, and 500 mg/kg). URBANČÍK et al. (1963)

this must be taken into account in any evaluation of therapeutic studies. Guinea pigs, rabbits, and primates produce in granulomas the specific epitheloid and giant cells of the Langerhans type, even though the organs are attacked by the infection with species – specific differences. For example, in guinea pigs the lungs are less involved than the spleen and the liver after subcutaneous or intramuscular infection, in contrast to rabbits in which the kidneys are the most susceptible organ. The course of the experimental tuberculosis in mice is determined mainly by disease in the lungs. The morphological picture in this species is characterized by necrosis; the bacilli multiply mainly in macrophages. In mice and in rats cellular immunity mechanisms are the major factor of resistance to tuberculosis. Macrophages play a central role.

In principle, all infection models can be used for testing antituberculotics. Despite the fact that the severity of the disease can be quantified by a scoring system, as has been done in the early classical investigations with guinea pigs by FELDMAN (1943) and by FELDMAN and HINSHAW (1945), or as could be done with X-rays in monkeys, at present those techniques are preferred that provide numerical values directly, e.g., survival times, weights, or counts of culturable bacilli per unit organ weight. Often-used criteria for biometric evaluations are the survival times or the mortality rates in treated and untreated groups. The simplest evaluation is a graphical representation of the times of death. It is intuitive, but provides no numerical values and does not allow calculations of significance. Figure 2 demonstrates a typical example of the influence exerted by the dose on the course of murine tuberculosis. Simple numerical values are obtained by calculating the arithmetic mean or the median value of the times of death (DONOVICK et al. 1949). In general the median values are lower than the arithmetic means, and they differ less because they are not influenced by a few unusually longsurviving animals (WAGNER 1975).

The arithmetic means and medians allow a quantitative comparison of treated and untreated groups or of groups treated in different ways. A significance test often used is the method of LITCHFIELD (1949) and LITCHFIELD and WILCOXON (1949). On the assumption that the time distribution of the mortality is log-normal, cumulative death rates (in percent) are plotted versus time. The ordinate scale is given by the cumulative distribution function of the normal distribution (probability scale), while the abscissa has a logarithmic scale. The best-fit straight line drawn through the cloud of points allows the mean time of death (50% lethal time, LT_{50}), the standard deviation, and the slope of the line to be read off. From these parameters the significance of differences between the mean and between slopes (test for parallelism) can be calculated. The method is applicable only if the values are normally (or log-normally) distributed, though this is often not true for death curves (WAGNER 1975). To avoid such difficulties a non-parametric test can be used, e.g., the rank U-test of MANN and WHITNEY (1947). The test is sensitive to differences between the medians.

GEBELEIN and WAGNER (1956) have developed a method which, for relatively small groups of animals, allows one to say whether a given substance has any measurable influence on the course of the disease. The technique consists in testing for a normal distribution of the death times and for significance of their differences. KRADOLFER and SCHNELL (1967) have used the survival time of untreated control groups as the basis for an evaluation. In principle, the aim is to determine what dose of the drug is capable of prolonging the survival of 50% of the animals (mice) as compared with the survival time in the bulk of the untreated controls. This dose (ED_{50}) is established on the basis of dose-effect curves. It is also possible to specify what dosage yields some other survival rate (e.g., ED_{95}). Evaluations of this type are possible only if data are obtained from experimental series under identical conditions. It should be borne in mind that the death times are influenced not only by the treatment but also by immunity to the infection. A less effective treatment, allowing the development of a stronger infection immunity, can lead to longer survival times (BARTMANN et al. 1958).

In some laboratories techniques are preferred in which the death times and the severity of the pulmonary lesions are integrated into a pathological index. If the lesions are always evaluated by the same person, the values are reliable. A statistical comparison of inter-experimental values is hardly possible, but the method is useful for intraexperimental group comparisons (WAGNER 1975). Evaluation of the pathological lesions by the same person is also necessary for all other methods based on a scoring system.

Numerical values can be obtained, however, directly with intradermal infections of guinea pigs by measuring the area of the developing local lesion (URBANČÍK et al. 1963). Table 3 presents an example and shows the dynamics of progress in untreated animals and of the healing under treatment with INH.

Another criterion that may be used is the average body weight, though this needs a cautious interpretation, because other factors (like toxicity of the drugs

Table 3. Average areas (in mm^2) of skin ulcers (4 per animal) in guinea pigs infected with M. tuberculosis H 37 Rv, in the presence and absence of treatment with 10 mg/kg INH. (After URBANČÍK et al. 1963)

Group	Animal no.	Weeks after infection					
		3	4	5	6	7	8
Controls	875	20.5	25.2	25.7	28.0	29.7	–[1]
	873	23.0	34.6	39.0	42.7	41.5	36.0
	870	30.2	29.0	36.9	42.5	41.5	52.5
	872	18.7	23.2	30.5	45.5	44.7	–[1]
	$\bar{x}$	23.1	28.1	33.9	39.6	39.3	44.2
INH 10 mg/kg	815	14.5	14.2	10.5	5.5	–[2]	
	802	19.6	19.3	12.6	10.6	–[2]	
	817	22.7	18.5	11.5	13.5	–[2]	
	$\bar{x}$	18.9	17.3	11.5	9.8	–[2]	

–[1] = died from tuberculosis.
–[2] = lesions healed with scars.

applied) can also influence the weight. More specific is the determination of the weight of diseased organs like the lungs or the spleen.

Counting of culturable bacilli found in the organs of small laboratory animals, especially mice, is the method preferred in the last years, because it provides direct information on the drug's action on the microbe. Standardized techniques have been developed (FENNER et al. 1950; MCCUNE and TOMPSETT 1956; MCCUNE et al. 1966; TRNKA and ŠTAFLOVÁ 1974). Animals are killed at certain time intervals and the organs are removed aseptically and carefully homogenized, keeping the procedure as undamaging as possible for the bacilli. The homogenates – mainly of the lungs and the spleens – are diluted serially and samples are planted on culture media. After appropriate incubation the numbers of colonies are counted and calculated per unit organ weight or per organ. Differences between the numbers of culturable bacilli can be tested for significance by various statistical methods. The disadvantage is that each animal provides only one value, because it has to be killed. Study of the dynamics over time requires the sacrifice of treated and untreated groups of animals (3 to 5) at certain intervals. By using such groups the interanimal variations can be satisfactorily balanced. Figure 3 presents the typical course of the counts of bacilli in the lungs and the spleen of mice with a chronic tuberculosis. The bacillary content of the spleen is lower than that in the lungs during the later course of the disease. This can be explained by a stronger local resistance of the spleen. The activity of antituberculotics becomes manifest as retardation of multiplication in comparison to untreated animals at the same point in time, or as a fall in the number of culturable bacilli in relation to the time to which the treatment started. Decreasing numbers of bacilli under treatment may reflect a bactericidal type of action in vivo, as has been substantiated for INH by BARTMANN (1960). Figure 4 shows an experiment in which groups of mice were infected intravenously with M. tuberculosis, strain H 37 Rv. After one day treatment started in one group with INH, in a second with RMP,

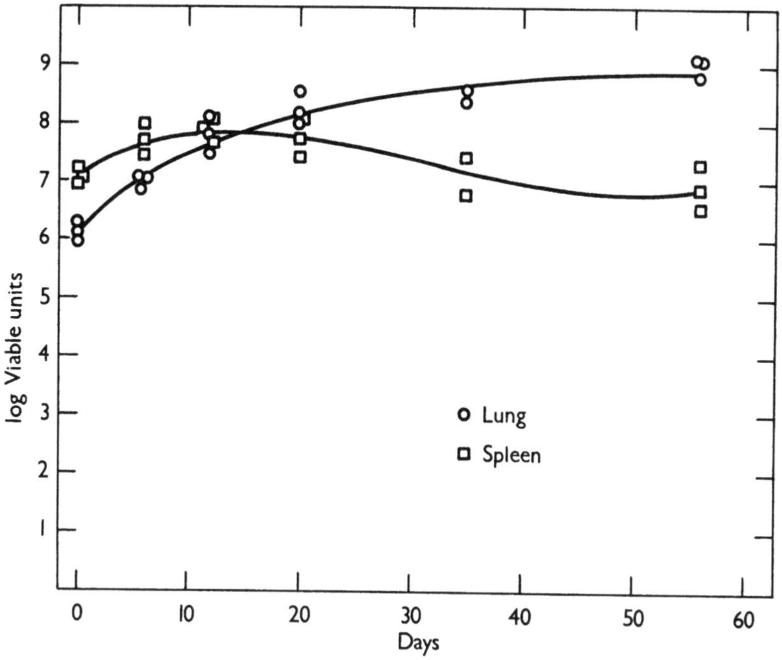

Fig. 3. Time course of culturable bacilli in the lung and spleen of mice with chronic tuberculosis. McCune and Tompsett (1956)

and in a third with PAS. The drugs were given daily and per os. A fourth group served as an untreated control. On day 3, 6, 9, and 12 five animals from each group were killed and the numbers of culturable bacilli in the lungs were determined. From the different course of the curves it can be concluded that within this short period RMP has a marked effect, in contrast to PAS.

The count of the bacilli may differ considerably between individual animals killed at the same time. This is due first of all to differences in natural and acquired resistance to the infection, and secondly – especially after long treatment periods – to the irregular occurrence of resistant mutants able to multiply under treatment.

To improve the reproducibility of the microbial counting technique, which is a sensitive indicator of therapeutic effects, the influence of many experimental details has been studied. Recommendations for standardization were given, regarding the selection of age, sex, and strain of the animals, their diet, the route and dose of the infection, the techniques of homogenization, decontamination, cultivation, reading of the results, etc. (Youmans and Raleigh 1948; Raleigh and Youmans 1948a, b; Dubos and Pierce 1948; Ilavsky 1954; Youmans et al. 1959; Uesaka and Oiwa 1956; Crowle 1958; Trnka and Urbančík 1962; Urbančík and Trnka 1962; Huempfner and Deuschle 1966). Paying attention to all these variables assures reliable results. Unfortunately, in many publications the description of the technical details is insufficient. Therefore, care has to be taken when comparing in-vivo experiments. The efficacy of drugs should be demon-

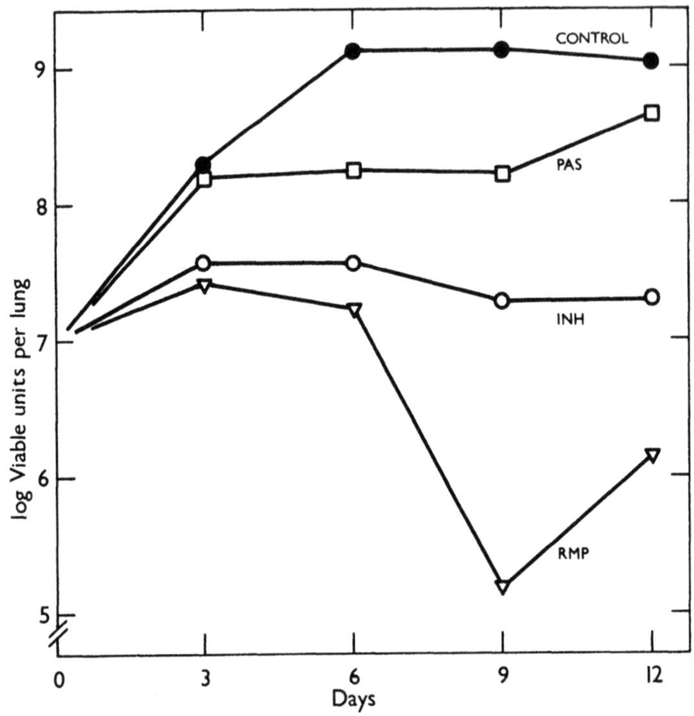

Fig. 4. Comparison of antituberculosis activity of isoniazid (*INH*, 10 mg/kg), rifampicin (*RMP*, 10 mg/kg), and p-aminosalicylic acid (*PAS*, 150 mg/kg) on the culturable bacilli in the lungs of mice treated 12 days after the infection. TRNKA et al. (1974)

strated by standardized techniques, using known antituberculotics as a reference.

There are many variables in drug administration, which can all be studied in each of the infection models: route of administration, dosage, continuous or intermittent treatment, duration of treatment, combinations of antituberculotics, treatment in phases (combined therapy followed by monotherapy), treatment for prophylaxis of the infection, for the prevention of spread, or for the therapy of manifest disease.

III. Cell Cultures

The effectiveness of antituberculotics depends on the possibility of a sufficient contact between the drug and the microbes. If the extracellular space is the site of contact, sufficient exposure will depend on the pharmacokinetic and pharmacodynamic effects of the substance, since untoward effects limit the dosage and thereby influence the kinetics (BARTMANN 1974). Tubercle bacilli, however, are phagocytosed after invasion by cells of various types, mainly those of the macrophage series. As facultatively intracellular parasites, they are able to survive and multiply within these cells, and even to destroy them (YOUMANS 1957).

Table 4. Summary of cell cultures used for the study of intracellular parasitism of tubercle bacilli

Cell type	Donor	Authors	Special objects of study
Macrophages from peritoneal cavity	Guinea pig	ABE (1958); BERTHRONG and HAMILTON (1958, 1959)	Virulence and immunobiology
		FONG et al. (1956)	Immunity
		HSU and KAPRAL (1960)	Influence of triiodothyronine
		SUTER (1953)	Immunity
		FREERKSEN and SCHELLENBERG (1956)	
		BONVENTRE and IMHOFF (1970)	
		SCHELLENBERG (1957)	
		LYANG (1960)	
	Rabbit	MACKANESS (1952, 1954a, b); MACKANESS and SMITH (1953)	Virulence, factors isolated from tubercle bacilli, surface-active substances
	Mouse	SUTER (1961); BOVENTRE and IMHOFF (1970)	Immunity
Fibroblasts	Rat	BROWN (1970); HANKS (1947)	Lepra
Fibrocytes	Rabbit	HANKS (1958)	
HeLa cells	Man	CLARK and FORREST (1959); SHEPARD (1955, 1957a, b, 1958, 1959); UTAGAWA (1962)	Immunity, etc.
Leucocytes	Man	HANKS (1958)	Lepra
Epithelial cells, embryonal cells, lung cells, spindle cells	Guinea pig	LYANG (1960)	
Kidney tissue	Monkey	SHEPARD (1959)	
Amniotic cells	Man	SHEPARD (1959)	
Spleen cells	Mouse	PAVLOV (1970); PAVLOV et al. (1974)	

From this it is evident that any potential antituberculotic should act not only on the extracellularly located bacilli but also on intracellularly located ones. It has been shown, however, that some antituberculosis drugs, like streptomycin, scarcely penetrates into the cells of the host in sufficient concentrations. Furthermore, the intracellular conditions, e.g., the pH, may antagonize the drug's action. This may have farreaching consequences, like the phenomenon of persisters. It is therefore necessary to investigate each new antituberculotic for its activity on intracellular bacilli.

The conditions of intracellular multiplication of the tubercle bacilli have been studied. The development of appropriate techniques and the results obtained with antituberculosis drugs are the subject of several reviews (FREERKSEN and KRÜGER-

THIEMER 1956; HANKS 1958; WAGNER 1975; BARTMANN 1975). The techniques are based on the in-vitro culture of cells derived from the host (animal or man). These techniques form a link between pure in-vitro and pure in-vivo methods and allow an assessment of the efficacy and the type of action of antituberculotics on bacilli located within cells.

Macrophages from guinea pigs, mice, and rabbits are mainly used as host cells. They are cultured in monolayers by techniques that allow long-term cultivation and suppress extracellular multiplication of the bacilli (e.g., by the addition of low concentrations of SM). Intracellular multiplication of the bacilli is followed either by counting stained preparations or by quantitative culture after disruption of the cells, though both these techniques are not free from technical difficulties (cf. BARTMANN 1975). These methods can also be used to see whether a substance can activate the bacteriostatic and bactericidal potency of macrophages. Activation of macrophages as effector cells is an expression of cell-mediated immunity which plays a dominant role in the defence of the host against tubercle bacilli. In activated macrophages the lysosomal apparatus becomes larger enabling intracellular killing of the tubercle bacilli. The observation of intracellular tubercle bacilli provides useful information on the immunocompetence of the macrophage donor. The immune mechanism may act synergistically with, or antagonistically to the chemotherapy.

Not only macrophages but also other cell types have been used. Table 4 presents the data from the literature. The activity of antituberculotics against intracellular bacilli can be higher, the same as, or lower than the activity against extracellular bacilli (CLINI and GRASSI 1970). The respective data for each antituberculosis drug are mentioned in Part C.

References

Abe S (1958) Studies on the intraperitoneal cells of a guinea pig and the multiplication of tubercle bacilli in the intraperitoneal mononuclear cells cultured in vitro. Sci Rep Res Inst Tohoku Univ (Med) 8:161–178

Armstrong AR (1960) Time-concentration relationship of isoniazid with tubercle bacilli. Am Rev Respir Dis 81:498–503

Armstrong AR (1965) Further studies on the time-concentration relationships of isoniazid and tubercle bacilli in vitro. Am Rev Respir Dis 91:440–443

Barclay WR, Winberg E (1964) Bactericidal effect of isoniazid as a function of time. Am Rev Respir Dis 90:749–753

Bartmann K, Villnow J, Schwarz C (1958) Tierexperimentelle Untersuchungen zu einer intermittierenden Chemotherapie und -prophylaxe der Tuberkulose. VII. Der Erfolg kontinuierlicher und intermittierender Gaben von INH und der Tripelkombination INH, Streptomycin, PAS im therapeutischen Versuch an Meerschweinchen. Beitr Klin Tuberk 118:297–313

Bartmann K (1960) Die experimentellen Grundlagen einer Chemoprophylaxe der Tuberkulose mit Isonicotinsäurehydrazid (INH). Adv Tuberc Res 10:127–215

Bartmann K, Abel U, Hart R (1966) Die Abhängigkeit des Hemmtiters von der Bebrütungsdauer bei der Bestimmung der Resistenz von *M. tuberculosis* gegen Antituberkulotika auf Löwenstein-Jensen Medium. Zentralbl Bakteriol Mikrobiol Hyg (A) 201:538–548

Bartmann K, Gálvez-Brandon J (1968) Towards an international standardization of resistance tests on mycobacteria. Scand J Respir Dis 49:141–152

Bartmann K (1974) Antimikrobielle Chemotherapie. Springer, Berlin Heidelberg New York Tokyo
Bartmann K (1975) Biometrie der Mykobakterien. In: Meissner G, Schmiedel A, Nelles A (Hrsg) Mykobakterien und mykobakterielle Krankheiten. III. Bakteriologische Grundlagen der Chemotherapie der Tuberkulose. Fischer, Jena, pp 19–57
Bartmann K (1980) Mikrobiologische Grundlagen. In: Jentgens H (Hrsg) Atmungsorgane. Lungentuberkulose. Springer, Berlin Heidelberg New York Tokyo, pp 1–45 (Handbuch der inneren Medizin Bd IV/3)
Beggs WH, Jenne JW, Hall WH (1968) Isoniazid uptake in relation to growth inhibition of *Mycobacterium tuberculosis*. J Bacteriol 96:293–297
Beggs WH, Jenne JW (1970) Growth inhibition of Mycobacterium tuberculosis after single pulsed exposure to streptomycin, ethambutol and rifampicin. Infect Immun 2:479–483
Beggs WH, Williams NE (1971) Streptomycin uptake by *Mycobacterium tuberculosis*. Appl Microbiol 21:751–753
Berthrong M, Hamilton MA (1958) Tissue culture studies on resistance in tuberculosis. I. Normal guinea pig monocytes with tubercle bacilli of different virulence. Am Rev Tuberc Pulm Dis 77:436–449
Berthrong M, Hamilton MA (1959) Tissue culture studies on resistance in tuberculosis. II. Monocytes from normal and immunized guinea pigs infected with virulent human tubercle bacilli. Am Rev Tuberc Pulm Dis 79:221–231
Bonventre PF, Imhoff JG (1970) Uptake of ^{3}H-dihydrostreptomycin by macrophages in culture. Infect Immun 2:89–95
Brown CA (1970) Association of lysozomal enzymes in cultured fibroblasts with the intracellular growth of *Mycobacterium lepraemurium*. Br J Exp Pathol 51:203–209
Canetti G, Froman S, Grosset J, Hauduroy P, Langerová M, Mahler HT, Meissner G, Mitchison DA, Šula L (1963) Mycobacteria: laboratory methods for testing drug sensitivity and resistance. Bull WHO 29:565–578
Canetti G, Rist N, Grosset J (1963) Mesure de la sensibilité du bacille tuberculeux aux drogues antibacillaires par la méthode des proportions. Méthodologie, critères de résistance, résultats, interprétation. Rev Tuberc 27:217–272
Canetti G (1965) Present aspects of bacterial resistance in tuberculosis. Am Rev Respir Dis 92:687–703
Canetti G, Fox W, Khomenko A, Mahler HT, Menon NK, Mitchison DA, Rist N, Šmelev NA (1969) Advances in techniques of testing mycobacterial drug sensitivity, and the use of sensitivity tests in tuberculosis control programmes. Bull WHO 41:21–43
Clark ME, Forrest E (1959) Growth characteristics of acid-fast microorganisms other than tubercle bacilli in HeLa cells. Am Rev Respir Dis 80:744–746
Clini V, Grassi C (1970) The action of new antituberculous drugs on intracellular tubercle bacilli. Antibiot Chemother 16:20–26
Crowle AJ (1958) Lung density as a measure of tuberculous involvement in mice. Am Rev Tuberc Pulm Dis 77:681–693
Deutsches Zentralkomitee zur Bekämpfung der Tuberkulose (1966) Empfehlungen zur Methodik und Bewertung von Resistenz-Bestimmungen bei Tuberkulose-Bakterien
Dickinson JM (1969) The suitability of new drugs for intermittent chemotherapy of tuberculosis. An experimental study. Scand J Respir Dis (Suppl) 96:91–98
Dickinson JM, Mitchison DA (1970) Suitability of rifampicin for intermittent administration in the treatment of tuberculosis. Tubercle 51:82–94
Donovick R, McKee CM, Jambor WP, Rake G (1949) The use of the mouse in a standardized test for antituberculous activity of compounds of natural or synthetic origin. I. Choice of mouse strain. Am Rev Tuberc 60:109–120
Dubos RJ, Pierce C (1948) The effect of diet on experimental tuberculosis of mice. Am Rev Tuberc 57:287–293
Feldman WH (1943) A scheme for numerical recording of tuberculous changes in experimentally infected guinea pigs. Am Rev Tuberc 48:248–255
Feldman WH, Hinshaw HC (1945) Chemotherapeutic testing in experimental tuberculosis; suggested outlines of laboratory procedures for testing antituberculous substances in experimentally infected guinea pigs. Am Rev Tuberc 51:582

Fenner F, Martin SP, Pierce CH (1950) The enumeration of viable tubercle bacilli in cultures and infected tissues. Ann NY Acad Sci 52:751–764
Fink H, Schröder KH (1973) Sensibilitätsbestimmung von Mykobakterien mit der Diffusionsmethode. Prax Pneumol 27:509–513
Fong J, Schneider P, Elberg SS (1956) Studies on tubercle bacillus – monocyte relationship. I. Quantitative analysis of effect of serum of animals vaccinated with BCG upon bacterium – monocyte system. J Exp Med 104:455–465
Freerksen E, Schellenberg H (1956) Die Vermehrung von Tuberkelbakterien in Monozyten gesunder Tiere. Z Hyg 142:554–571
Freerksen E, Krüger-Thiemer E (1956) Mycobakterien in der Gewebekultur. A. Gegenwärtiger Kenntnisstand. Jahrber Borstel 3:66–93
Gálvez-Brandon J, Bartmann K (1969) Statistical aspects of the proportion method for determining the drug-resistance of tubercle bacilli. Scand J Respir Dis 50:1–18
Gebelein H, Wagner WH (1956) Statistische Prüfung des chemotherapeutischen Reihenversuchs bei der experimentellen Mäusetuberkulose. Beitr Klin Tuberk 116:253–267
Grumbach F, Canetti G, LeLirzin M (1970) Caractère durable de la stérilisation de la tuberculose expérimentale de la souris par l'association rifampicine – isoniazide: épreuve de la cortisone. Rev Tuberc Pneumol 34:312–319
Hanks JH (1947) The fate of leprosy bacilli in fibroblasts cultivated from macular and tuberculoid lesions. Int J Lepr 15:48–60
Hanks JH (1958) Assay of the fate of mycobacteria in cell and tissue cultures. Am Rev Tuberc 77:789–801
Havel A, Trnka L, Kuška J (1965) Comparison of antituberculous effects of morphazinamide and pyrazinamide in chronic experimental tuberculosis. II. The emergence of resistance and its retardation in the course of monotherapy and combinations of antituberculous drugs. Chemotherapia 9:168–175
Hejný J, Melichar J (1965) Inhibitory concentrations of antituberculosis drugs for strains of Mycobacterium tuberculosis on Löwenstein-Jensen and ATS media. Acta Tuberc Pneumol Scand 46:51–56
Hsu HS, Kapral FA (1960) The suppressed multiplication of tubercle bacilli within macrophages derived from triiodothyronine-treated guinea pigs. Am Rev Respir Dis 81:881–887
Hussels HJ, Kroening U, Wundschock M (1981) Biophotometrische Schnellbestimmung der Empfindlichkeit von Mykobakterien. Prax Pneumol 35:609–611
Huempfner HR, Deuschle KW (1966) Experimental tuberculosis in germ-free and conventional mice. Am Rev Respir Dis 93:465–467
Ilavsky J (1954) A new procedure for screening antituberculous agents. Effect of chemotherapeutic agents on mice infected with massive doses of tubercle bacilli intraperitoneally. Am Rev Tuberc 69:280–286
Kradolfer F, Schnell R (1967) Analyse der Wirksamkeit von Rifamycin-Derivaten und bekannten Therapeutika erster Ordnung an der murinen Tuberkulose. In: Spitzy KH, Haschek H (eds) Proc Vth Int Congr Chemotherapy Wien, Vol II/2:525–532
Krebs A (1975) Mykobakterielle Resistenz und Resistenzbestimmungen. In: Meissner G, Schmiedel A, Nelles A (Hrsg) Mykobakterien und mykobakterielle Krankheiten. III. Bakteriologische Grundlagen der Chemotherapie der Tuberkulose. Fischer, Jena, pp 183–250
Kunze M, Sanabria de Isele T, Vogt A (1977) Über die Möglichkeit einer Schnellmethode zur Resistenzbestimmung von Mykobakterien durch Einbau von Uracil-5-H_3. Zentralbl Bakteriol Mikrobiol Hyg (A) 239:87–94
Laboratory Subcommittee of the Tuberculosis Chemotherapy Trials Committee, Medical Research Council (1953) Laboratory techniques for the determination of sensitivity of tubercle bacilli to isoniazid, streptomycin, and P.A.S. Lancet II:213–217
Litchfield JT Jr (1949) A method for rapid graphic solution of time-percent effect curves. J Pharmacol Exp Ther 97:399–408
Litchfield JT Jr, Wilcoxon F (1949) A simplified method of evaluating dose-effect experiments. J Pharmacol Exp Ther 96:99–113
Lyang KW (1960) Studies on the interaction between host cell and parasite. I. Morphologic studies of lung cultured in vitro. Am Rev Respir Dis 81:200–205

Mackaness GB (1952) The action of drugs on intracellular tubercle bacilli. J Pathol Bacteriol 64:429–446
Mackaness GB (1954a) Artificial cellular immunity against tubercle bacilli. An effect of polyoxyethylene ethers (Triton). Am Rev Tuberc 69:690–704
Mackaness GB (1954b) The growth of tubercle bacilli in monocytes from normal and vaccinated rabbits. Am Rev Tuberc 69:495–504
Mackaness GB, Smith N (1953) The bactericidal action of isoniazid, streptomycin and terramycin on extracellular and intracellular tubercle bacilli. Am Rev Tuberc 67:322–340
Mann HB, Whitney DR (1947) On a test of whether one of two random variables is stochastically larger than the other. Ann Math Statist 18:50–60
McCune RM, Tompsett R (1956) Fate of Mycobacterium tuberculosis in mouse tissues as determined by the microbial enumeration technique. I. The persistence of drug-susceptible tubercle bacilli in the tissues despite prolonged antimicrobial therapy. J Exp Med 104:737–762
McCune RM, Feldmann FF, Lambert HP, McDermott W (1966) Microbial persistence. I. The capacity of tubercle bacilli to survive sterilization in mouse tissue. J Exp Med 123:445–486
Meissner G (1965) Häufigkeit der Resistenz für Conteben und deren Bedeutung für das Auftreten der Resistenz für Isoxyl (4-4′-Diisoamyloxythiocarbanilid) bei Tuberkelbakterien. Prax Pneumol 19:387–395
Mitchison DA, Dickinson JM (1971) Laboratory aspects of intermittent drug therapy. Postgrad Med 47:737–741
Pavlov EP (1970) Some factors influencing the activity of streptomycin, kanamycin and isoniazid with respect to intracellularly seated Myco. tuberculosis (in Russian). Probl Tuberk 48, issue 9:72–76
Pavlov EP, Tushov EG, Kotlyarov LM (1974) The action of rifampicin on the extra- and intracellularly located Myco. tuberculosis (in Russian). Probl Tuberk 52, issue 12:64–67
Raleigh GW, Youmans GP (1948a) The use of mice in experimental chemotherapy of tuberculosis. I. Rationale and review of the literature. J Infect Dis 82:197–204
Raleigh GW, Youmans GP (1948b) The use of mice in experimental chemotherapy of tuberculosis. II. Pathology and pathogenesis. J Infect Dis 82:205–220
Reutgen H (1973) Zur Resistenzbestimmung von *Mycobacterium tuberculosis* gegenüber INH, Streptomycin, PAS, Äthionamid, Ethambutol und Rifampicin mittels ^{32}P-Inkorporationstest. Acta Biol Med Ger 30:309–316
Schellenberg H (1957) Die Gewebekultur in der Tuberkuloseforschung unter besonderer Berücksichtigung immunobiologischer Fragen. Jahrber Borstel 4:700–722
Schmiedel A (1958) Der Vertikaldiffusionstest als Methode zur Resistenzbestimmung von Tuberkelbakterien und zur INH-Spiegeltestung. Z Tbk 112:48–56
Shepard CC (1955) Phagocytosis by HeLa cells and their susceptibility to infection by human tubercle bacilli. Proc Soc Exp Biol Med 90:392–398
Shepard CC (1957a) Growth characteristics of tubercle bacilli and certain other mycobacteria in HeLa cells. J Exp Med 105:39–48
Shepard CC (1957b) Use of HeLa cells infected with tubercle bacilli for the study of antituberculous drugs. J Bacteriol 73:494–498
Shepard CC (1958) A study of the growth in HeLa cells of tubercle bacilli from human sputum. Am Rev Tuberc Pulm Dis 77:423–435
Shepard CC (1959) A comparison of the growth of selected mycobacteria in HeLa, monkey kidney, and human amnion cells in tissue culture. J Exp Med 107:237–246
Snider DE Jr, Good RC, Kilburn JO, Laskowski LF Jr, Lusk RH, Marr JJ, Reggiardo Z, Middlebrook G (1981) Rapid drug-susceptibility testing of Mycobacterium tuberculosis. Am Rev Respir Dis 123:402–406
Stottmeier KD, Woodley CL, Kubica GP (1969) New approach for the evaluation of antimycobacterial drug combinations in vitro (the laboratory model man). Appl Microbiol 18:399–403

Suter E (1953) Multiplication of tubercle bacilli within mononuclear phagocytes in tissue cultures derived from normal animals and animals vaccinated with BCG. J Exp Med 97:235–245

Suter E (1961) Passive transfer of acquired resistance to infection with Mycobacterium tuberculosis by means of cells. Am Rev Respir Dis 83:535–543

Trnka L, Urbančík R (1962) Comparative study on the sensitivity of mice strain H and CF_1 to experimental tuberculous infection (in Czech). Rozhl Tuberk 22:187–192

Trnka L, Havel A, Urbančík R (1966) Neueste Tuberkulostatika, ihre Bedeutung und Möglichkeiten der Wertbestimmung im Reagenzglas. Chemotherapia 11:121–134

Trnka L, Štaflová S (1974) Experimental principles on the use of rifampicin in the intermittent chemotherapy of tuberculosis. Ain Shams Med J 25 (Suppl):157–159

Trnka L, Mišoň P, Štaflová S (1974) Interaction aspects of antimycobacterial drugs in the chemotherapy of tuberculosis. II. The role of rifampicin and other drugs in the dependent or independent action of drug associations in vitro. Chemotherapy 20:82–91

Uesaka I, Oiwa K (1956) Studies on experimental tuberculosis in mice. 1. Factors affecting the survival time of mice experimentally infected with human type tubercle bacilli. Jpn J Tuberc 4:64–72

Urbančík R, Trnka L (1962) Preliminary observations on the increase in isoniazid resistance of *M. tuberculosis* H 37 Rv after exposure to an extract of tuberculous tissue. Am Rev Respir Dis 85:596–598

Urbančík R, Trnka L (1963) Report on the antimicrobial activity of Isoxyl on *M. tuberculosis* "in vitro" and "in vivo". Acta Tuberc Pneumol Belg 54:66–86

Urbančík R, Trnka L, Polenská H (1963) The suitability of intracutaneous infection in guinea pigs induced by virulent tubercle bacilli for the use in chemotherapeutic trials. Experientia 19:23–24

Utagawa K (1962) Intracellular multiplication of tubercle bacilli in HeLa cells. Sci Rep Res Inst Tohoku Univ (Med) Ser C10:302–309

Wagner WH (1964) Experimentelle Infektionen mit Tubercelbakterien. In: Eichler O (Hrsg) Erzeugung von Krankheitszuständen durch das Experiment. Springer, Berlin Göttingen Heidelberg, pp 354–430 (Handbook of Experimental Pharmacology, vol 16, Teil 9)

Wagner WH (1975) Die Wertbestimmung tuberkulostatischer Substanzen in vivo. In: Meissner G, Schmiedel A, Nelles A (Hrsg) Mykobakterien und mykobakterielle Krankheiten. III. Bakteriologische Grundlagen der Chemotherapie der Tuberkulose. Fischer, Jena, pp 129–158

Youmans GP (1957) Acquired immunity to tuberculosis. J Chronic Dis 6:606–632

Youmans GP, Raleigh G (1948) The use of mice in experimental chemotherapy of tuberculosis. III. The histopathologic assay of chemotherapeutic action. J Infect Dis 82:221–226

Youmans GP, Youmans AS, Kanai K (1959) The difference in response of four strains of mice to immunization against tuberculous infection. Am Rev Tuberc 80:753–756

Zebrowski T (1966) A new method for investigating the dynamic aspects of antibacterial properties of chemical compounds in vitro by the use of the dialyser tubing. Am Rev Respir Dis 93:111–113

C. Drugs and Treatment Regimens

I. p-Aminosalicylic Acid (PAS)

L. TRNKA and P. MIŠOŇ

1. Antimicrobial Spectrum in Vitro

PAS does not exert a bacteriostatic activity against non-acid-fast microorganisms (SIEVERS 1946). DICZFALUZI (1947) found that PAS had no effect against *Escherichia coli, Staphylococcus aureus,* or *Streptococcus haemolyticus.* WYSS et al. (1943) tested the biological action of substituted p-aminobenzoic acids and found that they had no action on *E. coli.* Similar results have been obtained with *Staphylococcus albus, Salmonella typhi, Aerobacter aerogenes, Streptococcus viridans, Streptococcus pneumoniae,* and *Bacillus anthracis* (SIEVERS 1947; RAGAZ 1948; TOBIE and JONES 1949). Generally speaking, non-acid fast bacteria require for their inhibition a concentration of 12,5 mg to 25 mg PAS/ml (SIEVERS 1946). Nonpathogenic Actinomycetales were inhibited by a concentration of 350 µg to 750 µg PAS/ml (WAKSMAN and LECHEVALIER 1953).

2. Antimycobacterial Activity

a) Activity in Artificial Media in Vitro

Several reports have demonstrated that PAS inhibits the growth of pathogenic mycobacteria (*M. tuberculosis* and *M. bovis*) including SM resistant variants (BLOCH et al. 1949) strongly and specifically. The bacteriostatic concentrations vary from about 1 µg/ml to 10 µg/ml in the case of different strains and under different conditions. The early works on the antimycobacterial activity of PAS were reviewed by ROBSON and KEELE (1956). Some of these results are summarized in Table 1.

As with other antituberculotic drugs, the inhibition is reduced by increasing the number of mycobacteria in the inoculum, but in the case of PAS this effect is particularly pronounced. According to YOUMANS and RALEIGH (1947), and to HEDGECOCK (1956) the inhibitory action is indirectly proportional to the size of the inoculum. The dependence is obviously non-linear: 10 times the volume of inoculum causes a 100-fold reduction in sensitivity (VENNESLAND et al. 1948). Otherwise, the results indicate that inhibitory concentrations on solid or liquid media are generally similar if small inocula are used (BOGEN et al. 1950).

M. avium strains and the so-called atypical mycobacteria seem to be more resistant to the bacteriostatic activity of PAS, although also some strains of *M. bovis* have been said to be resistant (BOGEN et al. 1950) and some strains of *M. phlei, M. fortuitum* (WOLINSKY et al. 1957; VELLUTI 1967), *M. kansasii, M. avium* and *M. aquae* (TOBIE and JONES 1949; WOLINSKY et al. 1957; HEDGECOCK 1965; GERNEZ-RIEUX and DEVULDER 1970; BURJANOVÁ and DORNETZHUBER 1975) have proved to be susceptible. It should be mentioned that when PAS is tested there is a small "initial growth", which must not be mistaken for a resistance. With a period of action more than 24 h on mycobacteria even a 1% PAS solution does not show any inhibition. The phenomenon is analogous to the lag-phase of bac-

Table 1. Minimal inhibitory concentrations of p-aminosalicylic acid (PAS) for mycobacteria in vitro

Myco-bacterium	Medium	Inoculum	Incu-bation time (days)	Minimal inhibitory conc. (MIC) (μg/ml)	Ref.
tuberculosis H37Rv	YS	0.01 mg ww	?	1.5	YOUMANS et al. (1947a)
	D	?	?	1.2	VENNESLAND et al. (1948)
	D	0.001 mg dw	14	0.49	GOODACRE et al. (1948)
	HO	?	21	4.0	HEILMEYER (1950)
	HO	0.01 mg ww	28+42	1.0	WALTER (1950)
	KT			0.25	MAYER et al. (1958)
	TAM	?	21	1.0	FURESZ (1970)
	KI	?	21	0.5	
	YS	1 mg ww	21+28	0.32	JANOWIEC et al. (1977)
tuberculosis				0.48	LEHMANN (1946a)
tuberculosis (14)[a]	S	?	20	0.25–0.25–2.5[a]	KLEBANOVA (1954)
	GD-Slide culture	?	?	1.53	SIEVERS (1946)
	LJ	?	21	3.3	DOMAGK (1950)
bovis (3)[a]	S	?	20	25	
avium	S	?	20	500	
kansasii	Šula	10^4–10^6 cells	24	1–10	BURJANOVÁ and DORNETZHUBER (1975)
kansasii	YS	1 mg ww	21+28	19.0	JANOWIEC et al. (1977)
smegmatis	KTA			125	MAYER et al. (1958)
battey	YS	1 mg ww	21+28	250.0	JANOWIEC et al. (1977)

Abbreviations of media: LJ = Löwenstein-Jensen; HO = Hohn; ATS = American Trudeau Society; OG = Ogawa; OAA = solid semi-synthetic medium with oleic acid and albumin; 7H9–7H10–7H11 = Middlebrook media; D-OAA = modification of OAA according to Dubos; HE = Herrold; D = Dubos; GB = glycerin bouillon; KI = Kirchner; KTA = Kirchner with Tween and albumin; TAM = Tween-albumin-medium; TB = broth with Tween; Y = Youmans synthetic liquid medium; YS = Youmans with serum; PB = Proskauer-Beck; PBS = Proskauer-Beck with serum; PBA = Proskauer-Beck with albumin; ST = Sauton; FS = Fisher; FGS-FSS = Fisher with glycerol, event. with serum.
ww = wet weight; dw = dry weight.
[a] The numbers in parentheses represent the numbers of strains tested.
MIC: lowest value – most common value – highest value observed.

teriostasis with many organisms, e.g., in the case of sulphonamides (DOMAGK 1950; YEGIAN and VANDERLINDE 1950).

According to TSUKAMURA and MIZUNO (1980), PAS belongs to the group of antituberculotics showing a straight line-relationship between the growth of mycobacteria and the drug concentration. Low PAS concentrations produce only partial inhibition of the growth and even higher concentrations often yield incomplete bacteriostasis. In liquid medium this has also been found by MITCHISON (1970). The fraction of mycobacteria inhibited varies from below 50% to over 95% depending on the concentration (BOGEN et al. 1950).

α) Factors Affecting the Activity in Vitro. The free acid is very slightly soluble in water (about 0.2%), but it is moderately soluble in alcohol (1.5%) and ether (1.2%) and readily soluble in alkaline solutions forming the highly soluble monosodium salt (ROSDAHL 1948; BOGEN et al. 1950). When protected from light, aqueous solutions are stable for 24 h at 4 °C. PAS in solution is altered at 80 °C and rapidly destroyed above this temperature. The decomposition, and especially decarboxylation with the release of m-aminophenol also occurs readily under the influence of moisture, light, or simply on standing, especially on exposure to air. PAS solutions cannot be boiled or autoclaved. According to some reports, PAS undergoes partial decomposition in egg media upon heating for coagulation (LORIAN 1966), but the degradation in the media during incubation at 37 °C has proved to be negligible (TSUKAMURA and MIZUNO 1980). It appears preferable to sterilize PAS solutions without risk of absorption by filtration through membrane or Seitz filters. For some purposes it is advisable to carry out sterilization simply by treating the dry sodium PAS powder with 75% ethyl alcohol and shaking, after which the salt is allowed to settle and the alcohol is removed prior to preparation of the solution under sterile conditions. If solutions are made up beforehand, they should be stored in a dark container at a low temperature and tightly closed in containers completely filled to prevent oxidation or loss of carbon dioxide. Completely dry, freshly prepared, pure PAS is thermostable, and may thus be sterilized by dry heat (LORIAN 1966).

As in the case of sulphonamides, the antimycobacterial activity of PAS is antagonized by the presence of structurally related p-aminobenzoic acid (PABA) (YOUMANS et al. 1947; HURNI 1949a, b; DOMAGK 1950; TOBIE and JONES 1949; BÖNICKE and REIF 1950/51; DONOVICK et al. 1952; HEDGECOCK 1956; KAKEMI et al. 1967). The antagonistic action is competitive (LEHMANN 1949) and the inhibition index (molar ratio of PABA to PAS necessary for inhibition) is equal to unity (HURNI 1949; HEDGECOCK 1956). The action of PAS is not antagonized by PABA in other bacterial species (DICZFALUZY 1947).

By the addition of calcium succinate (DOMAGK 1950), methionine (HURNI 1949b), salicylate (IVÁNOVICS 1949) or other substances (KAKEMI et al. 1967) it is possible in vitro to eliminate, at least in part, the deleterious effect of PABA. The inhibition indices vary from 0.01 to 0.02 in the case of methionine and from 0.08 to 0.25 in the case of salicylic acid. This effect of salicylate was shown to be highly specific and not shared by related compounds. On the other hand, PAS has a moderate antisulphonamide action. This action is slighter than that of PABA in the same concentration (DICZFALUZY 1947).

The inhibitory effect of PAS is apparently not reduced by the presence of serum or plasma in amounts as usually added to media (YOUMANS and RALEIGH 1947; YOUMANS et al. 1947; BOGEN et al. 1950; BÖNICKE 1950/51; ZEYER et al. 1960; OGAWA and OTANI 1961a, b), and may even be increased by the presence of surface-active agents such as Tween 80, or by copper ions (BOGEN et al. 1950; BÖNICKE and REIF 1950/51; SORKIN et al. 1951).

β) Resistance of Mycobacteria to PAS

Development of PAS Resistance in Vitro and Its Type: There are some differences in the reports regarding the development of mycobacterial strains resistant to PAS. It had been thought that it is apparently much more difficult to obtain strains resistant to PAS than to streptomycin. After repeated culture in vitro on nutrient media with gradually increasing PAS concentrations, several authors failed to observe resistant mycobacteria (LEHMANN 1947; GOODACRE and SEYMOUR 1949; HURNI 1949a), but their development in vitro has also been reported (BOGEN et al. 1950; YEGIAN and VANDERLINDE 1950). The possibility of rapid resistance development has also been confirmed (IVÁNOVICS 1950). The discrepancies may be due to the sensitivity tests used (KREBS 1975).

The pattern of PAS resistance development has been described as a so-called facultative single-step process (DEMEREC 1955, in a 1955 listing of literature; TSUKAMURA et al. 1956b). The colonies obtained by the first selection are characterized by an average resistance level that may be slight, indermediate, or high. Using *M. tuberculosis* strain H 37 Rv and Aoyama B, TSUKAMURA (1961) showed that a high resistance type was obtained by the second step, and that this level was the highest. Accordingly, there are only two phenotypes with respect to PAS resistance, and the pattern is a two-step pattern. However, in contrast to the case of the H 37 Rv strain, in Aoyama B strain the highest resistance was obtained in one step (facultative single-step pattern). When the mycobacteria reach the highest resistance further selection becomes ineffective, and no more stable resistant clones can be detected.

The upper limit of the resistance varies depending on the strain. In the case of *M. tuberculosis* H37Rv it is 20 mg/ml, in Aoyama B strain 1 mg/ml.

The proportion of resistant mutants ranges from approximately 10^{-5} to 10^{-9}. Some results obtained with initially sensitive strains of *M. tuberculosis* are summarized in Table 2, which is taken from KREBS (1975). The frequency of mutations from sensitivity to low resistance is higher than that of mutations to high

Table 2. Frequency of PAS-resistant mutants in strains of *M. tuberculosis* from untreated tuberculosis patients (KREBS 1975)

Medium	PAS (μg/ml)	Frequency	Ref.	Remarks
TAM	1	2×10^{-8}	YEGIAN and VANDERLINDE (1950)	H37Rv strain
LJ	1	3×10^{-5} to 10^{-7}	GROSSET and CANETTI (1962)	
LJ	1	5×10^{-6}	KREBS and KALICH (1964)	
OG	100	1.7×10^{-8}	TSUKAMURA et al. (1956a)	Aoyama B strain
OG	1–2	10^{-5}	TSUKAMURA et al. (1959a)	Aoyama B strain
	5–100	10^{-8}		
OG	1	1.6×10^{-9}	TSUKAMURA et al. (1959c)	H37Rv strain
OG	1–2	10^{-5}	TSUKAMURA et al. (1961)	Aoyama B strain
	5–100	10^{-8}		
	1–2	10^{-7} to 10^{-8}		H37Rv strain

Abbreviations of media: see Table 1

resistance. In addition to direct mutation from a sensitive to a highly resistant cell, cumulative mutations of a few to several genes are assumed, each of which can give rise to a low resistance or modify the degree of resistance, producing a highly resistant phenotype. The possible frequencies of mutants of this type have been reported to be about 10^{-13} to 10^{-14} (TSUKAMURA 1961). Heterogenic populations, characteristic for PAS-resistant strains, have been ascribed to fluctuation of the phenotype resistance, which is unstable and non-inheritable. Such resistance is interpreted as due to fluctuation within the same genotype (TSUKAMURA et al. 1959b, c).

An obligatory single-step pattern of PAS resistance (the bacterium being either sensitive or fully resistant) has been observed in *Bacillus megaterium* (SZYBALSKI and BRYSON 1953; SZYBALSKI 1954; BRYSON and SZYBALSKI 1955), but owing to the high primary insensitivity of this organism to PAS (about 400 µg/ml), it is difficult to compare the situation with the development of resistance in originally sensitive mycobacterial strains.

Features of Resistant Populations: The definition of PAS resistance depends on the evaluation method, the criteria used, and the clinical importance. With the aid of an indirect proportion method for the resistance evaluation, the critical level of PAS resistance has been found to be 1% of cells growing on Löwenstein-Jensen media containing 0.5 µg PAS/ml (DEUTSCHES ZENTRALKOMITEE 1966; CANETTI et al. 1969; GÁLVEZ-BRANDON and BARTMANN 1969; STANDARD METHODS 1980). The incubation time is usually 4 weeks (BARTMANN et al. 1966). The frequency of initial PAS resistance (i.e., resistance of *M. tuberculosis* strains isolated from untreated patients), according to the above mentioned methods or a method of the British Medical Council (resistance-ratio method) (MARKS 1961), is summarized on the basis of some representative communications in Table 3.

The prevalence of initially PAS-resistant strains is relatively low, even in the developing countries, and from the epidemiological point of view it is not a menace to treatment (TOMAN 1979).

Table 3. Frequency of initial PAS resistance in patients' strains reported in 1953–1979

Region	Percentages of resistant strains isolated		
	Minimum	Maximum	Median
North America	0.7	6.3	3.0
Asia (India and Korea)	8.0	12.5	
Europe	0.1	6.3	1.7
Africa	0.6	9.0	4.8

References: BJARTVEIT (1978); BURJANOVÁ et al. (1979); CANETTI et al. (1967); East African / British Medical Research Council Tanzania Tuberculosis Survey (1975); East African / British Medical Research Council Second Tanzania Tuberculosis Survey (1978); GOMI et al. (1979); HERSHFIELD et al. (1979); HOBBY et al. (1966); HOBBY et al. (1974); HORNE (1969); HUSSELS (1977); HUSSELS et al. (1978); JANOWIEC et al. (1979); KHALIE and SATHIANATHAN (1978); KIM (1971); KOK-JENSEN and TØRNING (1969); KOPANOFF et al. (1978); KUČANDA (1977); MATTHIESSEN et al. (1977); MILLER et al. (1966); PAGON and JAKŠIĆ (1979); PORVEN et al. (1978); PORVEN (1980); STEINER et al. (1974); STEINER et al. (1979); TOMAN (1979).

The development of PAS resistance does not imply any substantial changes in the mycobacteria, especially concerning the virulence. In contrast to sensitive strains, the resistant mutants bind PAS rapidly and strongly (REUTGEN 1975). Some controversial results have also been reported (WACKER 1956a, b; ZEYER et al. 1960). The binding depended on the temperature and practically ceased at 5 °C. Owing to the resistance, the inhibition index (PAS/PABA ratio) increased from 16 to 1024 (HEDGECOCK 1958). A similar increase has been observed in *M. kansasii* primarely insensitive to the action of PAS (HEDGECOCK 1965).

Cross-Resistance: With the exception of thiacetazone, there is no report of cross-resistance between PAS and other antituberculosis drugs. The cross-resistance appears only in PAS-highly-resistant mutants, which are 5 times as resistant to thiacetazone as parent sensitive organisms. PAS-low-resistant strains remain sensitive to thiacetazone (TSUKAMURA 1977). All thiacetazone-resistant mutants, on the other hand are sensitive to PAS.

Although p-aminobenzoic acid antagonizes both PAS and sulphonamides, no cross-resistance between PAS and the sulphonamides has been detected (RAGAZ 1948; YEGIAN and LONG 1951; TSUKAMURA et al. 1959a).

γ) Type of Action. The inhibitory effect of PAS is only bacteriostatic, not bactericidal, and does not affect the staining properties of mycobacteria (BOGEN et al. 1950; SINGH and MITCHISON 1954; KANAI and YANAGISAWA 1955; KANAI et al. 1963; KRÜGER-THIEMER and BÜNGER 1965, 1966; KREBS 1967, 1968). Some morphological changes occur only after exposure of 4–8 weeks (DOMAGK 1950). In an electron microscope the rods appear longer, with slightly thickened ends. Only about 1% of the mycobacteria are lysed (ROHAN and ROSENBERG 1950; WINDER 1964).

Because of the purely bacteriostatic action of PAS it is generally held that fully inhibitory concentrations should be maintained over the day as long as possible in order to prevent proliferation of the bacilli by "steady-state" treatment. The action of PAS is really reversible. However, it does not cease immediately with the removal of the drug. A contact of 10 µg/ml PAS for 2 h per day is sufficient to inhibit growth in liquid media. If the interval is prolonged to 3 days, slight growth occurs (KREBS 1967, 1968). This effect undoubtly depends on the uptake of PAS by mycobacteria, but little is known about the diffusion of PAS and of its metabolites into the bacterial cells. The pronounced hydrophilic properties of PAS make it seem unlikely that PAS could cross the lipid cover of the "full-grown" bacillus. PAS does not accumulate specially in the area of activity. Both in the bacteria and in the focus its concentration decreases from the outside inwards where the maximum is reached after approximately 3–4 days (WACKER 1956a, b; SUZUKI 1958; ZEYER et al. 1960; LAUBER et al. 1962; PROTIVINSKY 1971). Part of the drug becomes protein-bound (WAY et al. 1948; RAGAZ 1948), and is only released from this binding and becomes active again when the concentration of free PAS in the cell decreases (LEHMANN 1969).

b) Effects on Mycobacteria in Cell and Tissue Cultures

The rate of entry into and the concentration of PAS in the tissues are determined by the concentration gradient between the extracellular and the intracellular medium. The process is relatively slow, and therefore mycobacteria located within macrophages are for a time largely protected from the action of PAS. For a virulent strain of *M. bovis* parasitizing rabbit macrophages in vitro, the concentration of 100 μg PAS/ml in culture broth was insufficient to inhibit the intracellular mycobacteria (MACKANESS 1952; MACKANESS and SMITH 1953). The sensitivity of the same strain in Dubos-Davis broth has been shown to correspond to 1.56 μg PAS/ml. Similar results have been obtained in tissue cultures infected with *M. tuberculosis* susceptible in vitro to 0.6 μg PAS/ml (FREERKSEN 1954a; FREERKSEN and KRÜGER-THIEMER 1954, 1955). This can explain some discrepancies between the activity of PAS in vitro and in vivo.

c) Activity of PAS in Experimental Tuberculosis and Development of Resistance in Vivo

The main efforts have been aimed at finding the most effective regimen, whether continuous treatment is optimal or whether an intermittent mode or a treatment consisting of the administration of large single doses would be preferable. The problem was complicated by the almost exclusively bacteriostatic activity of the drug and by the pharmacological properties of PAS and its metabolites (LAUENER et al. 1957; LEHMANN 1969). Most of the studies on the effect of PAS monotherapy in experimental tuberculosis have been done in guinea pigs and in mice. Studies using other animal species are rare and deal mostly with special problems, including non-pulmonary tuberculosis.

α) Guinea Pigs. Owing to severe local reactions after subcutaneous administration of PAS, it is difficult to check out a wide range of doses in experimental chemotherapy. Apart from this, there is a dependence of efficacy upon the concentration of the injected solution. Thus, guinea pigs treated with 30 mg to 100 mg PAS/day s.c. in a dilution of 1:100 still showed extensive macroscopic tuberculous lesions in the spleen, liver and lungs after 30 days, in contrast to those cured with the same dose, diluted only 1:5. In this case the lesions were much less pronounced, especially in the lungs (SOLOMIDES and BOULAUD 1949). In therapeutic experiments a single daily dose of 125 mg PAS/animal (approximately 210 mg/kg) showed a pronounced effect on advanced tuberculosis when given for only 50 days. Furthermore, single daily injections of 250 mg and 500 mg were no more effective than 125 mg (FELDMAN et al. 1949). Comparison of the regimen with single injections of 200 mg PAS showed that the latter dose was as effective as 100 mg given twice a day, and moreover, 200 mg once daily appeared to be as beneficial as giving 200 mg twice a day (KARLSON and CARR 1958).

Most of the experiments were therefore done with oral PAS administration (in the feed or using a stomach tube). According to early experimental studies, when PAS was given mixed in with the feed, a high daily intake of the drug and a prolonged treatment were necessary to achieve a marked therapeutic effect (BLOCH et al. 1949). For example, only questionable results were obtained in an exploratory study in which tuberculous guinea pigs had been given a diet containing 2%–3% of PAS for 48 days (FELDMAN et al. 1949). Similarly uncertain results were reported after 5% of PAS in the feed (LEHMANN 1946a, b; SWEDBERG and WIDSTRÖM 1948). When, however, the PAS concentration in the feed was 4% (approximately 1600 mg PAS given daily) and the treatment was continued for 119 days, the effect on the tuberculosis was impressive. Subsequent studies showed that the administration of 4% of PAS in the feed had to be continued for a minimum of 60 days to achieve any significant therapeutic effect (KARLSON and CARR 1958).

More information has been obtained after the use of defined oral doses given directly and not in the feed. Single daily doses of 100 mg PAS/day (about 150 mg/kg) were found to be ineffective (BOGEN et al. 1950). Some positive results have been obtained in a therapeutic study with 150 mg/day (i.e., approximately 225 mg/kg) (YASHCHENKO 1954). Single daily oral doses of 200 mg (about 333 mg/kg) for 66 days resulted in a pronounced regression and even in disappearance of the lesions. Some therapeutic effect was also achieved with the same dose given 3 times a week, but the results were inferior to those produced by daily administration. No apparent benefit was derived from fractionating the 200 mg dose into 100 mg doses given twice daily (KARLSON and CARR 1958).

These results demonstrate clearly that, although PAS is rapidly absorbed and excreted, a single daily dose of 200 mg PAS/animal is strikingly effective in the treatment of experimental tuberculosis in guinea pigs (CARR and KARLSON 1961).

On the other hand, even a higher dose of PAS (400 mg/animal/day) is not sufficient to control highly letal experimental tuberculous meningitis in guinea pigs. The lesions in animals treated with PAS alone from the day of intracerebral infection were essentially the same as in the untreated controls. These findings are in accord with the poor results reported on PAS therapy of tuberculous meningitis in man. Evidently the drug cannot reach the brain tissue in adequate concentrations (WAY et al. 1948; STEENKEN et al. 1951).

β) Mice. The efficacy of PAS in experimental tuberculosis is considered to be somewhat lower in mice (or rats) than in other animal species. The effect may be explained by the characteristics of murine tuberculosis, the predominantly intracellularly localized mycobacteria being inaccessible to adequate PAS concentrations (GRUMBACH 1965; CANETTI 1968). The lower effectiveness of PAS has also been attributed to its solely bacteriostatic action (KREIS and FOURNAUD 1965a, b). The importance of both effects has been confirmed experimentically by BARTMANN (1960). In order to eliminate the influence of phagocytosis, BARTMANN used bacilli incorporated in agar blocks which were implanted subcutaneously into mice. The animals were treated with 1.7 g PAS/kg/day (in the feed) for a period of 14 days. The bacteriostatic effect of PAS on the extracellular mycobacteria was strongly pronounced in comparison with the controls. The numbers of culturable mycobacteria in the agar blocks remained unchanged in the course of the treatment.

In tuberculous mice lower PAS doses were found to be ineffective, even in prophylactic experiments. Doses of 0.125 – 0.25% of PAS in the feed (i.e., approximately 234 mg/kg/day–530 mg/kg/day) given for 14 days were only slightly effective. A prolongation of the median survival time has been observed after 0.5% –2.0% of PAS in the diet (i.e., about 1000 mg/kg/day–3800 mg/kg/day) (YOUMANS and YOUMANS 1951). 4% of PAS in the diet proved to be highly toxic to mice (YOUMANS et al. 1947). The slight effect of 5 mg PAS/animal (i.e., about 250 mg/kg) was also confirmed in therapeutic experiments with subcutaneous administration (YASHCHENKO 1954). Even 500 mg PAS/kg proved to be insufficient in advanced tuberculosis – the prolongation of survival was only a few days compared to the untreated controls (GRUMBACH 1965).

Summarizing the effects, it has been concluded that the median survival time of tuberculous mice treated orally with PAS is directly proportional to the dose administered in the range of some 400 mg/kg/day–2000 mg/kg/day for a minimum of 35 days (i.e., 2.77 mmol/kg–12.77 mmol/kg). Below 400 mg/kg the activity falls off rapidly (RAKE et al. 1949; YOUMANS and YOUMANS 1951). From the point of view of toxicity, a sufficient effective dose is about 750 mg/kg, given either subcutaneously (YASHCHENKO 1954) or orally (KREBS 1969). Mice suffering from advanced tuberculosis survived 3 months–5 months, in contrast to the 1-month survival of the controls. The bacteriostatic effect of the drug was pronounced. During 105 days of treatment the number of viable mycobacteria in the lungs remained unchanged. A similar effect was achieved with the same dose divided into 3 daily fractions or administered intermittently, i.e., twice a week in an amount of 2250 mg/kg (KREBS 1967, 1968).

γ) Other Animal Species. In a therapeutic study rabbits infected with *M. bovis* were treated with 600 mg PAS/day for 4 months without any significant results. All the animals died in the course of the treatment (FREERKSEN 1954b). In chickens PAS in a dose of 1 g/kg/day had also only slight effect against pronounced avian tuberculosis (CARMICHAEL and MACLAY 1950).

Rabbits were used to evaluate the influence of PAS on experimental ocular tuberculosis. An acute but not destructive inflammation developed subsequent to inoculation of *M. tuberculosis* into the anterior chamber of the eye. The therapeutic results depended largely on the time between the start of the treatment and the inoculation of mycobacteria into the eye and on the size of inoculum. In well-established cases, i.e., of more than 2 weeks' duration, PAS in a dose of 200 mg/kg/day failed to alter the ocular lesions and the subsequent course of ocular tuberculosis (ADAIR et al. 1951).

The resistance of mycobacteria in animals treated with PAS appears slowly, with the development of only partly resistant populations (BOGEN et al. 1950; KREBS 1968). Otherwise, in clinical studies the development of resistance is considered to be as high as in the case of other antituberculotics (KARLSON et al. 1949; RIST et al. 1951a; VERAN et al. 1951), especially during monotherapy. Strains with very high resistance have also been detected (ICHIOKA and OKAWA 1962). The suggestions that the development of PAS resistance in vivo is rare and slow may be ascribed to the shortcomings of the sensitivity-testing methods (KREBS 1975) (Table 4).

Table 4. Therapeutic activity of p-aminosalicyclic acid (PAS) in experimental tuberculosis

Animal species	Infection		Therapy			Total duration of exp. (days)	Evaluation method	Success of treatment (%)	Ref.
	Strain and route	Dose	Start after infection (days)	Route and dose[a]	Duration (days)				
Guinea pig	M. tbc i.v.	?	16	200 mg daily i.m. 7 days + 200 mg/day per os, 35 days	42	42	TB index[b]	55.0	[1]
	M. tbc SM-res.							13.3	
Guinea pig	M. bovis s.c.	1 µg	7	150 mg/day per os 40 mg/day per os	210	217	Autopsy, mortality	50.0 33.3	[2]
Guinea pig	M. tbc H37Rv s.c.	0.1 mg ww	21	s.c. 125 mg/day 125 mg twice daily 200 mg/day 100 mg twice daily 200 mg twice daily	70	91	Autopsy, TB index	 66.7 74.7 69.0 67.8	[3]
Guinea pig	M. tbc H37Rv intracerebrally	0.1 µg dw	0	200 mg twice daily, per os	26	26	Mortality, autopsy, histology	0.0	[4]

Mouse	M. tbc H37Rv i.v.	1 mg ww	− 1	1% in diet 0.5 % in diet 0.25% in diet 0.125% in diet	14	120	Prolongation of median survival time	326.0 215.0 185.0 159.0	[5]
Mouse	M. tbc H37Rv i.v.	4.4×10^6 cells 6.6×10^6 cells	15	Per os 750 mg/kg/day 750 mg/kg in 3 daily doses 2250 mg/kg twice weekly per os 750 mg/kg/day	237	252	Quantitative culture of lung homogenate	See text	[6]
Mouse	M. bovis i.v.	0.1 mg ww	3	S.c. 5 mg/day 15 mg/day	45–75	48–78	Autopsy, mortality	 28.6 78.6	[2]
Rabbit	M. bovis Vossloch i.v.	0.02 mg	16	Per os 0.6 g/kg/day in 2 doses	120	136	Survival time	0	[7]
Rabbit	M. tbc H37Rv intraocul.	0.005–0.01 mg dw	0	In diet 200 mg/kg/day	49	49	Suppressive effect on ocular lesions	25	[8]

Abbreviations: dw = dry weight; ww = wet weight.

References: [1]Maral and Blandin (1950); [2] Yashchenko (1954); [3] Karlson and Carr (1958); [4] Steenken et al. (1951); [5] Youmans and Youmans (1951); [6] Krebs (1968); [7] Freerksen (1954b); [8] Adair et al. (1951).

[a] Dose per animal unless otherwise stated.

[b] TB index (infection index) – a relative value compared to the same index in an untreated group.

3. Concluding Remarks

In general, the success of the antituberculotic action of PAS is determined by the duration of therapy and by the dosage used. Because of the exclusively bacteriostatic activity of the drug, the lesions cannot be completely eliminated by monotherapy and there is a risk of progression after the end of administration. On the other hand, the strong bacteriostatic action, the absence of cross-resistance, and its other properties make PAS highly suitable for use in combination with other antituberculotics. These combinations, some of them well established in clinical practice, will be discussed in turn in what follows.

References

Adair CV, Drobeck B, Bunn PA (1951) Use of rabbit eye as a tissue to study tuberculosis. II. Effect of certain antituberculous agents upon ocular tuberculosis. Am Rev Tuberc 64:207–217

Bartmann K (1960) Die experimentellen Grundlagen der Chemoprophylaxe der Tuberkulose mit Isonicotinsäurehydrazid (INH). Adv Tuberc Res 10:127–215

Bartmann K, Abel U, Hart R (1966) Die Abhängigkeit des Hemmtiters von der Bebrütungsdauer bei der Bestimmung der Resistenz von *M. tuberculosis* gegen Antituberkulotika auf Löwenstein-Jensen Medium. Zentralbl Bakteriol Mikrobiol Hyg (A) 201:538–548

Bjartveit K (1978) Tuberculosis situation in the Scandinavian countries. Norway. Scand J Respir Dis Suppl No 102:28–35

Bloch RG, Vennesland K, Ebert RH, Gomori G (1949) The effect of streptomycin, para-aminosalicylic acid (PAS) and their combination on the tubercle bacillus in vitro and in vivo. Am Rev Tuberc 59:554–561

Bogen E, Loomis RN, Will DW (1950) Para-aminosalicylic acid treatment of tuberculosis. A review. Am Rev Tuberc 61:226–246

Bönicke R (1950/51) Ernährung und tuberkulostatische Aktivität der PAS in vivo. Jahrber Borstel 1:255–258

Bönicke R, Reif W (1950/51) Untersuchungen über die tuberkulostatische Wirksamkeit und die Schwermetallkomplexbildung der PAS und ihrer Derivate. Jahrber Borstel 1:243–251

Bryson V, Szybalski W (1955) Microbial drug resistance. Adv Genet 7:1–46

Burjanová B, Dornetzhuber V (1975) Empfindlichkeit der Stämme des *M. kansasii* auf verschiedene Antibiotika und Chemotherapeutika in vitro und in vivo. Z Erkr Atmungsorgane 142:68–77

Burjanová B, Turzová M, Grígelová R (1979) Bacteriological tuberculosis diagnostics in the Slovak Socialist Republic during the period 1968–1977 (in Czech). Stud Pneumol Phtiseol Cechoslov 39:81–87

Canetti G, Kreis B, Thibier R, Gay P, LeLirzin M (1967) Données actuelles sur la résistance primaire dans la tuberculose pulmonaire de l'adulte en France. Deuxieme enquête du Centre d'Etudes sur la résistance primaire; années 1965–1966. Rev Tuberc 31:433–474

Canetti G (1968) Experiments on long-term intermittent chemotherapy in advanced tuberculosis in mice. Tubercle 49 (Suppl):70–74

Canetti G, Fox W, Khomenko A, Mahler HT, Menon NK, Mitchison DA, Rist N, Šmelev NA (1969) Advances in techniques of testing mycobacterial drug sensitivity, and the use of sensitivity tests in tuberculosis control programmes. Bull WHO 41:21–43

Carmichael J, Maclay MH (1950) The use of chicks in evaluation of anti-tuberculous agents. J Pathol Bacteriol 62:363–370

Carr DT, Karlson AG (1961) Optimal regimens of antituberculous drugs. Am Rev Respir Dis 84:90–92

Demerec M (1955) Genetic basis of acquired drug resistance. Public Health Rep 70:817–821

Deutsches Zentralkomitee zur Bekämpfung der Tuberkulose (1966) Empfehlungen zur Methodik und Bewertung von Resistenz-Bestimmungen bei Tuberkulose-Bakterien
Diczfaluzy E (1947) Action of salicylic acid derivatives. I. Investigations on the action of PAS. Ark Kemi 24B:1–8
Domagk G (1950) Investigations on the antituberculous activity of the thiosemicarbazones in vitro and in vivo. Am Rev Tuberc 61:8–19
Donovick R, Bayan A, Hamre D (1952) The reversal of the activity of antituberculous compounds in vitro. Am Rev Tuberc 66:219–227
East African/British Medical Research Council Tanzania Tuberculosis Survey (1975) Tuberculosis in Tanzania: a national sampling survey of drug resistance and other factors. Tubercle 56:269–294
East African/British Medical Research Council Second Kenya Tuberculosis Survey (1978) Tuberculosis in Kenya: a second national sampling survey of drug resistance and other factors, and a comparison with the prevalence data from the first national sampling survey. Tubercle 59:155–177
Feldman WH, Karlson AG, Carr DT, Hinshaw HC (1949) Parenteral administration of PAS in experimental tuberculosis. Proc Staff Meet Mayo Clin 24:220–224
Freerksen E (1954a) Wirkungsmöglichkeiten tuberkulostischer Stoffe im Makroorganismus. Beitr Klin Tuberk 111:17–34
Freerksen E (1954b) Über die experimentelle Grundlagen der Kombinationstherapie. Beitr Klin Tuberk 111:574–585
Freerksen E, Krüger-Thiemer E (1954/55) Mycobakterien in der Gewebekultur. A. Gegenwärtiger Kenntnisstand. Jahrber Borstel 3:66–93
Furesz S (1970) Chemical and biological properties of rifampicin. Antibiot Chemother 16:316–351
Gálvez-Brandon J, Bartmann K (1969) Statistical aspects of the proportion method for determining the drug-resistance of tubercle bacilli. Scand J Respir Dis 50:1–18
Gernez-Rieux C, Devulder B (1970) Comparative investigation in vitro of the sensibility of atypical mycobacteria to cycloserine and to other antibacterial substances. Scand J Respir Dis Suppl 71:22–34
Gomi J, Chiba Y, Yanagisawa K (1979) A study on prevalence of resistance to primary and secondary drugs among newly admitted pulmonary tuberculosis patients in 1977. Kekkaku 54:549–555
Goodacre CL, Mitchell BW, Seymour DE (1948) Para-aminosalicylic acid. Part II. The in vitro tuberculostatic behaviour of para-aminosalicylic acid and related compounds. Quart J Pharmacol 21:301–305
Goodacre CL, Seymour DE (1949) Attempts to induce resistance to P.A.S. in strains of Mycobacterium tuberculosis. J Pharm Pharmacol 1:788–789
Grosset J, Canetti G (1962) Teneur de souches sauvages de Mycobacterium tuberculosis en variants résistants aux antibiotiques mineurs (acide para-amino-salicylique, éthionamide, cyclosérine, viomycine, kanamycine). Ann Inst Pasteur 103:163–184
Grumbach F (1965) Etudes chimiothérapeutiques sur la tuberculose avancée de la souris. Adv Tuberc Res 14:31–96
Hedgecock LW (1956) Antagonism of the inhibitory action of aminosalicylic acid on *M. tuberculosis* by methionine, biotin and certain fatty acids, amino acids, and purines. J Bacteriol 72:839–846
Hedgecock LW (1958) Mechanisms involved in the resistance of Mycobacterium tuberculosis to para-aminosalicylic acid. J Bacteriol 75:345–350
Hedgecock LW (1965) Comparative study of the mode of action of para-aminosalicylic acid on Mycobacterium kansasii and Mycobacterium tuberculosis. Am Rev Respir Dis 91:719–727
Heilmeyer L (1950) Weitere Erfahrungen mit Streptomycin, PAS und TB I (Conteben) in der Behandlung der internen Tuberkulosen. Dtsch Med Wochenschr 75:473–477
Hershfield ES, Eidus L, Hlebecque DM (1979) Canadian survey to determine the rate of drug resistance to isoniazid, PAS and streptomycin in newly detected untreated tuberculosis patients and retreatment cases. Int J Clin Pharmacol Biopharm 17:387–393

Hobby GL, Johnson PM, Crawford-Gagliardi L, Boytar V, Johnson GE (1966) Primary drug resistance: a continuing study of drug resistance in tuberculosis in a veteran population within the United States. Am Rev Respir Dis 94:703–708
Hobby GL, Johnson PM, Boytar-Papirnyik V (1974) Primary drug resistance: a continuing study of drug resistance in tuberculosis in a veteran population within the United States. X. September 1970 to September 1973. Am Rev Respir Dis 110:95–98
Horne NW (1969) Drug-resistant tuberculosis: a review of the world situation. Tubercle 50 (Suppl):2–12
Hurni H (1949a) Gibt es eine Gewöhnung an p-Amino-salicylsäure (PAS)? Experientia 5:128
Hurni H (1949b) Über die quantitativen Verhältnisse beim Antagonismus zwischen p-Aminosalicylsäure (PAS) und p-Aminobenzoesäure (PABA). Schweiz Z Pathol Bakteriol 12:282–286
Hussels H (1977) Die Häufigkeit der primären Resistenz von Tuberkulosebakterien in der Bundesrepublik Deutschland einschließlich Berlin (West) im Beobachtungszeitraum 1972 bis 1975. Prax Pneumol 31:664–670
Hussels H, Mathiessen W, Kind A, Göbel D (1978) Frequency and epidemiology of primary drug-resistance in tuberculosis in the Federal Republic of Germany including Berlin (West). Partial result of study of the W.A.T.L. Scand J Respir Dis Suppl 79:65–67
Ichioka M, Okawa H (1962) Studies on Mycobacterium tuberculosis showing extremely high resistance to SM, PAS, and INH (in Japanese). Kekkaku 37:621–624
Ivánovics G (1949) Antagonism between effects of p-aminosalicylic acid and salicylic acid on growth of *M. tuberculosis*. Proc Soc Exp Biol Med 70:462–463
Ivánovics G (1950) Über die p-Aminosalicylsäure-Festigkeit von Tuberkelbakterien. Experientia 6:108–109
Janowiec M, Zwolska-Kwiek Z, Wiśniewska A, Wróblevska H (1977) Interakcja leków przeciwopratkowych. I. Skojarzone działanie rifampicyny s hydrazydem kwasu izonikotynowego, streptomycyna i kwasem paraaminosalicylowym na wzrost szcepów prątków gruźlicy. Pneumol Pol 45:425–430
Janowiec M, Zwolska-Kwiek Z, Bek E (1979) Drug resistance in newly discovered untreated tuberculosis patients in Poland, 1974–1977. Tubercle 60:233–237
Kakemi K, Sezaki H, Kitazawa S (1967) Studies on the pharmaceutical potentiation of drugs. III. Antagonistic effect of PABA on antitubercular activities of PAS derivatives. Chem Pharm Bull (Tokyo) 15:925–931
Kanai K, Yanagisawa K (1955) Antibacterial action of streptomycin against tubercle bacilli of various growth phase. Jpn J Med Sci Biol 8:63–76
Kanai K, Okamoto S, Murohashi T (1963) The in vitro effect of antituberculous agents in relation to the exposure time on Ogawa glycerol egg medium (in Japanese). Kekkaku 38:512–516
Karlson AG, Delaude A, Carr DT, Pfuetze KH, Feldman WH (1949) The occurrence of tubercle bacilli resistant to p-aminosalicylic acid (PAS). Dis Chest 16:667–675
Karlson AG, Carr DT (1958) Effect of single and of double daily doses of para-aminosalicylic acid in tuberculosis of guinea pigs. Am Rev Tuberc 78:753–759
Khalil A, Sathianathan S (1978) Impact of anti-tuberculosis legislation in Libya on the prevalence of primary and acquired resistance to the three main drugs at a major tuberculosis centre. Tubercle 59:1–12
Kim SC (1971) Primary drug resistance of Mycobacterium tuberculosis isolated from untreated patients with pulmonary tuberculosis in Korea (in Japanese). Kekkaku 46:165–171
Klebanova AA (1954) Action of PAS on the tubercle bacillus (in Russian). In: Shebanov FV (ed) Therapy of tuberculous patients by PAS. Medgiz, Moscow, pp 22–33
Kok-Jensen A, Tørning K (1969) Aspects of the tuberculosis situation in Denmark. Especially chemoresistance. Scand J Respir Dis (Suppl) 69:17–20
Kopanoff DE, Kilburn JO, Glassroth JL, Snider DE Jr, Farer LS, Good RC (1978) A continuing survey of tuberculosis primary drug resistance in the United States: March 1975 to November 1977. A United States Public Health Service cooperative study. Am Rev Respir Dis 118:835–842

Krebs A (1967) The action of antituberculous drugs. Tuberkuloza (Beograd) 19:329–337
Krebs A (1968) Die Wirkungsweise der „Tuberkulostatika". Konsequenzen für die Therapie. Z Tbk 128:208–217
Krebs A (1969) Experimentelle Chemotherapie der Tuberkulose. Z Erkr Atmungsorgane 130:417–448
Krebs A (1975) Mykobakterielle Resistenz und Resistenzbestimmungen. In: Meissner G, Schmiedel A, Nelles A (Hrsg) Mykobakterien und mykobakterielle Krankheiten. Teil III. Bakteriologische Grundlagen der Chemotherapie der Tuberkulose. Fischer, Jena, pp 183–250
Krebs A, Kalich R (1964) Unpublished data; cited from Krebs A (1975) p 238
Kreis B, Fournaud S (1965a) Les traitements antituberculeux de très courte durée chez le souris. I. Méthode d'étude et de comparison des médicaments antibacillaires. Ann Inst Pasteur 108:113–117
Kreis B, Fournaud S (1965b) Les traitements antituberculeux de très courte durée chez la souris. II. Résultats. Ann Inst Pasteur 108:117–120
Krüger-Thiemer E, Bünger P (1965/66) The role of the therapeutic regimen in dosage design. Chemotherapia (Basel) 10:61–73
Kučanda F (1977) Primary drug resistance in pulmonary tuberculosis (from 1966 till 1975). Plucne Bolesni Tuberk 29:229–233
Lauber E, Hurni H, Schmidt U, Aebi H (1962) Aufnahme und Retention von p-Aminosalicylsäure (PAS) und Benzoyl-p-aminosalicylsäure (B-PAS) durch *M. tuberculosis*. Z Naturforsch (B) 17:663–670
Lauener H, Hodler J, Favez C, Dettwiler E, Hadorn L (1957) Bildung und Ausscheidung der Stoffwechselprodukte von p-Aminosalicylsäure. Klin Wochenschr 35:393–401
Lehmann J (1946a) Kemoterapi av tuberkulos: p-Aminosalicylsyra (PAS) och närstående derivats bakteriostatiska effekt på tuberkelbacillen jämte djurexperimentella och kliniska försök med PAS. Sven Läkartidn 43:2029–2041
Lehmann J (1946b) Para-aminosalicylic acid in treatment of tuberculosis: preliminary communication. Lancet I:15–16
Lehmann J (1947) Recherches sur le bacille tuberculeux: Action bactériostatique, différentiation in vivo. Rev Gen Sci Pures Appl 54:222–230
Lehmann J (1949) On the effect of isomers of PAS and related substances on the tuberculostatic effect of PAS. Experientia 5:365–367
Lehmann J (1969) The role of the metabolism of p-amino-salicylic acid (PAS) in the treatment of tuberculosis. Scand J Respir Dis 50:169–185
Lorian V (1966) Antibiotics and chemotherapeutic agents in clinical laboratory practice. Thomas, Springfield, USA
Mackaness GB (1952) The action of drugs on intracellular tubercle bacilli. J Pathol Bacteriol 64:429–436
Mackaness GB, Smith N (1953) The bactericidal action of isoniazid, streptomycin, and terramycin on extracellular tubercle bacilli. Am Rev Tuberc 67:322–340
Maral R, Blandin A (1950) Étude in vitro de l'action du para-amino-salicylate de sodium (P.A.S.). I. Sur la sensibilité des souches de B.K. à la streptomycine. Ann Inst Pasteur 78:681–684
Marks J (1961) The design of sensitivity tests on tubercle bacilli. Tubercle 42:314–316
Matthiessen W, Kind A, Göbel D (1977) Epidemiologie der Primärresistenz von Tuberkulosebakterien in der Bundesrepublik Deutschland einschließlich Berlin (West) im Beobachtungszeitraum 1972 bis 1975. Prax Pneumol 31:890–899
Mayer FL, Eisman PC, Gisi TA, Konopka EA (1958) The chemotherapeutic activity upon chromogenic mycobacteria of certain derivatives of thiocarbanilide (SU-1906), thiazoline (SU-3068), and thiazolidinone (SU-3912). Am Rev Tuberc 77:694–702
Miller AB, Tall E, Fox W (1966) Primary drug resistance in pulmonary tuberculosis in Great Britain: Second national survey, 1963. Tubercle 47:92–107
Mitchison DA (1970) Bacteriological mechanisms in recent controlled chemotherapy studies. Bull Inter Un Tuberc 43:322–331
Ogawa T, Otani N (1961a) Studies on inactivation of antituberculous agents in media. 1st report: The relationship between the amount of incorporated activated carbon and inactivation of antituberculous agents (in Japanese). Kekkaku 36:32–37

Ogawa T, Otani N (1961 b) Studies on inactivation of antituberculous agents in media. 2nd report: Influence of p-aminobenzoic acid on inactivating effect of activated carbon (in Japanese). Kekkaku 36:67–72
Pagon S, Jakšsić A (1979) Auswertung der Mykobakterienbefunde, einschließlich Resistenzlage in den Jahren 1973 bis 1977. Tuberk Lungenkr No 5, pp 74–87
Porven G, Piccolo R, Padin L (1978) Primary resistance observed in 974 strains of *M. tuberculosis* isolated from adult pulmonary patients (in Spanish). Medicina (B Aires) 38:497–501
Porven GH (1980) Primary resistance observed in 974 strains of Mycobacterium tuberculosis isolated from adult lung patients. Medicina (B Aires) 40:490–492
Protivinsky R (1971) Chemotherapeutics with tuberculostatic action. Antibiot Chemother 17:101–121
Ragaz L (1948) p-Aminosalicylsäure in der Chemotherapie der Tuberkulose. Schweiz Med Wochenschr 78:1212–1232
Rake G, Jambor WP, McKee CM, Pansy F, Wiselogle FY, Donovick R (1949) The use of the mouse in a standardized test for antituberculous activity of compounds of natural or or synthetic origin. III. The standardized test. Am Rev Tuberc 60:121–130
Reutgen H (1975) p-Aminosalicylsäure. In: Meissner G, Schmiedel A, Nelles A (Hrsg) Mykobakterien und mykobakterielle Krankheiten. Teil III. Bakteriologische Grundlagen der Chemotherapie der Tuberkulose. Fischer, Jena, pp 319–336
Rist N, Véran P, Ballet B, Grumbach F, Trichereau R (1951 a) La résistance du bacille tuberculeux à l'acide para-amino-salicylique. Sem Hôp Paris 27:1823–1830
Rist N, Véran P, Ballet B, Grumbach F, Trichereau R (1951 b) L'abaissement du risque de résistance au PAS par l'association sulfones au PAS. Sem Hôp Paris 27:1830–1833
Robson JM, Keele CA (1956) Recent advances in pharmacology, 2nd ed. Churchill, London, pp 266–501
Rohan P, Rosenberg M (1950) Influence of p-aminosalicylic acid on Mycobacterium tuberculosis followed by electron microscope (in Czech). Lék listy 5:8
Rosdahl KG (1948) Some properties and derivatives of para-aminosalicylic acid (PAS). Sven Kemi Tid 60:12–14
Sievers O (1946) Experimental trials with p-aminosalicylic acid (PAS) against various bacteria (in Swedish). Sven Läkartidn 43:2041–2047
Sievers O (1947) Experimentella försök med para-aminosalicylsyra (PAS) och olika slag av bakterier. Nord Med 33:145–147
Singh B, Mitchison DA (1954) Bactericidal activity of streptomycin and isoniazid against tubercle bacilli. Br Med J 1:130–132
Solomides J, Boulaud E (1949) Essai de traitement de la tuberculose expérimentale du cobaye par les formes hyperactives du PAS (para-amino-salicylate de sodium). Ann Inst Pasteur 77:310–318
Sorkin E, Roth W, Kocher V, Erlenmeyer K (1951) Über die Wirkung von Metallionen auf die tuberkulostatische Aktivität des Oxins und der PAS. Experientia 7:257–258
Standard methods in the microbiology of tuberculosis and lepra (in Czech) (1980). Institute for Hygiene and Epidemiology, Prague
Steenken W Jr, Wolinsky E, Pratt PC (1951) Streptomycin and PAS in experimental tuberculosis of guinea pigs infected intracerebrally with virulent tubercle bacilli. Am Rev Tuberc 64:87–101
Steiner P, Rao M, Goldberg R, Steiner M (1974) Primary drug resistance in children. Drug susceptibility of strains of *M. tuberculosis* isolated from children during the years 1969–1972 at the Kings County Hospital Medical Center at Brooklyn. Am Rev Respir Dis 110:98–100
Steiner P, Rao M, Victoria MS, James P, Steiner M (1979) Primary drug resistance in children. Drug susceptibility of strains of Mycobacterium tuberculosis isolated from children during the years 1973 through 1977 at the Kings County Hospital Center of Brooklyn. Am Rev Respir Dis 119:680–682
Suzuki O (1958) On the mechanism of the bacteriostatic activity of p-aminosalicylic acid (in Japanese). Med Biol (Tokyo) 47:173–176

Swedberg B, Widström G (1948) Treatment of experimental tuberculosis in mice and guinea pigs with PAS and streptomycin. Acta Med Scand 131:116–128

Szybalski W, Bryson V (1953) One step resistance development to isoniazid and sodium-p-aminosalicylate. J Bacteriol 66:468–469

Szybalski W (1954) Genetic studies on microbial cross resistance to toxic agents. IV. Cross resistance of Bacillus megaterium to forty-four antimicrobial drugs. Appl Microbiol 2:57–63

Tobie WC, Jones MJ (1949) Para-aminosalicylic acid in the metabolism of bacteria. J Bacteriol 57:573

Toman K (1979) Tuberculosis. Case-finding and chemotherapy. WHO, Geneva, p 240

Tsukamura M (1961) Variation and heredity of mycobacteria with special reference to drug resistance. Jpn J Tuberc 9:43–64

Tsukamura M (1977) Cross-resistance of tubercle bacilli (a review II). Kekkaku 52:47–49

Tsukamura M, Miura K, Noda Y (1956a) On the mutation to streptomycin resistance and isoniazid resistance in PAS-resistant *Mycobacterium tuberculosis* var. hominis. J Antibiot (Tokyo) 9A:210–217

Tsukamura M, Noda Y, Miura K (1956b) A quantitative analysis of the resistance of *Mycobacterium tuberculosis* to streptomycin, isoniazid and PAS (in Japanese). Kekkaku 31:107–110

Tsukamura M, Noda Y, Yamamoto M (1959a) Studies on the kanamycin resistance in *Mycobacterium tuberculosis*. V. Sensitivity of kanamycin resistant mutants to various antituberculous drugs and mutation frequency to various drug resistance in kanamycin-resistant mutants. J Antibiot (Tokyo) A 12:323–327

Tsukamura M, Noda Y, Yamamoto M, Hayashi M (1959b) Genetic considerations of the mechanisms involved in PAS-resistant tubercle bacilli. Am Rev Tuberc 79:371–373

Tsukamura M, Noda Y, Yamamoto M, Hayashi M (1959c) A genetic study on the PAS-resistance-system of *Mycobacterium tuberculosis*. Jpn J Genet 34:43–54

Tsukamura M, Mizuno S (1980) A comparative study of the relationship between the growth rate of tubercle bacilli and the concentration of antituberculous agents (in Japanese). Kekkaku 55:365–370

Velluti G (1967) Observations on the acquired resistance of *Mycobacterium tuberculosis* to ethambutol. Riv Patol Clin Tuberc 40:815–822

Vennesland K, Ebert RH, Bloch RG (1948) In vitro effect of streptomycin and para-aminoalicylic acid (PAS) on the growth of tubercle bacilli. Proc Soc Exp Biol Med 68:250–255

Véran P, Rist N, Ballet B, Grumbach F, Trichereau R (1951) La résistance du bacille de Koch à l'acide paraamino-salicylique (PAS) au cours de la tuberculose pulmonaire cavitaire. Rev Tuberc 15:87–92

Wacker A (1956a) Wirkungsmechanismus der Sulfonamide und anderer Chemotherapeutika: Untersuchungen mit radioaktiv markierten Verbindungen. Pharmazie 11:562–563

Wacker A (1956b) Ursachen der Bakterienresistenz: Untersuchungen mit radioaktiv markierten Verbindungen. Angew Chem 68:388–389

Waksman SA, Lechevalier HA (1953) Sensitivity of actinomycetales to isonicotinic acid hydrazide, compared to other synthetic and antibiotic antituberculosis agents. Am Rev Tuberc 67:261–264

Walter A (1950) Die tuberkulostatische Wirksamkeit verschiedener PAS-Präparate in vitro. Dtsch Med Wochenschr 75:587

Way EL, Smith PK, Howie DL, Weiss R, Swanson R (1948) The absorption, distribution, excretion and fate of para-aminosalicylic acid. J Pharmacol Exp Ther 93:368–382

Winder F (1964) The antibacterial action of streptomycin, isoniazid and PAS. In: Barry VC (ed) Chemotherapy of tuberculosis. Butterworths, London, pp 111–149

Wolinsky E, Smith MM, Steenken W Jr (1957) Drug susceptibilities of 20 "atypical" as compared with 19 selected strains of mycobacteria. Am Rev Tuberc Pulm Dis 76:497–502

Wyss O, Rubin M, Strandskov FB (1943) Biological action of substituted p-aminobenzoic acids. Proc Soc Exp Biol Med 52:155–164

Yashchenko TN (1954) PAS in therapy of experimental tuberculosis (in Russian). In: Shebanov FV (ed) Therapy of tuberculous patients with PAS. Medgiz, Moscow, pp 34–48
Yegian D, Vanderlinde RJ (1950) The resistance of tubercle bacilli to chemotherapeutic agents. A review of basic biological considerations. Am Rev Tuberc 61:483–507
Yegian D, Long RT (1951) The specific resistance of tubercle bacilli to para-aminosalicylic acid and sulfonamides. J Bacteriol 61:747–749
Youmans GP (1946) The effect of para-aminosalicylic acid in vitro and in vivo on virulent human type bacilli. Bull Northwestern Un Med School 20:420–428
Youmans GP, Raleigh GW, Youmans AS (1947a) The tuberculostatic action of para-aminosalicylic acid. J Bacteriol 54:409–416
Youmans GP, Raleigh GW (1947b) The effect of para-aminosalicylic acid on tubercle bacilli. J Bacteriol 54:65–66
Youmans GP, Youmans AS (1951) The assessment of antituberculous chemotherapeutic activity in mice, using virulent human-type tubercle bacilli. Am Rev Tuberc 64:541–550
Zeyer J, Hurni H, Fischer R, Lauber E, Schönholzer G, Aebi H (1960) Versuche mit verschieden ^{14}C-markierter Benzoyl-PAS in Kulturen von *M. tuberculosis*. Z Naturforsch 15b:694–701

II. Streptomycin (SM) – Dihydrostreptomycin (DHSM)

L. TRNKA and P. MIŠOŇ

1. Antimicrobial Spectrum in Vitro

The antimicrobial spectrum of streptomycin (SM) covers gram-negative bacteria, mycobacteria, and some strains of gram-positives and cocci (WAKSMAN and SCHATZ 1945; LORIAN 1966; MODR et al. 1969). A division according to effectiveness in vitro is used. While such a division is purely arbitrary, it is at least partly justified by the fact that marked differences do exist in the microbial sensitivity to streptomycin in vitro. What is more important is that clinical observations tend to confirm the validity of a classification of this kind.

Among the most sensitive microorganisms are *Pasteurella, Brucella, Shigella, Klebsiella, Haemophilus* (except *H. influenzae*), and *Listeria* organisms, most of which are completely inhibited by less than 10 µg/ml.

The growth of moderately sensitive microorganisms is inhibited by SM concentrations of between 10 µg/ml and 100 µg/ml. This group comprises *Aerobacter, Alcaligenes, Corynebacterium, Diplococcus pneumoniae, Escherichia coli, Haemophilus influenzae, Staphylococcus, Streptococcus viridans, Proteus,* and *Salmonella* organisms.

Anaerobes, fungi, protozoa, rickettsia, and viruses are insensitive or resistant. Although streptomycin is inactive against filterable viruses, it can activate *E. coli* and *S. aureus* bacteriophage strains (YOUMANS and FISHER 1949; GOODMAN and GILMAN 1965).

Dihydrostreptomycin is essentially equal to streptomycin in its inhibitory action and is only less active especially against *Salmonella schottmülleri* and *S. typhosa*. The action of both mannosidostreptomycin and dihydromannosidostreptomycin is significantly weaker than that of streptomycin and dihydrostreptomycin on all the organisms, with the exception of the two Salmonella species mentioned (YOUMANS and FISHER 1949).

2. Antimycobacterial Activity

a) Activity in Artificial Media in Vitro

The first official announcement of the in-vitro bacteriostatic activity of streptomycin against *M. tuberculosis* was published soon after the discovery of this antibiotic (SCHATZ et al. 1944; SCHATZ and WAKSMAN 1944). The minimal inhibitory concentrations for *M. tuberculosis* and *M. bovis* on artificial media range between 0.05 µg/ml and 10 µg/ml depending on the mycobacterial strain, the composition of the broth, and other experimental conditions. It has also been proved that *M. bovis* is in general more streptomycin-sensitive. Some representative results are summarized in Table 1.

Approximately the same concentrations of SM are necessary to inhibit the growth of *M. tuberculosis* H37Rv whether the test is carried out in Dubos me-

Table 1. Minimal inhibitory concentrations of streptomycin for mycobacteria in vitro

Mycobacterium[a]	Medium	Inoculum	Incubation time (days)	Minimal inhib. conc. (MIC) (µg/ml)	Ref.
tuberculosis H37Rv	PB	0.2 mg/10 ml	16	0.4	WOLINSKY and STEENKEN (1974)
	D	0.1 ml of 6-day culture	20	0.4	
	Y	0.25 mg/5 ml	14	0.78	WILLISTON and YOUMANS (1947)
	PB	0.1 mg	14	0.78	WILLISTON and YOUMANS (1949)
	PBS	0.1 mg	14	1.56	
	D	0.1 mg	14	1.56	
	D+Tween	0.1 mg	14	0.39	
	KTA	?	14	2.0 DHSM	RAKE et al. (1948)
bovis Ravenel	KTA	?	14	0.58	
bovis BCG	KTA	?	14	0.52	
tuberculosis human strains (14)	Y	0.25 mg/5 ml	14	0.09–1.56–3.12[a]	WILLISTON and YOUMANS (1947)
(131)	PB	0.1 mg ww		0.09–0.39–12.5	YOUMANS and KARLSON (1947)
(20)	D	0.01 mg	14	Less than 1	FISHER (1948a)
(32)	PB	0.1 mg	14	0.095–0.19–0.78	WILLISTON and YOUMANS (1949)
(26)	HE	0.1 mg	14	1.56–3.12–12.5	
bovis (16)	PB	0.1 mg ww		0.095–0.19–3.12	YOUMANS and KARLSON (1947)
avium (14)	PB	0.1 mg ww		0.39–3.12–50.0	

Highly resistant mutants not included.

[a] The numbers in parentheses indicate the numbers of strains tested. MIC: Lowest value – most common value – highest value observed. For abbreviations of media see table 1, p. 52.

dium, in Proskauer and Beck's synthetic medium with surface growth, or in Proskauer and Beck's medium with subsurface growth, provided that the pH of the medium is kept between 7.1 and 7.4 (WOLINSKY and STEENKEN 1947). Strains freshly isolated from tuberculotic patients are susceptible to 0.1 µg/ml–12 µg/ml.

According to TSUKAMURA and MIZUNO (1980), streptomycin shows an inverse straight-line relationship between the growth rate of mycobacteria and the agent's concentration. An increase in the SM concentration is believed to produce a linearly increased activity in the lesions. In terms of SM-sensitivity, therefore, classical mycobacteria thus represent a relatively homogeneous group (HEJNÝ 1982).

The *M. avium-intracellulare* group is somewhat more resistant to the action of streptomycin in vitro (YOUMANS and KARLSON 1947; HEJNÝ 1982), but it has been suggested that this group also belongs to the SM-susceptible mycobacteria (URBANCZIK 1982). The so called atypical mycobacteria are in general less sensitive and markedly heterogeneous than the typical species. The minimal inhibitory concentrations are in the range of 0.2 µg/ml to 15 µg/ml (WOOD et al. 1956; MANTEN 1957; WOLINSKY et al. 1957; STEENKEN et al. 1958; BURJANOVÁ and DORNETZHUBER 1975; NEUBERT 1976; KUZE et al. 1977a, b; TSANG et al. 1978).

Dihydrostreptomycin is closely comparable with streptomycin in its antimycobacterial activity on a weight-for-weight basis, including *M. avium* strains (EDISON et al. 1948).

α) Factors Affecting the Activity in Vitro. At pH 3–7 streptomycin solutions are stable for 3 months at room temperature. At pH lower than 2 or higher than 10 inactivation occurs within 5 h to 10 h. The activity of SM is maximal at approximately pH 7.8 (7.7–8.0) and decreases markedly below pH 7.0 (ABRAHAM and DUTHIE 1946; MURRAY and FINLAND 1948; HENRY and HOBBY 1949; HURWITZ and MILLER 1950; LORIAN 1966). On the other hand, as the initial pH of a medium decreases below 6.5, dihydrostreptomycin stimulates the growth of drug-resistant strains (HURWITZ 1951).

SM is adsorbed by various substances including the unknown constituents of certain culture media and unidentified constituents of blood serum, plasma, or pus (HENRY et al. 1947; SCHOENBACH and SHANDLER 1947). This effect affects the activity of the drug only insofar as it reduces the concentration of free SM in the medium. Since these reactions are only partial, other variables must be critical for antimycobacterial activity. This may account in part for the conflicting reports on the antagonistic action of serum (HENRY and HOBBY 1949). The phospholipids in eggyolk media may inhibit the antimycobacterial activity of SM by up to 50%. Since the inhibitory factor of this substance is thermoresistant, there is no difference in the SM activity before and after egg-medium coagulation (LORIAN 1966). KREBS et al. (1962) have shown that SM mixed with egg medium prior to coagulation is not inactivated by coagulation. The activity decreases to one-half after this medium has been kept at 37 °C for a period of one month. No inactivation occurs if the medium has been stored at 4 °C.

The activity of SM is extremely sensitive to the salt concentrations in the environment. Both the salts of monovalent cations such as sodium, potassium, ammonium, and lithium (BERKMAN et al. 1947; DONOVICK et al. 1948; GREEN and WAKSMAN 1948; HENRY and HOBBY 1949) and those of divalent cations such as magnesium, calcium, and barium (DONOVICK et al. 1948; BEGGS and WILLIAMS 1971; ZIMELIS and JACKSON 1973) have been reported to be antagonistic to SM, but the divalent cations generally seem to be most effective. The positively doubly charged metal ions appear to play the primary role in this inhibitory activity. Experiments with radiolabelled SM have shown that salts interfere with drug's uptake or binding by susceptible organisms (BEGGS and WILLIAMS 1971). Two different mechanisms of the SM antagonism by salts have been suggested, one being divalent-cation- and concentration-dependent and the other being non-specific and dependent on the ionic strength (BEGGS and ANDREWS 1975 a, b).

Other important factors reducing the antimycobacterial activity of SM are reducing agents. The reduction can be due either to endogeneous reducing activity developed within the organism itself (SELIGMANN and WASSERMANN 1947) or to externally added reducing agents such as cysteine and other sulphhydryl compounds, ascorbic acid, stannous chloride, sodium bisulphite and sodium thiosulphate (DENKELWATER et al. 1945; BONDI et al. 1946; CAVALLITO 1946; BERKMAN et al. 1947; SIMON 1948). Anaerobiosis likewise decreases the activity of SM, although some authors have attributed this to a pH effect (GEIGER et al. 1946).

Surface-active agents enhance the antimycobacterial activity of SM. Tween 80, even in low concentrations, increases the sensitivity of most mycobacterial cultures to SM (FISHER 1948 b; WILLISTON and YOUMANS 1949). Triton A-20 has an enhancing effect on growth in lower concentrations and an inhibitory effect in higher concentrations. Triton A-20 becomes increasingly inhibitory to mycobacteria as the pH is raised above 7.0 (HURWITZ and MILLER 1950).

KREBS et al. (1962) have found that the MIC of SM is higher if the culture tubes are closed firmly, in contrast to tubes closed with caps allowing some gas exchange.

β) Resistance of Mycobacteria Against Streptomycin

Development of SM-Resistance in Vitro and Its Type: Like other types of microorganisms, mycobacteria can be made highly resistant to the action of SM in vitro. This is easily accomplished by repeated culture on nutrient media containing gradually increasing concentrations of SM. By using this method WILLISTON and YOUMANS (1947) were able to increase markedly the resistance of *M. tuberculosis, M. bovis,* and *M. avium.* The rate at which the resistance develops depends on a number of factors, mainly on the individual strain and the inoculum size. With large inocula strains resistant to more than 1000 μg/ml can develop after a few subcultures in SM-containing media (STEENKEN 1949; YOUMANS 1949; ALBERGHINA et al. 1973). The highest resistance levels, i.e., the upper limit of resistance, varied depending on the strain and is considered to be infinite (TSUKAMURA 1961).

It has now been demonstrated that the reason for the appearance of SM-resistant Mycobacteria is the presence of spontaneously occurring resistant mutants in the parent culture (PYLE 1947; VENNESLAND et al. 1947; YEGIAN and VANDERLINDE 1948; YOUMANS and WILLISTON 1948; YOUMANS 1949). This selection of re-

Table 2. Proportion of SM-resistant mutants among strains of *M. tuberculosis* isolated from untreated patients (KREBS 1975)

Medium	SM µg/ml	Frequency	Ref.	Remark
TAA	1	8×10^{-8}	YEGIAN and VANDERLINDE (1950)	
TAA	10	5×10^{-8}	YEGIAN and VANDERLINDE (1948)	
7H10	2	10^{-6}	COHN et al. (1959)	
Ditto	2	2×10^{-7}	RUSSELL and MIDDLEBROOK (1961)	
OAA	2	5×10^{-10}	MIDDLEBROOK (1952)	
Ditto	1	10^{-6}	MITCHISON (1953)	
	10	10^{-7}		
	40	2×10^{-8}		
Herrold Yolk Agar	10	10^{-5}	PYLE (1947)	Direct test
Ditto	0.25–0.5	10^{-6}	MITCHISON (1951)	
	1–2	10^{-7}		
	32	2×10^{-9}		
LJ	2	10^{-5}	GRUMBACH et al. (1964)	
Ditto	4	4×10^{-5}	CANETTI et al. (1963)	Average
Ditto	4	1.4×10^{-6}	KREBS and KALICH (1964)	Average
Ditto	10	10^{-7}	COLETSOS (1963)	
OG	10	6×10^{-7}	TSUKAMURA et al. (1956)	Strain Ayoama B
	50	10^{-8}		
	100	2×10^{-9}		
OG	20	4.6×10^{-6}	TSUKAMURA et al. (1959)	Strain H37Rv
OG	10	10^{-5}	TSUKAMURA (1961)	Strain H37Rv
	200	10^{-8}–10^{-9}		
	10	10^{-6}–10^{-7}		Strain Ayoama B
	200	10^{-8}		

sistant mutants plays a dominant role; adaptation processes are of negligible importance in this context (CANETTI 1959; COHN et al. 1959; CANETTI et al. 1963; MORDASINI and EULENBERGER 1971).

The frequency of SM-resistant mutants in mycobacterial populations varies within the probability limits for the occurrence of spontaneous mutants (HSIE and BRYSON 1950). The frequency of the mutation of sensitive strains in the direction of high resistance with single-step selection (a sign of chromosomal mutation) was found to be low (about $1:10^{-11}$). Higher concentrations of hydroxylamine increased the occurrence of resistant mutants 100-fold (KONÍČKOVÁ-RADOCHOVÁ and MÁLEK 1968). One of the factors giving rise to resistant mutants is ultraviolet light (STAKEMANN 1954). The results of principal in-vitro studies, derived from KREBS (1975), are presented in Table 2.

As already mentioned, SM-resistance develops by the "one-step" type of mechanism. Genetic control of this resistance was attributed to the action of one or more genes on the acquisition of drug resistance at several levels (TSUKAMURA

1961). A two-step mechanism has been confirmed only in the saprophytic *M. smegmatis* strain M 607 (USHIBA et al. 1957).

The type of the SM resistance in mycobacteria is very similar to that described in *E. coli* and other microorganisms (WITTMANN and APIRION 1975). One pattern includes a genetically stable component, caused by modified ribosomes, the other a genetically unstable component directed by plasmids. The latter is due to an enzymatic modification of SM (phosphorylation), which has been demonstrated in some strains of *M. fortuitum* and which is usually connected with low-level resistance (TRNKA, MIŠOŇ, and MORÁVEK, unpublished work). Moreover, the elimination of SM resistance by treatment with acridine dyes and ethidium bromide strongly suggests an existence of extrachromosomal genetic control in *M. tuberculosis* as well. The fact that the low-resistance mutants were not influenced by treatment with mutagenic agents has been explained by the hypothesis that these mycobacterial strains may be largely composed of phenotypic mutants (ALBERGHINA et al. 1973). A resistance factor transferred by transduction has been described for *M. smegmatis*. The transduction of the SM marker was not accompanied by the establishment of lysogeny by the transducing phage but was accompanied by an alteration in the phage pattern of the transduced cultures (JONES et al. 1974).

Features of Resistant Populations: A mycobacterial strain is classified as resistant if the resistant subpopulation exceeds certain agreed limits. The limits are established by experimentation, experience, and the methodology of resistance tests. Using the common indirect proportion method for resistance evaluation, the critical proportion of SM-resistance has been agreed as 1% of cells growing on Löwenstein-Jensen media containing 5 µg/ml (DEUTSCHES ZENTRALKOMITEE 1966) or 1% of ones growing in 4 µg/ml (CANETTI et al. 1969; GÁLVEZ-BRANDON and BARTMANN 1969; STANDARD METHODS 1980). The incubation times may vary between 3–10 weeks but the normal period is 4 weeks (BARTMANN et al. 1966). The frequencies of the initial SM-resistance in patients' strains determined by the above-mentioned methods are summarized in Table 3.

Table 3 indicates clearly the degree of efficacy of the antituberculous chemotherapy in a given region. The higher the figure for initial SM-resistance, the more inadequate the chemotherapy has been, since a correct use of drug combinations should prevent the development of SM-resistance.

Table 3. Frequencies of initial SM-resistance in patients' strains reported during 1953–1980

Region	Percentages of isolated resistant strains		
	Minimum	Maximum	Median
Africa	1.4	16.2	8.0
Asia	4.2	20.6	5.7
Europe	0	7.6	2.3
North and Central America	4.1	10.2	5.2
South America	3.8	43.3	9.1

(For references see PAS.)

SM-resistant mutants have in general the same features as SM-susceptible cells. Some authors, however, have reported changes in color and an increased tendency towards the formation of cytoplasmic granules (BENDA and URQUIA 1950). SM-resistance does not affect the degree of virulence (YOUMANS and WILLISTON 1946; STEENKEN 1949; MEISSNER 1953). Only some limited observations suggest that SM-resistant strains, though still capable of producing progressive disease, did so at a slower rate than the SM-sensitive strains (FELDMAN et al. 1948; FELDMAN and KARLSON 1949). It was also observed that the resistant strains grow comparatively slowly on media containing SM, although the rate of growth tends to increase as greater degrees of resistance are developed (PYLE 1947).

Once acquired, SM-resistance is generally irreversible (apart from exceptions mentioned in Part β) (MIDDLEBROOK and YEGIAN 1946; YOUMANS and WILLISTON 1946; FELDMAN and KARLSON 1949), and persists after passage through animals (TISON 1949). Most of the observed losses of resistance, especially in vivo (WOLINSKY et al. 1948; HOWLETT et al. 1949), are probably due to a change in the proportion of resistant mutants (BEEUWKES and VOS 1952; LINZ 1954).

Streptomycin Dependence: It has been observed that many types of bacteria produce variants dependent on SM for their growth. The first report concerning mycobacteria has been published by YEGIAN and BUDD (1948), who isolated such dependent variants in a culture of *M. ranae*. The observation has been repeatedly confirmed, inter alia with strains of *M. tuberculosis* (SPENDLOVE et al. 1948; PAINE and FINLAND 1948a, b; HOBBY and DOUGHERTY 1948; LENERT and HOBBY 1949; YEGIAN et al. 1949; YEGIAN and VANDERLINDE 1949; OWEN et al. 1950; YEGIAN and BUDD 1951; HURWITZ 1951).

Although guinea pigs injected with an SM-dependent strain showed rapid progression of the disease after administration of SM (TISON 1949), the SM-dependent variants have been found to be much less virulent than the parent strains. Other authors have reported that even when the animals have been inoculated with large numbers of the bacteria and treated with SM, the SM-dependent mycobacteria isolated in vitro do not produce a progressive disease in guinea pigs. SM-sensitive reverse mutants are fully virulent (VANDERLINDE and YEGIAN 1951; DOANE and BOGEN 1951).

Cross-Resistance: Because of the very close structural similarity, complete cross-resistance exists between streptomycin and dihydrostreptomycin (EDISON et al. 1948). Oneway cross-resistance exists between viomycin, kanamycin and streptomycin, in such a way that mycobacterial strains resistant to the first two drugs are usually insensitive to SM but not vice versa (YOUMANS and YOUMANS 1951; TSUKAMURA et al. 1959; HOK and SENG 1964; LUCCHESI 1970; MCCLATCHY et al. 1977). The reason lies in some naturally SM-resistant strains and in induced resistant strains with multistep selection that do not show cross-resistance to kanamycin, neomycin, and viomycin (ALBERGHINA et al. 1973). However, the SM resistance in kanamycin-resistant strains is only 2–4 times as high as the resistance levels of the parent strains (STEENKEN et al. 1959; TORIL et al. 1959). Cross-resistance between capreomycin and streptomycin has not been so far found, despite the fact that capreomycin is structurally closely related to viomycin (KOSEKI and OKAMOTO 1963).

SM-dependent strains of *M. smegmatis* and their revertants have remained resistant to kanamycin (TSUKAMURA 1961).

γ) Type of Action. The action of streptomycin on mycobacteria both in vitro and in vivo appears to be primarily bacteriostatic. This has been repeatedly shown by the fact that viable organisms could be recovered after exposure of mycobacteria to SM in vitro, even though multiplication had been prevented (YOUMANS 1949). However, like most other antibacterial agents, SM manifests both bacteriostatic and bactericidal effects (SCHATZ et al. 1944; BØE and VOGELSANG 1946; MACKANESS and SMITH 1953; GARROD 1950; KANAI and YANAGISAWA 1955). Predominance of one effect over the other in a particular instance appears to be determined, in part, by the time of contact with SM, by the organism involved, and by the SM concentration, as has been confirmed by intermittent applications of SM in vitro (BERNARD and KREIS 1951; KREBS 1967, 1968). Within certain limits the bacteriostatic action of SM appears to be independent of the mycobacterial count, a tenfold variation in the count having little significance (YOUMANS 1949).

In general, the inhibitory activity of SM depends largely on the metabolic activity of the mycobacterial cells; growing cells are much more susceptible. Even high concentrations of SM left in contact with virulent mycobacteria in a saline suspension for one week did not destroy the organisms, and had no effect after one week of contact with mycobacteria suspended in blood (CORPER and COHN 1946). The dependence of activity on the growth phase of mycobacteria has been repeatedly established, even if not ever fully accepted; cf. a review by KREBS (1969). Mycobacteria in the logarithmic phase of growth exposed to SM for 24 h are irreversibly damaged; the growth cannot be restored even after the removal of SM. In the stationary growth phase after 72-h exposure to SM, mycobacteria are still capable of multiplying when the antibiotic is removed (MIDDLEBROOK and YEGIAN 1946). Prolonged exposure leads again to bactericidal effects (BARTMANN 1960a), accompanied by structural changes typical of autolytic processes (BERNARD et al. 1954; LINZ 1954), namely loss of acid-fastness, increased granulation, shortening of the rods (SMITH and WAKSMAN 1947), clearing and vacuolation of cytoplasm and release of granular cytoplasmic material into media (RABUKHIN 1970).

δ) Effects in Combination with Other Antituberculotics in Vitro. Administration of SM simultaneously with some other drugs that are also effective in experimental tuberculosis was first reported by SMITH and MCCLOSKY (1945), and since then a number of other investigators have adopted this approach to obtain more effective therapeutic results than may be realized with SM alone. In this connection PAS received special attention, both in vivo and in vitro. It was found that PAS inhibited the growth of naturally occurring SM-resistant variants of *M. tuberculosis* completely in concentrations of 1.2 μg/ml and partly in a concentration of 0.6 μg/ml. Moreover, the inhibition of sensitive strains was markedly enhanced if a subinhibitory SM or PAS concentration was combined with a moderately inhibitory concentration of the other agent (BLOCH et al. 1949). This activity of PAS against *M. tuberculosis* when combined with SM in vitro has been reported to be additive (VENNESLAND et al. 1948; SAVARINO 1949), but contradictory results have also been published (MCCLOSKY et al. 1948; DIVATIA et al. 1951).

In view of the possibility that the SM-resistant variants were being inhibited by PAS in the combination, it was decided to check whether mycobacteria exposed to the action of both drugs subsequently retained their sensitivity to SM or to PAS alone (GRAESSLE and PIETROWSKI 1949). The results indicated that the PAS/SM combination had prevented or greatly retarded the in-vitro development of SM resistance and that repeated exposure of *M. tuberculosis* to PAS for 120 days had failed to produce any increase in the resistance of this strain to PAS. The addition of PAS to SM could prevent the development of an SM-resistant population by inhibiting the growth of SM-resistant mutants within the exposed mycobacterial population and it could enhance the inhibitory effect of the two drugs on the susceptible part of the mycobacterial population (DUNNER et al. 1949; KITAMOTO and RIST 1951). A similar effect in vitro was observed with the p-aminosalicylic acid salt of streptomycin or dihydrostreptomycin (HOBBY et al. 1949; VENNESLAND et al. 1950), but its activity was slightly inferior to that of an equivalent mixture of SM and PAS (LEVADITI et al. 1950).

Additive rather than synergistic action upon mycobacteria in vitro was observed when the SM was combined with streptothricin (SMITH and WAKSMAN 1947).

b) Effects on Mycobacteria in Cell and Tissue Cultures

SM is considerably less inhibitory in cell cultures than in artificial media. In peritoneal macrophages from guinea pigs the MIC on phagocytosed mycobacteria is 5 μg/ml (BERTHRONG and HAMILTON 1958), in macrophages from rabbits either 10 μg/ml (*M. bovis*) or 25 μg/ml (*M. tuberculosis*) (MACKANESS and SMITH 1953). SUTER (1952) has found that intracellularly localized mycobacteria were inhibited only be much higher SM concentrations (80 μg/ml to 100 μg/ml). The efficacy of SM on extracellularly localized mycobacteria exceeds 100-fold that on mycobacteria in phagocytes. This difference has been explained by the poor diffusion of SM into phagocytic cells.

However, experiments with long-term exposures have revealed that peritoneal macrophages from mice are capable of concentrating SM, so that after 7 days the cytoplasmic concentration exceeds by a factor of 5 the values estimated for an extracellular environment (BONVENTRE and IMHOFF 1970). A reappraisal of the problem by CROWLE et al. (1984) with a new experimental model using cultured human macrophages showed that 5 μg/ml and 50 μg/ml SM inhibited the bacilli strongly and killed some. The lowest concentration tested, 0.5 μg/ml, inhibited them weakly. A plausible explanation of the lower intracellular activity of SM on mycobacteria (EKZEMPLYAROW 1966) is therefore the presence of cytoplasmic zones of low pH surrounding the phagocytosed mycobacteria (PAVLOV 1970).

c) Activity of SM in Experimental Tuberculosis and Development of Resistance in Vivo

In-vivo studies of SM-activity against mycobacteria have been carried out mainly in guinea pigs and in mice. Other animal species that can be mentioned are rats, rabbits, chicks, and chick embryos. The studies have revealed important basic facts regarding the SM efficacy in vivo, applicable to clinical trials. In general, experimental tuberculous infections produced by *M. tuberculosis* or *M. bovis* respond to SM therapy irrespective of the animal species used.

α) Continuous Monotherapy

Guinea pigs: The ability of SM to suppress infections due to *M. tuberculosis* was first demonstrated on guinea pigs (FELDMAN and HINSHAW 1944). The effect was often very impressive. Many extensively diseased animals were apparently cured, if treatment was started simultaneously with infection, as evidenced by macroscopic inspection of the organs (FELDMAN et al. 1945, 1947). It was soon observed, however, that the therapeutic effect was definitely related to the duration of treatment (CORPER and COHN 1946; STEENKEN and WOLINSKY 1947; FELDMAN and KARLSON 1949), decreasing with increasing chronicity and, to a smaller degree, with increasing extent of the disease (JAMES et al. 1951). The antituberculotic potency of dihydrostreptomycin has been recognized as fully equal to that of SM (RAKE et al. 1948; FELDMAN et al. 1948a, b).

The daily doses of SM used in experimental tuberculosis in guinea pigs have varied widely. Some therapeutic results from curative experiments with well-established advanced tuberculosis in guinea pigs are summarized in Table 4.

It has been stated that 6 mg of SM per day will arrest the progress of tuberculosis in guinea-pigs when the treatment is continued for 54 days or longer (FELDMAN et al. 1945; FELDMAN and HINSHAW 1947; KARLSON et al. 1950; FELDMAN et al. 1947, 1948a). At the same time, the results indicated definitely that frequent administration of SM over 24 h is not essential to therapeutic success. Suppression of the disease was quite comparable whether the drug had been given every 6 h or once every 24 h. On the other hand, a shorter period of therapy (10 days) during an earlier phase of the infection had little deterrent effect on the disease (BERNARD and KREIS 1948). In an attempt to determine a subeffective dose of SM in experimental tuberculosis in guinea pigs, experiments were conducted in which the daily dose was varied over a wide range (KARLSON and FELDMAN 1948). The antituberculotic effects of 20, 6, and 4 mg were approximately the same. Each of these doses was sufficiently effective to bring about a striking suppression of the infection. In contrast, a daily dose of 2 mg resulted in only partial retardation of the disease, and the lowest doses of 0.5 mg–1.0 mg were markedly inferior. The dose of 8 mg markedly prolonged the survival of the animals (BLOCH et al. 1949), even if very high infectious doses had been used (FELDMAN et al. 1947a, b). Doses of about 20 mg were much more effective (STEENKEN and WOLINSKY 1947, 1948), but animals treated for 40 days still harbored virulent mycobacteria and developed a slowly progressive, chronic, type of tuberculosis when the treatment was stopped. Only some of the animals treated for 77–125 days harbored virulent mycobacteria (STEENKEN and WOLINSKY 1947; SMITH et al. 1948).

Particular attention was later also paid to the therapy of chronic necrotic lesions in guinea pigs allowing an experimental tuberculous infection to relapse for 105 days after a preliminary treatment with SM (90 days). With doses of up to 30 mg/day it was found that chronic necrotic tuberculous lesions responded less favorably to SM than did the acute type of disease (STEENKEN et al. 1952).

Table 4. Therapeutic activity of streptomycin on experimental tuberculosis in guinea pigs

Infection		Therapy			Total duration of exp.	Evaluation method	Success of treatment	Ref.
Strain and route	Dose	Start after infection (days)	Route and dose	Duration (days)	(days)		(%)	
M. tbc H37Rv s.c.	0.1 mg ww	21	2 mg DHSM s.c. daily	62	83	TB index	57.2	[1]
M. tbc H37Rv s.c.	0.1 mg	14	6 mg/kg s.c. in 4 daily doses	54	69	Mortality	75.0	[2]
						Histology	61.0	
M. bovis Ravenel						Mortality	75.0	
						Histology	63.0	
M. tbc H37Rv i.v.	1 mg ww	0	6 mg s.c. daily in 4 doses	60	193	Quant. cult.	83.0	[3]
						Autopsy	100.0	
M. tbc s.c.	0.1 mg ww	20	6 mg s.c. daily in 4 doses	146	166	Mortality	80.0	[4]
						Histology	20.0	
M. tbc H37Rv s.c.	0.001 mg	42	6 mg s.c. daily	119	161	TB index	95.4	[5]
			6 mg s.c. DHSM daily				93.3	
M. tbc H37Rv s.c.	0.1 mg ww	21	20 mg s.c. daily in 2 doses	56	77	TB index	97.1	[6]
			4 mg				97.8	
			2 mg				65.4	
			0.1 mg				22.5	
	0.0001 mg ww	42	6 mg s.c. daily	119	161	TB index	92.2	
			2 mg s.c. daily				60.6	
M. tbc H37Rv s.c.		23	8 mg/kg s.c. daily	60	83	Mortality	22.5	[7]
M. tbc H37Rv s.c.	0.1 mg ww	21	8 mg s.c. daily	24	45	TB index	42.7	[8]
				45	66		63.5	
M. tbc H37Rv s.c.	0.02 mg dw	28	18 mg s.c. daily in 4 doses	44	100	Mortality	100.0	[9]
H37Rv SM-R							25.0	
M. tbc H37Rv	0.021 mg dw	49	24 mg s.c. daily in 6 doses	40	89	Mortality	100.0	[10]
						Histology, culture	0.0	
				125	180	Mortality	100.0	
						Histology, culture	29.0	

TB index = a relative value compared with the TB index of an untreated group.
ww and dw = wet weight and dry weight.
References: [1] KARLSON et al. (1950); [2] FELDMAN and HINSHAW (1947); [3] FELDMAN et al. (1947a, b); [4] FELDMAN et al. (1948a); [5] FELDMAN et al. (1948b); [6] KARLSON and FELDMAN (1948); [7] FELDMAN et al. (1947a, b); [8] BLOCH et al. (1949); [9] STEENKEN and WOLINSKY (1948); [10] STEENKEN and WOLINSKY (1947); [11] SMITH et al. (1948).

Table 4 (continued)

Infection		Therapy			Total duration of exp. (days)	Evaluation method	Success of treatment (%)	Ref.
Strain and route	Dose	Start after infection (days)	Route and dose	Duration (days)				
M. tbc H37Rv i.p.	0.5 mg ww	0	40 mg/kg s.c.	7	133–148	TB index	3.4	[11]
			daily in 2 doses	14			16.4	
			each 5th day	28			51.4	
			80 mg	77			95.2	
		7		77	148–176	TB index	87.0	
		14					90.4	
		21					72.6	
		28					80.8	

Very large doses of SM are essential to control tuberculosis in intracerebrally infected guinea pigs (STEENKEN et al. 1949).

No successful results could be obtained in prophylactic trials. According to STEENKEN and PRATT (1949), SM therapy starting 48 h prior to an infection (18 mg/day) did not prevent the distribution of mycobacteria in the guinea pig organism. In the infected animals the treatment prevented only the development of specific lesions, but not the dissemination of mycobacteria into regional lymph nodes. An interruption of the SM after 40 days of daily treatment was followed by the development of progressive tuberculotic lesions (RABUKHIN 1970).

Summarizing the results, it may be concluded that the percentage reduction in mortality is definitely related to the dose of SM and to the duration of treatment (SMITH et al. 1948). The effective daily dose is considered to be 20 mg/kg or more. Intensive treatment during the incubation period of the disease does prolong life, but will do little to check the invasiveness of the mycobacteria, the progress of the disease, or the tissue destruction. Intensive treatment with SM during several phases of tuberculous infection in guinea pigs results in little evidence of chemotherapeutic activity when the treatment is restricted to the first 4 weeks of the infection (BERNARD and KREIS 1951; BURACZEWSKA 1952).

Mice and Rats: The first report on the ability of SM to suppress a tuberculous infection in experimentally infected mice was by YOUMANS and MCCARTER (1945). In the principally abortive experiments with 0.3 mg and 3 mg of SM per mouse and per day only some evidence of a favorable effect was observed. LEVADITI and VAISMAN (1950) used a minimal daily therapeutic dose of approximately 20 mg/kg. At this dosage the survival rate was 50%. No deaths occurred with doses of 40 mg/kg–80 mg/kg for 45 days. As regards viable counts in the lungs, it also appeared that doses from 20 mg/kg–80 mg/kg had an antibacterial effect, whereas doses below 20 mg/kg were almost ineffective. These results have been repeatedly confirmed (GRUMBACH 1965).

As CORPER and COHN (1946) have predicted, much higher doses of SM are necessary for a successful treatment of murine tuberculosis. The effective dose enabling a significant reduction in viable mycobacteria in mouse lungs during approximately 3 weeks to 2 months of therapy is about 200 mg/kg/day–300 mg/kg/day (BARTMANN 1960b; GRUMBACH 1965). From the point of long-term therapy even this dose is considered to be only bacteriostatic (MCCUNE and TOMPSETT 1956; BARTMANN 1960b). The explanation lies in the different pathology of tuberculosis in mice, where in contrast to the case of the guinea pigs the mycobacteria are localized predominantly intracellularly and are then less susceptible to SM.

Rats are generally considered to be highly resistant to experimental mycobacterial infections. However the effect of SM on such infections has been reported by SMITH et al. (1946). With daily doses of 50 mg/kg the results, though not striking, did indicate that SM had exerted a slight but favorable influence on the course of infection. Rats infected with Mycobacteria and treated with cortisone develop more severe tuberculosis than infected animals not receiving the hormone (CUMMINGS et al. 1952). Such animals treated with 10 mg SM/day survived the 60-day duration of the experiment, gained weight, and showed no sign of illness. The SM did not, however, prevent the formation of minimal lesions in the lungs, liver, and spleen.

Other Animal Species: The use of rabbits to study the activity of antituberculotic drugs including SM has been relatively rare. The effective dose of SM on well-established tuberculosis due to *M. bovis* was determined to be some 50 mg/day–100 mg/day (BLOCH et al. 1948). The effect of 5 mg/kg or 10 mg/kg is only limited. Out of 15 rabbits infected with *M. bovis* and treated so for 3 months only one animal survived the treatment period and died one week later (FREERKSEN 1954). On the other hand, rabbits sensitized by a subcutaneous injection of an avirulent strain of *M. tuberculosis*, infected intratracheally with a Ravenel strain of *M. bovis*, and treated with ACTH (to produce an extensive progressive tuberculosis) developed smaller lesions after treatment with SM (60 mg/day and 30 mg/day for 120 days) (BACOS and SMITH 1953). The experiments with rabbits were mainly devised so that the course of established acute tuberculosis could be closely followed by serial chest X-rays before, during, and after treatment (STEENKEN et al. 1953).

SM and DHSM (60 mg/kg/day) were also capable of a considerable modification of ocular tuberculotic lesions in rabbits when they were administered 24 h prior to the inoculation of mycobacteria (H37Rv) into the eye. Treatment after the inoculation failed to abort the course of the lesions completely, although a major slowing down of the disease and a reduction in its intensity were observed (ADAIR et al. 1951).

Chicks have occasionally been used, especially as the proper model for the chemotherapy of avian tuberculosis. Although *M. avium* was more resistant to the action of SM and DHSM, the massive infection in chicks was relatively sensitive to the action of both drugs (SOLOTOROVSKY et al. 1949). A marked activity of SM on tuberculosis in chicks (in a dose of 40 mg/kg/day) has been repeatedly confirmed (CARMICHAEL and MACLAY 1950).

Intravenous inoculation of chick embryos with *M. tuberculosis* was also tested, and resulted in a prompt establishment of the infection in the parenchymal organs. The infected embryos were exposed to SM by placing the antibiotic in solution on the allantoic membrane (2 mg/egg). Despite the absence of any visible histological response in the SM-treated embryos, viable mycobacteria were cultured from the organs in large numbers (LEE and STAVITSKY 1947).

β) Intermittent Monotherapy. SM was also found to be effective when it was used intermittently in experimental tuberculosis in mice (HOBBY and LENERT 1953), but the individual daily dose required was significantly greater than with daily administration.

This has been confirmed in guinea pigs (DICKINSON and MITCHISON 1966; DICKINSON 1968) by quantitative estimation of viable mycobacteria in organs. The same results could be achieved by giving the SM daily or at 2-, 4-, or 8-day intervals by elevating the SM dose in proportion. These experiments have opened the way to an extensive study of intermittent drug application, characteristic of the modern chemotherapy of tuberculosis.

γ) Development of Resistance. The regular occurrence of SM-resistant mycobacteria in a certain percentage of patients treated with streptomycin has been the subject of many papers since YOUMANS and WILLISTON (1946) first reported its occurrence in the early clinical trials on the drug. In experimental tuberculosis, however, SM-resistant mutants generally occur much less frequently. STEENKEN (1947) recovered no resistant forms in guinea pigs even after 125 days of treatment. After the use of 6 mg SM/day for 144–215 days only 8 cultures from 103 animals were found to be resistant (FELDMAN et al. 1947a, b; 1948a, b; FELDMAN and KARLSON 1949). Resistant mutants may also be recovered from mice treated for a prolonged period (on average 131 days) with 1.5 mg SM/day. Groups treated for shorter times with smaller doses yielded much lower percentages of resistant strains (LENERT and HOBBY 1947; YOUMANS and FISHER 1949).

Obviously, SM will not be therapeutically effective if the experimental tuberculosis has been induced with a highly SM-resistant mycobacterial strain. The results of SM therapy of guinea pigs infected with artificial mixtures containing various proportions of sensitive and resistant Mycobacteria indicate that the response to treatment improves when the percentage of resistant mutants falls under 10% (STEENKEN and WOLINSKY 1948).

δ) Combined Therapy: SM + PAS[1]. The problems connected with the development of resistance and with the not fully satisfactory results of SM monotherapy gradually attracted attention to drugs used concomitantly with SM. Among the previously discovered drugs tested in such combinations have been Promin (SMITH and MCCLOSKY 1945; SMITH et al. 1946), Diasone (CALLOMON et al. 1946), some sulphone derivatives (SMITH et al. 1947a, b; BROWNLEE and KENNEDY 1948; KOLMER 1951), and potassium iodide (HAMILTON and GEEVER 1952). Most of the

[1] Combinations of SM with other drugs will be mentioned in the sections on the respective drugs.

reports pertaining to the results of combined treatment showed evidence of various degrees of synergistic or additive chemotherapeutic activity, though of no practical consequence.

Special attention was paid to the combinations of SM with PAS as the second most promising antimycobacterial substance. YOUMANS and KARLSON (1947) reported a study on mice that confirmed the results of in-vitro studies, and showed that PAS in combination with SM is more effective than either of the drugs used alone. The results were considered as an additive effect rather than a potentiation. A similar favorable effect has been reported for experimental tuberculosis in guinea pigs (SWEDBERG and WIDSTRÖM 1948; BLOCH et al. 1949).

To ensure the effect a relatively high dose of PAS in the combination must be used. This became of particular importance in attempts to replace the combination by a single drug – the p-aminosalicylic acid salt of streptomycin (or dihydrostreptomycin). Owing to the small amount of PAS in the preparation (1 mg of the salt has a theoretical potency of 558 μg of pure SM or 560 μg of DHSM) there was no evidence of superiority over SM alone (KARLSON et al. 1950).

On the other hand, the combination therapy of experimental tuberculous meningitis was wholly unsuccessful, mainly because of the poor absorption of

Table 5. Therapeutic activity of streptomycin in combination with PAS in vivo

Infection		Therapy			Total duration of exp. (days)	Evaluation method	Success of treatment (%)	Ref.
Strain and route	Dose and animal	Start after infection (days)	Route and dose	Duration (days)				
M. tbc H37Rv s.c.	0.1 mg ww g.-pigs	21	8 mg SM daily s.c.	24	45	TB index	84.0	[1]
			250 mg PAS daily s.c.	45	66		86.6	
M. tbc H37Rv s.c.	0.1 mg ww g.-pigs	21	2 mg DHSM +100 mg PAS daily	62	83	TB index	77.3	[2]
			10.17 mg DHSM-PAS daily				73.0	
			3.39 mg DHSM-daily				54.0	
M. tbc H37Rv i.cer.	Mice	0	0.7 mg SM-PAS daily	30	30	Mortality	100.0	[3]
M. tbc H37Rv i.cer.	0.0001 mg dw g.-pigs	0	10 mg SM i.m. daily 150–200 mg PAS p.o. daily	147	221	See text		[4]

For explanations see Table 4.
References: [1] BLOCH et al. (1949); [2] KARLSON et al. (1950); [3] HOBBY et al. (1949); [4] STEENKEN et al. (1951).

PAS into cerebrospinal fluid or exudates (HOBBY et al. 1949). A group of guinea pigs infected intracerebrally with a small inoculum of *M. tuberculosis* H37Rv and treated with PAS behaved exactly like an untreated control group. In guinea pigs in which SM therapy had been discontinued after 58 or 147 days the infection relapsed and within 74 days all the animals died. Addition of PAS to the SM in animals treated for 147 days did not affect the rate of relapses (STEENKEN et al. 1951). The specific experimental conditions in some of the above-mentioned studies are summarized in Table 5.

In spite of these facts, prior to the discovery of further antituberculotics the combinations of SM with some form of PAS had been regarded as the best option available for the treatment of tuberculosis (AMERICAN TRUDEAU SOCIETY 1951) delaying the emergence of resistant organisms.

3. Concluding Remarks

Streptomycin and Dihydrostreptomycin need in vitro higher growth inhibiting concentrations than PAS. But they act, in contrast to PAS, bactericidal on growing bacilli and, to a certain extent, also on resting germs both in vitro and in animals. This is one of the reasons why the streptomycins are suited for intermittent treatment. They do not kill intracellularly located bacilli at concentrations attainable in the treatment of human beings. Their activity is markedly weakened at an acid pH, in artificial media and in inflammed lesions. Their distribution in the body is not uniform. Disease in compartments like the brain or the cerebrospinal fluid cannot be treated effectively by the systemic route. In the animal, the streptomycins are more efficient than PAS, even with lower dosage. It turned out later that the streptomycins, despite the disadvantages mentioned, are superior not only to PAS but to all other antituberculotics except INH and RMP.

References

Abraham EP, Duthie ES (1946) Effect of pH of the medium on activity of streptomycin and penicillin. Lancet I:455–459

Adair CV, Drobeck B, Bunn PA (1951) Use of rabbit eye as a tissue to study tuberculosis. II. Effect of certain antituberculous agents upon ocular tuberculosis. Am Rev Tuberc 64:207–217

Alberghina M, Nicoletti G, Torrisi A (1973) Genetic determinants of aminoglycoside resistance in strains of *Mycobacterium tuberculosis*. Chemotherapy 19:148–160

American Trudeau Society (1951) Current status of antimicrobial therapy in tuberculosis. Report of clinical subcommittee of committee on medical research and therapy. Am Rev Tuberc 63:617–623

Bacos JM, Smith DT (1953) The effect of corticotropin (ACTH), dihydrostreptomycin, and corticotropin-dihydrostreptomycin on experimental bovine tuberculosis in the rabbit. Am Rev Tuberc 67:201–208

Bartmann K (1960a) Langfristige Einwirkung von Isonicotinsäurehydrazid und Streptomycin auf ruhende Tuberkelbakterien in vitro. Beitr Klin Tuberk 122:94–113

Bartmann K (1960b) Tierexperimentelle Untersuchungen zu einer intermittierenden Chemotherapie und -prophylaxe der Tuberkulose. X. Mitteilung. Der Erfolg kontinuierlicher und intermittierender Gaben von INH und der Kombination INH-Streptomycin bei der Tuberkulose der Maus. Beitr Klin Tuberk 122:251–264

Bartmann K, Abel U, Hart R (1966) Die Abhängigkeit des Hemmtiters von der Bebrütungsdauer bei der Bestimmung der Resistenz von *M. tuberculosis* gegen Antituberkulotika auf Löwenstein-Jensen Medium. Zentralbl Bakteriol Mikrobiol Hyg (A) 201:538–548

Beeuwkes H, Vos H (1952) Résistance des bacilles tuberculeux a la streptomycine. Poumon 6:25–39

Beggs WH, Andrews FA (1971) Protection of Mycobacterium smegmatis from ethambutol and streptomycin inhibition by $MgSO_4$ and polyamines. Infect Immun 3:496–497

Beggs WH, Andrews FA (1975a) Nonspecificity in the divalent cation antagonism of dihydrostreptomycin action on Mycobacterium smegmatis. Res Comm Chem Pathol Pharmacol 10:185–188

Beggs WH, Andrews FA (1975b) Inhibition of dihydrostreptomycin action on Mycobacterium smegmatis by monovalent and divalent cation salts. Antimicrob Agents Chemother 7:636–639

Beggs WH, Williams NE (1971) Streptomycin uptake by *Mycobacterium tuberculosis*. Appl. Microb. 21:751–770.

Benda R, Urquia DA (1950) Essai de mesure rapide de la streptomycino-résistance. Rev Tuberc 14:343–347

Berkman S, Henry RJ, Housewright RD (1947) Studies on streptomycin. I. Factors influencing the activity of streptomycin. J Bacteriol 53:567–574

Bernard E, Kreis B (1948) Action d'un traitement streptomycinique immédiat, mais de courte durée, sur la tuberculose expérimentale du cobaye. Rev Tuberc 12:348–354

Bernard E, Kreis B (1951) Bases expérimentales de la streptomycino-thérapie en injections spacées (tous le deux ou trois jours). Bull Acad Nat Med 135:492–496

Bernard E, Kreis B, Lutier H (1954) Recherche expérimentale pour le pouvoir bactéricide des agents antibacillaires. Rev Tuberc 18:1010–1014

Berthrong M, Hamilton MA (1958) Tissue culture studies on resistance in tuberculosis. I. Normal guinea pig monocytes with tubercle bacilli of different virulence. Am Rev Tuberc Pulm Dis 77:436–449

Bloch RG, Gomori G, Sperry-Braude M (1948) The effect of iron on experimental tuberculosis. Am Rev Tuberc 58:671–674

Bloch RG, Vennesland K, Ebert RH, Gomori G (1949) The effect of streptomycin, paraaminosalicylic acid (PAS) and their combination on the tubercle bacillus in vitro and in vivo. Am Rev Tuberc 59:554–561

Bøe J, Vogelsang TM (1946) The sensitivity of BCG to streptomycin. Acta Tuberc Scand 20:158–163

Bondi A, Dietz CC, Spaulding EH (1946) Interference with the antibacterial action of streptomycin by reducing agents. Science 103:399–401

Bonventre PF, Imhoff JG (1970) Uptake of ^{3}H-dihydrostreptomycin by macrophages in culture. Infect Immun 2:89–95

Brownlee G, Kennedy CR (1948) The chemotherapeutic action of streptomycin, sulphetrone, and promin in experimental tuberculosis. Br J Pharmacol 3:37–43

Buraczewska M (1952) Wpływ streptomycyny na grúzlice doswiadczalna świnek morskich przy róźnym sposobie dawkowania i stosowania. Gruźlica 20:171–184

Burjanová B, Dornetzhuber V (1975) Empfindlichkeit der Stämme des *M. kansasii* auf verschiedene Antibiotika und Chemotherapeutika in vitro und in vivo. Z Erkr Atmungsorgane 142:68–77

Callomon FT, Kolmer JA, Rule AM, Paul AJ (1946) Streptomycin and diasone in the treatment of experimental tuberculosis of guinea pigs. Proc Soc Exp Biol Med 63:237–240

Canetti G (1959) Modifications des populations des foyers tuberculeux au cours de la chimiothérapie antibacillaire. Ann Inst Pasteur 97:53–79

Canetti G, Rist N, Grosset J (1963) Mesure de la sensibilité du bacille tuberculeux aux drogues antibacillaires par la méthode des proportions. Méthodologie, critères de résistance, résultats, interprétation. Rev Tuberc 27:217–272

Canetti G, Fox W, Khomenko A, Mahler HT, Menon NK, Mitchison DA, Rist N, Šmelev NA (1969) Advances in techniques of testing mycobacterial drug sensitivity, and the use of sensitivity tests in tuberculosis control programmes. Bull WHO 41:21–43

Carmichael J, Maclay MH (1950) The use of chicks in the evaluation of anti-tuberculous agents. J Pathol Bacteriol 62:363–370
Cavallito CJ (1946) Relationship of thiol structures to reaction with antibiotics. J Biol Chem 164:29–34
Cohn ML, Middlebrook G, Russell WF (1959) Prevention of emergence of mutant populations of tubercle bacilli resistant to both streptomycin and isoniazid in vitro. J Clin Invest 38:1349–1355
Coletsos PJ (1963) Données actuelles sur l'évaluation précise de la résistance du bacille de la tuberculose aux antibiotiques spécifiques. Poumon 19:109–127
Corper HJ, Cohn ML (1946) The tubercle bacillus and fundamental chemotherapeutic and antibiotic action. Yale J Biol Med 19:1–22
Crowle AJ, Sbarbaro A, Judson FN, Douvas GS, May MH (1984) Inhibition by streptomycin of tubercle bacilli within cultured human macrophages. Am Rev Respir Dis 130:839–844
Cummings MM, Hudgins PC, Whorton MC, Sheldon WH (1952) The influence of cortisone and streptomycin on experimental tuberculosis in the albino rat. Am Rev Tuberc 65:596–602
Denkelwater RG, Cook MA, Tishler M (1945) The effect of cysteine on streptomycin and streptothricin. Science 102:12
Deutsches Zentralkomitee zur Bekämpfung der Tuberkulose (1966) Empfehlungen zur Methodik und Bewertung von Resistenz-Bestimmungen bei Tuberkulose-Bakterien
Dickinson JM, Mitchison DA (1966) Short-term intermittent chemotherapy of experimental tuberculosis in the guinea pig. Tubercle 47:381–393
Dickinson JM (1968) In vitro and in vivo studies to assess the suitability of anti-tuberculosis drugs for use on intermittent chemotherapy regimens. Tubercle 49 (Suppl):60–70
Dickinson JM, Aber VR, Mitchison DA (1977) Bactericidal activity of streptomycin, isoniazid, rifampin, ethambutol, and pyrazinamide alone and in combination against *Mycobacterium tuberculosis*. Am Rev Resp Dis 116:627–635
Divatia KJ, Gardner G, Dufrenoy J, Pratt R (1951) Antagonism between streptomycin and para-aminosalicylic acid. Experientia 7:141–142
Doane EA, Bogen E (1951) Streptomycin-dependent tubercle bacilli. Am Rev Tuberc 64:192–196
Donovick R, Bayan AP, Canales P, Pansy F (1948) The influence of certain substances on the activity of streptomycin. III. Differential effects of various electrolytes on the action of streptomycin. J Bacteriol 56:125–137
Dunner E, Brown WB, Wallace J (1949) Effects of streptomycin with para-aminosalicylic acid on emergence of resistant strains of tubercle bacilli. Dis Chest 16:661
Edison AO, Frost BM, Graessle OE, Hawkins JE Jr, Kuna S, Mushett CW, Silber RH, Solotorovsky M (1948) An experimental evaluation of dihydrostreptomycin. Am Rev Tuberc 58:487–493
Ekzemplyarow ON (1966) Effect of tetracycline, chloramphenicol, monomycin, and streptomycin on S. typhimurium after phagocytosis by macrophages. Fed Proc (Suppl):T309–T312
Feldman WH, Hinshaw HC (1944) Effects of streptomycin on experimental tuberculosis in guinea pigs: a preliminary report. Proc Staff Meet Mayo Clin 19:593–599
Feldman WH, Hinshaw HC, Mann FC (1945) Streptomycin in experimental tuberculosis. Am Rev Tuberc 52:269–298
Feldman WH, Hinshaw HC (1947) Streptomycin in experimental tuberculosis. In vivo sensitivity to streptomycin of recently isolated strains of human tubercle bacilli and strains of bovine tubercle bacilli. Am Rev Tuberc 55:428–434
Feldman WH, Hinshaw HC, Karlson AG (1947 a) Frequency of administration of streptomycin. Its influence on results of treatment of tuberculosis in guinea pigs. Am Rev Tuberc 55:435–443
Feldman WH, Karlson AG, Hinshaw HC (1947 b) Streptomycin in experimental tuberculosis. The effects in guinea pigs following infection by intravenous inoculation. Am Rev Tuberc 56:346–359

Feldman WH, Karlson AG, Hinshaw CH (1948a) Streptomycin-resistant tubercle bacilli. Effects of resistance on therapeutic results in tuberculous guinea pigs. Am Rev Tuberc 57:162–174
Feldman WH, Karlson AG, Hinshaw HC (1948b) Dihydrostreptomycin: its effect on experimental tuberculosis. Am Rev Tuberc 58:494–500
Feldman WH, Karlson AG (1949) Streptomycin in experimental tuberculosis. In: Waksman SA (ed) Streptomycin. Nature and practical applications. Williams and Wilkins, Baltimore, pp 133–157
Fisher MW (1948a) Streptomycin resistant tubercle bacilli. Their development during streptomycin therapy of pulmonary tuberculosis. Am Rev Tuberc 57:53–57
Fisher MW (1948b) Sensitivity of tubercle bacilli to streptomycin. An in vitro study of some factors affecting results in various test media. Am Rev Tuberc 57:58–62
Freerksen E (1954) Über die experimentellen Grundlagen der Kombinationstherapie. Beitr Klin Tuberk 111:574–585
Gálvez-Brandon J, Bartmann K (1969) Statistical aspects of the proportion method for determining the drug-resistance of tubercle bacilli. Scand J Resp Dis 50:1–18
Garrod LW (1950) The nature of the action of streptomycin on tubercle bacilli. Am Rev Tuberc 62:582–585
Geiger WB, Green SR, Waksman SA (1946) The inactivation of streptomycin and its practical application. Proc Soc Exp Biol Med 61:187–192
Goodman S, Gilman A (1965) The pharmacological basis of therapeutics, 3rd edn. Macmillan, New York
Graessle OE, Pietrowski JJ (1949) The in vitro effect of para-aminosalicylic acid (PAS) in preventing acquired resistance to streptomycin by Mycobacterium tuberculosis. J Bacteriol 57:459–464
Green SR, Waksman SA (1948) Effect of glucose, peptone, and salts on streptomycin activity. Proc Soc Exp Biol Med 67:281–285
Grumbach F, Canetti G, Grosset J (1964) Further experiments on long-term chemotherapy of advanced murine tuberculosis with emphasis on intermittent regimes. Tubercle (Lond) 45:125–135
Grumbach F (1965) Etudes chimiothérapeutiques sur la tuberculose avancée de la souris. Progr Explor Tuberc 14:31–96
Hamilton MA, Geever EF (1952) The use of potassium iodide in combination with streptomycin in the treatment of experimental tuberculosis in guinea pigs. Am Rev Tuberc 66:680–698
Hejný J (1982) A drug sensitivity test strategy for atypical mycobacteria. Tubercle 63:63–69
Henry J, Henry RJ, Housewright RD, Berkman S (1947) On the mode of action of streptomycin. J Bacteriol 54:9–10
Henry RJ, Hobby GL (1949) The mode of action of streptomycin. In: Waksman SA (ed) Streptomycin. Nature and practical applications. Williams and Wilkins, Baltimore, pp 197–218
Hobby GL, Dougherty N (1948) Isolation of streptomycin-resistant organism capable of utilizing streptomycin for growth. Proc Soc Exp Biol Med 69:544–548
Hobby G, Regna P, Lenert T (1949) The chemotherapeutic action of streptomycin para-aminosalicylate in experimental tuberculosis in mice. Am Rev Tuberc 60:808–810
Hobby GL, Lenert TF (1953) The control of experimental mouse tuberculosis by the intermittent administration of streptomycin, viomycin, isoniazid, and streptomycylidene isonicotinyl hydrazine. Am Rev Tuberc 68:292–294
Hok TT, Seng TK (1964) A comparative study of the susceptibility to streptomycin, cycloserine, viomycin, and kanamycin of tubercle bacilli from 100 patients never treated with cycloserine, viomycin, or kanamycin. Am Rev Resp Dis 90:961–962
Howlett KS Jr, O'Connor JB, Sadusk JF Jr, Swift WE Jr, Beardsley FA (1949) Sensitivity of tubercle bacilli to streptomycin. The influence of various factors upon the emergence of resistant strains. Am Rev Tuberc 59:402–414
Hsie JY, Bryson V (1950) Genetic studies on the development of resistance to neomycin and dihydrostreptomycin in *Mycobacterium ranae*. Am Rev Tuberc 62:286–299

Hurwitz C, Miller JB (1950) Effect of Triton A-20 and pH value on the streptomycin sensitivity of a resistant strain of *M. tuberculosis*. Am Rev Tuberc 62:91–98
Hurwitz C (1951) The enhancement of growth of dihydrostreptomycin-resistant strains of tubercle bacilli by dihydrostreptomycin, a function of initial pH value of the medium. Am Rev Tuberc 63:568–578
James LA, Sides LJ, Dye WE, Deyke VF (1951) Intermittent streptomycin regimens. An analysis of ninety-seven patients with pulmonary tuberculosis treated with one or two grams of streptomycin every third day. Am Rev Tuberc 63:275–294
Jones WD Jr, Beam RE, David HL (1974) Transduction of a streptomycin R-factor from *Mycobacterium smegmatis* to *Mycobacterium tuberculosis* H37Rv. Tubercle 55:73–80
Kanai K, Yanagisawa K (1955) Antibacterial action of streptomycin against tubercle bacilli of various growth phase. Jap J med Sci Biol. 8:63–76.
Karlson AG, Feldman WH (1948) The subeffective dose of streptomycin in experimental tuberculosis of guinea pigs. Am Rev Tuberc 58:129–133
Karlson AG, Gainer JH, Feldman WH (1950) The effect of dihydrostreptomycin-para-aminosalicylate (DHS-PAS) on experimental tuberculosis in guinea pigs. Am Rev Tuberc 62:149–155
Kitamoto O, Rist N (1951) Sur le méchanisme d'action de l'association P.A.S.-streptomycine (étude bactériologique in vitro). Rev Tuberc 15:950–957
Kolmer JA (1951) Sulfone compounds and potassium iodide alone and in combination with streptomycin in the treatment of experimental tuberculosis of guinea pigs. Am Rev Tuberc 64:102–112
Koníčková-Radochová M, Málek I (1968) The mutagenic effect of hydroxylamine on *Mycobacterium phlei* strain PA. Fol Microbiol 13:226–230
Koseki Y, Okamoto S (1963) Studies on cross-resistance between capreomycin and certain other anti-mycobacterial agents. Jpn J Med Sci Biol 16:31–38
Krebs A, Käppler W, Ferreira OT (1962) Beitrag zur Behebung von Unstimmigkeiten bei der Resistenzbestimmung von Tuberkelbakterien gegenüber Streptomycin. Beitr Klin Tuberk 126:84–97
Krebs A (1967) The action of antituberculous drugs. Tuberkuloza 19:328–337
Krebs A (1968) Die Wirkungsweise der „Tuberkulostatika". Konsequenzen für die Therapie. Z Tbk 128:208–217
Krebs A (1969) Experimentelle Chemotherapie der Tuberkulose. Z Erkr Atmungsorg 130:417–448
Krebs A (1975) Mykobakterielle Resistenz und Resistenzbestimmungen. In: Meissner G, Schmiedel A, Nelles A (Hrsg) Mykobakterien und mykobakterielle Krankheiten. III. Bakteriologische Grundlagen der Chemotherapie der Tuberkulose. Fischer, Jena, pp 183–250
Krebs A, Kalich R (1964) Unpublished data; cited from Krebs A (1975) p 238
Kuze F, Takeda S, Maekawa N (1977a) Sensitivities of atypical mycobacteria to various drugs. III. Sensitivities of M. intracellulare to antituberculous drugs in triple combination. Kekkaku 52:331–338
Kuze F, Naito Y, Takeda S, Maekawa N (1977b) Sensitivities of atypical mycobacteria to various drugs. IV. Sensitivities of atypical mycobacteria originally isolated in the USA to antituberculous drugs in triple combinations (in Japanese). Kekkaku 52:505–513
Lee HF, Stavitsky AB (1947) Intravenous infection of the chick embryo with tubercle bacilli. Inhibitory effects of streptomycin. Am Rev Tuberc 55:262–280
Lenert TF, Hobby GL (1947) Observations on the action of streptomycin in vitro. (I). Proc Soc Exp Biol Med 65:235–242
Lenert TF, Hobby GL (1949) Streptomycin-dependent strains of *Mycobacterium tuberculosis*. Am Rev Tuberc 59:219–220
Levaditi C, Vaisman A (1950) Effets antituberculeux exercés par la streptomycine chez les souris contaminées par les souches de bacille acido-résistants H.512, BCG et 607. Ann Inst Pasteur 78:407–411
Levaditi C, Vaisman A, Chaigneau H, Henry-Eveno J (1950) Effets antituberculeux du p-amino-salicylate de streptomycine. Ann Inst Pasteur 79:886–890
Linz R (1954) La multiplication de *Mycobacterium tuberculosis* en présence de streptomycine. Ann Inst Pasteur 86:334–337

Lorian V (1966) Antibiotics and chemotherapeutic agents in clinical and laboratory practice. Thomas, Springfield
Lucchesi M (1970) The antimycobacterial activity of capreomycin. Antibiot Chemother 16:27–31
Mackaness GB, Smith N (1953) The bactericidal action of isoniazid, streptomycin, and terramycin on extracellular and intracellular tubercle bacilli. Am Rev Tuberc 67:322–340
Manten A (1957) Antimicrobial susceptibility and some other properties of photochromogenic mycobacteria associated with pulmonary disease. Antonie Van Leeuwenhoek 23:357–363
McClatchy JK, Kanes W, Davidson PT, Moulding TS (1977) Cross-resistance in *M. tuberculosis* to kanamycin, capreomycin and viomycin. Tubercle 58:29–34
McClosky WT, Smith MI, Frias JEG (1948) The action of p-aminosalicylic acid (PAS) in experimental tuberculosis. J Pharmacol 92:447–453
McCune RM, Tompsett R (1956) Fate of *Mycobacterium tuberculosis* in mouse tissues as determined by the microbial enumeration technique. I. The persistence of drug-susceptible tubercle bacilli in the tissues despite prolonged antimicrobial therapy. J Exp Med 104:737–742
Meissner G (1953) Zur Frage der Virulenz chemo-resistenter Tuberkelbakterien. I. Ein Fall mit Doppelresistenz gegen Streptomycin und Isoniazid. Beitr Klin Tuberk 110:219–226
Middlebrook G, Yegian D (1946) Certain effects of streptomycin on mycobacteria in vitro. Am Rev Tuberc 54:553–558
Middlebrook G (1952) Sterilization of tubercle bacilli by isonicotinic acid hydrazide and the incidence of variants resistant to the drug in vitro. Am Rev Tuberc 65:765–767
Mitchison DA (1951) The segregation of streptomycin-resistant variants of *Mycobacterium tuberculosis* into groups with characteristic levels of resistance. J Gen Microbiol 5:596–604
Mitchison DA (1953) The ecology of tubercle bacilli resistant to streptomycin and isoniazid. 3rd Symp Soc Gen Microbiol, London
Modr Z, Heřmanský M, Vlček V (1969) Antibiotics and their drug forms (in Czech). SZN Praha
Mordasini ER, Eulenberger J (1971) Tuberkulostatika. Teil 2. Spezifische Chemotherapeutika. Int J Clin Pharmacol 5:70–95
Murray R, Finland M (1948) Effect of pH on streptomycin activity. Am J Clin Pathol 18:247–252
Neubert R (1976) Sensibilitätsprüfungen von Mykobakterien gegenüber INH, SM, EMB und RMP im halbflüssigen Serum-Sauton-Agar. Z Erkr Atmungsorgane 144:63–68
Owen CR, Adcock J, Stow RM, Staudt LW, Devey WN (1950) Susceptible, resistant, and dependent tubercle bacilli isolated from patients treated with streptomycin. Am Rev Tuberc 61:705–718
Paine TF, Finland M (1948 a) Streptomycin-sensitive, -dependent, and -resistant bacteria. Science 107:143–144
Paine TF Jr, Finland M (1948 b) Observations on bacteria sensitive to, resistant to, and dependent upon streptomycin. J Bacteriol 56:207–218
Pavlov EP (1970) Some factors influencing the activity of streptomycin, kanamycin and isoniazid with respect to intracellularly seated Myco. tuberculosis (in Russian). Probl Tuberk 48, issue 9:72–76
Pyle MM (1947) Relative numbers of resistant tubercle bacilli in sputa of patients before and during treatment with streptomycin. Proc Staff Meet Mayo Clin 22:465–475
Rabukhin AE (1970) Chemotherapy of tuberculosis (in Russian). Medicina, Moscow
Rake G, Pansy FE, Jambor WP, Donovick R (1948) Further studies on the dihydrostreptomycins. Am Rev Tuberc 58:479–486
Rake G, Donovick R (1949) Tuberculostatic activity of aureomycin in vitro and in vivo. Am Rev Tuberc 60:143
Russell WF, Middlebrook G (1961) Chemotherapy of tuberculosis. Thomas, Springfield
Savarino S (1949) Action of streptomycin in vitro with p-aminosalicylic acid against tubercle bacilli. Minerva Med 2:19–20

Schatz A, Bugie E, Waksman SA (1944) Streptomycin, a substance exhibiting antibiotic activity against gram positive and gram negative bacteria. Proc Soc Exp Biol Med 55:66–69

Schatz A, Waksman SA (1944) Effect of streptomycin and other antibiotic substances upon *Mycobacterium tuberculosis* and related organisms. Proc Soc Exp Biol Med 57:244–248

Schoenbach EB, Chandler CA (1947) Activity of streptomycin in presence of serum and whole blood. Proc Soc Exp Biol Med 66:493–500

Seligmann E, Wassermann M (1947) Induced resistance to streptomycin. J Immunol 57:351–360

Simon RD (1948) Antagonization of the antibacterial action of neoarsphenamine, penicillin and streptomycin by – SH compounds. Br J Exp Pathol 29:202–215

Smith MI, McClosky WT (1945) The chemotherapeutic action of streptomycin and promin in experimental tuberculosis. Public Health Rep 60:1129–1138

Smith MI, McClosky WT, Emmart EW (1946) Influence of streptomycin and promin on proliferation of tubercle bacilli in the tissue of albino rat. Proc Soc Exp Biol Med 62:157–162

Smith DG, Waksman SA (1947) Tuberculostatic and tuberculocidal properties of streptomycin. J Bacteriol 54:253–261

Smith MI, McClosky WT, Jackson EL (1947a) Studies in chemotherapy of tuberculosis. VIII. The comparative action of four sulfones in experimental tuberculosis in guinea pigs and the combined action of streptomycin with one of the sulfones. Am Rev Tuberc 55:366–373

Smith MI, McClosky WT, Jackson EL, Bauer H (1947b) Chemotherapeutic action of streptomycin and of streptomycin with a sulfone or sulfadiazine on tuberculosis. Proc Soc Exp Biol Med 64:261–269

Smith MI, Emmart EW, McClosky WT (1948) Streptomycin in experimental guinea pig tuberculosis. Am Rev Tuberc 58:112–122

Solotorovsky M, Siegel H, Bugie EJ, Gregory FJ (1949) The evaluation of antituberculous agents with avian tuberculosis in chicks: a comparison of dihydrostreptomycin and streptomycin. Am Rev Tuberc 60:366–376

Spendlove GA, Cummings MM, Fackler WB, Michael M (1948) Enhancement of growth of a strain of *M. tuberculosis* (var. hominis) by streptomycin. Public Health Rep 63:1177–1179

Stakemann G (1954) Undersøgelser over de streptomycinresistente tubercelbacteriers oprindelse. Dansk Videnskabs Forlag, København

Standard methods in the microbiology of tuberculosis and lepra (1980) (in Czech). Institute for Hygiene and Epidemiology, Prague

Steenken W Jr, Wolinsky E (1947) Streptomycin in experimental tuberculosis. I. Its effect upon a well-established progressive tuberculous infection in guinea pigs. Am Rev Tuberc 56:227–240

Steenken W Jr, Wolinsky E (1948) Streptomycin in experimental tuberculosis. II. Response in guinea pigs infected with strains of varying degrees of streptomycin resistance. Am Rev Tuberc 58:353–362

Steenken W Jr (1949) Streptomycin and the tubercle bacillus. In: Riggins HM, Hinshaw HC (eds) Streptomycin and dihydrostreptomycin in tuberculosis. National Tuberculosis Association, pp 39–57

Steenken W Jr, Pratt PC (1949) Streptomycin in experimental tuberculosis. III. Effect on the pathogenesis of early tuberculosis in the guinea pig infected with streptomycin-sensitive H37Rv tubercle bacilli. Am Rev Tuberc 59:664–673

Steenken W, Wolinsky E, Reginster A, Pratt P (1949) La streptomycine et le bacille tuberculeux. Rev Belge Pathol Med Exp 19:225–227

Steenken W Jr, Wolinsky E, Pratt PC (1951) Streptomycin and PAS in experimental tuberculosis of guinea pigs infected intracerebrally with virulent tubercle bacilli. Am Rev Tuberc 64:87–101

Steenken W Jr, Wolinsky E, Pratt PC, Smith MM (1952) Streptomycin in guinea pigs with discrete chronic tuberculous lesions. Am Rev Tuberc 66:194–212

Steenken W Jr, Wolinsky E, Bristol LJ, Costigan WJ (1953) Use of the rabbit in experimental tuberculosis. I. A visual method of evaluation of antituberculous agents by serial chest roentgenograms. Am Rev Tuberc 68:65–74
Steenken W Jr, Smith MM, Montalbine V (1958) In vitro and in vivo effect of antimicrobial agents on atypical mycobacteria. Am Rev Tuberc 78:454–461
Steenken W Jr, Montalbine V, Thurston JR (1959) The antituberculous activity of kanamycin in vitro and in the experimental animal (guinea pig). Am Rev Tuberc Pulm Dis 79:66–71
Suter E (1952) Multiplication of tubercle bacilli within phagocytes cultivated in vitro, and effect of streptomycin and isonicotinic acid hydrazide. Am Rev Tuberc 65:775–776
Swedberg B, Widström G (1948) Treatment of experimental tuberculosis in mice and guinea pigs with para-aminosalicylic acid (PAS) and streptomycin. Acta Med Scand 131:116–128
Tison F (1949) Repartition des bacilles plus ou moins résistant à la streptomycine selon les organes et le type de lésion dans la tuberculose expérimentale du cobaye: action des traitements par l'antibiotique. Ann Inst Pasteur 77:767–769
Toril F, Yamamoto M, Hayashi M, Noda Y, Tsukamura M (1959) Studies on the kanamycin-resistance of *Mycobacterium tuberculosis*. II. Kanamycin-sensitivity of various drug-resistant strains. J Antibiot (Tokyo) Ser A12:103–104
Tsang AY, Bentz RR, Schork MA, Sodeman TM (1978) Combined vs. single-drug studies on susceptibilities of *Mycobacterium kansasii* to isoniazid, streptomycin, and ethambutol. Am J Clin Pathol 70:816–820
Tsukamura M, Noda Y, Miura K (1956) A quantitative analysis of the resistance of *Mycobacterium tuberculosis* to streptomycin, isoniazid and PAS (in Japanese). Kekkaku 31:107–110, 116–117
Tsukamura M, Noda Y, Yamamoto M (1959) Studies on the kanamycin resistance in Mycobacterium tuberculosis. V. Sensitivity of kanamycin resistant mutants to various antituberculous drugs and mutation frequency to various drug resistance in kanamycin-resistant mutants. J Antibiot (Tokyo) Ser A 12:323–327
Tsukamura M (1961) Variation and heredity of mycobacteria with special reference to drug resistance. Jpn J Tuberc 9:43–64
Tsukamura M, Mizuno S (1980) A comparative study of the relationship between the growth rate of tubercle bacilli and the concentration of antituberculous agents (in Japanese). Kekkaku 55:365–370
Urbanczik R (1982) Medikamentöse Therapie der Lungentuberkulose. In: Hein J, Ferlinz R (Hrsg) Lungentuberkulose, Pathogenese, Klinik, Therapie und Epidemiologie. vol 2, P. 8.1–8.65. Thieme, Stuttgart New York
Ushiba D, Hsu Y, Fukazawa T (1957) Spontaneity of the gradual increase of streptomycin resistance in Mycobacterium 607. Am Rev Tuberc 75:841–842
Vanderlinde RJ, Yegian D (1951) The pathogenicity of streptomycin-dependent tubercle bacilli. Am Rev Tuberc 63:96–99
Vennesland K, Ebert RH, Bloch RG (1947) The demonstration of naturally-occurring streptomycin-resistant variants in the human strain of tubercle bacillus H37Rv. Science 106:476–477
Vennesland K, Ebert RH, Bloch RG (1948) In vitro effect of streptomycin and para-aminosalicylic acid (PAS) on the growth of tubercle bacilli. Proc Soc Exp Biol Med 68:250–255
Vennesland K, Altona J, Bloch RG (1950) Comparative in vitro response of tubercle bacillus (H37Rv) to dihydrostreptomycin, para-aminosalicylic acid, and dihydrostreptomycin-para-aminosalicylate. Proc Soc Exp Biol Med 75:436–438
Waksman SA, Schatz A (1945) Streptomycin-origin, nature and properties. J Am Pharm Ass 34:273–280
Williston EH, Youmans GP (1947) Streptomycin resistant strains of tubercle bacilli. Production of streptomycin resistance in vitro. Am Rev Tuberc 55:536–539
Williston EH, Youmans GP (1949) Factors affecting the sensitivity in vitro of tubercle bacilli to streptomycin. Am Rev Tuberc 59:336–352

Wittmann HG, Apirion D (1975) Analysis of ribosomal proteins in streptomycin resistant and dependent mutants isolated from streptomycin independent Escherichia-coli strain. MGG 141:343–356
Wolinsky E, Steenken W Jr (1947) Effect of streptomycin on the tubercle bacillus. The use of Dubos' and other media in tests for streptomycin sensitivity. Am Rev Tuberc 55:281–288
Wolinsky E, Reginster A, Steenken W Jr (1948) Drug-resistant tubercle bacilli in patients under treatment with streptomycin. Am Rev Tuberc 58:335–343
Wolinsky E, Smith MM, Steenken W Jr (1957) Drug susceptibilities of 20 "atypical" as compared with 19 selected strains of mycobacteria. Am Rev Resp Dis 76:497–502
Wood LE, Buhler VB, Pollak A (1956) Human infection with the "yellow" acid-fast bacillus. Am Rev Tuberc 73:917–929
Yegian D, Budd V (1948) A variant of *Mycobacterium ranae* requiring streptomycin for growth. J Bacteriol 55:459–461
Yegian D, Vanderlinde RJ (1948) A quantitative analysis of the resistance of mycobacteria to streptomycin. J Bacteriol 56:177–186
Yegian D, Budd V, Vanderlinde RJ (1949) Streptomycin-dependent tubercle bacilli: a simple method for isolation. J Bacteriol 58:257–259
Yegian D, Vanderlinde RJ (1949) The biological characteristics of streptomycin-dependent *Mycobacterium ranae*. J Bacteriol 57:169–178
Yegian D, Vanderlinde RJ (1950) The resistance of tubercle bacilli to chemotherapeutic agents. Am Rev Tuberc 61:483–507
Yegian D, Budd V (1951) Heterogeneous character of streptomycin-dependent mutants of a Mycobacterium. J Bacteriol 61:161–165
Youmans GP, McCarter JC (1945) Streptomycin in experimental tuberculosis. Am Rev Tuberc 52:432–439
Youmans GP, Williston EH (1946) Effect of streptomycin on experimental infections produced in mice with streptomycin resistant strains of *M. tuberculosis* var. hominis. Proc Soc Exp Biol Med 63:131–134
Youmans GP, Karlson AG (1947) Streptomycin sensitivity of tubercle bacilli. Studies on recently isolated tubercle bacilli and the development of resistance to streptomycin in vivo. Am Rev Tuberc 55:529–535
Youmans GP, Williston EH (1948) Streptomycin-resistant variants obtained from recently isolated cultures of tubercle bacilli. Proc Soc Exp Biol Med 68:458–460
Youmans GP (1949) Some bacteriological aspects of streptomycin therapy in tuberculosis. In: Riggins HM, Hinshaw HC (eds) Streptomycin and dihydrostreptomycin in tuberculosis. National Tuberculosis Association, p 58–73
Youmans GP, Fisher MW (1949) Action of streptomycin on microorganisms in vitro. In: Waksman SA (ed) Streptomycin. Nature and practical applications. Williams and Wilkins, Baltimore, pp 91–111
Youmans GP, Williston EH, Osborne RR (1949) Occurrence of streptomycin-resistant tubercle bacilli in mice treated with streptomycin. Proc Soc Exp Biol Med 70:36–37
Youmans GP, Youmans AS (1951) The effect of viomycin in vitro and in vivo on *Mycobacterium tuberculosis*. Am Rev Tuberc 63:25–29
Zimelis VM, Jackson GG (1973) Activities of aminoglycoside antibiotics against *Pseudomonas aeruginosa:* specificity and site of calcium and magnesium antagonism. J Infect Dis 127:663–669

III. Thiosemicarbazones (TSC)

L. TRNKA

DOMAGK et al. reported in 1946 that some sulphathiazole and sulphathiodiazole compounds were weakly active against tubercle bacilli in vitro, this activity being independent of the simultaneous presence of the sulphonamide group or the thiazole or thiodiazole ring. Suitably substituted condensation products of thiosemicarbazides – thiosemicarbazones proved to be more active.

Several studies on the relationship between TSC modifications and their antimycobacterial activity have been published (DOMAGK 1949, 1950; HOGGARTH et al. 1949; BEHNISCH et al. 1950; BAVIN et al. 1950; CROSHAW and DICKINSON 1950; DONOVICK et al. 1950; STEINBACH and BAKER 1950).

It was recognized that the sulphur atoms in TSC played an essential role and that the TSC of aldehydes behaved more favorably than those of ketones, which were more toxic. Aromatic aldehyde derivatives were more active than those of the aliphatic series. The action was increased by the introduction of suitable substituents on the aromatic ring. The nature and the position of these substituents determined the magnitude of the activity against tubercle bacilli. TSC substituted with groups containing nitrogen, oxygen, and sulphur in the paraposition were advantageous.

From the large number of compounds studied, 4-acetylaminobenzaldehyde thiosemicarbazone TBI (698), further referred to as TSC, had proved to be the most active product which, after pharmacological examination, was studied extensively in the laboratory and in clinical practice.

1. Antimicrobial Spectrum in Vitro

Despite the fact that sulphathiazole and sulphathiodiazole compounds are active against a variety of microbial species, TSC and their derivatives exert inhibitory activity only against bacteria of the genus Mycobacterium. They were developed in this respect on purpose. Reports are so far available only on the inhibitory activity of TSC on tubercle bacilli.

2. Antimycobacterial Activity

a) Activity in Artificial Media in Vitro

A great variety of testing methods was used for the study of the in-vitro activity of TSC in the early fifties, and a comparison of the results is therefore rather difficult. In experiments performed in 1946–1947, DOMAGK (1950) found that the growth of *M. tuberculosis*, strain Karlshorst, on solid egg media was completely inhibited by TSC suspended in water diluted 2.5×10^{-4}, and partly in dilutions of 5×10^{-4} or 1×10^{-5}. SM and PAS exerted almost the same inhibitory activity. The results were in agreement with those of HOGGARTH et al. (1949), GEKS and WOLF (1950), and MALLUCHE (1952). TSC suspended in water inhibited the growth of tubercle bacilli in dilutions of 10^{-6}, PAS in dilutions of 10^{-6}, and SM in dilutions of 5×10^{-4}–1×10^{-5}.

In contrast to this, HURNI (1949) found that TSC was less active in comparison with SM or PAS. The dilutions of drug suspension which inhibited the growth of tubercle bacilli after 12 days of incubation at 37 °C to the extent of 50% (in comparison with the controls) were 2.11×10^{-5} for TSC, 5.93×10^{-6} for SM, and 1.63×10^{-6} for PAS.

TSC dissolved in ethylene or propylene glycol exerted higher activity, the inhibitory dilution being 5×10^{-6}.

The minimal inhibitory concentration (MIC) of TSC dissolved in propylene glycol was estimated by RUSSELL et al. (1950) for *M. tuberculosis* grown in liquid media (Dubos-Davis, Tween albumin) as 0.1 µg/ml–0.5 µg/ml. Approximately 10 times higher concentrations of TSC were required to prevent the growth of *M. tuberculosis* on solid egg media (5.0 µg/ml) and on medium 7H10 containing Tween 80 (10.0 µg/ml) (DICKINSON 1968).

RIST et al. (1951) discovered two types of strains of tubercle bacilli, namely one inhibited by 0.6 µg/ml even after 28 days of culture (complete inhibition) and one inhibited by 0.3 µg/ml after 7 days of incubation, but partially grown after 14 or 28 days of culture (partial inhibition). The phenomenon was confirmed 20 years later by OHSATO et al. (1971). In 27.5% of 40 strains of tubercle bacilli ("wild strains" isolated from tuberculosis patients) the MIC of TSC was 0.5 µg/ml, in 50% it was 1.0 µg/ml, and in the remaining 22% it exceeded 2.0 µg/ml. The authors used an inoculum of 10^{-6} g cultured on solid media for 4 weeks.

Other tubercle bacilli than *M. tuberculosis* were in general less susceptible to TSC. KUZE et al. (1979) estimated the MIC for 5 strains of *M. intracellulare* in liquid Dubos Tween medium (inoculum 10^{-5} g) as to 50 µg/ml. HEJNÝ (1978, 1979) found the MIC of TSC on solid Löwenstein-Jensen media seeded with an inoculum of 2×10^{-3} to 2×10^{-5} g for 85% of strains of *M. kansasii* to be below 2.0 µg/ml, and for 39% of strains *M. avium-intracellulare* and for all tested strains of *M. fortuitum* the MIC of TSC exceeded 2.0 µg/ml. Similar experience has been reported by BURJANOVÁ and URBANCZIK (1970).

However, it was soon discovered by HAMRE et al. (1950) that there was no obvious quantitative relationship between the in-vitro activities of TSC and its in-vivo efficacy. Although all compounds showing activity in vivo had MICs in vitro equal to or smaller than 1.5 µg/ml, one of the most active TSC compounds was also one of the least active in vivo. It was pointed out even at that time that in-vitro results can at best serve only as a guide for in-vivo screening. Similar conclusions can be drawn from the papers by DAVIS et al. (1950), MOLLOV et al. (1951), and BARTMANN (1974).

α) Factors Affecting the Activity in Vitro. The low solubility of TSC in water makes it necessary to use solvents in sensitivity tests, and consequently studies had to be carried out on the inhibitory activity of these solvents themselves. Propylene glycol in concentrations below 1% did not inhibit the growth of tubercle bacilli on solid or liquid media (RUSSELL et al. 1950). The omission of Tween 80 in liquid media resulted in an increase in the MIC to values similar to those on solid media.

The dependence of the MIC values on the size of the inoculum of tubercle bacilli was soon recognized. An increase in size from 2×10^{-7} to 10^{-4} g per 10 ml of liquid media resulted in a tenfold increase in the TSC concentration required to inhibit growth. On solid media the use of a heavy inoculum or a coarse suspension resulted in the growth of resistant colonies at higher concentrations of TSC (RUSSELL et al. 1950; BARTMANN 1954a).

The cultivation period of tubercle bacilli on artificial media with TSC also affected the MIC values as mentioned above (RIST et al. 1951; BARTMANN et al. 1966).

As noted by DOMAGK (1950), p-aminobenzoic acid (10^{-4}) had a smaller effect on the activity of TSC than on those of SM or PAS.

β) Resistance of Tubercle Bacilli to TSC

Development of Resistance in Vitro and Its Type: In the early clinical trials with TSC the development of TSC resistance was rarely encountered. MOLLOV et al. (1951) estimated that a TSC-resistant population of tubercle bacilli developed in 1 out of 15 patients treated by TSC monotherapy for 4–16 weeks. HOFMANN and NICKEL (1950) observed in 2 out of 27 patients treated for 2–12 months the development of TSC resistance from 2 μg/ml to 20 μg/ml.

Later on it was estimated that, in contrast to the case of PAS, the development of TSC resistance was very slow and probably followed a multistep pattern. Primarily TSC-resistant populations of tubercle bacilli were rare (in tuberculous patients not treated with TSC-initial resistance). Different results were obtained after administration of TSC to patients excreting initially TSC-resistant populations of tubercle bacilli (MALLUCHE 1952) and the performance of TSC sensitivity tests was therefore recommended.

Features of Resistant Populations: Soon after the introduction of in-vitro sensitivity tests it was found by THOMAS et al. (1961) that "wild strains" of tubercle bacilli isolated from patients in India were in general more resistant to TSC than those isolated from patients in the United Kingdom. MITCHISON and LLOYD (1964) delineated clearly the phenomenon of geographical variation in the TSC sensitivity of tubercle bacilli.

BARNETT et al. (1963) and OHSATO et al. (1970) reported that resistance to TSC is usually associated with low virulence in guinea pigs. A survey of papers dealing with this subject, taken from the review of GROSSET and BENHASSINE (1970), is presented in Table 1.

In the papers summarized in Table 1 the predominance of initially TSC-resistant strains in India (Madras) and Hong Kong is evident, accounting for more than half of the strains tested. In East, South, and North Africa the prevalence of TSC-resistant strains was lower than in South-East Asia, but exceeded the values estimated in the British Isles.

Two types of initial (pretreatment) resistance to TSC are distinguished: resistance associated with a reduced virulence in guinea pigs (occurring in India, Madagascar, and East Africa) and resistance associated with an unchanged virulence in guinea pigs (Hong Kong) (RAO et al. 1966; GROSSET and BENHASSINE 1970). In Japan no relation was detected between resistance to TSC and virulence in guinea pigs (OHSATO et al. 1971).

In view of the geographical variation in the prevalence of TSC-resistant strains CANETTI et al. (1969) concluded that laboratory TSC-sensitivity tests were

Table 1. Prevalence of initially TSC-resistant strains of tubercle bacilli in different countries or geographical regions. (After GROSSET and BENHASSINE 1970, Table 2)

Authors	Year	No. of strains	Country where isolated	% of initially TSC-resistant strains
THOMAS et al.	1961	66	UK	16.7
		225	India	64.0
East African/BMRC	1963	204	East Africa	14.2
	1966a	312	East Africa	35.5
	1966b	48	East Africa	33.3
	1968	544	Kenya	14.7
JOSEPH et al.	1964	66	UK	3.0
		209	India	47.3
MITCHISON et al.	1964	23	UK	26.0
		26	East Africa	8.0
		30	India (Madras)	47.0
		47	Hong Kong	54.0
GROSSET et al.	1968	38	UK	5.2
		44	Algiers	13.6
		26	India	65.0
		34	Hong Kong	70.6
Hong Kong/BMRC	1968	87	Hong Kong	73.5
BRIGGS et al.	1968	76	UK	13.0
		168	Rhodesia	53.0
CHICOU et al.	1968	32	India (Madras)	56.0
		58	Tanger	0

TSC resistance evaluated by the absolute method (>20 colonies growing at 2 µg TSC/ml), by the "resistance ratio" method (>4), or by the proportion method (>10% colonies growing at 1 µg TSC/ml).

of little prognostic value in parts of the world where a higher proportion of wild strains was naturally resistant to the drug. It was difficult to distinguish between strains with natural (initial) and acquired resistance, because there was no close correlation between TSC sensitivity of pretreatment strains (initial resistance) and the response of patients to treatment with regimens containing TSC.

For routine testing the proportion method (in its simplified and standard variants) was recommended, using as the criterion of resistance 10% of cells growing at a TSC concentration of 2 µg/ml or 50% growing at 1.0 µg/ml or 1% growing at 4 µg/ml.

TSC Dependence: No TSC dependence is mentioned in the papers available.

Cross-Resistance: On the basis of the existing structural similarities, the occurrence of cross-resistance between TSC and other thiosemicarbazones might well be assumed. In practice other derivatives were not used widely, and mainly in commercial combinations of heterocyclic thiosemicarbazones with INH.

Cross-resistance in vitro was detected between TSC and 4,4′-bis(isopentyloxy) thiocarbanilide or Isoxyl, belonging to the group of thiourea derivatives (MEISSNER 1955; TRNKA et al. 1966).

RIST et al. (1958) recognized that the strains of tubercle bacilli that developed TSC resistance after successive passaging on media containing TSC were almost invariably sensitive to ETH. In contrast to this, wild TSC-resistant strains (isolated from TSC-treated patients) proved to be ETH-resistant. BARTMANN (1960) reported ETH resistance in 68% of strains isolated from patients treated for a long time with TSC. EULE and WERNER (1967) observed ETH resistance in 81 out of 91 strains isolated from TSC-treated patients; 80 were resistant both to TSC and ETH, and one only to ETH. CHICOU et al. (1968) found cross-resistance between TSC and ETH in only 30% of the tested strains of tubercle bacilli.

GROSSET et al. (1968) came across TSC resistance in 53% out of 122 strains secondarily resistant to ETH (isolated from patients treated with ETH). SOJKOVÁ et al. (1965) reported TSC resistance in 82% of ETH-treated patients. In TSC-treated patients there was a partial TSC-ETH cross-resistance. Similar results have been published by AFANASIJEVA and MKRTCHJAN (1969).

γ) Type of Action: DICKINSON and MITCHISON studied the suitability of antimycobacterial drugs for intermittent chemotherapy, which depends on the drug's ability to inhibit bacterial multiplication in the times between doses, when an effective concentration is no longer present. The results have been reported in several papers (DICKINSON and MITCHISON 1966; DICKINSON 1968; MITCHISON 1971).

Tubercle bacilli (*M. tuberculosis* H37Rv) were cultivated in a liquid medium filled into the tops of all-glass membrane filters. When the organisms were judged to be in the logarithmic phase of the growth, and at viable counts of approximately $\log_{10}$ 4.5–5.5 units/ml, the TSC was added in a concentration equal to 10 times the MIC (100.0 μg/ml). After the desired exposure period the drug was washed off through the filter and viable counts were made at intervals until full growth had been obtained.

In these experiments no definite bactericidal activity of TSC was found even after exposure for 96 h. Multiplication of the organisms began immediately after removal of the drug. The rate of growth in the cultures after exposure to TSC was slower till a 100-fold increase in the counts than in the control cultures. TSC was thus evaluated as a bacteriostatic drug not suitable for intermittent use.

In electron-microscopic studies degenerative changes of the mycobacterial cells were found after exposure to TSC (RUZICKA and ORTH 1950; ROLLE and MAYR 1951). Despite extensive studies, the exact mode of action of TSC on tubercle bacilli was not definitely elucidated (WAGNER and VONDERBANK 1951; ARITA 1956; KLAPP 1956).

δ) Effects in Combination with Antimycobacterial Drugs in Vitro. The effects of combinations of PAS and TSC were studied already in the early experiments performed by HURNI in 1949. A combination of PAS with a subinhibitory dose of TSC was as effective as PAS alone, whereas a combination of PAS with one fifth of the bacteriostatic concentration of SM resulted in a higher inhibitory activity of the former drug. Subinhibitory concentrations of SM (1/5 and 1/25 of the bacteriostatic concentration) enhanced considerably (30-fold) the activity of TSC, whereas subinhibitory concentrations of TSC (1/20 to 1/200) exerted only a weak supportive effect on SM.

ULSTRUP (1950) performed in-vitro experiments in Dubos liquid medium, and found no evidence of a potentiating effect of TSC with PAS on *M. tuberculosis* (H37Rv). PAS produced 50% inhibition at dilutions between −6 and −7 log mol and TSC at dilutions of −4.2 to −5.2 log mol. TSC produced complete inhibition at −2.2 to −3.2 log mol. This was interpreted as a result of differences between the action mechanisms of the two antimycobacterial drugs.

Combinations of antimycobacterial drugs were also studied by BARTMANN (1954b). By the use of a chequerboard technique, the MICs for 3 strains of *M. tuberculosis* were determined on egg medium, inter alia, for double combinations of TSC with PAS, SM, and INH. The strains reacted individually. For one and the same combination synergistic as well as antagonistic effects could be observed dependent further on the proportions of the drugs in the combinations.

b) Effect on Mycobacteria in Cell and Tissue Cultures

No data on this type of TSC action are available.

c) Activity of TSC in Experimental Tuberculosis and Development of Resistance in Vivo

Surveying the animal studies, at least two groups of experiments can be distinguished. The first covers the period of the early fifties. Various TSC compounds were assessed for their antimycobacterial activity, using screening methods developed at that time in mice, guinea pigs, and rabbits. Acute tuberculosis and assessments for this type of disease were preferred.

Mice were infected either intravenously or intraperitoneally with high doses of *M. tuberculosis* (H37Rv). The animals were obligatorily treated from the date of the infection (prophylactic treatment), TSC being mixed in with the feed. Some workers (HOGGARTH et al. 1949; HOGGARTH and MARTIN 1951) preferred TSC suspended in water, given orally twice a day via a syringe or catheter at doses ranging downwards from the maximum tolerated. The efficacy of the test drugs was assessed by checking macroscopic lesions in the lungs and the spleen (CROSHAW and DICKINSON 1950) or on the basis of mortality curves, assuming that all untreated mice had died from tuberculosis within 2 months after the infection (LEVADITI 1949). The presence or absence of tubercle bacilli in organs was also followed by cultures. The mortality curves were quantified by the introduction of mouse survival tests (BAVIN et al. 1950). The drug was regarded as active if it produced a significant prolongation in the survival time of a group of 10 mice. The methods used in the mouse studies are described in detail by RALEIGH and YOUMANS (1948a, b).

Few authors used the method put forward by REES and ROBSON (1951), based on the effect of the drug on the development of tuberculous lesions in the mouse cornea (corneal test). The intracorneal infections were induced using 1000 viable organisms of *M. bovis*. A drug was regarded as active if its prophylactic application prevented the development of corneal lesions.

The methods of studies in guinea pigs were more uniform. Animals weighing 300 g–400 g were usually infected with 0.01 mg–0.2 mg of tubercle bacilli (preferably in the logarithmic phase of growth), given either intramuscularly or subcutaneously. Treatment was started after the appearance of signs of tuberculosis in the regional lymph nodes, usually 3–4 weeks after the infection (therapeutic type of treatment). The drugs were administered with the feed. The effect of drugs given for several weeks was assessed by their action in prolonging life and in limiting the spread of the disease by sacrificing the surviving animals at a specified time. A record was then made of the extent of tuberculosis observed at the autopsy. A numerical index of the average severity of the tuberculosis was used as the basis for calculating tuberculosis indices in treated and untreated animals or groups. The indices of treated and untreated (control) animals/groups were compared statistically (CROSHAW and DICKINSON 1950; DOMAGK 1949, 1950; SPAIN et al. 1950; KARLSON et al. 1950; SPAIN and CHILDRESS 1951).

The Brownlee test only was used for the evaluation of the inhibitory activity of TSC by CROSHAW and DICKINSON 1950. The blood of guinea pigs was collected 2 h after intraperitoneal injection of the drug, mixed with an equal volume of Long agar, and inoculated with *M. tuberculosis* (strain H.4+8). The inhibition thus produced was calculated.

In his screening experiments, DOMAGK (1950) used rabbits as tuberculosis models. The animals were infected intravenously with 1.0 mg of *M. tuberculosis*, and treatment was started after the tuberculin skin reaction had become positive. 3 months after the first infection a reinfection with the same dose was carried out. Shortly afterwards nearly all animals died. The extent of the lesions was assessed by methods similar to those described for guinea pigs.

Regarding the results of the screening procedures, a marked activity against acute infection with *M. tuberculosis* in mice was limited to the TSC of substituted benzaldehydes or heterocyclic aldehydes. For highest activity a para-substituent had to be present in the aromatic nucleus of benzaldehyde TSC (HOGGARTH et al. 1949; DOMAGK 1949, 1950). o-Nitrobenzaldehyde TSC was accordingly ineffective both in mice and in guinea pig systems in spite of its in-vitro activity (CROSHAW and DICKINSON 1950).

HOGGARTH and MARTIN (1951) confirmed the narrowness of the limits within which activity was observed among compounds related to TSC by testing of 60 compounds prepared from TSC by a variety of oxidative and reductive processes. In various test systems in vivo only p-acetamido-, p-dimethylamino-, p-ethylsulphonyl, and p-methoxybenzaldehyde TSC were found to be active.

Attention was thus focused on TSC, i.e., the 4-acetylaminobenzaldehyde derivative. DOMAGK (1950) reported that TSC in a dose of 100 mg given subcutaneously to guinea pigs for 50 days prevented the progress of tuberculosis. STEINBACH and BAKER (1950) confirmed these results by using TSC in the feed (1%) over a period of 30 days. DONOVICK and BERNSTEIN (1949) estimated that in mice the minimally effective and maximally tolerated TSC doses were respectively 32 mg/kg and 65 mg/kg. Similar results have been obtained by FRANCIS et al. (1950).

The virtual ineffectiveness of TSC on tuberculous mice was reported by STEENKEN et al. in 1958. After daily doses of 500 mg/kg given in the diet, the extent of macroscopic lung lesions were the same in treated and untreated animals. However, the white mice (strain CF_1) had been infected intravenously by a very high dose (4 mg dry weight, from an 8-day culture of 4 "wild" strains of *M. tuberculosis* grown on Steenken-Smith medium.

Using also the method of quantitative culture of mouse organs in the course of the treatment, GRUMBACH (1965) was likewise sceptical about the effect of TSC administered in the prophylactic-type studies for 20 days. TSC at a dose of 50 mg/kg produced an indefinite effect, the survival period of the mice was only slightly prolonged, and isolated tubercle bacilli retained TSC sensitivity. In the therapeutic-type studies (treatment started only when the disease had developed), TSC doses higher than 50 mg/kg (mouse) were needed to prolong survival, without any marked reduction in the viability of tubercle bacilli in organs.

The relationship between the efficacy of TSC and the doses and dose intervals has been studied in guinea pigs by DICKINSON (1966). The animals were infected with 1.0 mg (moist weight) of *M. tuberculosis*. The treatment was started 3 weeks after the infection, TSC being administered by a stomach tube either daily or every second, fourth, or eighth day for 6 weeks. At the end of the treatment period all the animals were sacrificed and the extent of tuberculosis was graded using a score system. The score was divided by the survival time in days to give an "index" that took into account the extent of the disease present at autopsy and the lenght of survival of the animal during treatment. In untreated controls this index was 0.81; in the treated animals the indices were as follows: after 20 mg/kg/day 0.81, after 40 mg/kg every other day 1.12, after 80 mg/kg every 4th day 1.13, and after 160 mg/kg every 8th day 1.09. Similar results were obtained if the daily dose comprised 40 mg/kg. From these experiments it was concluded that as the interval between the doses increased there was a reduction in the bacteriostatic activity of TSC. The results supported the assumption presented above, namely that, because of its pharmacodynamic properties, TSC is unsuitable for intermittent therapy.

A considerable amount of attention was paid to the effect of combinations of TSC with other antimycobacterial drugs. The results represent the other group of reviewed papers. DOMAGK (1950) drew attention to the combination of TSC with SM. In his guinea pig experiments this combination proved to be superior to related monotherapies. KARLSON et al. (1950) confirmed that guinea pigs treated for 60 days with TSC in monotherapy (50 mg/kg–100 mg/kg) and those treated with a combination of TSC and SM (2 mg/kg) had markedly less visible macroscopic tuberculosis lesions than untreated controls. Both macroscopically and microscopically there was evidence of greater regression and healing of the lesions than after 2 mg/kg of SM alone. According to SPAIN and CHILDRESS (1950, 1951) and to CHILDRESS et al. (1952), in guinea pigs TSC was as effective as SM and definitely superior to PAS. Combined therapy with TSC and SM in half-doses was as effective as TSC alone (50 mg/kg) and possibly more effective than SM (1 mg/kg) alone. In the second set of experiments, TSC in combination with a subeffective dose of SM proved to be more effective than a combination of PAS with a subeffective dose of SM.

Using the above-mentioned intracorneal method, REES and ROBSON (1951) discovered that a combination of TSC with PAS had no advantages over TSC alone, and that a combination of TSC with SM had a definite additive effect greater than that produced under the same experimental conditions by a combination of SM with PAS. Ulstrup (1950) found in guinea pigs that a combination of TSC (150 mg/kg) and PAS (500 mg/kg) was ineffective.

In mouse experiments published in 1965, Grumbach found, surprisingly, that the combination of TSC (50 or 100 mg/kg) with INH (5 or 25 mg/kg) had, after 2 months of administration, the same effect on the number of viable tubercle bacilli in the lungs as 5 mg/kg of INH alone. After 5 months of administration the inhibitory effect of combinations with higher doses of TSC was more pronounced. Elevated TSC doses of 250 to 500 mg/kg produced a delay in the development of isoniazid resistance (if applied in the combination with the latter drug). The author suggested poor absorption and poor penetration of TSC into mouse cells as the principal reasons for the relative ineffectiveness of TSC in combination with isoniazid in experimental murine tuberculosis.

3. Concluding Remarks

The growth inhibiting activity of TSC in vitro is of the same order as that of SM or PAS. The type of action of TSC is bacteriostatic in vitro. Guinea pig experiments with spaced dosage did not favor its intermittent use in man. In the guinea pig and rabbit antituberculosis activity can be clearly demonstrated but only by doses which cannot be applicated to man because of toxicity. In mice even higher doses are needed in order to produce an effect and to delay the emergence of INH resistance during combined treatment with INH + TSC. Combinations of TSC with SM were found to be superior to single drug treatment, but combination of TSC with PAS offered no advantage. Thus, the experimental evidence suggested TSC not to be a leading drug but suitable as a companion drug in continuous combined treatment, at least in some drug combinations.

References

Afanasijeva JP, Mkrtchjan SV (1969) Criteria of *M. tuberculosis* resistance to thiacetazone and of cross resistance to ethionamide (in Russian). Probl Tuberk 47, issue 3:66–69

Arita T (1956) Change of thiosemicarbazone in vivo. II. Colorimetric determination of thiosemicarbazone in urine and its excretion. III. Decomposition products of thiacetazone excreted in urine. IV. Decomposition of thiacetazone in the intestinal tract. J Pharm Soc Jpn 76:984–996

Barnett M, Bushby SRM, Dickinson JM, Mitchison DA (1963) The response to treatment with thiacetazone of guinea pigs and mice infected with tubercle bacilli obtained from untreated African patients. Tubercle 44:417–430

Bartmann K (1954a) Die Bildung gegen Conteben hochresistenter Varianten als stammesspezifische Eigenschaft bei Mycobact. tuberc. var. hom, Z Túberk 104:305–311

Bartmann K (1954b) Die wachstumshemmende Wirkung verschiedener Tuberkulostatika und ihrer Kombinationen in vitro. Tuberkulosearzt 8:276–282

Bartmann K (1960) Kreuzresistenz zwischen α-Äthylthioisonicotinamid (1314 Th) und Thiosemicarbazon (Conteben). Tuberkulosearzt 14:525–529

Bartmann K (1974) Antimikrobielle Chemotherapie. Springer, Berlin Heidelberg New York Tokyo

Bartmann K, Abel U, Hart R (1966) Die Abhängigkeit des Hemmtiters von der Bebrütungsdauer bei der Bestimmung der Resistenz von M. tuberculosis gegen Antituberkulotika auf Löwenstein-Jensen Medium. Z Bakteriol Mikrobiol Hyg (A) 201:538–548

Bavin EM, Rees RJW, Robson JM, Seiler M, Seymour DE, Suddaly D (1950) The tuberculostatic activity of some thiosemicarbazones. J Pharm Pharmacol Lond 2:764–771

Behnisch R, Mietzsch F, Schmidt H (1950) Chemical studies on thiosemicarbazones with particular reference to antituberculous activity. Am Rev Tuberc 61:1–7

Bekierkunst A (1968) Tubercle bacilli grown in vivo. Ann N Y Acad Sci 154:79–87

Burjanová B, Urbanczik R (1970) Experimental chemotherapy of mycobacterioses provoked by atypical mycobacteria. Adv Tub Res 17:154–188

Canetti G, Fox W, Khomenko A, Mahler HT, Menon NK, Mitchison DA, Rist N, Šmelev NA (1969) Advances in techniques of testing mycobacterial drug sensitivity, and the use of sensitivity tests in tuberculosis control programmes. Bull WHO 41:21–43

Chicou FJ, Hétrick G, Huet M, Radenac H, Rist N (1968) Essai comparatif de deux types de traitement oral de la tuberculose pulmonaire (éthionamide + isoniazide, thiacetazone + isoniazide). Bull WHO 39:731–769

Childress WG, Norman JW, Ott RH, Spain DM (1952) Observations on the effect of amithiozone (Tibione) in selected tuberculous pulmonary lesion. Am Rev Tuberc 65:692–708

Croshaw B, Dickinson L (1950) Experimental tuberculosis and its chemotherapy. Br J Pharmacol 5:178–187

Davis JD, Netzer S, Schwartz JA, Pattison EH (1950) Tibione: laboratory and clinical studies. Dis Chest 18:521–522

Dickinson JM, Mitchison DA (1966) In vitro studies on the choice of drugs for intermittent chemotherapy of tuberculosis. Tubercle 47:370–380

Dickinson JM (1968) In vitro and in vivo studies to assess the suitability of antituberculous drugs for use in intermittent chemotherapy regimens. Tubercle 49 (Suppl):66–70

Domagk G, Behnisch R, Mietzsch F, Schmidt H (1946) Über eine neue, gegen Tuberkelbakterien in vitro wirksame Verbindungsklasse. Naturwiss 33:315

Domagk G (1949) Die experimentellen Grundlagen einer Chemotherapie der Tuberkulose. Beitr Klin Tuberk 101:365–394

Domagk G (1950) Chemotherapie der Tuberkulose mit Thiosemikarbazonen. Thieme, Stuttgart

Domagk G (1950) Investigations of the antituberculous activity of the thiosemicarbazones in vitro and in vivo. Am Rev Tuberc 61:8–19

Donovick R, Bernstein J (1949) On the action of thiosemicarbazone in experimental tuberculosis in the mouse. Am Rev Tuberc 60:539

Donovick R, Pansy F, Stryker G, Bernstein J (1950) The chemotherapy of experimental tuberculosis. I. The in vitro activity of thiosemicarbazides, thiosemicarbazones and related compounds. J Bacteriol 59:667–674

Eule H, Werner E (1967) Die Resistenz des Mycobacterium tuberculosis gegen Ethionamid, Thiosemicarbazon und Isoxyl und ihre Beziehungen zueinander. Beitr Klin Tuberk 134:247–258

Francis J, Spinks A, Stewart GA (1950) The toxic and antituberculous effect of two thiosemicarbazones in dogs, monkeys and guinea pigs. Brit J Pharmacol 5:549–564

Geks FJ, Wolf J (1950) Experimentelle und klinische Untersuchungen mit Conteben. Dtsch Med Wochenschr 75:1293–1295

Grosset J, Rodrigues F, Benhassine M, Chaulet P, Larbaoui D (1968) Sensitivity to thiacetazone of strains of Mycobacterium tuberculosis isolated in Algiers: practical deductions. Tubercle 49 (Suppl):46–48

Grosset J, Benhassine M (1970) La thiacetazone (TB_1) donnée expérimentales et cliniques récentes. Adv Tub Res 17:107–153

Grumbach F (1965) Etudes chimiothérapiques sur la tuberculose avancée de la souris. Adv Tub Res 14:31–96

Hamre D, Bernstein J, Donovick R (1950) The chemotherapy of experimental tuberculosis. II. Thiosemicarbazones and analogues in experimental tuberculosis in the mouse. J Bacteriol 59:675–680

Hejný J (1978) Mycobacteriological aspects of the treatment of mycobacterioses. I. In vitro studies (in Czech). Stud Pneumol Phtiseol Cechoslovac 38:579–583

Hejný J (1979) The bacteriological aspect of the treatment of mycobacterial diseases with non-specific antibiotics and with sulphonamides. Bull Int Union Tuberc 54:342–343

Hofmann P, Nickel L (1950) Über die Resistenz von Tuberkelbakterien und den antibakteriellen Blutspiegel bei Lungentuberkulösen während der Behandlung mit Conteben, PAS und Streptomycin. Tuberkulosearzt 4:695–702
Hoggarth E, Martin AR, Storey NE, Young EHP (1949) Studies on the chemotherapy of tuberculosis. Part V. Thiosemicarbazones and related compounds. Br J Pharmacol 4:248–253
Hoggarth E, Martin AR (1951) Studies on the chemotherapy of tuberculosis. Part VII. The oxidation and reduction products of thiosemicarbazones. Br J Pharmacol 6:454–458
Hurni H (1949) Die tuberkulostatische Wirkung von Kombinationen einiger bekannter Chemotherapeutica. Schweiz Z Path Bakter 12:596–601
Karlson AG, Gainer JH, Feldman WH (1950) The therapeutic effect on experimental tuberculosis in guinea pigs of 4-acetylamino-benzaldehyde thiosemicarbazone (TB I) alone and in combination with streptomycin. Proc Mayo Clin 25:160–164.
Klapp A (1956) Contebengehalt gesunder und kranker Meerschweinchenorgane. Ein Beitrag zur Frage der Contebenwirkung. Beitr Klin Tuberk 115:135–144
Kuze F, Lee Y, Maekawa N, Suzuki Y (1979) A study on experimental mycobacterioses provoked by atypical mycobacteria. Combined antituberculous chemotherapy against conventional mice infected intravenously with *M. intracellulare* (in Japanese). Kekkaku 54:453–460
Levaditi C (1949) Effets curatifs du thiosémicarbazone (Tb I) dans la tuberculose expérimentale de la souris. Presse Med 57:519
Malluche H (1952) Die Thiosemicarbazon-Therapie der Tuberkulose. Fortschr Tbk Forsch 5:152–254
Meissner G (1955) Häufigkeit der Resistenz für Conteben und deren Bedeutung für das Auftreten der Resistenz für Isoxyl (4-4′-Diisoamyloxythiocarbanilid) bei Tuberkelbakterien. Prax Pneumol 19:387–395
Mitchison DA, Lloyd J (1964) Comparison of the sensitivity to thiacetazone of tubercle bacilli from patients in Britain, East Africa, South India and Hong Kong. Tubercle 45:360–369
Mitchison DA (1971) The principles of intermittent chemotherapy (in Czech). Stud Pneumol Phtiseol Cechoslovac 31:288–296
Moeschlin S, Demiral B (1950) Vergleich der Kombinationstherapie von Streptomycin mit TB 1 (Thiosemicarbazon) oder PAS (Paraaminosalicylsäure) sowie zwei neuen PAS-Derivaten bei der experimentellen Tuberkulose. Schweiz Med Wochenschr 80:373–374
Mollov M, Hill I, Kott ThJ (1951) Sensitivity of tubercle bacilli to amithiozone (myvizone). Am Rev Tuberc 63:487–489
Ohsato T, Tsukagoshi K, Shimizu H (1970) Studies on thiacetazone resistance of tubercle bacilli. Part I. Thiacetazone sensitivity of tubercle bacilli isolated from previously untreated tuberculous children (in Japanese). Kekkaku 46:65–70
Ohsato T, Tsukagoshi K, Shimizu H (1971) Studies on thiacetazone resistance of tubercle bacilli. Part II. The relation between virulence in guinea pigs and thiacetazone sensitivity of tubercle bacilli isolated from previously untreated tuberculous children (in Japanese). Kekkaku 46:83–87
Raleigh GW, Youmans GP (1948a) The use of mice in experimental chemotherapy of tuberculosis. I. Rationale and review of literature. J Infect Dis 82:197–204
Raleigh GW, Youmans GP (1948b) The use of mice in experimental chemotherapy of tuberculosis. II. Pathology and pathogenesis. J Infect Dis 82:205–209
Rao KP, Nair SS, Naghanathan N, Rao R (1966) An in vitro study on sensitivity of tubercle bacilli to thiacetazone (TB_1). Ind J Tuberc 13:147–157
Rees RJW, Robson JM (1951) The activity of thiosemicarbazones alone and in combination with other drugs in experimental corneal tuberculosis. Br J Pharmacol 6:83–88
Rist N (1968) Thiacetazone sensitivity and resistance: introductory remarks. Tubercle 49, suppl: 36
Rist N, Cals S, Jullien W (1951) Aspect variés de la sensibilité du bacille tuberculeux à la para-acétylbenzaldehydethiosemicarbazone (Tb_1) en milieu de Youmans. Ann Inst Pasteur 81:324–328

Rist N, Grumbach F, Libermann D, Moyeux M, Cals S, Clavel S (1958) Un noveau médicament antituberculeux actif sur les bacilles isoniazido-résistants: le thioamide de l'acide alpha-ethylisonicotinic. Rev Tuberc 22:278–283
Rist N, Grumbach F, Libermann D (1959) Experiments on the antituberculous activity of alpha-ethyl-thioisonicotinamide. Am Rev Tuberc Pulm Dis 79:1–5
Rolle M, Mayr A (1951) Die Veränderungen der Tuberkelbakterien nach Einwirkung von Streptomycin und TB I/698. Arch Hyg Bakt 134:23–32
Russell M, Bush D, Hurwitz C (1950) Studies on methods for determining sensitivities of tubercle bacilli to Tibione. Am Rev Tuberc 62:638–644
Ruzicka O, Orth E (1950) An Tuberkelbakterien elektronoptisch dargestellte Wirkung von Thiosemicarbazonen (TB I, TB VI). Wien Med Wochenschr 100:95–102
Shephard CC (1957) Use of HeLa cells infected with tubercle bacilli for the study of antituberculous drugs. J Bacteriol 73:494–498
Sojková M, Toušek J, Trnka L (1965) Zur Frage der Kreuzresistenz zwischen Äthionamid, Thiosemikarbazonen und Thioharnstoffderivaten. Prax Pneumol 19:522–527
Spain DM, Childress WG, Fishler JS (1950) The effect of 4-acetylaminobenzal thiosemicarbazone (Tibione) on experimental tuberculosis in guinea pigs. Am Rev Tuberc 62:144–148
Spain DM, Childress WG (1951) The therapeutic effect on experimental tuberculosis in guinea pigs of 4-acetylaminobenzal thiosemicarbazone (Tibione) in combination with dihydrostreptomycin as compared with the effect of para-aminosalicylic acid in combination with dihydrostreptomycin. Am Rev Tuberc 63:339–345
Steenken W Jr, Smith MM, Montalbine V (1958) In vitro and in vivo effect of antimicrobial agents in atypical mycobacteria. Am Rev Tuberc 78:454–461
Steinbach MM, Baker H (1950) p-Anisaldehyde-thiosemicarbazone in treatment of experimental murine tuberculosis. Proc Soc Exp Biol Med 74:595–596
Thomas KL, Joseph S, Subbaiah TV, Selkon JB (1961) Identification of tubercle bacilli from Indian patients with pulmonary tuberculosis. Bull WHO 25:747–758
Trnka L, Havel A, Urbančík R (1966) Neueste Tuberkulostatika, ihre Bedeutung und Möglichkeiten der Wertbestimmung im Reagenzglas. Chemotherapia 11:121–134
Ulstrup JC (1950) Treatment of experimental tuberculosis of guinea pigs by a combination of PAS and TB 1/698. Acta Pathol Microbiol Scand 27:487–491
Wagner WH, Vonderbank H (1951) Zur Wirkungsweise von 4-Acetylbenzaldehydthiosemicarbazon, Streptomycin und p-Aminosalicylsäure bei Tuberkelbakterien. Arb Paul Ehrlich Inst 49:98–109

IV. Pyrazinamide (PZA) and Morphazinamide (MZA)

L. Trnka

Nicotinamide was found by Chorine (1945) to retard the development of tuberculosis in experimental animals. McKenzie et al. (1948) confirmed the activity of this substance in murine tuberculosis. In the search for effective analogues PZA was synthesized by Kushner et al. (1952). Intensive clinical trials were conducted, following the discovery of the antimycobacterial properties of PZA, and their results stimulated a worldwide interest in designing more effective and/or better tolerated derivatives. MZA, a PZA with an attached N-morpholinomethyl group, was synthesized by Felder et al. (1962) and later put on the market with the claim for a better tolerability than that of PZA.

1. Antimicrobial Spectrum in Vitro

PZA has been found to be active only against tubercle bacilli, perhaps because it possesses an enzyme pyrazinamidase, which transforms PZA into pyrazinoic acid believed by some authors to be the intracellularly active substance. MZA has been reported to have detectable bacteriostatic activity against a fairly wide range of pathogenic microorganisms, such as *Pseudomonas*, *Proteus vulgaris*, and *Staphylococcus aureus* on agar as well as in liquid media (BONATI and BERTONI 1962). This difference may be due to degradation products of MZA appearing during incubation (see 2.a.α).

2. Antimycobacterial Activity

a) Antimycobacterial Activity in Artificial Media

The results of several investigations with PZA are summarized in Table 1. At neutral pH only a very weak activity against laboratory or wild strains of *M. tuberculosis* is apparent. MCDERMOTT and TOMPSETT (1954), however, observed that acidification of the media down to pH 5.0–5.5 resulted in a considerable increase in efficacy. In Tween® albumin liquid medium the MIC after 2 weeks of incubation was 500 μg/ml at pH 6.0 and 16 μg/ml at pH 5.5; in an oleic acid albumin liquid medium, the respective figures were 450 μg/ml and 6.25 μg/ml. On solid egg media acidified to pH 4.8–5.5 before inspissation the activity of PZA is also markedly higher. STEENKEN et al. (1957) have observed that strains of *M. bovis*, *M. avium-intracellulare* and fast-growing strains of mycobacteria were highly resistant to PZA. WOLINSKY (1979) and TELLIS and PUTNAM (1980) found PZA to be inactive against most strains not belonging to the species *M. tuberculosis*.

The in-vitro activities of PZA and MZA have been compared by several authors. BONATI and BERTONI (1962) and LUCCHESI (1963) reported MZA to be more active than PZA. BÖNICKE (1963) determined the antimycobacterial activity

Table 1. Antimycobacterial activity of pyrazinamide on *M. tuberculosis* in artificial media

Author	Strain of *M. tuberculosis*	Type of media	MIC[a] in μg/ml
SOLOTOROVSKY et al. (1952)	H37Rv	Dubos-albumin-Tween pH 6.8	150
		Proskauer-Beck pH 6.8	120
STEENKEN and WOLINSKY (1954)	H37Rv	Dubos-albumin-Tween pH 6.8	>200
		Proskauer-Beck with 10% serum pH 6.8	>200
TARSHIS and WEED (1953)	Wild strains	ATS[b]	100
MCDERMOTT and TOMPSETT (1954)	H37Rv	Dubos-albumin-Tween pH 6.0	503
		Dubos-albumin-Tween pH 5.5	16
		Oleic acid-albumin pH 6.0	450
		Oleic acid-albumin pH 5.5	6.25
GRUMBACH (1958)	H37Rv	Dubos-albumin-Tween pH 7.0	400
		Dubos-albumin-Tween pH 6.0	125
		Dubos-albumin-Tween pH 5.5	25

[a] Minimal inhibitory concentration of PZA.
[b] American Trudeau Society.

in serial dilution tests using Lockemann liquid medium, enriched with 0.05% of pyruvate and 2% of bovine serum, at pH 5.6, 6.2, and 6.8. At pH 5.6 MZA was as active as PZA, whereas at pH 6.8 it became more active than the latter.

No differences in the MICs of MZA and PZA were observed by TRNKA et at. (1964) for *M. tuberculosis*, strain H37Rv, and wild strains sensitive or resistant to INH, SM, or PAS. The experiments were performed in a liquid Šula medium at pH 5.6. The MICs were 8 μg/ml–16 μg/ml. The MIC values of MZA for photochromogenic, atypical mycobacteria were above 32 μg/ml. With regard to *M. tuberculosis*, similar results have been reported by DISSMANN (1963). BARTMANN (1963) found MZA to be slightly more active than PZA, as did CARRADA BRAVO et al. (1975) (see also the following section).

It may thus be concluded that the antimycobacterial spectrum of MZA and PZA in vitro is the same, and that there are no substantial differences in the antimycobacterial activity.

α) Factors Affecting the Activity in Vitro. KONNO et al. (1967) reported that the growth of tubercle bacilli in acid media could be inhibited by 50 μg/ml of pyrazinoic acid, the substance released from PZA by bacterial amidase. A correlation between the pyrazinamidase activity of tubercle bacilli and their sensitivity or resistance to PZA was established. The destruction of PZA by pyrazinamidase is a phenomenon estimated as unlikely to be of importance in human tuberculous lesions, because fresh PZA would always diffuse rapidly to the bacilli in the lesions (DICKINSON and MITCHISON 1970). The disproportional increase in the MIC of PZA with larger inoculum sizes has also been explained as an effect of pyrazinamidase with a consequent shift in the pH of the medium to the alkaline side, thereby reducing the activity of PZA (DICKINSON and MITCHISON 1970; TRIPATHY et al. 1970).

MZA likewise undergoes enzymatic destruction in liquid media. According to BÖNICKE (1963) and FELDER et al. (1964), the reaction products are PZA, formaldehyde, and morpholine. In contrast to formaldehyde, morpholine has no antimycobacterial activity. The effect of formaldehyde on the MIC of MZA has been studied by CASTELLI et al. (1966) and the question was later taken up again by CARRADA BRAVO et al. (1975). The MICs of PZA, MZA, and formaldehyde were determined in high-citrate medium without Tween 80 at pH 5.6 for 35 strains. The titres were read after incubation at 37 °C for 7 days. The geometric means of the MICs expressed in μg/ml were 9.1 for PZA, 6.3 for MZA, 4.7 for formaldehyde, and 1.6+0.4 for PZA + formaldehyde. On an equimolar basis, MZA appeared to be about 3 times as active as PZA. Since PZA + formaldehyde had an MIC about half that of MZA, the apparent activity of MZA could be due to MZA itself or to its hydrolysis products. To decide between these two alternatives, slide cultures were set up and exposed successively at intervals of 1 h to freshly prepared medium with various concentrations of MZA, PZA, formaldehyde, and PZA + formaldehyde. Chemical estimates indicated that the stock solutions of MZA did not contain cleavage products and that during an exposure time of 1 h at 37 °C only 15% of the MZA would be decomposed. Thus, the inhibitory effect of MZA had to be ascribed largely to MZA itself. Nevertheless, the growth-retarding effect of MZA was very similar to those of PZA and PZA + formaldehyde. It was therefore concluded that the apparent activity of MZA is due to the substance itself.

β) Sensitivity Testing and Resistance to PZA. Routine sensitivity testing of PZA is associated with considerable technical difficulties due mainly to the necessary acidification of the medium to an exact pH, the limited hardening of egg media at acid pH, retardation or arrest of bacterial growth under these conditions, and the marked effect of the size of inoculum. Technical details have been discussed briefly by BARTMANN (1966) and at length by TRIPATHY et al. (1970, 1971). The proportion method has been found to be particularly useful. The critical concentration selected by many investigators is 100 μg/ml, the critical proportion, depending on the initial pH, varying between 1% and 50% (CANETTI et al. 1963; TRIPATHY et al. 1970; NOVÁK et al. 1970).

STOTTMEIER et al. (1967) and BUTLER and KILBURN (1982) observed satisfactory growth of tubercle bacilli on Middlebrook and Cohn 7H10 media at pH 5.5 if an albumin-dextrose-catalase supplement was used rather than an oleic acid-albumin-dextrose-catalase complex. They found this medium to be suitable for sensitivity testing.

To avoid the technical problems, BRANDER (1972) proposed to replace the testing of PZA at acid pH by testing of nicotinamide at neutral pH on solid media. This is possible because of the complete cross-resistance between PZA and nicotinamide. The feasibility of this technique has been confirmed by TATAR (1974) and by KALICH et al. (1978).

Another approach was used by MCCLATCHY et al. (1981). Having confirmed the correlation between pyrazinamidase activity and PZA sensitivity reported by KONNO et al. (1967), these authors compared a thin-layer chromatographic method for the detection of pyrazinoic acid with a technique described by WAYNE (1974) and found close correlation between the two methods. JAKSCHIK (1985) found excellent agreement between a slight modification of WAYNE's technique and sensitivity tests using nicotinamide, and DE KANTOR et al. (1985) obtained 96% agreement between WAYNE's technique and sensitivity tests using PZA at pH 5. The incidence of resistant mutants in wild strains of *M. tuberculosis* has been estimated by RIST (1962, 1964) to be approximately 10^{-4}, with considerable variations between strains. This is a fairly high rate compared to other antituberculotics.

According to the criteria reported above, initial resistance to PZA or MZA is very rare. Only 0.3%–3% of the wild strains of *M. tuberculosis* tested were regarded as resistant to PZA (WASZ HÖCKERT et al. 1956; BATTEN 1968; KREBS 1969; TRIPATHY et al. 1970; CITRON 1975).

Secondary resistance seems to develop by the multistep pattern in vitro (BONATI and BERTONI 1962) as well as in patients (TRIPATHY et al. 1970). During daily treatment with PZA 8%–9% of the cultures obtained in the first 3 months were resistant, 43%–52% of those obtained at 4–6 months, and 44%–49% of those obtained at 7–12 months. With MZA no increase in the MIC was noted during 4 passages in subinhibitory concentrations (BONATI and BERTONI 1962).

Cross-resistance exists, as already mentioned, between PZA and nicotinamide (KONNO et al. 1967) and between PZA and MZA (BÖNICKE 1963; TRNKA et al.

1964; CARRADA BRAVO et al. 1975), but not with other antituberculotics. Normal PZA sensitivity of INH-resistant strains has been reported by PERRY and MORSE (1955) and by GRUMBACH (1958), and normal sensitivity of strains resistant to PAS, SM, TSC, INH, VM, CS, or ETH by TRNKA et al. (1964).

γ) Type of Action. The type of action of PZA can be deduced from in-vitro studies of DICKINSON and MITCHISON (1970) on the suitability of PZA for intermittent application. PZA (50 μg/ml) was added to a growing culture of *M. tuberculosis* in liquid medium and removed after 6 h, 24 h, or 96 h of exposure. Viable counts showed that multiplication of a small inoculum was prevented for 40 days even after a single 6 h exposure. After exposure for 96 h no growth occured within 76 days, when the experiment was terminated. The authors summarize all their experiments by saying that PZA was bactericidal to small inocula in moderately acid media.

b) Antimycobacterial Activity Against Phagocytosed Bacilli

MACKANESS (1956) studied the activity of PZA and nicotinamide on tubercle bacilli, strain H37Rv, taken up by isolated rabbit monocytes. Real multiplication was virtually completely prevented by 12.5 μg/ml nicotinamide or PZA. After incubation of the monocytes for 30 h or 72 h in a medium containing 25 μg/ml PZA, the washed cell residues were planted onto oleic-acid-albumin agar. After incubation for 30 h the proportion of monocytes yielding colonies of tubercle bacilli was the same in the controls and the PZA-exposed cells, and after 72 h of incubation the PZA-exposed cells yielded a third to a quarter of that registered for the controls. A slight bactericidal effect was thus demonstrated. Many authors have confirmed that the MIC of PZA and MZA for phagocytosed tubercle bacilli is definitely lower than that in artificial media (BASILICO 1959, CASALONE et al. 1962; SOLOVIEV and PAVLOV 1966). BERTONI and BREGA (1965) compared the activities of PZA and MZA against tubercle bacilli located in rabbit peritoneal monocytes. On a molar basis, MZA was twice as effective as PZA. The killing of macrophage-ingested tubercle bacilli was again studied by CARLONE et al. (1985). Unstimulated resident peritoneal mouse macrophages harboring tubercle bacilli of a recently isolated strain were exposed inter alia to 30 μg/ml PZA or 8 μg/ml pyrazinoic acid. The concentrations correspond to peak serum concentrations in man after the administration of therapeutic doses. After an incubation time of 24 h the highest rates of killing noted were 93% for PZA and 92% for pyrazinoic acid, as opposed to 59% in the controls. On the second and third days the numbers of viable bacilli increased in the controls as well as in drug-containing cell cultures, indicating that a complete killing of the ingested bacilli was not achieved.

c) Activity of PZA and MZA in Experimental Tuberculosis and Development of Resistance in Vivo

α) PZA and MZA in Monotherapy. The first studies with PZA were done, as was usual at that time, in guinea pigs. DESSAU et al. (1952) infected the animals intraperitoneally. Treatment by various routes and with different doses started 14 days

Table 2. Tuberculostatic guinea pig unit[a] of different substances with antituberculous activity. (After DESSAU et al. 1952)

Substance	Form of administration			
	In the diet	Subcutaneously	Intraperitoneally	Orally
Streptomycin	–	15 mg	–	–
4,4′-Diaminodiphenylsulfone	50 mg	–	–	50 mg
PAS	300 mg	–	–	–
Nicotinamide	200 mg	200 mg	–	200 mg
Pyrazinamide	75 mg	30–45 mg	50 mg	50 mg

[a] Guinea pig unit = minimal dose of any substance with tuberculostatic activity equal to the standard preparation of 50 mg DDS daily.

after inoculation and lasted 3 weeks. The results were evaluated on the basis of postmortem findings. PZA was compared against DDS, PAS, SM, and nicotinamide; the relative activities are presented in Table 2. The authors concluded that PZA was slightly less effective than DDS, more effective than PAS and nicotinamide, and less effective than SM. The activities of PZA and nicotinamide were independent of the route of administration (oral or parenteral). PZA had the same efficacy on an SM-resistant strain as on SM-sensitive ones. A bovine strain, however, gave a rather poor response to PZA, as could be expected. In curative experiments on guinea pigs carried out by STEENKEN and WOLINSKY (1954), PZA produced only a slight beneficial effect when given orally in a dose of 145 mg/kg per day. In contrast, INH had a marked effect at the dose of 5 mg/kg.

In mice, results turned out to be more clear-cut, though not so much in the first experiments, in which the survival time and the change in the body weight were used as indicators of efficacy (MALONE et al. 1952). According to time/percentage survival curves, evaluated by LITCHFIELD's method PZA was superior to PAS but inferior to SM. Likewise, SOLOTOROVSKY et al. (1952) found PZA to be superior to nicotinamide and PAS when the drugs were given to intravenously infected mice in the diet or subcutaneously at the same dosage. The effect was evaluated by scoring the gross involvement of the organs. MCCUNE and TOMPSETT (1956) and MCCUNE et al. (1956) then demonstrated, by the microbial counting technique, the strong killing effect of PZA. The drug was administered in the diet at 2%, either from the day of the infection or after lesions had developed. Mice were sacrificed at specified intervals, and homogenates prepared from the lungs and the spleen were cultured quantitatively. PZA dramatically reduced the number of culturable bacilli during the first 2 months of the treatment. At 2 months the cultures of many specimens remained negative. After 3 months there was a marked increase in the bacterial population in part of the animals, which could be explained by the development of PZA resistance. These results were subsequently confirmed in therapeutic-type experiments carried out by GRUMBACH (1958). Mice (14 g–16 g) were infected massively by the intravenous route, so that the controls died in 20 days–24 days. Treatment started 2 weeks after the infection and lasted 8 weeks. PZA was given by a gastric tube. After the end of the treatment cultures were made from the lungs and the spleens. PZA at a daily dose of 10 mg per mouse reduced the viable counts from the lungs to the same extent as 0.1 mg INH per mouse. In the spleen, on the other hand, PZA reduced the number of culturable bacilli by 80 times as much as INH. In a preventive type of treatment the drugs were administered from the next day after the infection. Criteria based on macroscopic organs' changes indicated that PZA at a dose of 10 mg/mouse/day was equal in effect to INH at a daily dose of 0.05 mg/mouse, but even 5 mg and 3 mg PZA/mouse had some activity. The drug was furthermore shown to be effective against INH-resistant bacilli. In later experiments (GRUMBACH 1965) it was observed that higher doses of PZA (1500 mg/kg/day) caused a faster development of PZA resistance. KREIS and FOURNAUD (1965) postulated that the degree of PZA activity in mice was a function of its early bactericidal action. The duration of treatment, i.e., the total dose, seems to be more important than the individual doses. With the same total dose, a longer survival time was achieved if the drug had been given intermittently once or twice a week.

FREERKSEN et al. (1963) compared MZA against PZA in guinea pigs and in mice, treating the animals for 10 days with 300 mg/kg and 500 mg/kg of either drug or with 1 mg INH/kg and then measuring the survival rates. PZA prolonged survival clearly in comparison with the controls, but less than 1 mg INH/kg; MZA had no effect. It must be admitted, however, that the conditions of this test are probably not sensitive enough to reveal a weak activity. In guinea pigs, MZA at daily doses of between 60 mg/kg and about 240 mg/kg delayed the progress of disease when therapy was started shortly after the infection (COCCIANTE et al. 1962; LUCCHESI 1963; CATENA et al. 1963; MULARGIA and PICCALUGA 1964; CASTORINA et al. 1964), whereas treatment of an established infection had little or no effect (D'ALFONSO et al. 1962; MULARGIA and PICCALUGA 1964). TRNKA et al. (1964) compared PZA and MZA in a chronic mouse model. The strain of *M. tuberculosis* used for the infection had a relatively low virulence in mice, so that during the 6 months of the experiment in any animal group no more than half of the mice died from tuberculosis. Treatment with 500 mg/kg/day of either drug, given subcutaneously, started 1 month after the infection and lasted 20 weeks. On the basis of the relative spleen and lung weights, MZA differed very little from the control group, whereas PZA exerted a clear effect. The microbial census of the lungs and the spleens, determined by culture, was reduced by MZA to about 10% and to a level of the order of 0.1% by PZA.

Thus, MZA proved to be much inferior to PZA on the basis of the various parameters used. HAVEL et al. (1964) demonstrated for this experiment a 42% incidence of resistant bacterial populations in the organs of PZA-treated mice, in contrast to one of 0% in MZA-treated mice. This also reflects the weak activity of MZA. The absence of any significant antimycobacterial activity of MZA in laboratory animals was reported by BLASI (1963), and subsequently confirmed by VERBIST (1966) and by DRABKINA and GINSBURG (1971). Since CARRADA BRAVO et al. (1975) have shown that in vitro MZA is active by itself, and even more so than PZA, it is tempting to speculate that the poor efficacy of MZA in animals might be due to some special features of its pharmacokinetics or metabolism. In contrast, a definite antimycobacterial activity of PZA in laboratory animals has been detected without exception. Microbial counts show PZA to have the same pattern of action as other effective drugs: an initial reduction in the bacterial organ population, followed by a secondary increase due to the development of bacterial resistance.

β) PZA in Combined Therapy. Following their studies on microbial persistence during chemotherapy, McCUNE et al. (1956) mentioned without providing further details that the irregular but marked sterilizing action of PZA alone could be made to occur regularly by association with another drug. Constant results were obtained not only by the addition of INH, but also with SM (4 mg/mouse) and even with very weak drugs like PAS (0.75% in the diet) or oxytetracycline. The very remarkable sterilizing capacity of PZA in combination with other antituberculotics, especially with INH and RMP, turned out to be one of the cornerstones of short-course therapy and will be dealt with in the respective sections.

3. Concluding Remarks

It took a long time for PZA to find its definite place in the treatment of tuberculosis. During the early years its fate was threatened by discrepancies in the experimental data, the liver toxicity of the doses originally used, and the introduction of the highly active and well tolerated INH. The uncertainties in the interpretation of the experimental data were due to the differences between the MICs for extracellular bacilli at neutral and acid pH, between the MICs for extra- and intracellularly located bacilli, and to the difference between the low efficacy in guinea pigs and the high and sometimes sterilizing activity in mice. Only in later years was it realized how important a role PZA could play in short-course chemotherapy when it was combined with other bactericidal antituberculotics.

MZA, the semisynthetic PZA derivative, is even more difficult to evaluate experimentally than PZA. All one can say is that it could not be shown to be superior to PZA in antimycobacterial activity.

References

Bartmann K (1963) Orientierende Untersuchungen über Morphazinamid. G Ital Chemioter 10:158–160
Bartmann K (1966) Discussion remark. Bull Int Union Tuberc XXXVII:215
Basilico F (1959) Attività antitubercolare della pirazinamide nella monocito-coltura. Atti Soc Lombarda Sci Med-Biol 14:430–433
Batten J (1968) Experimental chemotherapy of tuberculosis. Br Med J 3:75–82
Bertoni Z, Brega A (1965) Effect of pyrazinamide and morpholine-methyl-pyrazinamide on the intracellular multiplication of tubercle bacilli in monocytes. Clin Medicine 72:1006–1012
Blasi A (1963) Experimental "in vivo" results on the antimycobacterial activity of morphazinamide (in Italian). G Ital Chemioter 10:51–55
Bönicke R (1963) Der ursächliche Zusammenhang zwischen der tuberkulostatischen Wirksamkeit des Morphazinamids und seiner Instabilität. G Ital Chemioter 10:190–195
Bonati F, Bertoni L (1962) Basic derivatives of pyrazino-2-carboxylic acid possessing antimycobacterial activity. Microbiological and pharmacological study. Min Med 53:1704–1708

Brander E (1972) A simple way of detecting pyrazinamide resistance. Tubercle 53:128–131
Butler WR, Kilburn JO (1982) Improved method for testing susceptibility of *Mycobacterium tuberculosis* to pyrazinamide. J Clin Microbiol 16:1106–1109
Canetti G, Rist N, Grosset J (1963) Mesure de la sensibilité du bacille tuberculeux aux drogues antibacillaires par la méthode des proportions. Rev Tuberc Pneumol 27:217–272
Canetti G, Fox W, Khomenko A, Mahler HT, Menon NK, Mitchison DA, Rist N, Šmelev NA (1969) Advances in technique of testing mycobacterial drug sensitivity, and the use of sensitivity tests in tuberculous control programmes. Bull WHO 41:21–43
Carlone NA, Acocella G, Cuffini AM, Forno-Pizzoglio M (1985) Killing of macrophage-ingested mycobacteria by rifampicin, pyrazinamide, and pyrazinoic acid alone and in combination. Am Rev Respir Dis 132:1274–1277
Carrada Bravo T, Ellard GA, Mitchison DA, Horsfall PAL (1975) Reappraisal of the activity of morphazinamide against M. tuberculosis. Tubercle 56:211–217
Casalone G, Ganzetti G, Mangiarotti S, Rimoldi R (1962) Ricerche sperimentali e cliniche sull'attività antitubercolare della N-(morfolino-4-metil)-amide dell'acido pirazincarbonico. Minerva Med 53:1709–1711
Castelli D, Vercellino E, Vercellino A (1966) The role of formaldehyde in the antimicrobial action of morphazinamide in vitro (in Italian). G Ital Mal Torace 20:261–267
Castorina S, Battaglia B, Di Stefano L (1964) La morfazinamide nella tubercolosi sperimentale delle cavie. G Med Tisiol 13:69–82
Catena A, Aliperta A, Rocco V (1963) Il focolaio da inoculazione in cavie in trattamento con morfazinamide. (Infezioni con ceppi sensibili e resistenti ai chemioantibiotici). Arch Tisiol Mal App Resp (Sez Sci) 18:366–377
Chorine MV (1945) Action de l'amide nicotinique sur les bacilles du genre Mycobacterium. C R Acad Sci 220:150–156
Citron KM (1975) Problems of drug resistance in pulmonary tuberculosis. Abstracts of World Medicine 38:1–11
Cocciante B, Miglio M, Mori G, Piazza R (1962) Prime osservazioni cliniche e rilievi sperimentali sull'impiego della Piazofolina nei processi tubercolari. Minerva Med 53:1711–1718
D'Alfonso G, Bariffi F, Giuliano V (1962) Indagini sperimentali sull'attività antitubercolare della morfazinamide. Arch Tisiol 17:919–928
De Kantor IN (1985) Discussion remark. Bull Int Union Tuberc 60:66
Dessau FI, Yeager RL, Burger FJ, Williams JH (1952) Pyrazinamide (Aldinamide) in experimental tuberculosis of the guinea pig. Am Rev Tuberc 65:519–522
Dickinson JM, Mitchison DA (1970) Observations in vitro on the suitability of pyrazinamide for intermittent chemotherapy of tuberculosis. Tubercle 51:389–396
Dissmann E (1963) Erfahrungen mit Morphazinamid (MZA) (in Italian). G Ital Chemioter 10:161–163
Drabkina RD, Ginzburg TS (1971) Tuberculostatic activity of the 2nd line drugs (in Russian). Probl Tuberk 49 issue 8:67–81
Felder E, Pitrè D, Tiepolo U (1962) N-morpholinometilpirazinamide: caratteristiche chimio-fisiche e determinazione nei liquidi biologici. Minerva Med 53:1699–1704
Felder E, Pitrè D, Tiepolo V (1964) Hydrolyse und Bildung von Morpholinomethylpyrazinamid. Arzneimittelforsch 14:1227–1230
Freerksen E, Bönicke R, Rosenfeld M (1963) Vergleichende Untersuchungen zur tuberkulostatischen Aktivität von N-morpholino-methyl-pyrazinamid und Pyrazin-2-carboxamid (Pyrazinamid) in vitro und in vivo. Arzneimittelforsch 13:722–724
Grumbach F (1958) Activité antituberculeuse expérimentale du pyrazinamide (P.Z.A.). Ann Inst Pasteur 94:694–708
Grumbach F (1965) Etudes chimiothérapiques sur la tuberculose avancée de la souris. Adv Tuberc Res 14:31–96
Havel A, Trnka L, Kuška J (1964) Comparison of antituberculous effects of morphazinamide and pyrazinamide in chronic experimental tuberculosis. II. The emergence of resistance and its retardation in the course of treatment by single drugs and by combination of antituberculous drugs. Chemotherapia (Basel) 9:168–175
Jakschik M (1985) Discussion remark. Bull Int Union Tuberc 60:66

Kalich R, Gerloff W, Neubert R, Ulber U (1978) Resistenzbestimmung von Mykobakterien gegenüber Pyrazinamid und Nikotinamid. Z Erkr Atmungsorgane 151:102–112

Konno K, Feldmann FM, McDermott W (1967) Pyrazinamide susceptibility and amidase activity of tubercle bacilli. Am Rev Respir Dis 15:461–469

Krebs A (1969) Experimentelle Chemotherapie der Tuberkulose. Z Erkr Atmungsorgane 130:417–448

Kreis B, Fournaud S (1965) Les traitements antituberculeux de très courte durée chez la souris. II. résultats. Ann Inst Pasteur 108:117–121

Kushner S, Dalalian H, Sanjurjo JL, Bach FL Jr, Safir SR, Smith VK Jr, Williams JH (1952) Experimental chemotherapy of tuberculosis. II. The synthesis of pyrazinamide and related compounds. J Am Chem Soc 74:3617–3621

Lucchesi M (1963) Ricerche sperimentali sull'azione antitubercolare della morfazinamide. G Ital Chemioter 10:58–64

Mackaness GB (1956) The intracellular activation of pyrazinamide and nicotinamide. Am Rev Tuberc Pulm Dis 74:718–728

Malone L, Schurr A, Lindh H, McKenzie D, Kiser JS, Williams JH (1952) The effect of pyrazinamide (Aldinamide) on experimental tuberculosis in mice. Am Rev Tuberc 65:511–518

McClatchy J, Tsang AY, Cernich M (1981) Use of pyrazinamidase activity in Mycobacterium tuberculosis as a rapid method for determination of pyrazinamide susceptibility. Antimicrob Agents Chemother 20:556–557

McCune RM Jr, Tompsett R (1956) Fate of Mycobacterium tuberculosis in mouse tissues as determined by the microbial enumeration technique. I. The persistence of drug-susceptible tubercle bacilli in the tissues despite prolonged antimicrobial therapy. J Exp Med 104:737–762

McCune RM Jr, Tompsett R, McDermott W (1956) The fate of Mycobacterium tuberculosis in mouse tissues as determined by the microbial enumeration technique. II. The conversion of tuberculous infection to the latent state by the administration of pyrazinamide and a companion drug. J Exp Med 104:763–802

McDermott W, Tompsett R (1954) Activation of pyrazinamide and nicotinamide in acidic environments in vitro. Am Rev Tuberc 70:748–754

McKenzie D, Malone L, Kushner S, Oleson JJ, SubbaRow Y (1948) The effect of nicotinic acid on experimental tuberculosis of white mice. J Lab Clin Med 33:1249–1253

Mulargia A, Piccaluga A (1964) Contributo sperimentale e clinico sull'attività antitubercolare della morfazinamide. G Pneumol 8:156–166

Novák M, Krátký J, Feitová F (1970) Assessment of the sensitivity and resistance of *M. tuberculosis* to pyrazinamide (in Czech.). Stud pneumol phtiseol cechoslovac 30:22–28

Perry CR, Morse WC (1955) The pyrazinamide susceptibility of isoniazid-resistant mutants of tubercle bacilli. Am Rev Tuberc Pulm Dis 72:840–842

Rist N (1962) Le pyrazinamide. Rev Tuberc Pneumol (Paris) 26:752–754

Rist N (1964) Nature and development of resistance of tubercle bacilli to chemotherapeutic agents. In: Barry VC (ed) Chemotherapy of tuberculosis. Butterworth, London, p 199

Solotorovsky M, Gregory FJ, Ironson EJ, Bugie EJ, O'Neill RC, Pfister K (1952) Pyrazinoic acid amide – an agent active against experimental murine tuberculosis. Proc Soc exp Biol 79:563–569

Soloviev VN, Pavlov EP (1966) Significance of intracellular medium for antimycobacterial activity of some pyrazin-2-carbonic acid derivates. Chemotherapia 11:345–354

Steenken W Jr, Wolinsky E (1954) The antituberculous activity of pyrazinamide in vitro and in the guinea pig. Am Rev Tuberc 70:367–369

Steenken W Jr, Wolinsky E, Smith MM, Montalbine V (1957) Further observations on pyrazinamide alone and in combination with other drugs in experimental tuberculosis. Am Rev Tuberc Pulm Dis 76:643–659

Stottmeier KD, Beam RE, Kubica GP (1967) Determination of drug susceptibility of Mycobacteria to pyrazinamide in 7H10 agar. Am Rev Respir Dis 96:1072–1075

Tarshis MS, Weed WA Jr (1953) Lack of significant in vitro sensitivity of *Mycobacterium tuberculosis* to pyrazinamide on three different solid media. Am Rev Tuberc 67:391–395

Tatar J (1974) Sensitivity of tubercle bacilli to pyrazinamide determined on the basis of their sensitivity to nicotinamide (in Polish). Gruzlica 42:773–777
Tellis CLJ, Putnam JS (1980) Pulmonary disease caused by nontuberculous mycobacteria. Med Clin North Am 64:433–446
Tripathy SP, Mitchison DA, Nair NGK, Radhakrishna S, Subbammal S (1970) A comparison of various measures of sensitivity of *M. tuberculosis* to pyrazinamide. Tubercle 51:375–381
Tripathy SP, Mitchison DA, Nair NGK, Radhakrishna S (1971) A comparison of various measures of sensitivity of *M. tuberculosis* to PZA. Ind J Med Res 59:175–189
Trnka L, Kuška J, Havel A (1964) Comparison of the antituberculous activity of morphazinamide and pyrazinamide on chronic experimental tuberculosis. I. The antimycobacterial efficacy made in vitro and in vivo. Chemotherapia (Basel) 9:158–167
Verbist L (1966) Tuberculostatic activity of N-morpholine-4'methylamide pyrazinecarbonic acid on experimental tuberculosis of mice. Acta Tuberc Pneumol Belg 57:211–217
Wasz-Höckert O, McCune RM Jr, Lee SH, McDermott W, Tompsett R (1956) Resistance of tubercle bacilli to pyrazinamide in vivo. Am Rev Tuberc Pulm Dis 74:572–580
Wayne LG (1974) Simple pyrazinamidase and urea tests for routine identification of mycobacteria. Am Rev Respir Dis 74:147–151
Wolinsky E (1979) "State of the Art": Nontuberculous mycobacteria and associated disease. Am Rev Respir Dis 119:107–159

V. Isoniazid (INH)

K. Bartmann

Since the antimycobacterial activity of INH was detected independently at practically the same time in 3 pharmaceutical companies (Domagk et al. 1952; Grunberg and Schnitzer 1952; Bernstein et al. 1952), the results of many preclinical and clinical studies were already published in 1952. By 1953 Fust was able to review 677 papers, nearly 90 of them dealing with microbiological aspects. In the following years the numbers of publications increased still further, and it is therefore impossible to cover all published work. The present account will accordingly be confined to a selection of what seems to the writer to be most representative and most relevant to clinical application.

1. Antimicrobial Spectrum in Vitro

The antimicrobial activity of INH is restricted to mycobacteria (Grunberg and Schnitzer 1952; Fust et al. 1952; Pansy et al. 1952; Heilmeyer et al. 1952; Lembke et al. 1952; Knox et al. 1952; Rist and Grumbach 1952a; Tison 1952a; Linz and Lecocq 1952; Cattaneo and Morellini 1952; Waksman and Lechevalier 1953).

2. Antimycobacterial Activity

a) Activity in Artificial Media in Vitro – Continuous Exposure

In 22 early investigations the MICs were determined with large variations in the type of the medium, the inoculum size, and the incubation period. Nevertheless, the range of MIC values for *M. tuberculosis* was only between 0.01 µg/ml and 0.25 µg/ml, with a 50th percentile of 0.06 µg/ml and an 80th percentile of 0.1 µg/ml (GRUNBERG and SCHNITZER 1952; FUST 1952; DOMAGK et al. 1952; STEENKEN and WOLINSKY 1952; PANSY et al. 1952; RIST and GRUMBACH 1952a; HEILMEYER et al. 1952; CATTANEO and MORELLINI 1952; BARONI 1952; LUTZ 1952; LINZ and LECOCQ 1952; KNOX et al. 1952; MITCHISON 1952; EIDUS and LANYI 1953; SCHRIEVER and HOFFMANN 1953; DISSMANN and IGLAUER 1953a; BALOGH 1953; WAKSMAN and LECHEVALIER 1953; PANSY et al. 1953; KIMMIG 1953; FUST and BÖHNI 1953; BÜNGER and LASS 1953).

Among the *M. bovis* species there are strains less sensitive to INH than *M. tuberculosis* (KNOX et al. 1952; RIST and GRUMBACH 1952a; CATTANEO and MORELLINI 1952; FUST and BÖHNI 1953; SCHRIEVER and HOFFMANN 1953; MEISSNER 1962). The so-called atypical mycobacteria are more or less resistant (KNOX et al. 1952; LUTZ 1952; KRÜGER-THIEMER et al. 1952; CATTANEO and MORELLINI 1952; LEMBKE et al. 1952) except *M. xenopi* where a part of the strains is moderately sensitive (see Chap. 4).

α) Factors Affecting the Activity in Vitro. The clustering of the MIC values of *M. tuberculosis* in the early papers mentioned indicates that the composition of the media used (liquid: Proskauer and Beck, Kirchner, Youmans, Šula, Dubos with or without albumin and Tween 80; solid: oleic acid albumin agar, egg media according to Löwenstein, Hohn or modified Gottsacker) had little or no influence, as the inoculum size, varied 1:100 (by MITCHISON 1952), and the addition of 10% serum (STEENKEN and WOLINSKY 1952). The most critical factor in the tests in liquid media is incubation time (KNOX et al. 1952; MITCHISON 1952; FUST and BÖHNI 1953). Prolongation of the incubation beyond 2 weeks allows outgrowth of resistant mutants regularly present in sensitive-strain populations (see the section on resistance). On a solid egg medium, however, the MIC does not change for sensitive strains if the incubation period is extended from 3 weeks to 10 weeks; only for INH-resistant strains does the MIC increase with the passage of time (BARTMANN et al. 1966).

In aqueous solutions at 37 °C the antimycobacterial activity of INH remains unchanged for at least 1 week (KNOX et al. 1952; PANSY et al. 1953). In liquid Dubos medium no activity is lost for several weeks at 4 °C, though at 37 °C INH becomes inactivated with a half-life of about a week (GOULDING et al. 1952; MITCHISON 1952; KNOX et al. 1952). This loss of activity, ascribed to ferric ions at alkaline pH by PANSY et al. (1953), may contribute to the increase in the MICs observed on prolonged incubation in liquid media. In Löwenstein-Jensen egg medium too the activity of incorporated INH decreases at 37 °C within 4 weeks, but at 4 °C it remains unchanged for several months (COLWELL and HESS 1957; WALLACE 1964). Tubes with drug-containing media can be stored for sensitivity testing at 4 °C for up to 2 months (CANETTI et al. 1969). The stable MIC obtained with a Löwenstein-Jensen medium on prolonged incubation can be explained by the type of action of INH, its killing of proliferating bacilli within the first week of contact (see below).

INH in media is fairly stable to heat. To produce a slight loss a Dubos medium has to be autoclaved for 30 min (MITCHISON 1952).

The MIC is virtually unaffected by pH in the range between 5 to 8 (MITCHISON 1952; MCDERMOTT and TOMPSETT 1954). This is also true for the growth-dependent bactericidal activity of INH, tested at pH values between 6.6 and 5.4 (DICKINSON and MITCHISON 1981).

The in-vitro experiments on INH derivatives, predominantly hydrazones, strongly suggest that their inhibitory activity is due to their INH content (KOCH-WESER and EBERT 1955; COLWELL and HESS 1956; ORLOWSKI et al. 1976).

The publications on INH-antagonizing substances have been reviewed by BARTMANN (1963), YOUATT (1969), and KRÜGER-THIEMER et al. (1975). For details the reader is referred to these reviews. Suffice it to say here that these substances can be divided into the following groups:

1. Nicotinic acid hydrazide may displace INH in the oxidation by peroxidase, and its oxidation product, nicotinic acid, may in turn prevent isonicotinic acid from incorporation into NAD.
2. All other carboxylic acid hydrazides are able to displace INH in the oxidation by peroxidase.
3. Acetone, pyridoxal, and pyruvic and α-ketoglutaric acids may form hydrazones with INH which cannot be attacked by peroxidase but which hydrolyse readily following a change in the INH concentration.
4. O_2 and H_2O_2 outside the bacterial cell are able to oxidize INH to isonicotonic acid in the presence of catalysts like heavy metal ions, heminchloride, peroxidase, and perhaps catalase. Manganese dioxide and potassium ferricyanide do so in the absence of aerial oxygen.
5. All substances that can destroy H_2O_2 in culture media reduce the damaging effect of INH. To this class belong some substances of groups 3 and 4, like pyruvic acid, α-ketoglutaric acid, catalase, peroxidase, heminchloride, and cobaltphthalocyanine.
6. Substances with other or unknown action mechanism: active charcoal, condensed milk, tyrosine (HERMAN and WEBER 1980), Youmans anti-isoniazid substance, and extracts of tuberculous tissue (URBANČÍK and TRNKA 1962).

In 1955, Youmans and Youmans reported that filtrates and extracts from the cultures of various mycobacteria could inactivate or destroy INH in vitro. In 1956 they found that filtrates and extracts were able to antagonize INH appreciably when administered parenterally to infected, INH-treated mice. Later the authors extended their experiments to a larger group of strains and observed that unclassified mycobacteria and INH-susceptible strains of *M. tuberculosis* produced more anti-isoniazid than INH-resistant *M. tuberculosis* strains (YOUMANS and YOUMANS 1960). Their in-vitro data have been confirmed by KUBALA (1960) and by KRAUS et al. (1961). The chemical nature of the substance or substances is still unknown.

URBANČÍK and TRNKA (1962) prepared a filtrate from murine lung homogenate of tuberculous mice. Exposure to this cell-free filtrate for 180 min made tubercle bacilli, when tested after several washings in a medium with INH, less sensitive to the drug than a control. A single subculture of the exposed bacteria resulted in a complete recovery of sensitivity. No clear-cut difference in INH activity could be found in mice between animals infected with exposed and with unexposed tubercle bacilli.

The MIC of wild strains of *M. tuberculosis* on Löwenstein-Jensen media inoculated with about 10^4 colony-forming units has been found to be 0.05 μg/ml INH in many laboratories, without any geographic variation, taking as the end-point either 20 colonies (when using the absolute concentration method) or 1% of the control tubes (when using the proportion method). 0.2 μg/ml INH has been accepted as the critical concentration at which growth indicates resistance, and 1% of the inoculum has been defined as growth, i.e., as the critical proportion (CANETTI et al. 1969).

β) Resistance

Clinical Criteria and Development of Resistance: The quantitative studies carried out by TOMPSETT (1954) on the pattern of emergence of INH resistance revealed quite different types of resistance development in patients treated in monotherapy. In some cases high degrees of resistance of the majority of bacilli were observed very early in the course of therapy. In other patients the proportion of resistant bacilli and also the degree of resistance increased in steps, and in a third subgroup both the proportion of resistant bacilli and the degree of resistance reached a plateau.

Despite this diverse behavior of the bacilli, all studies correlating the results of treatment with the initial sensitivity of the bacilli have shown that even low degrees of resistance – to 0.2 μg/ml–1 μg/ml INH – involve an elevated risk of therapeutic failure, even in the event of combined therapy (DEVADATTA et al. 1961; RAMAKRISHNAN et al. 1962; JANČIK 1963; EAST AFRICAN/BRITISH MEDICAL RESEARCH COUNCIL PRETREATMENT DRUG RESISTANCE REPORT 1963; STEWART and CROFTON 1964; TRIPATHY et al. 1969; CHAULET et al. 1976). Thus, the clinical criteria of bacterial resistance are very close to the biological criteria on the basis of the frequency distribution of the MICs for wild strains. MITCHISON (1962) calculated an MIC of 0.23 μg/ml INH for the 1% confidence limits. In studies where, for technical reasons, the MIC for wild strains was found to be lower, the clinically relevant MIC was also correspondingly lower (AUERSBACH et al. 1961). This clinical experience corresponds closely to the results of INH treatment of experimental animals infected with bacteria exhibiting various degrees of INH-resistance. The data of GOULDING et al. (1952), BARNETT et al. (1953a; b), MITCHISON (1954), and FREERKSEN et al. (1969) can be summarized by saying that the efficacy even of high doses – up to 20 mg/kg/day or 75 mg/kg/day – is reduced if the bacilli are completely resistant to 0.1 μg/ml INH or partly resistant to 1 μg/ml. FREERKSEN et al. (1969) have observed that the addition of INH to two other fully effective drugs prolonged the survival of animals infected with INH-resistant bacilli.

The proportion of resistant variants in wild strain populations growing at 0.1 μg/ml–0.2 μg/ml INH is of the order of 10^{-3} and that of variants growing at 1 μg/ml of the order of 10^{-5} to 10^{-7} (AUERSBACH et al. 1961; KREBS 1975).

Serial transfer in media with increasing INH concentrations selects more or less rapidly resistant bacterial populations. As in patients the rate and the degree of resistance development may vary between strains of *M. tuberculosis* (LECOCQ 1952; HOBBY et al. 1953; LIEBERMEISTER 1953; BARNETT et al. 1953a). After investigating more than 50 wild strains RIST (1964) states that, in general, wild strains contain single-step mutants highly resistant to INH. The maximal resistance found among single-step mutants was to 50 µg/ml of INH. HOBBY and LENERT (1952) observed variants resistant to 100 µg/ml as did RIST and GRUMBACH (1952b).

As can be seen from Table 1, acquired resistance to INH develops rapidly in patients with pulmonary tuberculosis treated with INH alone.

The frequency of initial resistance differs in time and according to the geographic area, reflecting the quality of antituberculosis chemotherapy. The latest worldwide data collected by KLEEBERG and OLIVIER (1984), are shown in Table 2.

Features of Resistant Populations: The regularly observed biological and biochemical alterations correlating with the degree of INH resistance have been reviewed by MEISSNER (1956) and by KREIS (1958).

In stored cultures the INH-resistant subpopulation does not as a rule survive as long as the sensitive fraction (BARNETT et al. 1953a, b; DISSMANN 1954; MEISSNER 1956). It is common bacteriological experience that mixed bacterial populations tend to become more sensitive to INH on storage. The initial lag phase in fluid culture media may be prolonged (DISSMANN 1954). The metabolism of some resistant strains of *M. tuberculosis* becomes similar to that of *M. bovis*. They grow dysgonically on glycerol-containing egg media, are intolerant to glycerol (KREBS and KÄPPLER 1956), prefer pyruvate as the source of carbon, and grow better at lower O_2 and higher CO_2 partial pressures. Pyruvate media have been found especially useful for the isolation of INH-resistant *M. tuberculosis* (STONEBRINK 1958; GERLOFF 1960). The growth requirements for many special substances have been studied using synthetic basal media for the cultures. Most of these requirements are obviously related to the higher sensitivity of INH-resistant bacilli to hydrogen peroxide. Low virulence – the first aberration of INH-resistant strains noted (STEENKEN and WOLINSKY 1953; BARNETT et al. 1953b) – is associated with sensitivity to H_2O_2 in native and isoniazid-resistant strains, but not in the laboratory-attenuated strain H37Ra, and is only partly related to the catalase content (JACKETT et al. 1978). The activity of peroxidase is lost earlier, and more regularly, than the activity of catalase (ANDREJEW and TACQUET 1957; TIRUNARAYAN and VISCHER 1957; HEDGECOCK and FAUCHER 1957; DUNBAR et al. 1959). The reduced virulence of INH-resistant strains, correlating with the degree of resistance and to a smaller extent with catalase activity, has been widely confirmed and was encountered in various animal species (see MEISSNER 1956), including monkeys (SCHMIDT et al. 1958). The observations in man are not conclusive; some speak for and some against a reduced virulence in man (MEISSNER 1956; KREIS 1958; CANETTI 1965; KESSLER and BARTMANN 1971). Many clinical studies aimed at making the bacilli highly resistant in chronic cases by further treatment with INH, in the hope of achieving a cure because of reduced virulence. All these efforts were unsuccessful – see, for example, BERNARD et al. (1957), SIMON (1958), ECKLEY and WILSON (1960), RAMAKRISHNAN et al. (1962), and WERNER et al. (1963). Some authors (DOMAGK 1953; BARRY et al. 1954; BRIGGS et al. 1968) have reported an increase in TSC sensitivity of INH resistant strains, a fact not observed in patient strains from Germany (BARTMANN 1960a).

Table 1. Development of secondary bacterial resistance to INH during monotherapy of pulmonary tuberculosis with INH

Authors	Year of publ.	Type of disease	Number of cult[a] tested	Number of pat. treated	INH daily dose	Critical concn.[b] (mg/l)	% of pos. cultures res. after months 2–3	4–5	6–8	9–12	% of patients treated with res. bacilli after months of therapy 2–3	4–5	6–8	9–12
Br Med Res Council	1952	Mixed	173		200 mg	0.2	45.9							
Br Med Res Council	1952	Mixed	189		200 mg	0.2	54.5							
Coates et al.	1953	Predom. cavernous		42	4 mg/kg	0.2		63				79		
Claus	1953	Mixed		181	5–8 mg/kg	0.1			53.5				22.6	
Lotte and Poussier	1953	Mixed	32		5 mg/kg	0.1	94							
USPHS Coop Invest	1953	Mixed	28		150 mg–300 mg	0.1	89	94	100		47	60	49	
Schwartz and Moyer	1954	Chronic, pretreated	59		150 mg	0.2	51	73	93		32	43	72	
Meissner and Berg	1954	Mixed		883	Not stated	0.1	64	87	92	100				
Tompsett	1954	Difficult to treat	37			0.1	83		71	100				
Jenney and Landis	1954	Mixed	26	29	150 mg				65				59	
		Mixed	21	35	300 mg				95				57	
Chemotherapy Centre, Madras	1960	Mixed	27		1 × 400 mg	0.2	78		100	100	30		28	26
			28		2 × 200 mg	0.2	79		100	100	33		37	38
			48		2 × 100 mg	0.2	75		97	100	43		51	54
East African – BMRC Isoniazid Invest.	1960	Recent	30		200 mg	0.2	83		100	100	66		61	64
			22		20 mg/kg	0.2	73		100	100	46		47	55
Chicou et al.	1961	Recent	10		400 mg	0.1		100				50		
Le Hir et al.	1964	Prob. mixed	29			0.1		93	96			66	68	

[a] Number of results available at the first term of investigation.
[b] Growth at critical concentration indicates resistance.

Table 2. Initial resistance to INH and SM according to KLEEBERG and OLIVIER (1984). Latest data.

	Percentage of initial resistance (range)		
	INH	SM	INH+SM
Africa	2 –24.9	<1 –20	1.3–23
America North and Central	1.8–15.1	1.8–13.9	0.2– 2.2
South	1.5–32.6	3.5–43.3	1.4–17.4
Asia	9.4–27	4.7–20.6	0.3–10.1
Europe	<1 –10.2	<1 –12.8	<1 – 2.6

INH-Dependence: No reports are known on INH-dependent mycobacteria.

Cross-Resistance: There is no cross-resistance between INH and other antituberculotics with a different chemical structure. Low degrees of INH resistance are associated with an increased resistance to other acid hydrazides (KRÜGER-THIEMER et al. 1975). In a substrain of H37Rv with a very high INH resistance KAKIMOTO et al. (1961) observed a reduced sensitivity to ETH. However, INH-resistant patient strains are normally ETH-sensitive.

γ) *Type of Action*

The Effect on Resting Bacteria: Concentrations of up to 100 µg/ml or more at the most slightly reduce O_2 consumption or the activity of transhydrogenases during an incubation period of several hours (ARONSON et al. 1952; KIMMIG 1953; WAGNER and SAAR 1953; KOCH-WESER 1956).

The technical difficulties in excluding rigorously all possibilities of multiplication have been discussed by BARTMANN (1960b). It is therefore difficult to say whether INH reduces the viable count of really resting bacilli within 1 week or 2 weeks. In any event, the decrease in viable counts was small if the bacilli were tested at 37 °C suspended in water (FUST et al. 1952), in a phosphate buffer (HOBBY and LENERT 1957), in a synthetic medium without a major carbon source (SCHAEFER 1954), in a complete medium under anaerobic conditions or with addition of INH to bacilli in the stationary phase (MITCHISON and SELKON 1956), in a phosphate buffer at 22 °C (HOBBY and LENERT 1957), or in a complete medium at 8 °C (DICKINSON and MITCHISON 1981). HOBBY and LENERT (1957) have also shown that the killing kinetics of proliferating tubercle bacilli in INH-containing media slows down the more the generation time of the bacilli increases after the phase of exponential growth has been passed.

BARTMANN (1960b) incubated 3 strains in dialysed albumin fraction V for up to 4 months at 37 °C or in non-dialysed albumin fraction V at room temperature (20 °C–25 °C) in the dark for up to 6 months. INH or SM were added at final concentrations of respectively 1 µg/ml and 10 µg/ml. The drugs were renewed several times and their concentrations checked. The bacilli remained completely sensitive to both drugs. At the end of the investigation the viable counts of the INH-exposed bacilli amounted to about 10% of the control and to about 0.1% with

SM. From these experiments it can be concluded that INH damages resting bacilli irreversibly, provided the bacilli are exposed to the drug for a long time. The necessary concentration can be achieved in the tuberculosis lesions in man (BARTMANN and FREISE 1963).

Effect on Proliferating Bacteria on Continuous and Intermittent Exposure: The influence of initially added INH on the viable count in liquid media allowing fairly homogenous growth has been studied by many authors and with remarkably uniform results. At a concentration of 1 µg/ml–2 µg INH/ml the viable count falls to about 1% after 3 days–4 days of incubation at 37 °C and, on average, to 0.1% after 7 days (MACKANESS and SMITH 1953; HOBBY et al. 1953; SINGH and MITCHISON 1954; SCHAEFER 1954; MITCHISON and SELKON 1956; HOBBY and LENERT 1957; BARTMANN 1960b, 1963; DICKINSON and MITCHISON 1966, 1976, 1981; DICKINSON et al. 1977). The number of culturable units may be reduced to a few percent after only 24 h of incubation (MIDDLEBROOK 1952; LINZ 1952; TISON 1952b; DICKINSON and MITCHISON 1966), but sometimes the count begins to fall only after 1 day–2 days (MACKANESS and SMITH 1953; WAGNER and SAAR 1953; SINGH and MITCHISON 1954). DICKINSON and MITCHISON (1981) compared the killing activity of INH and RMP under various conditions. The results were the same for both drugs if a uniform slowing down of the growth rate had been produced. However, if the cultures were held dormant at 8 °C and then allowed to metabolize briefly by increasing the temperature for 1 h or 6 h per day, RMP appeared to be considerably more bactericidal than INH. These experiments show also the delay in the killing effect INH. It was observed by MIDDLEBROOK (1952) and by RIST et al. (1952), and later confirmed by KOCH-WESER et al. (1955) and by DUNBAR (1957) that proliferating bacilli exposed to INH rapidly lose their acid-fastness. The morphological changes observable by scanning electron microcopy have been described by TAKAYAMA et al. (1973). Eventually the cells fragmented and coalesced into an amorphous mass. Using a slide culture technique, DISSMANN and IGLAUER (1953b) have shown that the MIC of INH (0.06 µg/ml) already kills 98% of the bacterial populations; 4 µg/ml is not more effective than 1 µg/ml. Many of the papers cited above report a remarkable reduction in viable counts at low INH concentrations (0.1 µg/ml or 0.2 µg/ml). The fact that concentrations above 1 µg/ml have no higher killing activity on continuous exposure has also been found by other authors: WAGNER and SAAR (1953) compared 1 µg/ml and 10 µg/ml and BARTMANN (1963) 1 µg/ml, 10 µg/ml, and 100 µg/ml.

Thus, the survival kinetics display the same pattern as has been observed with penicillin for rapidly growing gram-positives: the killing effect is growth-dependent and, above a certain optimal concentration, concentration-independent. It could be expected, by analogy, that a time-limited exposure, as in the case of penicillin, will be sufficient to produce a delay before growth restarts after removal of the drug, and this has indeed been observed by BEKIERKUNST and SZULGA (1954) and by DICKINSON and MITCHISON (1966). In the experiments of the last-mentioned authors an exposure of the H37Rv strain to 1 µg/ml INH in a liquid medium for 24 h produced a growth delay of 2.5 days to 6.9 days, and an exposure for 96 h a delay of 6.2 days to 19 days. Exposure periods from 2 h to 12 h did not cause any retardation of the lag phase.

It is this delay in the resumption of multiplication that forms the basis for intermittent treatment with INH. Pulsed exposure to INH in vitro has been studied by several authors using different techniques (BOURGEOIS et al. 1958; ARMSTRONG 1960, 1965; GANGADHARAM et al. 1963; DICKINSON and MITCHISON 1966; KREBS 1968; BEGGS and JENNE 1969; AWANESS and MITCHISON 1973). The results concerning the relationships between the time-concentration product and the bacteriostatic, bactericidal, and multiplication-delaying effect are not uniform. As has been suggested by AWANESS and MITCHISON (1973), this may be due to differences in the physiological state of the organisms exposed to the pulses. In any event, the data taken together show that an exposure for a few hours to concentrations attainable in man is sufficient to produce a bactericidal effect and a marked delay in the resumption of multiplication, at least if the exposures are repeated several times. In some experiments even a single exposure was in fact sufficient to elicit these phenomena.

It has been asked whether the bacilli that are made non-culturable by INH are merely in a latent state or genuinely dead in the sense that both multiplication and metabolism have been irreversibly damaged. Many procedures and substances have been tried for their revival, and have been described in detail by BARTMANN (1960c, 1963). Suffice it to say at this point that all efforts have been unsuccessful. Substances able to bind INH chemically, or physically to destroy the drug or to destroy hydrogen peroxide have been added to various protein-containing media without any success. Likewise, the many attempts to obtain growth of bacilli from sputum or tissue specimens which were positive on microscopy but negative in standard cultures ended in failure: washing of homogenates, addition of detoxifying substances, incubation for up to 2 years under various atmospheres, biphasic cultures, inoculation into normal or silicotic or cortisone-treated guinea pigs.

The question of the type of action exerted by INH on tubercle bacilli in experimental animals has been dealt with by BARTMANN (1960c). The leading idea was to alter the balance between the host and the bacillus and to follow the consequences in INH-treated infected animals by viable counts from organs. It was shown that alteration of the balance had no influence on the reduction in viable counts. The number of culturable bacilli falls off during immediate treatment in the guinea pig, which is highly sensitive to infection, as in the resistant mouse, and in the mouse to the same extent for virulent and non-virulent strains, in non-immunized animals as in immunized ones. The bactericidal activity of INH in mice also depends on their multiplication rate (Fig. 1). If the mice are infected with hypovirulent bacilli the organisms multiply for about 2 weeks, after which the number of culturable bacilli begins to fall slowly on account of infection immunity. If INH treatment is started immediately at the time of the infection, the viable count will be reduced markedly; if the treatment is started after 14 days, the decrease is minimal despite the fact that the tissues are histologically unchanged. These results show clearly that the reduction in the viable count that is found in the tissues of INH-treated animals is due largely to the killing effect of the drug on multiplying bacteria and not to the host's defense mechanisms acting on bacteria held in stasis by the drug. Similar results have been obtained by KONDO and KANAI (1977a), who used mice infected with an SM-dependent strain, whose multiplication in organs was regulated by giving or omitting SM besides INH. In their

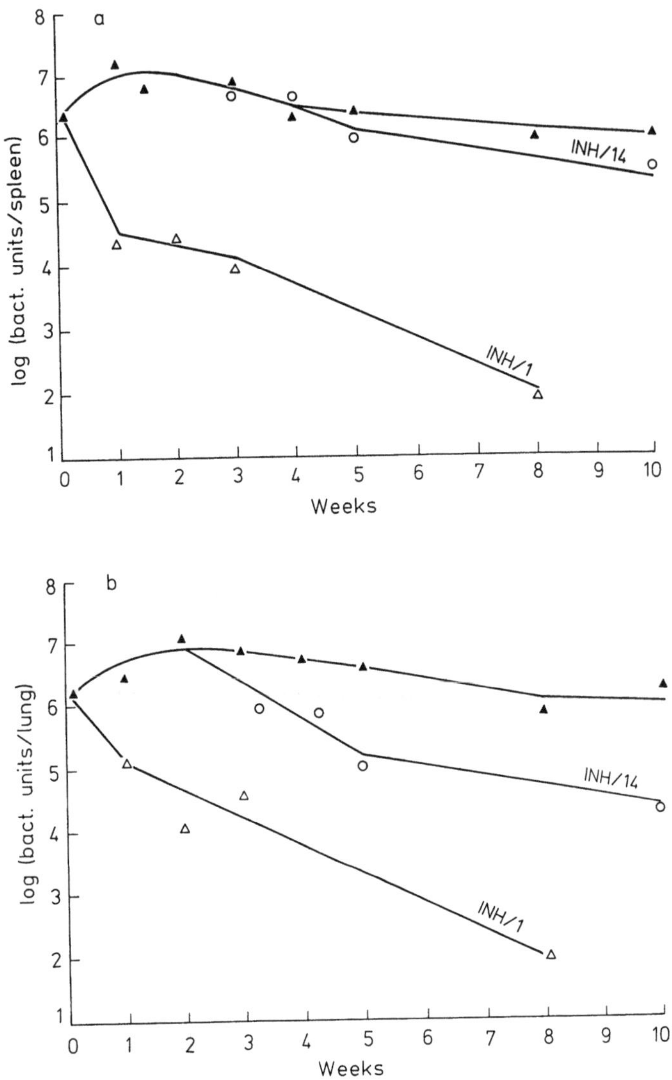

Fig. 1 a, b. Reduction in the bacterial counts in the spleen (**a**) and lungs (**b**) in infections with hypovirulent tubercle bacilli, strain H37Ra. ▲–▲ controls; △–△ INH/1 (therapy started 1 day after infection); ○–○, INH/14 (ditto 14 days after infection). 5 animals were used together for each point plotted. (After BARTMANN 1960c)

second paper (1977b), KONDO and KANAI reported that INH was less effective in previously immunized mice, in which the multiplication of the challenge strain was reduced; INH was also less effective when the infecting bacilli had been preexposed in vitro to a low concentration of SM, and it was remarkably bactericidal despite accelerated multiplication due to administration of cortisone. This last observation confirms the findings of BATTEN and MCCUNE (1957). Thus, the type of action is the same in vivo as in vitro.

δ) Effects in Combination with Antituberculotis Drugs in Vitro. Various media and various principles of mixing the drugs (using one or both substances in constant or varied concentrations) have been used. In most experiments only the inhibitory concentrations were determined, in a few the killing kinetics.

INH and PAS: Synergism with regard to the MIC has been observed by MORELLI and DADDI (1952), AITOFF (1952), and by EIDUS and LÁNYI (1953), only additive effects by COLETSOS (1952) and by BARTMANN (1954). The bactericidal activity of 2 μg INH/ml + 100 μg PAS/ml was slightly synergistic in the experiments reported by SINGH and MITCHISON (1955). Emergence of resistance was prevented. Suppression of secondary resistance by combining INH with PAS was also reported by RIST and GRUMBACH (1952 b).

INH and TSC: BARTMANN (1954) determined the MICs for 3 strains by the checkerboard technique. For the first strain the combination was synergistic over the whole range of concentrations tested, for the second strain antagonistic, and for the third strain partially synergistic and partially antagonistic. BARRY et al. (1954) could restrain the outgrowth of INH resistant variants in INH containing medium by addition of 1 or 10 μg/ml TSC.

INH and SM: Bacteriostatic synergism has been found for this combination by MORELLI and DADDI (1952), ILAVSKY (1952), and AITOFF and SALAS (1952). Slight antagonism has been reported by PANSY et al. (1952), COLETSOS (1952), EIDUS and LÁNYI (1953), and BARTMANN (1954). Additivity was reported by HOBBY et al. (1953). In contrast to the different results obtained with regard to bacteriostasis, all the investigators observed synergism with regard to bactericidal effects (MACKANESS and SMITH 1953; SINGH and MITCHISON 1954, 1955; BARTMANN 1963; DICKINSON et al. 1977). By combining INH with SM the development of resistance is suppressed (RIST and GRUMBACH 1952 b; COHN et al. 1959) or at least delayed (HOBBY et al. 1953). RIST and GRUMBACH (1952 b) observed that tubercle bacilli exposed to INH + SM under growth conditions remain acid-fast.

INH and PZA: Tests at pH 5.6 causing a lowered growth rate without drugs, showed the occurrence of antagonism (DICKINSON et al. 1977).

b) Effects of INH in Cell and Tissue Cultures

The MIC of INH for intracellulary located tubercle bacilli is practically the same as for extracellular bacilli in artificial media (SUTER 1952; MACKANESS and SMITH 1952; SHEPARD 1957; PAVLOV 1970; STOICA and NITZULESCO 1971). INH at a concentration of 1 μg/ml kills the intracellular bacilli, whereas 10 μg SM/ml exerts only a static effect (MACKANESS and SMITH 1953). The combinations of INH + SM (MACKANESS and SMITH 1953) and of INH + PZA (MACKANESS 1956) had a higher killing activity than any of these drugs alone.

c) Effects of INH in Embryonated Eggs

This technique was used by KLOSE and KNOTHE (1952). INH injected at a dose of 25 μg together with 0.02 mg tubercle bacilli prevented the development of tuberculosis of the chorioallantois.

d) Activity of INH in Experimental Tuberculosis and Development of Resistance in Vivo

Here INH is considered mainly with regard to its therapeutic efficacy in experimentally infected animals. Chemoprophylaxis with INH and treatment of naturally infected animals is dealt with in Chap. 3 by KLEEBERG and in his paper, published in 1967 (KLEEBERG 1967). There is some overlap between prophylactic and therapeutic aspects in experiments aiming at the prevention of spread of the disease. Some of these investigations are therefore considered in both chapters.

α) Dose-Response Relationship of INH with Continuous Administration. This topic will be discussed first, because it provides information useful for the evaluation of the curative experiments.

In the following species daily doses of 50 mg/kg–100 mg/kg are no more active than 10 mg/kg:

monkey	(SCHMIDT 1956a, 1959; SCHMIDT et al. 1963)
rabbit	(FREERKSEN 1957)
guinea pig	(FUST et al. 1952; DOMAGK et al. 1952; KARLSON and FELDMAN 1953; HOBBY et al. 1953; VELTMAN 1955; FEREBEE and PALMER 1956; NASTA et al. 1957; SPIESS 1959; BARTMANN 1959; BARTMANN and BLISSE 1967). Depending on the experimental design, even 2.5 mg/kg–3 mg/kg may be equivalent to 10 mg/kg.

In mice, some investigators found doses up to 100 mg/kg to be no more effective than 10 mg/kg (FUST et al. 1952; GRUNBERG and SCHNITZER 1952; MCCUNE et al. 1957; BARTMANN 1960d) while other investigators reported an increase in efficacy with increasing doses [up to 100 mg/kg on parenteral administration (NOUFFLARD and BERTEAUX 1960); up to 250 mg/kg on a medicated diet (GRUNBERG and SCHNITZER 1952; NOUFFLARD 1954)]. The differences might be due to differences in the experimental design. With the most specific technique, i.e. quantative culture of organs, no increase in efficacy has been observed with doses exceeding 10 mg/kg (MCCUNE et al. 1957; BARTMANN 1960d).

The rat acetylates INH very rapidly and therefore requires a therapeutic dose higher than 10 mg/kg (GRUMBACH et al. 1960).

Within the range of well effective doses, the therapeutic differences between the same daily dose given orally or parenterally, in single or divided doses, in the diet, or in the drinking water are very small and slightly in favor of a daily dose given all at once (BARTMANN 1959, 1960d; GENAZZANI et al. 1966; BJERKEDAL and PALMER 1967).

Comparative determinations of INH concentrations in animal and human serum and tissues carried out by BARTMANN and FREISE (1963), have shown that the optimal effective dose of 10 mg/kg in animals corresponds to a dose of 5 mg/kg in man.

INH definitely eradicates a minimal infection in 2 months–3 months when given prophylactically. For an established infection the situation is quite different. Here too the therapeutic action sets in immediately. The viable count in the organs fell markedly within the first few days in mice (MCCUNE and TOMPSETT

1956; many other investigations, see also Fig. 1) and in guinea pigs (MITCHISON and SELKON 1956; NITTI and NINNI 1969). The first change in the histological picture of murine lungs due to the treatment was detectable after 5 days (MAYER and SALAMANDRA 1967; MAUSS 1968). The spread of corneal tuberculosis stopped immediately in mice (ROBSON and SULLIVAN 1959) and in rabbits (GOULDING and ROBSON 1952). Recovery proceeds during the next weeks and months. This can be judged continuously on skin ulcers (URBANCIK and TRNKA 1963), abscesses and regional lymph nodes (BARTMANN et al. 1958), eye lesions (GOULDING and ROBSON 1952; ROBSON and SULLIVAN 1959), and by X-ray clearing of pulmonary lesions in rabbits (GERNEZ-RIEUX et al. 1952/53; 1953/54 and in monkeys (SCHMIDT 1956a, b; SCHMIDT et al. 1963). Histological examinations carried out after various treatment periods in mice (STUDER and FUST 1952; Vischer and ROULET 1963), guinea pigs (FINKELDEY 1952), and monkeys (SCHMIDT 1956a) correspond well to the continual observation of signs and symptoms. The dissemination of an established primary infection into organs is nearly completely prevented (UEHLINGER et al. 1952; FINKELDEY 1952; BARON 1952; BARTMANN et al. 1955, 1956). The viable counts fall slower after the first 2 or 3 weeks, as shown in mice and in guinea pigs. From the second to the third month the number of culturable bacilli stabilizes more or less at a low level and may finally rise again. The evaluation of treatment becomes difficult, because now secondary bacterial resistance comes into play.

This has been observed in mice by MCCUNE and TOMPSETT (1956), BARTMANN (1960), CANETTI et al. (1960), VISCHER and ROULET (1963), GRUMBACH (1965), and KRADOLFER (1970), in rabbits by FREERKSEN (1957), and in monkeys by SCHMIDT (1956a). The speed and the degree of the development of resistance depend on the size of the bacterial population at the start of the treatment and also on the dosage. The larger the population, and the higher the dosage, the earlier does the resistance become manifest and the higher is the level it reaches (CANETTI et al. 1960). Since INH treatment is ineffective or insufficient in infections with INH-resistant tubercle bacilli as reported above, failure of further treatment after the emergence of secondary resistance in an originally sensitive bacterial population is easy to understand. But there are also well documented cases of relapses with sensitive bacilli after INH treatment for 1 year in rabbits (FREERKSEN 1957) and in monkeys (SCHMIDT 1956a). It could be that in some of these relapsed animals the isolated sensitive bacilli were reverters from INH resistance to sensitivity, since SCHMIDT et al. (1958) have demonstrated that INH-sensitive bacilli can be isolated from the organs of monkeys infected with a purified, homogenously INH-resistant culture which must therefore have arisen by back mutation. VELTMAN (1955) was able to isolate INH-sensitive bacilli from histologically normal organs of guinea pigs after termination of treatment lasting 5 months.

It emerges from the above picture of the situation that there is no clear relationship between the duration of treatment and efficacy. Depending on the experimental model, secondary resistance to INH interferes from the second month onwards with increasing frequency. On the other hand, the phenomenon of persisting bacilli which are not genetically resistant but refractory to killing because of their more or less resting metabolism makes their eradication irregular even after treatment for a period of 1 year. As Table IV in BARTMANN (1960c) shows, there is a certain correlation between the duration of treatment and the proportion of protected or cured animals if many experiments are evaluated. For therapeutic experiments with treatment periods ranging from 9.5 weeks to 17 weeks (n=6) the median level of success is 41.5%, and for treatment periods from 20 weeks to 64 weeks (n=9) the median is 72.5%. Since the percentage of animals carrying resistant bacilli increases with increasing time, while the chances of eradication decrease, the increasing proportion of cured animals with time can be interpreted as showing that killing of sensitive bacilli prevails over the emergence of resistant ones. Whether this balance can be changed in favor of eradication by combined treatment will be discussed below.

β) Efficacy of INH in Special Animal Models. Ocular infections producing keratitis and iriditis have been studied in mice (GOULDING and ROBSON 1952; ROBSON and SULLIVAN 1959; ROBSON et al. 1960) and in rabbits (GOULDING and ROBSON 1952; LEPRI and CAPALBI 1952; ZINTZ and WEGNER 1953). The mouse model studied by ROBSON's group is a self-limiting disease. Multiplication of the bacilli is much lower than in internal organs, and the increases in lesions cease after a 2 weeks, probably as a result of immunity processes. The lesions then stabilize in size and the number of viable bacteria falls off dramatically. Thus, the model is not well suited to demonstrating the capabilities of a growth-dependent bactericidal drug. The only clear effects of INH that could be demonstrated were the prevention of bacterial multiplication in the eye when treatment was started immediately and the prevention of systemic spread. Contrary to the natural course of corneal disease in mice, in rabbits the infection is progressive not only with *M. bovis,* but locally also with *M. tuberculosis*. Immediate treatment of an acute infection for 8 weeks to 15 weeks with 5 mg/kg–15 mg/kg suppressed the development of the disease without relapses (GOULDING and ROBSON 1952) or with relapses (ZINTZ and WEGNER 1953) after the end of treatment. GOULDING and ROBSON found INH to be clearly superior to 100 mg SM/kg/day. According to their preliminary report, LEPRI and CAPALBI (1952) were likewise able to suppress the infection. They considered the efficacy of INH superior to that of PAS, SM, and TSC. Established disease was treated by GOULDING and ROBSON (1952) for 8 weeks with 10 mg/kg/d with rapid clinical improvement and no relapse within an 8 weeks' post treatment period, and by ZINTZ and WEGNER (1953), using 5 mg/kg/d–15 mg/kd/d for 100 days. The lesions had healed clinically 4 weeks–13 weeks after start of treatment. Within 6 months after the end of treatment relapse was observed in 5 of 10 animals.

Intracerebral infection of guinea pigs was used by LEVADITI et al. (1953) and by WOLINSKY et al. (1954). When treatment started up to 8 days after infection all animals could be saved during treatment (up to 6 months). Begin of treatment 16 days after infection could protect 4 of 6 guinea pigs, but in the post-treatment period all animals died from tuberculosis independent of the day of starting therapy (WOLINSKY et al. 1954). TAKAHASHI (1959), too, was unable to cure the animals by INH or SM, or a combination of both. FUST et al. (1952) stated shortly that rabbits with manifest meningitis could not be saved with 10 mg/kg INH.

SUGIMOTO (1970) produced a silicotuberculosis or talcotuberculosis in guinea pigs, which were then treated from the day of infection with INH, 2 mg per animal or SM, 10 mg per animal. INH was superior to SM but less effective than in animals with simple tuberculosis. These results were confirmed by FUJISAWA (1972), who also started treatment at an advanced stage of disease. In this case INH was much less effective.

γ) Efficacy of INH Derivatives. Animal studies have been published on glucuronic acid derivatives of isonicotinoylhydrazone, the glucuronic acid lactone (INH-G) Gluronazid®, Gatalone®, and INH sodium glucuronide. CROWLE (1958) treated mice for 7 or 9 days, beginning 5 days after the infection with equimolar doses. Using the lung density technique he concluded that INH-G was equi-effective with INH, that glucurolactone alone was in-effective, and that therefore the activity of INH-G was due to its INH content. The results were the same with enteral and parenteral administration. ORLOWSKI et al. (1976) treated intravenously infected rabbits for 70 days with equimolar doses of INH and both derivatives. On the basis of the survival curves, the derivatives and INH had equal activity.

δ) Concurrent Administration of Isoniazid and Pyridoxine. In man pyridoxine has been used successfully for the prevention or cure of peripheral neuritis and disturbances of the central nervous system due to high doses of INH (ZIERSKI and ROTERMUND 1984). As antagonism between pyridoxine/pyridoxal and INH has been observed in vitro (e.g., by POPE 1953, 1956) the question arose whether in vivo the therapeutic effect of INH would be reduced by concurrent administration of vitamin B_6 products. Animal experiments in guinea pigs (BRUN et al. 1954) and in mice (UNGAR et al. 1954; GRUNBERG and BLENCOWE 1955; WASZ-HÖCKERT et al. 1956) showed that even very high doses of pyridoxine did not produce a manifest antagonism.

ε) INH in Combined Therapy. As it gradually became evident that the efficacy of INH monotherapy was limited by the development of secondary resistance and by the persistence of sensitive bacilli, two questions received increasing interest: 1) Could combination of INH with other antituberculotics prevent or retard the development of drug resistance and 2) would combined treatment increase the bactericidal effect?

GRUMBACH's model of advanced murine tuberculosis was found to be particularly well suited to the study of these questions. The model is similar to the situation in pulmonary cavities in the large size of the bacterial population and the correspondingly elevated risk of secondary drug resistance. Its treatment conditions are harder than those in human tuberculosis with regard to the proportion of intracellularly located and/or resting bacilli and with regard to pharmakokinetics because of the shorter half-life of many antituberculotics in rodents (for a discussion of the model see GRUMBACH et al. 1967; GROSSET 1978a).

It is not surprising, therefore, that neither PAS nor TSC at doses up to 500 mg/kg/day, by themselves practically ineffective, can, when added to INH, prevent the development of INH resistance or influence the viable count (GRUMBACH 1965). Likewise, MCCUNE and TOMPSETT (1956) could not significantly increase the effect of INH by the addition of PAS (1.5 g/kg in the diet).

The situation with SM is quite different. The antibiotic must be applied in high dosage to overcome its drawbacks of a short half-life, poor penetration into cells, and a reduced activity at acid pH prevailing at the site of the bacilli within the macrophage. The publications of GRUMBACH (1953), HOBBY et al. (1953), BARTMANN (1960d), GRUMBACH (1965, summary of several papers in Tables II and IV), GRUMBACH et al. (1969), and GRUMBACH et al. (1970) show that appropriate daily doses of SM can largely delay or prevent the development of secondary INH resistance.

Furthermore, it has been found that the addition of SM to maximally active doses of INH improves the therapeutic effect in mice (GOULDING and ROBSON 1952; GRUMBACH 1953; SIEBENMANN 1953; MCCUNE and TOMPSETT 1956; MCCUNE et al. 1956; BARTMANN 1960d; GRUMBACH 1965; GRUMBACH et al. 1969, 1970) and in guinea pigs (BESTA et al. 1955).

Nevertheless, in the murine model the combination of 25 mg INH/kg + 200 mg SM/kg given daily for 18 months, i.e. the duration of treatment in man, was unable to sterilize the organs of mice in a reliable manner. 35% of the animals still had culturable bacilli at the end of the treatment and 75% after a post-treatment period of 3 months (GRUMBACH et al. 1970; GROSSET 1978a). Antagonism between INH and SM has been reported by GRUNBERG and SCHNITZER (1953) in murine tuberculosis, but only if not fully active doses of the 2 drugs were combined.

The combination of INH + PZA was found to have, in the murine model, a much higher organ-sterilizing potency than INH + SM. This was first detected by MCCUNE and TOMPSETT (1956) and was subsequently confirmed by BATTEN and MCCUNE (1957) and by GRUMBACH (1958). MCCUNE et al. (1956) spoke of a conversion of the infection to the latent state as contrasted to a dormant infection. In the case of non-PZA containing regimens, the infection could be made inactive, but persisting bacilli could always be detected; this situation was called "dormant" infection. In the case of PZA-containing regimens, especially in combination with INH, the infection was inactive at the end of the treatment; viable bacilli could not be demonstrated, but were only hidden beyond the reach of the available methods of detection. The presence of persisters could only be shown in a fraction of the animals retrospectively, after a 90 day treatment-free interval. This situation was called "latent" infection. (In later years, the technique for discovering latent bacilli was refined by prolonging the after-treatment period and giving cortisone during that time). An observation reported by MCCUNE et al. (1956) may have some bearing for short-course chemotherapy developed in the last decade: If INH and PZA are not given simultaneously but sequentially to mice, PZA acts on the resting bacilli that have survived treatment with INH, but INH does not eradicate the bacilli that were first under the influence of PZA. GRUMBACH (1965) has shown that the secondary resistance that develops when INH or PZA are given alone, does not occur when the drugs are administered in combination.

In contrast to the results in mice, a combination of a large dose of INH (26 mg/kg) with 52 mg/kg TSC applicated for the treatment of an established tuberculosis in guinea pigs was more effective than 25 mg/kg INH alone as measured by macroscopic disease index and cultures from regional lymph nodes (BARRY et al. 1954).

In rabbits, GERNEZ-RIEUX et al. (1952/1953) observed an additive effect for the combination of INH + SM, which when given at a high dosage, prevented relapse for more than 400 days even after a treatment period of 30 days only. In a later report (GERNEZ-RIEUX et al. 1953/1954) the authors stated that a treatment from the first to the 28th day after infection with 50 mg/kg INH + 50 mg/kg SM daily could definitely heal some of the rabbits.

The effects of INH in combination with PAS or SM in intravenously infected rabbits have been studied by FREERKSEN (1954). Treatment started 16 days after infection and lasted for 4 months. Thereafter, the animals were observed until their natural death. 14 of 15 rabbits treated with 5 mg/kg SM died during treatment as did 4 of 14 treated with 5 mg/kg INH, but no animal treated with 5 mg/kg INH + 5 mg/kg SM died during this period. The same effect as this combination had INH alone in a dose of 10 mg/kg/d.

For combinations of INH with antituberculotics that were tested clinically later than INH the reader is referred to the respective sections dealing with those drugs. Here it remains to be mentioned that, according to VISCHER and ROULET (1963), when the antileprosy drug B 663, a phenazine derivative active against some species of mycobacteria, is combined with INH it prevents the development of secondary resistance and may enhance the killing effect of INH.

Triple Combinations: Very few investigations are available on triple combinations. In 2 of them, one in mice (MCCUNE and TOMPSETT 1956) and one in guinea pigs (BARTMANN et al. 1958), INH + SM + PAS was compared against INH alone. The triple combination was found to be superior. It is difficult to say to what extent PAS contributed to this effect. MCCUNE et al. (1956) compared INH + SM + PAS to INH + PZA in mice by viable counts in the lungs and the spleens. In early as well as in delayed treatment the bactericidal activity of INH + PZA was clearly higher than that of INH + SM + PAS. A long-term study was undertaken by GROSSET (1978 b), in which an established mouse infection was treated for up to 12 months with either INH (25 mg/kg) + SM (200 mg/kg) or with this combination + PZA (150 mg/kg). After 6 months the percentage of negative cultures from lungs or spleens was 0 for INH + SM and 10 for INH + SM + PZA. However, thereafter the difference became marked: at 9 months 20% of the cultures were negative with INH + SM as opposed to 90% with INH + SM + PZA, and at 12 months 30% as opposed to 100%. These results again demonstrate the unique activity of PZA in mice.

e) Efficacy of INH Alone and in Combinations with Intermittent Treatment Throughout

α) Daily Dose Kept Constant, Total Dose Varied in Mice. BARTMANN (1960 d) used early and late treatment with daily doses of 20 mg/kg INH, 300 mg/kg SM, and the same doses in combination. Monotherapy and combined treatment were given 6 or 2 days (every third or fourth day) a week. According to the viable counts, the rank order was as follows:

$$\mathrm{INH}_6 + \mathrm{SM}_6 > \mathrm{INH}_2 + \mathrm{SM}_2 \simeq \mathrm{INH}_6 > \mathrm{SM}_6 > \mathrm{INH}_2 \ .$$

GRUMBACH (1965) states that INH at a dose of 100 mg/kg given twice weekly for 3 months had a disastrous effect. From her 1968 publication it can be seen that the combination of INH (25 mg/kg) + SM (200 mg/kg) given twice weekly remains inferior to daily administration even if the treatment period is extended to 6 months–12 months. Using survival as the criterion, and administering INH in the diet (0.05%), BLOCH (1961) observed that treatment once a week preserved life as well as daily treatment when the therapy was started 3 or 6 days after the infection. When it was started after 10 days, however, the daily treatment was clearly superior. In this experiment the therapy lasted about 4 months. If this period was reduced to 3 weeks, continuous treatment was superior to intermittent administration once or twice a week.

In Guinea Pigs: KARLSON and FELDMAN (1953) compared continuous with trice weekly dosage in early treatment given for 9 weeks. In a daily dose of 10 mg or 15 mg per animal (800 g), continuous and intermittent treatments were equieffective. At lower doses, tested in another experiment, 1 mg 3 times a week was equivalent to 0.25 mg/day of the experiment first-mentioned. ŻEBROWSKI et al. (1954) tried late treatment in reinfected, previously immunized animals with 5 mg/kg/day or 5 mg/kg or 10 mg/kg every third day. According to the survival times, the rank order was 10 mg/kg every third day > 5 mg/kg every third day > 5 mg/kg/day. It is doubtful whether this result reflects the antimicrobial activity of the various regimens, and it is more likely that a less effective intermittent treatment allowed a stronger immunity to develop, which in turn then became decisive for survival. It has been demonstrated by BARTMANN et al. (1958) that a less effective therapy can indeed produce longer survival times if the experimental conditions are appropriately selected. Likewise, PALMER et al. (1956) have shown that immunity against a superinfection is higher in intermittently treated guinea pigs than in ones which had received continuous therapy before the re-challenge. BARTMANN et al. (1958) treated an already generalized tuberculosis for 3 months with either 10 mg INH/kg 6 times or 2 times a week or with INH (10 mg/kg + SM (20 mg/kg) + PAS (0.2 g/kg) also given either 6 or 2 times per week. Measured by the rate of the healing of abscesses, regression of regional lymph nodes, gross and microscopic autopsy findings, cultures from spleen and the primary complex, the rank order of these regimens was as follows: triple combination 6 times a week > triple combination twice a week > INH 6 times a week > INH twice a week. DICKINSON et al. (1968) treated an established tuberculosis for 6 weeks at various dose levels and intervals. The results were evaluated by scores assigned to the macroscopic findings and viable counts from the spleens. The therapeutic efficacy increased from the lowest mean daily dose (0.5 mg/kg) to the highest (4 mg/kg) and was practically the same for treatment intervals from 1 day to 4 days. An interval of 8 days was significantly less effective. Essentially the same results were obtained in later experiments, using 1 mg/kg, 2 mg/kg, and 4 mg/kg as the daily doses and 1, 2, 4, 7, 10, and 14 days as the intervals. When guinea pigs were treated with higher doses at weekly intervals the best response was obtained with 20 mg/kg–30 mg/kg, given either as single or as repeated doses. Any further increase in the dosage did not improve the results. The best responses obtained with doses given at intervals of 10.5 days were inferior to those obtained with weekly doses, which were in turn less satisfactory than ones in animals treated twice a week (DICKINSON et al. 1973).

β) Daily Dose Varied, Total Dose Kept Constant or Nearly Constant

In Mice: GRUMBACH et al. (1952) treated the animals daily with 2.5 mg/kg INH or 50 mg/kg SM or INH + SM at the same dosage, every other day with 5 or 100 or 5 + 100, and every third day with 7.5 or 150 or 7.5 + 150. After 40 days of the therapy the mice were killed and the results assessed by a macroscopic index and standardized microscopic counting of bacilli in the lungs and the spleens. With INH alone the index was the same for all treatment schedules, but the microscopic count was higher after the intermittent regimes. With SM the therapeutic activity decreased with increasing intervals between the doses. Combined treatment was similarly effective with all schedules, and may have been slightly better than either drug alone. HOBBY and LENERT (1953) compared daily and twice weekly (every 3rd or 4th day) treatments on the basis of the survival rates and calculations of the CD_{50}. This value increased in twice weekly application by a factor of 3.7 for SM, by one of 6.4 for INH, and by one of 4.9 for INH + SM given in a fixed combination. BATTEN (1968) states shortly in a summary that after 9 weeks of treatment, according to the viable counts made from lungs and spleens, an increase in the intervals from 1 day to 8 days did not reduce the activity of SM, but it did have this effect with INH (using 6.25 mg/kg to 25 mg/kg). KREBS (1968) found similar activity for 5 mgINH/kg/day or 50 mgINH/kg/day and 150 mg/kg twice a week as long as the bacilli remained sensitive; 15 mg/kg was inferior (viable counts in lungs). In a later experiment KREBS (1970) compared 15 mg/kg/day with 45 mg/kg twice a week and 90 mg/kg once a week. After treatment for 2 ½ months the viable counts in the 2 × 45 mg/kg-group were nearly as low as that in the group treated daily; 90 mg/kg once a week was distinctly less active.

In Guinea Pigs: PALMER et al. (1956) varied the dose and the frequency of early administration of INH. The animals were treated for periods of 10 to 20 weeks. The survival rates were the same as in non-infected controls for the groups treated with 3 mg/kg/day, 4 mg/kg/day, or 5 mg/kg/day or with 5 mg/kg or 10 mg/kg 3 times a week. The groups treated with 4 mg/kg 3 times a week or 5 mg/kg once a week or 2 mg/kg daily had increasingly shorter survival rates. ENGBAEK et al. (1959) used weekly doses of 7 mg/kg or 70 mg/kg. Single doses were spaced out to every other, third, or seventh day. The treatment started a month after the infection and lasted 5 months. The survival rates were then noted. At both drug levels the survival-times decreased with increasing drug-free intervals.

GENAZZANI et al. (1966) found in early as well as in late treatment of guinea pigs, both given for one month, that the mean number of caseous lesions increased in the following order: 2 × 6 mg/kg/day or 1 × 12 mg/kg/day < 40 mg/kg every third day < 40 mg/kg every sixth day.

γ) Development of INH Resistance During Intermittent Treatment. In guinea pigs no resistant cultures have been found by KARLSON and FELDMAN (1953), ŻEBROWSKI et al. (1954), BARTMANN et al. (1958), and DICKINSON et al. (1968, 1973). Only ENGBAEK et al. (1959), who used a longer treatment period than the other investigators, encountered resistant strains. These were found predominantly in the groups treated with a small dose daily or every other day or with a large dose once a week.

A similar picture emerges from the combined data on mice. Bartmann (1960d) observed the emergence of resistance only during continuous monotherapy with INH or SM, and not with intermittent monotherapy (twice weekly) or with daily or twice-weekly combined administration of INH and SM. Grumbach's mice (1965) treated once a week with 100 mg/kg all harbored resistant bacilli. The following sequence of secondary resistance development can be read off from Fig. 4 in Krebs (1968): First 50 mg/kg/day, then 150 mg/kg twice a week at the same time as 5 mg/kg/day, and finally 15 mg/kg twice a week. In general, the risk is lowest in groups treated intermittently with relatively low doses of INH. This has also been observed for therapy in phases (Grumbach 1965).

δ) Comment on Intermittent Treatment Throughout. If one takes into account that the results of survival experiments depend only in part on the efficacy of the treatment applied, and also in part on the infection immunity, it seems fair to say that at least in mice, intermittent administration is inferior to continuous treatment not only in the earlier months but also after 9 months of therapy. Increasing the INH dosage can compensate spacing out of the intervals only within certain limits. Combinations of INH + SM in fully effective doses given twice weekly every third and fourth day seem to be equivalent to continuous application of INH alone, but are clearly less effective than daily doses of INH + SM.

f) Treatment in Phases

When it became obvious that intermittent chemotherapy from the very beginning could not achieve the desired result, the question arose whether an initial intensive treatment phase in which the size of the bacterial population would be drastically reduced could be followed by a less intensive phase, and therefore also one less costly and perhaps less toxic. The observations made by Bloch (1961), that even a week of initial continuous therapy with INH could improve the results of subsequent intermittent INH treatment, suggested that this approach was promising.

The potentialities of treatment in phases were systematically explored by the research group at the Pasteur Institute in Paris, using established murine tuberculosis as the model. The early experiments have been reviewed by Grumbach (1965) and may be summarized here as follows:

1. All phase treatment schedules are compared to the combination of 25 mg INH/kg + 200 mg SM/kg administered daily for up to 9 months or longer. Standard treatment results, after 9 months to 12 months, in negative cultures form the organs of 30%–50% of the animals, and in very low viable counts in the remaining 50%. Resistance to INH may be found in about 10% of the positive cultures.
2. The same results as with the standard regimen can be obtained by 3 months on INH + SM at the same dosage, followed by 25 mg INH/kg daily for 6 months or 9 months. Initial treatment with SM every other day in combination with daily INH or continuous application of INH + SM in standard doses followed by only 5 mg INH/kg daily for up to 9 months yields unsatisfactory results.

3. INH alone or INH + SM given intermittently once or twice a week after a standard treatment of 3 months' duration are insufficient.
4. Certain types of intermittent therapy do, however, give satisfactory results if they are given only in the third 3-month period. These are INH + SM or INH alone twice a week (not once a week). Treatment during months 1–3 was INH + SM daily at a standard dosage, followed by daily INH in months 4–6.
5. The initial intensive phase may be made shorter, but then needs a more intensive second phase. About equal efficacy has been found for the following regimens: 3 months on INH + SM daily followed by 3 months on daily INH; 2 months on INH + SM daily followed by 4 months on INH + SM twice a week or INH daily, and 1 months on INH + SM daily followed by 5 months on INH + SM 3 times a day. However, follow-up data (GRUMBACH et al. 1967) showed that the shortening of the initial intensive phase from 3 to 2 months resulted in a higher proportion of INH-resistant cultures among the surviving animals.
6. Doubling of the doses of INH and SM allows a reduction in the daily initial intensive phase to about 15 days, provided that the following phase fulfils certain conditions (GRUMBACH et al. 1967).

Later studies (GRUMBACH and GROSSET 1975; GROSSET 1978b) included PZA and yielded the following results:

1. Addition of 200 mg SM/kg daily to 25 mg INH/kg + 1.5 g PZA/kg improves the reduction in the viable count slightly during the first month. Thereafter, both regimens are equal: at 6 months cultures from 80% or more of the animals are negative, while the remaining grow sensitive bacilli.
2. 3 months on INH + PZA daily at the dosage stated above followed by daily INH is as effective as INH + PZA daily throughout. Shortening of the period of combined treatment to 2 months or to 1 month results in increasingly worse results.
3. Of various intermittent regimens in the second phase (months 3–6), only INH + PZA twice weekly was satisfactory. The first phase consisted of daily INH + PZA.
4. INH + SM + PZA given daily for 12 months resulted in 100% of negative cultures, whereas with daily INH + SM for the same treatment period only 30% were negative. INH + SM + PZA daily for 2 months may be followed by INH + PZA daily without loss of efficacy, but not by INH + PZA twice weekly or by INH daily alone.

Summarizing, treatment in phases developed into a clinically fruitful concept, gaining new impetus with the advent of RMP.

3. Concluding Remarks

The minimal inhibitory concentrations of INH for *M. tuberculosis* and *M. bovis* in vitro compare favorably with those of the antituberculotics known before and becoming known later, except RMP. INH is growth-dependently bactericidal with respect to extracellularly and intracellularly located bacilli at concentrations near the MIC. It does not exhibit cross-resistance with the other antituberculotics. In experimental animals INH has been found to be more active than the other antituberculotics except RMP. In the animal, as in vitro, INH kills proliferating but not resting bacilli. This killing action can be enhanced by combining INH with other bactericidal drugs. Combination with other antituberculotics is necessary to prevent or delay the development of secondary INH resistance. Evaluation of intermittent administration of INH alone or in combination has shown this type of treatment to be effective, but inferior to the respective continuous regimens. The concept of treatment in phases was developed on the basis of these facts and corresponding clinical experience. An initial intensive phase aiming at a rapid reduction in the bacterial organ populations by daily administration of INH in combination with other bactericidal drugs like SM and/or PZA can then be followed by certain types of less intensive, and therefore less costly and perhaps less toxic, continuous or intermittent treatment schedules.

Over the years INH remained the leading antituberculotic drug until the advent of RMP. The combination of INH with RMP then formed the indispensable core of all socalled short-course regimens of the present day, which need a total duration of treatment of 6 months–9 months instead of 18 months–24 months.

References

Aitoff M (1952) Action *in vitro* de l'hydrazide de l'acide isonicotinique seul et combiné avec l'autres produits. Ann Inst Pasteur 83:130–134

Aitoff M, Salas A (1952) Action combinée *in vitro* de l' I.N.H. et de la streptomycine sur le bacille de Koch. Ann Inst Pasteur 83:273–275

Andrejew A, Tacquet A (1957) Métabolisme des mycobactéries sensibles et résistantes à l'INH. Activité amino-acide oxydasique (production d'eau oxygénée). Ann Inst Pasteur 93:695–704

Armstrong AR (1960) Time-concentration relationships of isoniazid with tubercle bacilli in vitro. Am Rev Respir Dis 81:498–503

Armstrong AR (1965) Further studies on the time/concentration relationships of isoniazid and tubercle bacilli in vitro. Am Rev Respir Dis 91:440–443

Aronson JD, Ehrlich SL, Flagg W (1952) Effects of isonicotinic acid derivatives on tubercle bacilli. Proc Soc Exp Biol Med 80:259–262

Auersbach K, Bartmann K, Kauffmann GW, Krebs A, Schütz I, Steinbrück P (1961) Die frühe Erkennung des ungenügenden Effekts der konservativ-chemischen Behandlung bei kavernöser Lungentuberkulose. Adv Tuberc Res 11:122–192

Awaness AM, Mitchison DA (1973) Cumulative effects of pulsed exposures of *Mycobacterium tuberculosis* to isoniazid. Tubercle 54:153–158

Balogh A (1953) Zur Tuberkelbazillenresistenz gegenüber Isonikotinsäurehydrazid. Wien Klin Wochenschr 65:287–289

Barnett M, Bushby SRM, Mitchison DA (1953 a) Isoniazid-resistant strains of tubercle bacilli. Their development and stability. Lancet I:314–320

Barnett M, Bushby SRM, Mitchison DA (1953 b) Tubercle bacilli resistant to isoniazid: virulence and response to treatment with isoniazid in guinea-pigs and mice. Br J Exp Pathol 34:568–581

Baroni V (1952) Expériences cliniques et de laboratoire avec l' H.I.N. Schweiz Z Tuberk 9:283–292

Barry VC, Conalty ML, Gaffney EE (1954) Amithiozone as an adjuvant to isoniazid therapy. Irish J Med Sci 1954:299–303

Bartmann K (1954) Die wachstumshemmende Wirkung verschiedener Tuberkulostatika und ihrer Kombinationen in vitro. Tbk Arzt 8:276–282

Bartmann K (1959) Isoniazid-prophylaxis in exposed or minimally infected animals. Bull Int Union Tuberc XXIX:214–226
Bartmann K (1960a) Die Empfindlichkeit INH-resistenter Tuberkelbakterien gegen Thiosemicarbazon (Conteben). Tbk Arzt 14:450–452
Bartmann K (1960b) Langfristige Einwirkung von Isonicotinsäurehydrazid und Streptomycin auf ruhende Tuberkelbakterien in vitro. Beitr Klin Tuberk 122:94–113
Bartmann K (1960c) Die experimentellen Grundlagen der Chemoprophylaxe der Tuberkulose mit Isonicotinsäurehydrazid (INH). Adv Tuberc Res 10:127–215
Bartmann K (1960d) Tierexperimentelle Untersuchungen zu einer intermittierenden Chemotherapie und -prophylaxe der Tuberkulose. X. Mitteilung. Der Erfolg kontinuierlicher und intermittierender Gaben von INH und der Kombination INH-Streptomycin bei der Tuberkulose der Maus. Beitr Klin Tuberk 122:251–264
Bartmann K (1963) Isoniazid. Möglichkeiten und Grenzen seiner Wirkung. Thieme, Stuttgart
Bartmann K, Villnow J, Schwarz C (1955) Tierexperimentelle Untersuchungen zu einer intermittierenden Chemotherapie und -prophylaxe der Tuberkulose. I. Mitteilung. Der Erfolg intermittierender Gaben von 10 mg INH je Kilogramm Körpergewicht im Simultanversuch an Meerschweinchen. Beitr Klin Tuberk 115:79–86
Bartmann K, Villnow J, Schwarz C (1956) Tierexperimentelle Untersuchungen zu einer intermittierenden Chemotherapie und -prophylaxe der Tuberkulose. II. Mitteilung. Der Erfolg zweimal wöchentlich verabfolgter Gaben von INH in verschiedener Dosierung beim Simultanversuch an Meerschweinchen. Beitr Klin Tuberk 115:269–275
Bartmann K, Villnow J, Schwarz C (1958) Tierexperimentelle Untersuchungen zu einer intermittierenden Chemotherapie und -prophylaxe der Tuberkulose. VII. Mitteilung. Der Erfolg kontinuierlicher und intermittierender Gaben von INH und der Tripelkombination INH, Streptomycin, PAS im therapeutischen Versuch an Meerschweinchen. Beitr Klin Tuberk 118:297–313
Bartmann K, Freise G (1963) Mikrobiologisch bestimmte Isoniazid-Konzentrationen im Gewebe von Tier und Mensch. Beitr Klin Tuberk 127:546–560
Bartmann K, Abel U, Hart R (1966) Die Abhängigkeit des Hemmtiters von der Bebrütungsdauer bei der Bestimmung der Resistenz von *M. tuberculosis* gegen Antituberkulotika auf Löwenstein-Jensen Medium. Z Bakteriol Mikrobiol Hyg (A) 201:538–548
Bartmann K, Blisse A (1967) Kurzfristige, primäre INH-Prophylaxe mit hohen Dosen bei minimal infizierten Meerschweinchen. Beitr Klin Tuberk 135:351–356
Batten JC (1968) Intermittent chemotherapy in murine tuberculosis. Tubercle (Lond) 49, Suppl:70
Batten JC, Mc Cune RM Jr (1957) The influence of corticotrophin and cortisone with antituberculous drugs on populations of *Mycobacterium tuberculosis* in tissues of mice. Br J Exp Path 38:424–437
Beggs WH, Jenne JW (1969) Isoniazid uptake and growth inhibition of *Mycobacterium tuberculosis* in relation to time and concentration of pulsed drug exposures. Tubercle (Lond) 50:377–385
Bekierkunst A, Szulga T (1954) A new method for determining the growth rate of *M. tuberculosis* and its application to the study of the toxic effects of streptomycin and isonicotinic hydrazide acid on tubercle bacilli. Schweiz Z Allg Path 17:47–71
Bernard E, Kreis B, Le Joubioux E (1957) Evolution clinique de 31 cas de tuberculose cavitaire avec bacilles isoniazido-résistants de faible virulence expérimentale. Rev Tuberc (Paris) 21:429
Bernstein J, Lott WA, Steinberg BA, Yale HL (1952) Chemotherapy of experimental tuberculosis. V. Isonicotinic acid hydrazide (Nydrazid) and related compounds. Am Rev Tuberc 65:357–364
Besta B, Lucchesi M, Pana C, Spina G (1955) Ann Inst Forlanini 15:3–39, cited from: Bartmann K, Villnow J, Schwarz C (1958). Beitr Klin Tuberk 118:297–313
Bjerkedahl T, Palmer CE (1967) Effect of isoniazid on tuberculosis in guinea pigs. Comparison of single versus multiple daily doses. Scand J Respir Dis 48:94–108
Bloch H (1961) Intermittent isoniazid therapy for mice. Am Rev Respir Dis 84:824–836

Bourgeois P, Dubois-Verlière Mlle, Maëll Mlle (1958) Étude de l'action discontinue de l'isoniazide sur le bacille de Koch par la méthode des cultures sur lames. Rev Tuberc (Paris) 22:108–111
Briggs IL, Rochester WR, Shennan DH, Riddell RW, Fox W, Heffernan JF, Miller AB, Nunn AJ, Stott H, Tall R (1968) Streptomycin plus thiacetazone (thioacetazone) compared with streptomycin plus PAS and with isoniazid plus thiacetazone in the treatment of pulmonary tuberculosis in Rhodesia. Tubercle (Lond) 49:48–69
British Medical Research Council (1952) The treatment of pulmonary tuberculosis with isoniazid. An interim report to the Medical Research Council by their Tuberculosis Trials Committee. Br Med J II:735–746
British Medical Research Council (1953) Isoniazid in the treatment of pulmonary tuberculosis. Second report to the Medical Research Council by their Tuberculosis Trials Committee. Br Med J I:521–536
Brun J, Cayré RM, Viallier J (1954) Influence de la vitamine B_6 sur l'activité antituberculeuse de l'isoniazide. CR Soc Biol 148:1817–1818
Bünger P, Lass A (1953) Beitrag zur Resistenzentwicklung der Tuberkelbakterien unter Isoniazidbehandlung. Dtsch Med Wochenschr 78:1193–1194
Canetti G (1965) Present aspects of bacterial resistance in tuberculosis. Am Rev Respir Dis 92:687–703
Canetti G, Grumbach F, Grosset J (1960) Studies of bacillary populations in experimental tuberculosis of mice treated by isoniazid. Am Rev Respir Dis 82:295–313
Canetti G, Fox W, Khomenko A, Mahler HT, Menon NK, Mitchison DA, Rist N, Šmelev NA (1969) Advances in techniques of testing mycobacterial drug sensitivity, and the use of sensitivity tests in tuberculosis control programmes. Bull WHO 41:21–43
Cattaneo C, Morellini M (1952) Sulle proprietà antitubercolari dell'idrazide dell'acido isonicotinico. Minerva Med 43:1081–1086
Chaulet P, Abderrahim K, Oussedik N, Amrane R, Mercer M, Si Hassen C, Bouhlabal F (1976) Résultats d'un traitement standardisé chez les tuberculeux pulmonaires porteurs d'une résistance primaire à Alger. Rev Fr Mal Resp 4:5–14
Chicou FJ, Hétrick G, Lahlou M, Le Hir M, Mercier A, Neel R, Rist N, Vincent J (1961) Enquête contrôlée sur trois types de traitement per os de la tuberculose pulmonaire réalisée au Maroc, à Tanger (I.N.H. + éthionamide; I.N.H. + P.A.S.; I.N.H. seul). Premiers résultats après un an d'observation. Rev Tuberc (Paris) 25:1031–1056
Claus H (1953) Beitrag zur Resistenzfrage bei INH-Therapie der Lungentuberkulose. Tbk Arzt 7:452–456
Coates EO Jr, Meade GM, Steenken W Jr, Wolinsky E, Brinkman GL (1953) The clinical significance of the emergence of drug-resistant organisms during the therapy of chronic pulmonary tuberculosis with hydrazides of isonicotinic acid. N Engl J Med 248:1081–1087
Cohn ML, Middlebrook G, Russell WF Jr (1959) Combined drug treatment of tuberculosis. I. Prevention of emergence of mutant populations of tubercle bacilli resistant to both streptomycin and isoniazid *in vitro*. J Clin Invest 38:1349–1355
Coletsos PJ (1952) De l'association I.N.H. – streptomycine – P.A.S. Rev Tuberc (Paris) 16:670–678
Colwell CA, Hess AR (1956) Stability and antibacterial effect of D-glucurolactone isonicotinyl hydrazone and isoniazid. Am Rev Tuberc Pulm Dis 73:892–906
Colwell CA, Hess AR (1957) The effect of inspissation and storage on isoniazid concentrations in culture media. Am Rev Tuberc Pulm Dis 75:678–683
Crowle AJ (1958) Comparison of the chemotherapeutic activities of INH, "Gatalone" and glucurolactone in tuberculous mice by the lung density technique. Tubercle (Lond) 39:41–44
Devadatta S, Bhatia AL, Andrews RH, Fox W, Mitchison DA, Radhakrishna S, Ramakrishnan CV, Selkon JB, Velu S (1961) Response of patients infected with isoniazid-resistant tubercle bacilli to treatment with isoniazid plus PAS or isoniazid alone. Bull WHO 25:807–829
Dickinson JM, Mitchison DA (1966) In vitro studies on the choice of drugs for intermittent chemotherapy of tuberculosis. Tubercle (Lond) 47:370–380

Dickinson JM, Ellard GA, Mitchison DA (1968) Suitability of isoniazid and ethambutol for intermittent administration in the treatment of tuberculosis. Tubercle (Lond) 49:351–366

Dickinson JM, Aber VR, Mitchison DA (1973) Studies on the treatment of experimental tuberculosis of the guinea pig with intermittent doses of isoniazid. Tubercle 54:211–224

Dickinson JM, Mitchison DA (1976) Bactericidal activity *in vitro* and in the guinea-pig of isoniazid, rifampicin and ethambutol. Tubercle 57:251–258

Dickinson JM, Aber VR, Mitchison DA (1977) Bactericidal activity of streptomycin, isoniazid, rifampin, ethambutol, and pyrazinamide alone and in combination against *Mycobacterium tuberculosis*. Am Rev Respir Dis 116:627–635

Dickinson JM, Mitchison DA (1981) Experimental models to explain the high sterilizing activity of rifampin in the chemotherapy of tuberculosis. Am Rev Respir Dis 123:367–371

Dissmann E (1954) Unterschiede der Wachstumsgeschwindigkeit und Wachstumseffekt subminimaler Hemmungsmengen von Isoniacid (INH) bei INH-resistenten und -sensiblen Tuberkelbakterienpopulationen. Naturwissenschaften 41:218–219

Dissmann E, Iglauer E (1953a) Die normale Sensibilität gegenüber Streptomycin, Dihydrostreptomycin, PAS, TB I und Isonicotinsäurehydracid bei unbehandelten Tbb-Populationen in der Objektträgermikrokultur. Beitr Klin Tuberk 109:89–97

Dissmann E, Iglauer E (1953b) Untersuchungen über den bakteriostatischen und bactericiden Effekt von Streptomycin, PAS, TB I und Rimifon, im Verlaufe der Behandlung der Tuberkulose. Beitr Klin Tuberk 109:8–26

Domagk G (1953) Zu welchen Erwartungen berechtigt uns die Chemotherapie der Tuberkulose? Dtsch Med J 4:473–480

Domagk G, Offe HA, Siefken W (1952) Ein weiterer Beitrag zur experimentellen Chemotherapie der Tuberkulose (Neoteben). Dtsch Med Wochenschr 77:573–578

Dunbar JM (1957) L'apparition de formes non acido-résistantes de *Mycobacterium tuberculosis* en présence d'isoniazide, de cyclosérine et du thioamide de l'acide α-éthyl isonicotinique. Ann Inst Pasteur 92:451–458

Dunbar FP, Mc Allister E, Jefferies MB (1959) Catalase and peroxidase activities of isoniazid-susceptible and -resistant strains of M. tuberculosis. Am Rev Tuberc Pulm Dis 79:669–671

East African/British Medical Research Council Isoniazid Investigation (1960) Comparative trial of isoniazid alone in low and high dosage and isoniazid plus PAS in the treatment of acute pulmonary tuberculosis in East Africans. Tubercle (Lond) 41:83–102

East African/British Medical Research Council Pretreatment Drug Resistance Report (1963) Influence of pretreatment bacterial resistance to isoniazid, thiacetazone or PAS on the response to chemotherapy of African patients with pulmonary tuberculosis. Tubercle (Lond) 44:393–416

Eckley GM, Wilson JL (1960) Comparative study of isoniazid versus no chemotherapy in the prevention of relapse of chronic cavitary tuberculosis. Am Rev Respir Dis 82:242–243

Eidus L, Lányi MR (1953) Experimentelle Erfahrungen mit Isonikotinsäurehydrazid und anderen Hydrazidderivaten. Z Tbk 102:193–196

Engbaek HC, Jespersen A, Rasmussen KN (1959) Isoniazid treatment of tuberculosis in guinea pigs. A study on the effect of varying dosage regimens. Acta Tuberc Scand Suppl 47:62–76

Ferebee SH, Palmer CE (1956) Prevention of experimental tuberculosis with isoniazid. Am Rev Tuberc Pulm Dis 73:1–18

Finkeldey W (1952) Der Ablauf der experimentellen Meerschweinchentuberkulose unter dem Einfluß des INH (Isonikotinylhydrazid) Rimifon (Roche). Z Tbk 101:166–169

Freerksen E (1954) Grundlagen, Möglichkeiten und Grenzen einer Chemotherapie der Tuberkulose. Arch Gynäkol 186:262–277

Freerksen E (1957) Discussion remark. Bull Int Union Tuberc XXVII:245–247

Freerksen E, Rosenfeld M, Matsumiya T (1969) Isoniazid-Wirkung trotz INH-Resistenz? Prax Pneumol 23:450–464

Fujisawa Y (1972) Studies on treatment with isoniazid and ethambutol in experimental silicotuberculosis due to pertracheal intrapulmonary vinyl tube infusion of tubercle bacilli with free silica particles. J Nara Med Ass 23:253–277
Fust B (1952) Orientierung über das Antituberculoticum Rimifon „Roche“. Schweiz Med Wochenschr 82:333–335
Fust B (1953) Therapie der Tuberkulose mit Isoniazid (Rimifon). In: Gordonoff T (Hrsg) Hdb der Therapie in Einzeldarstellungen, Lieferung 4. Huber, Bern, pp 467–535
Fust B, Studer A, Böhni E (1952) Experimentelle Erfahrungen mit dem Antituberculoticum „Rimifon“. Schweiz Z Tuberk 9:226–242
Fust B, Böhni E (1953) Sensibilität und Resistenz von Tuberkelbazillen gegenüber Rimifon. Schweiz Med Wochenschr 83:377–383
Gangadharam PRJ, Cohn ML, Middlebrook G (1963) Dynamic aspects of the sterilizing action of isoniazid on *M. tuberculosis*. Am Rev Respir Dis 88:558–562
Genazzani E, Ninni A, Pacilio G (1966) Effects of isonicotinic acid hydrazide administered to tuberculous guinea-pigs at different doses and at different space intervalls. Med Thorac 23:225–239
Gerloff W (1960) Entwicklung und heutiger Stand der Kultivierung des *Mycobacteriums tuberculosis* unter besonderer Berücksichtigung des Pyruvateffektes. Z Ärztl Fortbild (Jena) 54:623–627
Gernez-Rieux C, Tacquet A, Fabre M (1952/1953) Étude de l’action de diverses substances antibacillaires utilisées seules ou en association au cours de la tuberculose expérimentale du lapin. Ann Inst Pasteur Lille 5:32–55
Gernez-Rieux C, Tacquet A, Voisin C, Fabre M (1953/1954) La tuberculose expérimentale du lapin peut-elle guerir définitivement par l’emploi de diverses substances antibacillaires administrées seules et en association? Ann Inst Pasteur Lille 6:145–154
Goulding R, Robson JM (1952) Isoniazid in the control of experimental corneal tuberculosis. Lancet II:849–853
Goulding R, King MB, Knox R, Robson JM (1952) Relation between in-vitro and in-vivo resistance to isoniazid. Lancet II:69–70
Grosset J (1978a) The sterilizing value of rifampicin and pyrazinamide in experimental short course chemotherapy. Tubercle 59:287–297
Grosset J (1978b) Chemotherapy of tuberculosis. In: Siegenthaler W, Lüthy R (eds) Proc 10th Intern Congr Chemother I, pp 43–44
Grumbach F (1953) Chimiothérapie antituberculeuse expérimentale. Etude comparée des traitements prolongés par la streptomycine et par l’isoniazide. Conditions d’apparition des résistants. Atti del VI ° Congresso internazionale di Microbiologia (Rome) Vol 1:553–558
Grumbach F (1958) Activité antituberculeuse expérimentale du pyrazinamide (P.Z.A.). Ann Inst Pasteur 94:694–708
Grumbach F (1962) Treatment of experimental murine tuberculosis with different combinations of isoniazid/streptomycin followed by isoniazid alone. Am Rev Respir Dis 86:211–215
Grumbach F (1965) Etudes chimiothérapiques sur la tuberculose avancée de la souris. Adv Tuberc Res 14:31–96
Grumbach F (1968) Chimiothérapie intermittente de longue durée dans la tuberculose expérimentale de la souris. Bull Int Union Tuberc XLI:303–308
Grumbach F, Rist N, Riebel J (1952) Traitement discontinu de la tuberculose expérimentale de la souris par l’hydrazide isonicotinique (isoniazide). Ann Inst Pasteur 83:397–399
Grumbach F, Grosset J, Canetti G (1960) L’inactivation de l’isoniazide chez le rat. Son incidence sur les résultats de la chimiothérapie de la tuberculose dans cette espèce. Ann Inst Pasteur 98:642–656
Grumbach F, Canetti G, Grosset J, Le Lirzin M (1967) Late results of long-term, intermittent chemotherapy of advanced, murine tuberculosis: limits of the murine model. Tubercle (Lond) 48:11–26
Grumbach F, Canetti G, Le Lirzin M (1969) Rifampicin in daily and intermittent treatment of experimental murine tuberculosis with emphasis on late results. Tubercle 50:280–283

Grumbach F, Canetti G, Le Lirzin M (1970) Caractère durable de la stérilisation de la tuberculose expérimentale de la souris par l'association rifampicine-isoniazide. Epreuve de la cortisone. Rev Tuberc Pneumol 34:312–319
Grumbach F, Grosset J (1975) Le pyrazinamide dans le traitement de courte durée de la tuberculose murine. Rev Fr Mal Respir 3:5–18
Grunberg E, Schnitzer RJ (1952) Studies on the activity of hydrazine derivatives of isonicotinic acid in the experimental tuberculosis of mice. Quart Bull Sea View Hosp 13:3–11
Grunberg E, Schnitzer RJ (1953) Antagonism of isoniazid and streptomycin in experimental infection of mice with *M. tuberculosis* H37Rv. Am Rev Tuberc 68:277–279
Grunberg E, Blencowe W (1955) The influence of pyridoxine on the in vitro antituberculous activity of isoniazid. Am Rev Tuberc Pulm Dis 71:898–899
Hedgecock LW, Faucher IO (1957) Relation of pyrogallol-peroxidative activity to isoniazid resistance in *Mycobacterium tuberculosis*. Am Rev Tuberc Pulm Dis 75:670–674
Heilmeyer L, Schaich W, Buchegger G, Kilchling H, Schmidt F, Walter AM (1952) Vorläufiger Bericht über Isonikotinsäurehydrazid (Rimifon, Neoteben) auf Grund experimenteller und klinischer Untersuchungen. MMW 94:1303–1308
Herman RP, Weber MM (1980) Isoniazid interaction with tyrosine as a possible mode of action of the drug in mycobacteria. Antimicrob Agents Chemother 17:170–178
Hobby GL, Lenert TF (1952) Resistance to isonicotinic acid hydrazide. Am Rev Tuberc 65:771–774
Hobby GL, Lenert TF (1953) The control of experimental mouse tuberculosis by the intermittent administration of streptomycin, viomycin, isoniazid, and streptomycilidene isonicotinyl hydrazine. Am Rev Tuberc 68:292–294
Hobby GL, Lenert TF, Rivoire ZC, Donikian M, Picula D (1953) In vitro and in vivo activity of streptomycin and isoniazid singly and in combination. Am Rev Tuberc 67:808–827
Hobby GL, Lenert TF (1957) The in vitro action of antituberculous agents against multiplying and non-multiplying microbial cells. Am Rev Tuberc Pulm Dis 76:1031–1048
Ilavsky J (1952) Synergistic action of isonicotinic acid hydrazide and streptomycin in vitro. Am Rev Tuberc 65:777–778
Jackett PS, Aber VR, Lowrie DM (1978) Virulence and resistance to superoxide, low pH and hydrogen peroxide among strains of *Mycobacterium tuberculosis*. J Gen Microbiol 104:37–45
Jančik E (1963) Comparative evaluation of the results obtained through the use of major chemotherapeutic combinations in cases discharging bacilli with low resistance and cases discharging bacilli with high resistance to the same drug. Bull Int Union Tuberc XXXIII:98–117
Jenney FS, Landis RE (1954) A study of the development of resistance to isoniazid during the treatment of pulmonary tuberculosis. Trans 13th Conf Chemother Tuberc VAAF:231–233
Kakimoto S, Seydel JK, Wempe E (1961) Zusammenhänge zwischen Struktur und Wirkung bei Carbothionamiden. Jber Borstel 5:233–239
Karlson AG, Feldman WH (1953) Effective therapeutic dose of isoniazid for experimental tuberculosis of guinea pigs. Am Rev Tuberc 68:75–81
Kessler R, Bartmann K (1971) Primäre Isoniazid-Resistenz bei tuberkulösen Kindern in West-Berlin. Pneumonologie 145:400–406
Kimmig J (1953) Klinische und experimentelle Untersuchungen zur Therapie der Hauttuberkulose. Z Haut-Geschlechtskr 14:69–77; 103–108
Kleeberg HH (1967) The use of chemotherapeutic agents in animal tuberculosis. The Veterinarian 4:197–211
Kleeberg HH, Olivier MS (1984) A world atlas of initial drug resistance published by the Tuberculosis Research Institute of the South African Medical Research Council, 2nd revised edition
Klose F, Knothe H (1952) Über die Einwirkung von Antibiotica und Chemotherapeutica auf *Mycobacterium tuberculosis* Typ humanus im bebrüteten Hühnerei. 3. Mitteilung: Das Verhalten von Tuberkelbakterien gegenüber Isonikotinsäurehydrazid (Rimifon, Neoteben, Sauterazid). Ärztliche Wochenschr 7:893–895

Knox R, King MB, Woodroffe RC (1952) In-vitro action of isoniazid on Mycobacterium tuberculosis. Lancet II:854–858
Knox R, Meadow PM, Worssam ARH (1956) The relationship between the catalase activity, hydrogen peroxide sensitivity and isoniazid resistance of mycobacteria. Am Rev Tuberc 73:726–734
Koch-Weser D (1956) The usefulness of C^{14} labeled compound in tuberculosis research. IVth Intern Congr Chest Diseases, Cologne, p 557
Koch-Weser D, Ebert RH (1955) The use of differential C^{14} labeling for the investigation of the in vitro antituberculous activity of isonicotinyl hydrazide of glucuronolactone. J Lab Clin Med 44:711–716
Koch-Weser D, Barclay WR, Ebert RH (1955) The influence of isoniazid and streptomycin on acid-fastness, tetrazolium reduction, growth, and survival of tubercle bacilli. Am Rev Tuberc Pulm Dis 71:556–565
Kondo E, Kanai K (1977a) Studies on the relationship between the proliferation rate of infecting tubercle bacilli and the effectiveness of chemotherapy. I. Observations in a mouse experimental model using a streptomycin-dependent strain. Kekkaku 52:411–415
Kondo E, Kanai K (1977b) Studies on the relationship between the proliferation rate of infecting tubercle bacilli and the effectiveness of chemotherapy. II. Observations in various types of infection experiment. Kekkaku 52:475–479
Kradolfer F (1970) Rifampicin, isoniazid, ethambutol, ethionamide and streptomycin in murine tuberculosis: comparative chemotherapeutic studies. Antibiot Chemother 16:352–360
Kraus P, Urbančík R, Šimánĕ Z, Reil I (1961) A contribution to the problem of the anti-isoniazid factor. Am Rev Respir Dis 84:684–689
Krebs A (1968) Mikro- und Makroorganismus unter dem Einfluß tuberkulosewirksamer Mittel. Z Tbk 128:208–217
Krebs A (1969) Experimentelle Chemotherapie der Tuberkulose. Z Erkr Atmungsorgane 130:417–448
Krebs A (1970) Experimentelle Untersuchungen zur intermittierenden Chemotherapie der Tuberkulose. Z Erkr Atmungsorgane 133:411–418
Krebs A (1975) Mykobakterielle Resistenz und Resistenzbestimmungen. In: Meissner G, Schmiedel A, Nelles A (Hrsg) Mykobakterien und mykobakterielle Krankheiten. III. Bakteriologische Grundlagen der Chemotherapie der Tuberkulose. Fischer, Jena, pp 183–250
Krebs A, Käppler W (1956) Intoleranz INH-resistenter TBB-Stämme gegenüber Glycerin. Klin Wochenschr 34:873
Kreis B (1958) Les déficiences enzymatiques des bacilles isoniazido-résistants. Adv Tuberc Res 9:178–247
Krüger-Thiemer E, Kuhn RB, Lembke A (1952) Die Hemmung von Mykobakterien durch Isonicotinsäurehydrazid. Klin Wochenschr 30:613
Krüger-Thiemer E, Kröger H, Nestler HJ, Seydel K (1975) In: Meissner G, Schmiedel A, Nelles A (Hrsg) Mykobakterien und mykobakterielle Krankheiten. Teil III. Bakteriologische Grundlagen der Chemotherapie der Tuberkulose. Wirkungsmodi antituberkulöser Chemotherapeutika. Isoniazid. Fischer, Jena, pp 257–288
Kubala E (1960) Beitrag zur Existenz eines Anti-INH-Faktors bei den Mykobakterien. Z Tbk 115:66–69
Lecocq E (1952) Apparition de la résistance à l'hydrazide de l'acide isonicotinique parmi les Mycobactéries soumises à son action. CR Soc Biol 146:1447–1449
Le Hir M, Chicou J, Hétrick G, Mercier A, Neel R, Rist N (1964) Essai clinique contrôlé de trois types de traitement oral de la tuberculose pulmonaire. Bull WHO 30:701–732
Lembke A, Kuhn RB, Krüger-Thiemer E (1952) Über die antimikrobielle Wirkung von Isonicotinsäurehydrazid. Klin Wochenschr 30:717–718
Lepri G, Capalbi S (1952) Studio sulla chemioterapia della tubercolosi: idrazide dell'acido isonicotinico ed associazioni chemio-antibiotiche nella tubercolosi oculare sperimentale. Minerva Med 43:1113–1118

Levaditi C, Vaisman A, Chaigneau-Erhard H (1953) Effets thérapeutiques de l'isonicotinhydrazide (INH) dans l'infection tuberculeuse provoquée chez le cobaye par l'inoculation intra-névraxique de *Mycobacterium tuberculosis*. Ann Inst Pasteur 84:630–633
Liebermeister K (1953) Bakteriologische Befunde mit Neoteben. Z Hyg 137:461–470
Linz R (1952) Irréversibilité de l'action inhibitrice de l'hydrazide de l'acide isonicotinique sur *Mycobacterium tuberculosis*. CR Soc Biol 146:1449–1451
Linz R, Lecocq E (1952) La sensibilité *in vitro* de *Mycobacterium tuberculosis* à l'hydrazide de l'acide isonicotinique. CR Soc Biol 146:1444–1447
Lotte A, Poussier J (1953) Traitement de 414 tuberculeux pulmonaires par l'isoniazide. Rev Tuberc (Paris) 17:1–29
Lutz A (1952) Recherches sur l'action comparée *in vitro* de l'hydrazide de l'acide isonicotinique sur diverses souches de Mycobactéries pathogènes et saprophytes. CR Soc Biol 146:1368–1372
Mackaness GB (1956) The intracellular activation of pyrazinamide and nicotinamide. Am Rev Tuberc 74:718–728
Mackaness GB, Smith N (1952) The action of isoniazid (isonicotinic acid hydrazide) on intracellular tubercle bacilli. Am Rev Tuberc 66:125–133
Mackaness GB, Smith N (1953) The bactericidal action of isoniazid, streptomycin, and terramycin on extracellular and intracellar tubercle bacilli. Am Rev Tuberc 67:322–340
Mauss H (1968) Effet de l'isoniazide sur les lésions précoces de la tuberculose de la souris. Rev Immunol (Paris) 32:357–371
Mayer E, Salamandra IA (1967) Conversion by isoniazid of hyperacute to chronic pulmonary tuberculosis in mice. Am Rev Respir Dis 96:220–228
Mc Cune RM Jr, Tompsett R (1956) Fate of Mycobacterium tuberculosis in mouse tissue as determined by the microbial enumeration technique. I. The persistence of drug-susceptible tubercle bacilli in the tissues despite prolonged antimicrobial therapy. J Exp Med 104:737–762
Mc Cune RM Jr, Tompsett R, Mc Dermott W (1956) The fate of *Mycobacterium tuberculosis* in mouse tissue as determined by the microbial enumeration technique. II. The conversion of tuberculous infection to the latent state by the administration of pyrazinamide and a companion drug. J Exp Med 104:763–802
Mc Cune R, Lee SH, Deuschle K, Mc Dermott W (1957) Ineffectiveness of isoniazid in modifying the phenomenon of microbial persistence. Am Rev Tuberc Pulm Dis 76:1106–1109
Mc Dermott W, Tompsett R (1954) Activitation of pyrazinamide and nicotinamide in acidic environment. Am Rev Tuberc 70:748–754
Meissner G (1956) Isoniazid-resistente Tuberkelbakterien. Adv Tuberc Res 7:52–100
Meissner G (1962) Primary drug resistance of the tubercle bacillus. Bacteriological, therapeutic and epidemiological aspects. Bull Int Union Tuberc XXXII:15–35
Meissner G, Berg G (1954) Ein Jahr Therapie mit Isoniacid. Beitr Klin Tuberk 111:340–352
Middlebrook G (1952) Sterilization of tubercle bacilli by isonicotinic acid hydrazide and the incidence of variants resistant to the drug in vitro. Am Rev Tuberc 65:765–767
Mitchison DA (1952) Titration of strains of tubercle bacilli against isoniazid. Lancet II:858–860
Mitchison DA (1954) Tubercle bacilli resistant to isoniazid. Virulence and response to treatment with isoniazid in guinea pigs. Br Med J I:128–131
Mitchison DA (1962) Primary drug resistance. Bull Int Union Tuberc XXXII, No 2:81–99
Mitchison DA, Selkon JB (1956) The bactericidal activities of antituberculous drugs. Am Rev Tuberc Pulm Dis 74, Suppl:109–116
Morelli E, Daddi G (1952) G Ital Tbc VI:117; cited from: Bartmann K. (1954) Tbk Arzt 8:276–282
Nasta M, Algeorgi G, Arhiri M, Negulescu V (1957) Recherches sur la chimioprophylaxie de la tuberculose expérimentale du cobaye. Rev Tuberc (Paris) 21:1013–1017
Nitti V, Ninni A (1969) *In vivo* bactericidal activity of rifampicin in combination with other antimycobacterial agents. Chemotherapy 14:356–365

Noufflard H (1954) Traitement par l'isoniazide à différentes doses d'une tuberculose expérimentale très avancée de la souris. Influence des doses élevées. CR Soc Biol 148:1757–1759
Noufflard H, Berteaux S (1960) An increased effect with increased dosage of isoniazid in experimental tuberculosis. Am Rev Respir Dis 82:561–563
Orlowski EH, Rosenfeld M, Wolter H, Schunk R (1976) Experimentelle vergleichende Untersuchung der tuberkulostatischen Wirksamkeit und Toxizität von INH, INHG und INHG-Na. Arzneimittelforsch 26:409–416
Palmer CE, Ferebee SH, Hopwood L (1956) Studies on prevention of experimental tuberculosis with isoniazid. II. Effects of different dosage regimens. Am Rev Tuberc 74:917–939
Pansy F, Stander H, Donovick R (1952) In vitro studies on isonicotinic acid hydrazide. Am Rev Tuberc 65:761–764
Pansy FE, Koerber WL, Stander H, Donovick R (1953) The inactivation of isoniazid by Dubos medium. Am Rev Tuberc 68:284–285
Pavlov EP (1970) Some factors influencing the activity of streptomycin, kanamycin and isoniazid with respect to intracellulary seated *Myco. tuberculosis*. Probl Tuberk 48, issue 9:72–76 (in Russian)
Pope H (1953) Antagonism of isoniazid by certain metabolites. Am Rev Tuberc 68:938–939
Pope H (1956) The neutralization of isoniazid activity in *Mycobacterium tuberculosis* by certain metabolites. Am Rev Tuberc Pulm Dis 73:735–747
Ramakrishnan CV, Bhatia AL, Devadatta S, Fox W, Narayana ASL, Selkon JB, Velu S (1962) The course of pulmonary tuberculosis in patients excreting organisms which have acquired resistance to isoniazid. Bull WHO 26:1–18
Rist N (1964) Nature and development of resistance of tubercle bacilli to chemotherapeutic agents. In: Barry VC (ed) Chemotherapy of tuberculosis. Butterworths, London, pp 192–227
Rist N, Grumbach F (1952a) Sur l'activité antituberculeuse expérimentale de l'hydraside de l'acide iso-nicotinique. C R Soc Biol 146:564–566
Rist N, Grumbach F (1952b) La résistance du bacille tuberculeux à l'hydrazide isonicotinique. Rev Tuberc (Paris) 16:665–669
Rist N, Grumbach F, Cals S, Riebel J (1952) L'hydrazide de l'acide isonicotinique (INH). Activité antituberculeuse chez la souris. Création de souches résistants *in vitro*. Ann Inst Pasteur 82:757–760
Robson JM, Sullivan FM (1959) The effect of treatment with a large dose of isoniazid on an established tuberculous infection in mice. Br J Pharmacol 14:222–228
Robson JM, Smith JT, Thomas CGA (1960) Multiplication of *Mycobacterium tuberculosis* in the cornea and its modification by immunity and by isoniazid. Am Rev Respir Dis 82:195–201
Schaefer WB (1954) The effect of isoniazid on growing and resting tubercle bacilli. Am Rev Tuberc 69:125–127
Schmidt LH (1956a) Some observations on the utility of simian pulmonary tuberculosis in defining the therapeutic potentialities of isoniazid. Am Rev Tuberc Pulm Dis 74, part 2:138–159
Schmidt LH (1956b) Studies on the therapeutic properties of cycloserine. Trans 15th Conf Chemother Tuberc VAAF:353–365
Schmidt LH (1959) Observations on the utility of isoniazid in the prophylaxis of experimental tuberculosis. Bull Int Union Tuberc XXIX:276–284
Schmidt LH, Grover AA, Hoffmann R, Rehm J, Sullivan R (1958) The emergence of isoniazid-sensitive bacilli in monkeys inoculated with isoniazid-resistant strains. Trans 17th Conf Chemother Tuberc VAAF:264–269
Schmidt LH, Good RC, Mack HP, Zeek-Minning P, Schmidt IG (1963) An experimental appraisal of the therapeutic potentialities of ethambutol. Trans 22nd Research Conf Pulm Dis VAAF:262–274
Schriever O, Hoffmann K (1953) Zur Ermittlung des Resistenzwertes von Tuberkelbakterien gegen Neoteben. Beitr Klin Tuberk 109:53–56

Schwartz WS, Moyer RE (1954) The use of isoniazid alone in the treatment of pulmonary tuberculosis. Am Rev Tuberc 70:924–925
Shepard CC (1957) Use of Hela cells infected with tubercle bacilli for the study of antituberculous drugs. J Bacteriol 73:494–498
Siebenmann CO (1953) Isoniazid in combined chemotherapy of experimental tuberculosis in mice. Am Rev Tuberc 68:411–418
Simon K (1958) INH-Resistenz, ihre Auswirkung auf Prognose und Therapie beim Jugendlichen. Tbk Arzt 12:493–500
Singh B, Mitchison DA (1954) Bactericidal activity of streptomycin and isoniazid against tubercle bacilli. Br Med J I:130–132
Singh B, Mitchison DA (1955) The bactericidal activities of combinations of streptomycin, isoniazid, p-aminosalicylic acid (PAS), oxytetracycline (terramycin) and viomycin against *Mycobacterium tuberculosis*. J gen Microbiol 13:176–184
Spiess H (1959) Chemoprophylaxe und präventive Chemotherapie gegen die Tuberkulose. Dtsch Med Wochenschr 84:1410–1415
Steenken W Jr, Wolinsky E (1952) Antituberculous properties of hydrazines of isonicotinic acid (Rimifon, Marsilid). Am Rev Tuberc 65:365–375
Steenken W Jr, Wolinsky E (1953) Virulence of tubercle bacilli recovered from patients treated with isoniazid. Am Rev Tuberc 68:548–556
Stewart SM, Crofton JW (1964) The clinical significance of low degrees of drug resistance in pulmonary tuberculosis. Am Rev Respir Dis 89:811–829
Stoica E, Nitzulesco G (1971) Etude comparative de l'action de l'isoniazide (INH) et de la tuberculoprotéine (PPD) sur le sort des mycobactéries phagocytées par les macrophages alvéolaires „in vitro". Acta Tuberc Pneumol Belg 62:48–61
Stonebrink B (1958) The use of pyruvate containing egg medium in the culture of isoniazid resistant strains of *Mycobacterium tuberculosis* var hominis. Acta tuberc scand 35:67–80
Studer A, Fust B (1952) Protrahierte und therapeutische Wirkung von Rimifon bei experimenteller Mäusetuberkulose. Schweiz Z Allg Pathol Bakteriol 15:612–622
Sugimoto J (1970) Studies on the effects of chemotherapy with streptomycin and isoniazid in experimental pneumoconiotuberculosis. J Nara Med Ass 21:253–266
Suter E (1952) Multiplication of tubercle bacilli within phagocytes cultivated in vitro, and effect of streptomycin and isonicotinic acid hydrazide. Am Rev Tuberc 65:775–776
Takahashi H (1959) Experimental tuberculous meningitis in guinea pigs. 3. The effect of the administration of SM or INH alone and of SM, INH and PAS in combination. Kekkaku 34:665–666
Takayama K, Wang L, Merkal RS (1973) Scanning electron microscopy of the H37Ra strain of *Mycobacterium tuberculosis* exposed to isoniazid. Antimicrob Agents Chemother 4:62–65
Tirunarayanan MO, Vischer WA (1957) Relationship of isoniazid to the metabolism of mycobacteria. Am Rev Tuberc Pulm Dis 75:62–70
Tison F (1952a) Sensibilité de divers germes et du bacille de Koch à l'hydrazide de l'acide isonicotinique. Ann Inst Pasteur 82:760–761
Tison F (1952b) Dissociation des pouvoirs bactériostatique et bactéricide de l'hydrazide isonicotinique *in vitro*. Ann Inst Pasteur 83:134–135
Tompsett R (1954) Quantitative observations on the pattern of emergence of resistance to isoniazid. Am Rev Tuberc 70:91–101
Tripathy SP, Menon NK, Mitchison DA, Narayana ASL, Somasundaram PA, Stott H, Velu S (1969) Response to treatment with isoniazid plus PAS of tuberculous patients with primary isoniazid resistance. Tubercle (Lond) 50:257–267
Tuberculosis Chemotherapy Centre, Madras (1960) A concurrent comparison of isoniazid plus PAS with three regimens of isoniazid alone in the domiciliary treatment of pulmonary tuberculosis in South India. Bull WHO 23:535–585
Uehlinger E, Siebenmann R, Frei H (1952) Erste Erfahrungen mit Rimifon „Roche" bei experimenteller Meerschweinchentuberkulose. Schweiz Med Wochenschr 82:335–338
Ungar J, Tomich EG, Parkin KR, Muggleton PW (1954) Effect of pyridoxine on the action of isoniazid. Lancet II:220–221

United States Public Health Service Cooperative Investigation (1953) The effect of streptomycin on the emergence of bacterial resistance to isoniazid. Am Rev Tuberc 67:553–567

Urbančík R, Trnka L (1962) Preliminary observations on the increase in isoniazid resistance of *M. tuberculosis* H37Rv after exposure to an extract of tuberculous tissue. Am Rev Respir Dis 85:596–598

Urbanczik R, Trnka L (1963) Report on the antimicrobial activity of Isoxyl on *M. tuberculosis* "in vitro" and "in vivo". Acta Tuberc Pneumol Belg 54:66–86

Veltman G (1955) Experimentelle Untersuchungen zur Chemotherapie der Tuberkulose. 1. Mitteilung. Z Bakteriol Mikrobiol Hyg (A) 63:177–209

Vischer WA, Roulet FC (1963) Kombinierte Chemotherapie bei der Maustuberkulose. Beitr Klin Tuberk 126:253–270

Wagner WH (1964) Experimentelle Infektionen mit Tuberkelbakterien. In: Eichler O (Hrsg) Erzeugung von Krankheitszuständen durch das Experiment. Springer, Berlin Göttingen Heidelberg, pp 354–430 (Handbook of Experimental Pharmacology, vol 16, Teil 9)

Wagner WH, Saar G (1953) Untersuchungen über die Wirkung von Isonicotinsäurehydrazid in vitro. Beitr Klin Tuberk 110:236–241

Waksman SA, Lechevalier HA (1953) Sensitivity of actinomycetales to isonicotinic acid hydrazide, compared to other synthetic and antibiotic antituberculosis agents. Am Rev Tuberc 67:261–264

Wallace A (1964) The stability of some antituberculosis drugs. Bull Int Union Tuberc XXXIV:191

Wasz-Höckert O, Mc Cune RM Jr, Tompsett R (1956) Concurrent administration of pyridoxine and isoniazid. Am Rev Tuberc Pulm Dis 74:471–473

Werner E, Drobny H, Ziesché K (1963) Ergebnisse einer fünfjährigen ambulanten INH-Langzeitbehandlung. Beitr Klin Tuberk 126:329–338

Wolinsky E, Pratt P, Steenken W Jr (1954) Experimental tuberculous meningitis in guinea pigs: results of treatment with isoniazid, iproniazid, streptomycin, and isoniazid-streptomycin. Am Rev Tuberc 70:714–727

Youatt J (1969) A review of the action of isoniazid. Am Rev Respir Dis 99:729–749

Youmans AS, Youmans GP (1955) The inactivation of isoniazid by filtrates and extracts of mycobacteria. Am Rev Tuberc Pulm Dis 72:196–203

Youmans AS, Youmans GP (1956) The effect of the „anti-isoniazid" substance produced by mycobacteria on the chemotherapeutic activity of isoniazid in vivo. Am Rev Tuberc Pulm Dis 73:764–767

Youmans AS, Youmans GP (1960) The production of „anti-isoniazid" substance by isoniazid-susceptible, isoniazid-resistant, and unclassified strains of mycobacteria. Am Rev Respir Dis 81:929–931

Żebrowski T, Pieniążek K, Borowiecka A (1954) Die Behandlung der chronischen Experimentaltuberkulose der Meerschweinchen mit Isoniazid jeden Tag und jeden dritten Tag. Beitr Klin Tuberk 111:335–339

Zierski M, Rotermund C (1984) Isoniazid – Wesentliches und Neues. Prax Klin Pneumol 38:201–216

Zintz R, Wegner W (1953) Über die Behandlung der tierexperimentellen und menschlichen Augentuberkulose mit Neoteben. Dtsch Med Wochenschr 78:433–435

VI. Tetracyclines

L. TRNKA

The group of tetracycline antibiotics as discussed here includes chlortetracycline (CTC), oxytetracycline (OTC), and tetracycline (TC). They have similar structures, almost identical antimicrobial spectra, and complete mutual cross-resistance, and they produce the same pattern of side effects. Where they do differ, however, is in some pharmacokinetic properties, and particularly in their distribution in tissues, organs, and body fluids. The group as a whole was discovered in the late "forties" and early "fifties" (for a review see MODR 1962; MODR et al. 1964; HLAVKA and BOOTHE 1985). Publications on the effectiveness of the later developed derivatives are nearly completely lacking as far as *M. tuberculosis* is concerned. Data on their activity against atypical mycobacteria are presented by BARTMANN in Chap. 4 of this book.

1. Antimicrobial Spectrum in Vitro

The results reported by FINLAY et al. (1950), HOBBY et al. (1950), and many subsequent authors emphasize the strong antimicrobial activity of CTC and OTC and of their salts against a broad spectrum of aerobic and anaerobic gram-positive and gram-negative bacteria and against certain rickettsiae. The minimal inhibitory concentrations in vitro are usually below 1 μg/ml: for the majority of the gram-positives they range between 0.2 μg/ml and 1.2 μg/ml and for the majority of gram-negatives between 0.4 μg/ml and 3.1 μg/ml, with individual strain variations. Strains of *K. pneumoniae, E. aerogenes, E. coli, S. dysenteriae* and *paratyphosa* are more sensitive to CTC than to OTC; the MIC values of CTC are about one-half of those of OTC.

Most strains of *P. vulgaris* and *Ps. aeruginosa* are rather insensitive to CTC and OTC. OTC in concentrations as high as 300 μg/ml of medium was incapable of inhibiting the growth of nine strains of fungi (*Nocardia asteroides, Sporotrichum schenckii, Microsporon canis, Trichophyton rubrum, Cryptococcus neoformans, Trichophyton mentagrophytes, Candida albicans, Epidermophyton floccosum*, and *Microsporum audouini*) (HOBBY et al. 1950).

The minimal inhibitory concentrations of TC are within the same range as those of the other tetracyclines, and its activity covers the same microbial spectrum. Because of the widespread use of the tetracyclines for many years the incidence of initially resistant strains is now much higher than in the early "fifties".

2. Antimycobacterial Activity

a) Activity in Artificial Media in Vitro

The antimycobacterial activity in artificial media in vitro was studied for the individual drugs soon after their discovery. The strains H37Rv of *M. tuberculosis* and BCG of *M. bovis* were generally used at first, and later experiments on larger numbers of strains of tubercle bacilli were performed comparatively for groups of tetracyclines.

Table 1. Antimycobacterial activity of CTC, OTC, and TC in vitro

Author	Strain	Minimal inhibitory concentration			Medium
		CTC	OTC	TC	
RAKE and DONOVICK (1949)	H37Rv	4.55			Kirchner with Triton without serum
	Ravenel	12.5			
	BCG	0.36			
	BCG	0.27–1.0			Kirchner with serum
STEENKEN and WOLINSKY (1949, 1950)	H37Rv		1.0–5.0		Dubos albumin with Tween
			5.0–10.0		Proskauer-Beck
			50.0–100.0		Proskauer-Beck with serum
	H37Rv SM-resistant		1.0–5.0		Dubos albumin with Tween
STEINBACH et al. (1950)	H37Rv	1.0			Dubos albumin with Tween
HOBBY et al. (1951)	H37Rv	10.0	10.0	8.0	Dubos albumin with Tween
	"wild strains"	8.0–12.0	3.0–8.0	4.0–16.0	Ditto
HOBBY and LENERT (1955)	H37Rv	31.0	31.0	1.6	Dubos albumin with Tween at pH 6.8
	–INH–R	31.0	31.0	6.3	
	–PAS–R	31.0	16.0	0.8	
	–SM–R	31.0	31.0	6.3	
	BCG	2.0	2.0	0.8	
	"wild strains"	2.0–63.0	2.0–63.0	0.2–6.3	
GUY and CHAPMAN (1961)	Non-tuberculous mycobateria	>20.0	>20.0	>20.0	
	photochromogenic, scotochromogenic	>20.0	>20.0	>20.0	
	fast-growing	>20.0	>20.0	>20.0	

The in-vitro tests were carried out in a conventional manner, usually with liquid media and incubation periods ranging from 5 days to 14 days. The results of the published studies are summarized in Table 1.

It is apparent that in vitro TC was more active than CTC and OTC against strains of *M. tuberculosis* and *M. bovis*. The activity of the drugs against *M. tuberculosis*, strain H37Rv, was the same irrespective of sensitivity or resistance to INH, SM, or PAS. On the other hand, the tetracyclines were rather ineffective against non-tuberculous (atypical) mycobacteria.

It may be concluded that, when tested under the conditions of in-vitro experiments summarized in Table 1, CTC and OTC possess the same antimycobacterial activity, which may be described as weak. The in-vitro activity of TC is somewhat higher, corresponding to that of viomycin.

α) Factors Affecting the Activity in Vitro. The activity of tetracyclines in vitro was found to be enhanced at pH 5.5, while that of SM and VM was frequently diminished in the acid range, and the activity of INH was unaffected by changes in pH (HOBBY and LENERT 1955). This might indicate that the antimycobacterial action of tetracyclines is enhanced in areas of inflammation or necrotic tissue or inside the host cells.

β) Resistance of Mycobacteria to Tetracyclines

Development of Resistance in Vitro and Its Type: STEENKEN and WOLINSKY (1950) attempted to develop OTC-resistant tubercle bacilli by serial transfer in Dubos albumin medium with Tween and various drug concentrations, but after 5 transfers at 10-day intervals no increase in resistance could be detected. HOBBY et al. (1951) found that tubercle bacilli resistant to OTC emerged from otherwise sensitive cultures at an extremely slow rate.

The development of tetracycline resistance probably follows the multiple-step pattern in tubercle bacilli, as has been described for other microorganisms (MODR et al. 1964).

Cross-Resistance: A complete cross-resistance of tubercle bacilli is found between CTC, OTC, and TC. Cross-resistance between tetracyclines and other antimycobacterial drugs has not, so far, been reported.

γ) Type of Action. The effect of the tetracyclines on tubercle bacilli is bacteriostatic. This has been established by MACKANESS and SMITH (1953), who studied the survival rates of *M. tuberculosis* (H37Rv) in Dubos-Davis medium during exposure to various tetracycline concentrations. HOBBY et al. (1950) observed that tetracyclines were highly bacteriostatic against a wide range of microorganisms, although under certain conditions there were indications of a bactericidal activity.

δ) Activity in Combination with Antimycobacterial Drugs in Vitro. Studying the interference of CTC and OTC with SM in vitro, JAWETZ et al. (1951) observed that both tetracyclines antagonized the bactericidal action of SM, the effect being most marked during the first 12 h of incubation of *Klebsiella pneumoniae*. The antagonism was most pronounced at bacteriostatic concentrations. This interference was observed only with organisms sensitive to SM; in the case of a bacterial strain resistant to SM tetracyclines might have a synergistic action.

MACKANESS and SMITH (1953) also used the in-vitro method outlined above. The inocula were prepared from shallow cultures grown in Dubos-Davis medium, containing 0.05% of Tween 80 and 0.25% of heat-inactivated bovine albumin fraction V. The cultures were shaken daily to promote dispersion and were harvested after 11 days. The growth was pooled and washed in fresh medium. The final suspension was lightly centrifuged to settle the larger aggregates, and the density of the supernatant was adjusted according to particular requirements. The survival rate of *M. tuberculosis* (H37Rv) during exposure to various drug concentrations could thus be followed. It was found that OTC (10 μg/ml) used in combination with INH (0.1 μg/ml) abolished the bactericidal activity of the latter. The results have been confirmed by SINGH and MITCHISON (1955), who extended the finding of the antagonistic action of tetracyclines also to VM. The reduced killing rate is probably due to a transformation of the bacilli into the resting state by tetracycline.

b) Effect on Mycobacteria in Cell and Tissue Cultures

MACKANESS and SMITH (1953) suggested that tetracyclines might have a free passage into cells. They studied the survival rate of *M. tuberculosis* (H37Rv) in isolated mammalian macrophage cultures during exposure to various drug concentrations. In comparison with INH, the effect of OTC was weak under these experimental conditions.

c) Activity of Tetracyclines in Experimental Tuberculosis

α) Monotherapy. PERRY (1949) tested the activity of CTC on tuberculosis in guinea pigs. The animals were inoculated with 0.02 mg of virulent tubercle bacilli and the treatment was started after 28 days. CTC was given subcutaneously in a daily dose of 10 mg/kg for 42 days. The same animal model was used by STEENKEN and WOLINSKY (1950). The animals were treated by CTC given intramuscularly in a daily dose of 3.2 mg/kg for 42 days. In both reports the results were evaluated as negative. It was shown that CTC given in much higher dosage than that used for other infections failed to influence favorably the course of guinea pig tuberculosis and produced definite toxicity.

RAKE and DONOVICK (1949) estimated that the maximal tolerated daily oral dose of CTC in albino mice was 250 mg/kg. No detactable effects upon the course of infection were found in mice infected with virulent tubercle bacilli and treated orally with a daily dose of 25 mg/kg–100 mg/kg. The ineffectiveness of CTC in mouse tuberculosis was later confirmed by STEINBACH et al. (1950), who injected the drug subcutaneously in daily doses of 1 mg/kg–5 mg/kg.

OTC proved to be somewhat more active than CTC in delaying the development of tuberculosis, but the activity was low (STEENKEN and WOLINSKY 1950). Guinea pigs infected subcutaneously with 0.1 mg *M. tuberculosis* (H37Rv) were treated 26 days after the infection with oral OTC in the dose of 10 mg/kg. The toxic dose for this route of administration was 100 mg/kg.

Preliminary studies carried out by HOBBY et al. (1950) indicated that OTC in a daily dose of 7.1 mg/kg administered subcutaneously was sufficient to exert a suppressive effect on tuberculosis in mice. After both oral and parenteral administration, the drug was absorbed rapidly into the circulatory system. Significant concentrations were detected in the urine of the injected animals in a biologically active form.

Later HOBBY et al. (1951) used lower doses of OTC, namely 1 mg/kg–3 mg/kg administered to tuberculous mice by the subcutaneous route. They reported a weak retarding effect. The effect of TC in vivo was reported by HOBBY and LENERT (1955). Despite its apparently greater activity in vitro, in murine tuberculosis TC appeared to be no more effective than OTC, which in turn was somewhat more effective than CTC, but only at higher doses. In view of this, no further studies on this drug were performed in experimental models.

β) Combination Therapy. No reports on experiments in animal models are available. One of the reasons is that tetracyclines have been found to have little therapeutic effect in patients with pulmonary tuberculosis (PFEFER et al. 1952; SÖDERHOLM 1952). However, MILLER et al. (1952, 1954) and ROTHSTEIN and JOHNSON (1954) have shown that OTC with SM was as effective as SM + PAS or as SM + INH in preventing the emergence of SM-resistant populations. Furthermore, STEWART et al. (1954) found that OTC + INH effectively suppressed the emergence of INH-resistant tubercle bacilli in patients who excreted bacilli with initial resistance to SM, to PAS, or to both.

d) Further Tetracycline Derivatives

FUSSGÄNGER (1958) mentioned that pyrrolidinomethyltetracycline, a derivative designed for parenteral use, gave the same MIC as TC for a strain of *M. tuberculosis* tested as representative of this bacterial species.

Minocycline was investigated by REDIN (1967) in mice infected intravenously with *M. tuberculosis*, strain H37Rv. The treatment was started on the day of the infection, the drug being applied for 2 weeks in the diet or once daily by gavage or by the subcutaneous route. The median effective doses, calculated from the 60-day survival rates, were 85 mg/kg/day for the subcutaneous route and 100 mg/kg/day–120 mg/kg/day for both forms of oral treatment. The maximal tolerated doses of TC and PAS (e.g., 1600 mg/kg/day of TC or 800 mg/kg/day of PAS when given by gavage) increased the survival time slightly, but not enough to permit a calculation of median effective doses.

3. Concluding Remarks

Tetracyclines inhibit *M. tuberculosis* in vitro at concentrations that would require high doses to be attained in the human body. The action is purely bacteriostatic. The activity in various animal models is weak. The experimental data suggested that tetracyclines would be useful only as reserve drugs, and this was indeed found to be true in the treatment of human tuberculosis.

References

Finlay AC, Hobby GL, P'an SY, Regna PP, Routien JB, Seeley DB, Shull GM, Sobin BA, Solomons IA, Vinson JW, Kane JH (1950) Terramycin, a new antibiotic. Science 111:85

Fussgänger R (1958) Vergleichende mikrobiologische Untersuchungen von Pyrrolidino-methyl-tetracyclin (Reverin®) mit Tetracyclin-hydrochlorid. MMW 100:665–670

Guy LR, Chapman JS (1961) Susceptibility in vitro of unclassified mycobacteria to commonly used antimicrobials. Am Rev Resp Dis 84:746–749

Hlavka JJ, Boothe JH (1985) The tetracyclines. Handbook of experimental pharmacology, vol 78. Springer, Berlin Heidelberg New York Tokyo

Hobby GL, Dougherty N, Lenert TF, Hidders E, Kiseluk M (1950) Antimicrobial action of terramycin in vitro and in vivo. Proc Soc Exp Biol Med 73:503–511

Hobby GL, Lenert TF, Donikian M, Pikula D (1951) The tuberculostatic activity of terramycin. Am Rev Tub 61:434–440

Hobby GL, Lenert TF (1955) Antituberculous activity of tetracycline and related compounds. Am Rev Tub 72:367–372

Jawetz E, Gunnison JB, Speck RS (1951) Interference of aureomycin, chloramphenicol and terramycin with the action of streptomycin. Am J Med Sci 222:404–410
Mackaness GB, Smith N (1953) The bactericidal action of isoniazid, streptomycin and terramycin on extracellular and intracelluar tubercle bacilli. Am Rev Tub 67:322–340
Miller FL, Sands JH, Walker R, Dye WE, Tempel CW (1952) Combined daily terramycin and intermittent streptomycin in the treatment of pulmonary tuberculosis. Am Rev Tub 66:534–542
Miller FL, Sands JH, Gregory LJ, Hightower JA, Weisser OL, Tempel CW (1954) Daily oxytetracycline (terramycin) and intermittent streptomycin in the treatment of pulmonary tuberculosis. Am Rev Tub 69:58–67
Modr Z (1962) Antibiotics their use in therapy (in Czech). Spofa, Prague
Modr Z, Heřmanský M, Vlček V (1964) Antibiotics and their pharmaceutical products (in Czech). Avicenum, Prague
Perry TL (1949) Failure of aureomycin in the treatment of experimental tuberculosis. Proc Soc Exp Biol Med 72:45–46
Pfefer LM, Hughes FJ, Dye WE (1952) Terramycin in the treatment of pulmonary tuberculosis: a pilot study. Dis Chest 21:123–124
Rake G, Donovick R (1949) Tuberculostatic activity of aureomycin in vitro and in vivo. Am Rev Tub 60:143
Redin GS (1967) Antibacterial activity in mice of minocycline, a new tetracycline. Antimicrob Agents Chemother 1966:371–376
Rothstein E, Johnson M (1954) Streptomycin and oxytetracycline (terramycin) in the treatment of pulmonary tuberculosis. Am Rev Tub Pulm Dis 69:65–70
Singh B, Mitchison DA (1955) The bactericidal activities of combinations of streptomycin, isoniazid, p-aminosalicylic acid (PAS), oxytetracycline (terramycin) and viomycin against Mycobacterium tuberculosis. J Gen Microbiol 13:176–184
Söderholm B (1952) Clinical experiments with terramycin in the treatment of pulmonary tuberculosis. Acta Tub Scand 27:109–116
Steenken W Jr, Wolinsky E (1949) Tuberculostatic activity of aureomycin in vitro and in vivo. Am Rev Tub 59:221–223
Steenken W Jr, Wolinsky E (1950) The tuberculostatic action of terramycin in vitro and in the experimental animal. Ann NY Acad Sci 53:309–318
Steinbach MM, Baker H, Duca CHJ (1950) A comparative study of susceptibility of tubercle bacillus (H37Rv) to aureomycin, streptomycin and para-aminosalicyclic acid. Proc Soc Exp Biol Med 74:596–598
Stewart S, Turnbull FWA, Crofton JW (1954) The use of oxytetracycline in preventing and delaying isoniazid resistance in pulmonary tuberculosis. Br Med J II:1508

VII. Viomycin (VM)

L. TRNKA

1. Antimicrobial Spectrum in Vitro and in Vivo

Soon after its isolation the antimicrobial activity of VM sulphate was tested in vitro. Almost identical minimal inhibitory concentrations of VM sulphate (in μg/ml) on various bacterial species were reported by BARTZ et al. (1951), EHRLICH et al. (1951), and HOBBY et al. (1951).

The minimal inhibitory concentration of VM sulphate on *Aerobacter aerogenes* was 10 μg/ml–25 μg/ml, on *B. subtilis* 25 μg/ml, on *Br. abortus* 50 μg/ml, on *E. coli* 10 μg/ml to >100 μg/ml, on *N. catarrhalis* 10 μg/ml–25 μg/ml, on *N. meningitidis* 25 μg/ml, on *K. pneumoniae* type A 10 μg/ml, on *P. vulgaris* >100 μg/ml, on *Ps. aeruginosa* >100 μg/ml, on *S. typhosa* 10 μg/ml–25 μg/ml, on *Str. pneumoniae* 50 μg/ml, etc.

These data thus show that VM is moderately active on gram-positive bacteria and less active on the gram-negatives.

In contrast, VM proved to be inactive on human and plant pathogenic fungi at concentrations as high as 250 µg/ml (EHRLICH et al. 1951). The same authors reported that the antibiotic had no activity against two protozoa and several small viruses. Antiphage activity of VM has been reported at inordinately high concentrations (5 mg/ml) (CALTRIDER 1967).

The antimicrobial activity of VM sulphate tended to increase with increasing initial pH in the range between pH 7.1 and 8.5, and the greater part of this activity was maintained in broth cultures for at least 6 days (EHRLICH et al. 1951).

Under comparable conditions, even at high doses, VM failed to protect mice against experimental infections due to *Str. hemolyticus, Str. pneumoniae, Ps. aeruginosa,* or *P. vulgaris*. It was, however, effective against these organisms after oral or subcutaneous administration, provided that a sufficiently high dose had been used (HOBBY et al. 1951).

2. Antimycobacterial Activity

a) Activity in Artificial Media in Vitro

The data on the antimycobacterial activity of VM sulphate on laboratory (H37Rv) or patient strains of *M. tuberculosis,* either sensitive or resistant to other antituberculotics, are summarized in Table 1.

It will be seen that VM inhibits the growth of the H37Rv strain at concentrations ranging from 2 µg/ml to 12 µg/ml and the growth of "wild" strains (isolated from tuberculous patients) at about the same concentrations. The inhibitory activity on solid egg media is lower than on media without egg-yolk.

In-vitro studies have shown that strains of tubercle bacilli resistant to SM, PAS, or neomycin are as sensitive to VM as the respective parent strains.

The activity of VM on other mycobacterial species (*M. bovis,* potentially pathogenic mycobacteria such as *M. kansasii,* etc.) in vitro was less evident (LEVADITI 1951; PLICHET 1951; TACQUET and CHENET 1951; BARTMANN et al. 1956).

α) Factors Affecting the Activity in Vitro. The inhibitory effect of VM in artificial media was evidently not antagonized by the presence of serum (STEENKEN and WOLINSKY 1951; YOUMANS and YOUMANS 1951). The influence of the incubation time was studied by BARTMANN et al. (1966). The MIC increases with increasing incubation time, as in the case of KM, but the critical level was not reached by any of the 50 sensitive strains tested. No other factors affecting the VM activity in vitro have so far been reported.

β) Resistance of Mycobacteria to VM

Development of Resistance in Vitro and Its Type: Resistance to VM may be due to several mechanisms, including the mutational alteration of ribosomal targets which prevent binding, enzymatic inactivation of the drug by covalent addition of acetyl, adenyl, or phosphoryl groups, and impermeability to the drug.

Table 1. Minimal inhibitory concentrations (MIC) of Viomycin for various strains of *M. tuberculosis* in vitro

Author	Species strain	MIC (μg/ml)	Remarks
COLETSOS (1951)	*M. tuberc.*		
	"wild"	10.0	Solid egg media
BARTZ et al. (1951)	*M. tuberc.*		
	H37Rv	6.25–12.5	
	H37Rv SM-R	6.25–12.5	
	"wild"	3.12– 6.25	
	ATCC 607	0.78	
	ATCC 607 SM-R	0.78	
	ATCC 607 Neo-R	0.78	
EHRLICH et al. (1951)	*M. tuberc.*		
	H37Rv	2.5 – 12.5	
FINLAY et al. (1951)	*M. tuberc.*		
	H37Rv	1.0 – 2.8	DAT[a] incub. 12 days
	"wild"	1.9 – 5.6	
HOBBY et al. (1951)	*M. tuberc.*		
	H37Rv	1.0 – 5.2	DAT
	"wild"	1.0 – 5.2	
STEENKEN and WOLINSKY (1951)	*M. tuberc.*		
	H37Rv	0.1	DAT incub. 10 days
		5.0	DAT incub. 14–21 days
		5.0	PB[b] liquid 10–21 days
		5.0	PB liquid with serum
	H37Rv SM-R	0.1	DAT incub. 10 days
		5.0	DAT incub. 14–21 days
KARLSON and GAINER (1951)	*M. tuberc.*		
	H37Rv	2.0	PB
		8.0	Solid egg-yolk medium
	H37Rv SM-R	8.0	ditto
	H37Rv PAS-R	8.0	ditto
YOUMANS and YOUMANS (1951)	*M. tuberc.*		
	H37Rv	3.12	PB
		6.25	PB with bovine serum
	"wild"	3.25– 6.25	PB
		6.25–12.5	PB with bovine serum
HOBBY et al. (1953)	*M. tuberc.*		
	H37Rv	0.4[c]	DAT
	H37Rv SM-R	0.4[c]	DAT
	"wild"	0.5 –80.0	
AOYAGI et al. (1975)	*M. tuberc.*		
	H37Rv	5.0	DAT semiliquid
		20.00–40.0	1% Ogawa solid

[a] Dubos albumin (0.5%) – Tween (0.02%) liquid medium.
[b] Proskauer-Beck liquid medium.
[c] Equivalent amount of pure VM base.

TSUKAMURA (1961) has suggested that the VM resistance of *M. tuberculosis* strain H37Rv follows a multistep pattern of development and that it is controlled by one gene. Slight differences in the degree of resistance could be due to additional factors. With the strain *M. Jucho* an obligatory single-step pattern of development and only one phenotype was observed. YAMADA et al. (1972, 1976) have reported that VM-resistant mutants of *M. smegmatis* may have mutations at two different genetic loci, one of which results in an altered 30s ribosomal subunit and the other in mutation at the 50s ribosomal subunit. The two mutants have different degrees of resistance to other aminoglycoside antibiotics. These results would thus confirm the earlier suggestions, made by MAC KENZIE and JORDAN in 1970.

EHRLICH et al. (1951) concluded that the resistance to VM, like that to streptomycin, seems to emerge suddenly, and that the rates of emergence of resistance of *M. tuberculosis* strain H37Rv to VM and SM are probably not significantly different.

According to GROSSET and CANETTI (1962), the proportion of variants resistant to VM is roughly 10 times as high as the proportion resistant to KM.

The results of YOUMANS and YOUMANS (1951) indicated that virulent strains of *M. tuberculosis* in vitro will become resistant to VM fairly rapidly (after 5–6 transfers in Dubos liquid medium containing low concentrations of VM).

Features of Resistant Populations: There is a considerable lack of knowledge on the features of VM-resistant populations of tubercle bacilli. HOK and SENG (1964) have suggested that the incidence of initial VM resistance is as low as that to SM, and it may therefore be assumed that other features of VM resistance are also rather similar to those of SM resistance.

Various methods and various critical concentrations were proposed for the laboratory testing of mycobacterial VM sensitivity/resistance. For a simplified variant of the proportion method a VM concentration of 30 µg/ml was recommended as critical (CANETTI et al. 1969). Below a critical proportion of 10% the strain was to be classified as sensitive, above 10% as resistant. The proportions are reported in percentages.

In the standard variant of the proportion method the criteria of VM resistance are as follows: 10% for the concentration of 20 µg/ml, 1% for the concentration of 30 µg/ml, and 50% for the concentration of 10 µg/ml (CANETTI et al. 1969).

In the method used by the Medical Research Council of Great Britain (Resistance Ratio method), three concentrations of VM above and below the usual endpoints for sensitive strains are tried, referred to as respectively the lower, the middle, and the upper concentration.

The sensitive strains are defined as those not growing on the lower concentration. Resistance means growth on the middle or upper concentration, or growth on the lower concentration followed by similar growth in a further test done on the control slope or on another culture from the same patient (CANETTI et al. 1969).

TSUKAMURA et al. (1975) recommended 200 µg VM/ml as the critical concentration on solid egg media. The high concentration is needed in the absolute-concentration method, where the size of the inoculum can easily influence the results.

VM Dependence: In contrast to the situation with SM, the phenomenon of VM dependence of tubercle bacilli has not so far been reported.

Cross-Resistance: MCCLATCHY et al. (1977) isolated mutants resistant to SM, KM, CM, RMP, and VM from four strains of *M. tuberculosis*. The mutants isolated from each parent strain were then tested for the development of cross-resistance to other drugs.

Complete cross-resistance was found for VM and CM, but not for other drugs. The cross-resistance between VM and KM was variable. VM inhibits the growth of tubercle bacilli already resistant to KM, but the opposite does not apply (ŠIMÁNĚ et al. 1966; BARTMANN 1970; KOHOUT 1973). VM-resistant strains are sometimes also resistant to SM, but not vice versa (BARTMANN 1970).

γ) Type of Action. After the original paper by GERNEZ-RIEUX et al. (1951) it was assumed that VM acts only bacteriostatically on tubercle bacilli, but SINGH and MITCHISON (1955) reported a bactericidal effect with 40 μg/ml. The killing rate was less than that produced by 20 μg/ml SM. HOBBY and LENERT (1957) also reported a killing of over 99% of the bacterial population after 4 days of incubation in a nutrient medium with 9 μg VM/ml at 37 °C. The viable count remained unaltered on incubation of tubercle bacilli in a phosphate buffer with 100 μg VM/ml. It can therefore be concluded that VM has a growth-dependent bactericidal effect, but weaker than that of SM.

δ) Effects in Combination with Antituberculotic Drugs in Vitro. SINGH and MITCHISON (1955) are the only authors to report results of experiments performed in vitro with combinations of VM and other antituberculotic drugs. The drugs were added to Tween/albumin cultures of the H37Rv strain of *M. tuberculosis*, so that the final concentration approximated to those found in the serum of patients treated with the usual therapeutic doses. Surface viable counts on oleic acid and albumin agar were then carried out at intervals from these cultures.

VM alone at a concentration of 40 μg/ml caused a decrease in $\log_{10}$ viable units from 6.5 to 3.5 within 14 days of incubation. After that time an increase in viable counts appeared in the next 2 weeks of incubation. This phenomenon was caused by the growth of VM-resistant organisms. SM at a concentration of 20 units/ml was more active in the depression of viable counts. A secondary increase was observed at about the same time as in VM cultures. In a combination, VM seemed to reduce the activity of SM, but the degree of antagonism was so slight as to be of doubtful significance. The combination was, however, more active than VM alone and prevented the appearance of a VM- or SM-resistant population.

In contrast, a combination of VM and INH (2 μg/ml) was distinctly more active than either of the two drugs alone. The appearance of a resistant population was also prevented. A triple combination of VM, SM, and INH was more active than any of the double combinations tested. Oxytetracycline (10 μg/ml) prevented the killing activity of VM during the first 7 days of incubation; PAS (100 μg/ml) had no demonstrable antagonistic or synergistic effect.

b) Effects on Mycobacteria in Cell and Tissue Cultures

MACKANESS (1952) studied the bacteriostatic effects of various antituberculotics on the Branch bovine strain in Dubos-Davis medium and in rabbit macrophage cultures. The MIC values were 6.25 μg/ml for extracellular bacilli and 100 μg/ml for intracellular. The respective concentrations of SM were 0.6 μg/ml and 10 μg/ml. SHEPARD (1957) found an MIC of 4 μg/ml for the H37Rv strain in a bacteriological medium, but one of 64 μg/ml to >2000 μg/ml for bacilli phagocytosed by Hela cells, the MIC being the higher, the later VM was added after ingestion of the bacilli by the cells. Taking into consideration the concentrations of VM that can be attained in vivo, at best a partial inhibition of intracellular bacilli can be expected.

c) Activity of VM in Experimental Tuberculosis

α) Monotherapy. Experiments on the activity of VM in experimental guinea pig tuberculosis were performed soon after the discovery of the drug. KARLSON and GAINER (1951) used the therapeutic type of treatment. Guinea pigs were infected with virulent strains of *M. tuberculosis* and treatment was started at the time of extensive organ involvement (on the 28th day). A daily dose of 25 mg/kg divided into two subcutaneous administrations was given for 62 days, and all treated and the untreated animals were then killed. Autopsy of VM-treated animals did not show any tuberculous involvement of the lungs, liver, and spleen. Subsequent histological studies revealed healed fibrotic lesions.

STEENKEN and WOLINSKY (1951) confirmed these results and discovered that VM at a daily dose of 80 mg/kg produced a beneficial effect approximately equal to that achieved with intramuscular administration of 20 mg/kg streptomycin. To obtain an equivalent effect a four times higher dose of VM was thus necessary.

CARR and KARLSON (1961) recommended the use of only single daily injections and found that similar therapeutic results were achieved in animals infected by tubercle bacilli sensitive and resistant to SM. There is no cross-resistance between VM and SM in vivo.

The results of preventive treatment of infected guinea pigs with VM (drug administration started on the day after the infection) were more promising because the disease had not been too extended. Sterilization of the lesions could not, however, be achieved even in these experiments. The suppressive action of VM was of limited duration, and soon after the end of the treatment tuberculosis proceeded further in the surviving animals (ŠIMÁNĚ et al. 1966).

The results obtained in the model of experimental guinea pig tuberculosis were confirmed and specified more closely in the model of experimental mouse tuberculosis (YOUMANS and YOUMANS 1951; FINLAY et al. 1951; HOBBY and LENERT 1953; AOYAGI et al. 1975). The effective doses in these models were, however, close to those already producing toxic effects. The absence of cross-resistance between VM and SM was confirmed. VM was evidently less active than streptomycin, and had the same bacteriostatic potency as tuberactinomycin.

β) Combination Therapy. VM was investigated in combination with ETH by GRUMBACH (1965). Mice with advanced tuberculosis were treated for 4 months with daily doses of 1 mg ETH, 4 mg SM, 4 mg KM, and 4 mg VM. In the combined treatments the same doses were used. In monotherapy the efficacy decreased in the sequence ETH>SM>KM>VM, for the combinations the sequence was ETH + SM>ETH + VM>ETH + KM. Whereas SM (but not VM and KM) prevented secondary resistance to ETH, VM and KM did not. ETH prevented the development of resistance to all three antibiotics.

3. Concluding Remarks

On the basis of its bacteriostatic and growth-dependent bactericidal activity, its efficacy against intracellular bacilli, and its effectiveness in animals, VM is inferior to SM. Furthermore, it is more toxic than SM in animals and in man. For those reasons VM could not replace SM. Its advantage was its full activity exerted on SM-resistant tubercle bacilli. This was then the indication for its clinical use until KM, and later CM, had become isolated. KM and CM were equal or superior in efficacy, and were better tolerated than VM, which was now no longer useful.

References

Aoyagi T, Kawai T, Yamada Y, Fujino T, Kaneko K, Aizawa Y (1975) Basic studies on viomycin and tuberactinomycin (in Japanese). Kekkaku 50:295–301

Bartmann K (1970) Discussion remark. Antibiotica et Chemotherapia 16:81–82

Bartmann K, Blisse A, Zander I (1956) Bakteriologische Untersuchungen über die Wirkung von Viomycin auf Tuberkelbakterien. Beitr Klin Tuberk 115:211–222

Bartmann K, Abel U, Hart R (1966) Die Abhängigkeit des Hemmtiters von der Bebrütungsdauer bei der Bestimmung der Resistenz von *M. tuberculosis* gegen Antituberkulotika auf Löwenstein-Jensen Medium. Zentralbl Bakteriol Mikrobiol Hyg (A) 201:538–548

Bartz QR, Ehrlich J, Mold JD, Penner MA, Smith RM (1951) Viomycin, a new tuberculostatic antibiotic. Am Rev Tuberc 63:4–6

Caltrider PG (1967) Viomycin. In: Gottlieb D, Shaw PD (eds) Antibiotics, vol I, Mechanism of action. Springer, Berlin Heidelberg New York

Canetti G, Fox W, Khomenko A, Mahler HT, Menon NK, Mitchison DA, Rist N, Šmelev NA (1969) Advances in techniques of testing mycobacterial drug sensitivity, and the use of sensitivity tests in tuberculosis control programmes. Bull WHO 41:21–43

Carr DT, Karlson AG (1961) Optimal regimens of antituberculous drugs. Am Rev Resp Dis 84:90–92

Coletsos P (1951) L'action synergique in vitro sur *Mycobacterium tuberculosis* de streptomycine-P.A.S.-viomycine-neomycine dans 11 types d'association. Rev Tuberc (Paris) 15:957–965

Ehrlich J, Smith RM, Penner MA, Anderson LE, Bratton AC Jr (1951) Antimicrobial activity of streptomyces floridae and of viomycin. Am Rev Tuberc 63:7–16

Finlay AC, Hobby GL, Hochstein F, Lees TM, Lenert TF, Means JA, P'an SY, Regna PP, Routien JB, Sobin BA, Tate KB, Kane JH (1951) Viomycin, a new antibiotic active against mycobacteria. Am Rev Tuberc 63:1–3

Gernez-Rieux CH, Tacquet A, Chenet C (1951) Étude expérimentale du pouvoir tuberculostatique de la viomycine. Rev Tuberc (Paris) 15:665–668

Grosset J, Canetti G (1962) Teneur des souches sauvages de *Mycobacterium tuberculosis* en variants résistants aux antibiotiques mineurs. Ann Inst Pasteur 103:163–184

Grumbach F (1965) Etudes chimiothérapiques sur la tuberculose avancée de la souris. Adv Tuberc Res 14:31–96

Hobby GL, Lenert TF (1953) The control of experimental mouse tuberculosis by the intermittent administration of streptomycin, viomycin, isoniazid and streptomycilidene isonicotinyl hydrazide. Am Rev Tuberc 68:292–306

Hobby GL, Lenert TF (1957) The in vitro action of antituberculous agents against multiplying and non-multiplying microbial cells. Am Rev Tuberc Pulm Dis 76:1031–1048

Hobby GL, Lenert TF, Donikian M, Pikula D (1951) The activity of viomycin against *Mycobacterium tuberculosis* and other microorganisms in vitro and in vivo. Am Rev Tuberc 63:17–24

Hobby GL, Lenert TF, Rivoire ZC, Donikian M, Pikula D (1953) In vitro and in vivo activity of streptomycin and isoniazid singly and in combination. Am Rev Tuberc 67:808–827

Hok TT, Seng TK (1964) A comparative study of the susceptibility to streptomycin, cycloserine, viomycin and kanamycin of tubercle bacilli from 100 patients never treated with cycloserine, viomycin and kanamycin. Am Rev resp Dis 94:961–962

Karlson AG, Gainer JH (1951) The effect of viomycin in tuberculosis of guinea pigs, including in vitro effects against tubercle bacilli resistant to certain drugs. Am Rev Tuberc 63:36–43

Kohout J (1973) Chemotherapie der Tuberkulose. Facultas, Wien

Levaditi C (1951) La viomycine, nouvel antibiotique tuberculostatique. Rev Immunol (Paris) 15:297–302

Mackaness GB (1952) The action of drugs on intracellular tubercle bacilli. J Pathol Bacteriol LXIV:429–445

Mac Kenzie CR, Jordan DC (1970) Cell wall phospholipid and viomycin resistance in Rhizobium meliloti. Biochem Biophys Res Comm 40:1008–1012

Mc Clatchy JK, Kanes W, Davidson PT, Moulding TS (1977) Cross-resistance in *M. tuberculosis* to kanamycin, capreomycin and viomycin. Tubercle 58:29–34

Plichet A (1951) Un nouvel antibiotic contre la tuberculose. La viomycine. Presse Méd 59:219–221

Shepard CS (1957) Use of HeLa cells infected with tubercle bacilli for the study of antituberculous drugs. J Bacteriol 73:494–498

Šimáně Z, Kraus P, Krausová E (1966) Antituberculotics (in Czech). Spofa, Prague, p 112

Singh B, Mitchison DA (1955) The bactericidal activities of combinations of streptomycin, isoniazid, p-aminosalicylic acid (PAS), oxytetracycline (terramycin) and viomycin against *Mycobacterium tuberculosis*. J gen Microbiol 13:176–184

Steenken W Jr, Wolinsky E (1951) Viomycin in experimental tuberculosis. Am Rev Tuberc 63:30–35

Tacquet A, Chenet C (1951) La viomycine. Rev Tuberc (Paris) 15:665–669

Tsukamura M (1961) Variation and heredity of mycobacteria with special reference to drug resistance. Jpn J Tuberc 9:43–64

Tsukamura M, Mizuno S, Murata H, Oshima T (1975) Critical concentrations for resistances of tubercle bacilli to tuberactinomycin-N, viomycin, capreomycin, and lividomycin in patients treated with these agents (cross-resistance relationship among resistances to aminoglycoside antibiotics found during chemotherapy for tuberculosis) (in Japanese). Kekkaku 50:123–130

Yamada T, Masuda K, Shoji K, Hori M (1972) Analysis of ribosomes from viomycin-sensitive and resistant strains of *Mycobacterium smegmatis*. J Bacteriol 112:1–6

Yamada T, Mizuguchi Y, Suga K (1976) Localization of co-resistance to streptomycin, kanamycin, capreomycin and tuberactinomycin, in core particles derived from ribosomes of viomycin-resistant *Mycobacterium smegmatis*. J Antib A29:1124–1126

Youmans GP, Youmans AS (1951) The effect of viomycin in vitro and in vivo on *Mycobacterium tuberculosis*. Am Rev Tuberc 63:25–29

VIII. Cycloserine (CS) and Terizidone (TZ)

H. OTTEN

1. Cycloserine (CS)

Its action spectrum makes cycloserine a broad-spectrum antibiotic. However, all in all it is only a moderately active drug, and in the clinical sector its use is confined practically exclusively to antituberculosis therapy. In individual cases its effect on gram-negatives can be of importance, where it is considered as an alternative medication. The activity detectable in vitro against gram-positive pathogens, some spirochetes (CUCKLER et al. 1955), Rickettsia (CUCKLER et al. 1955; MOULDER et al. 1963), Chlamydiaceae (GORDON and QUAN 1972) and various protozoa (NAKAMURA 1957; CUCKLER et al. 1955) is of no clinical relevance because of the many alternative and more effective drugs.

As a guide to its antibacterial activity, let us consider the following MIC values (given in µg/ml). The data have been collected from various reports (CUCKLER et al. 1955; FREERKSEN et al. 1958; FUST 1958a, b; FUST et al. 1958; MEIER 1962; NAKAMURA 1957; NEUHAUS 1967; STEENKEN and WOLINSKY 1956), and so to some extent they are based on different methods, which should be borne in mind in a comparative evaluation:

Gram-positive pathogens	
Staphylococcus aureus	(3–) 6.2 – 25 – 50 (–200)
Streptococcus faecalis	50 – 200 – >400
Streptococcus pneumoniae	6.2 – 50 – 100 – >300
Streptococcus pyogenes	50 – 100 – 200 – >400
Streptococcus viridans	50 – >100
Corynebacterium diphtheriae	6.2 – 12.5 – 50
Corynebacterium, various species	6.2 – 50
Erysipelothrix rhusiopathiae	50
Bac. anthracis	>100
Nocardia asteroides	(10–) – 50 – >200
Mycobacterium tuberculosis	Egg medium, e.g. Löwenstein-Jensen (3–) 6.2 – 12.5 – 25 (– >100) Semi-synthetic, liquid media (1.5–) 6.2 – 12.5 – 25 (– >50)
Mycobacterium bovis	Egg medium 6.2 – 12.5 (– >25) Semi-synthetic, liquid media 6.2 – 12.5 (– >25)
"Atypical" Mycobacteria, Runyon Groups I–IV	(1.5–3–) 12.5 – 50 – 200
Gram-negative pathogens	
E. coli	(6.2–) 25 – 100 – >200
Enterobacter aerogenes	100 – >400
Klebsiella pneumoniae	25 – 100 – >200
Neisseria gonorrhoeae	200
Proteus vulgaris	(12.5–) 100 – >400
Proteus species, various	100 – >400
Pseudomonas aeruginosa	100 – >400
Salmonellae	50 – 100 – 200 – >400
Shigellae	50 – >100

Other pathogens, such as fungi – e.g. *Candida albicans, Cryptococcus neoformans, Blastomyces dermatitidis, Trichophyton mentagrophytes, Microsporon audouini,* and *Epidermophyton floccosum* – are still resistant to concentrations higher than 100 μg/ml; by contrast, amoebas such as *Entamoeba histolytica* can be inhibited with concentrations as low as 1 μg/ml.

The information available on the sensitivity of mycobacteria varies, probably largely as a result of the use of different determination methods. In sensitivity tests in egg medium a sensitivity rate of more than 80%–90% can be expected at a threshold concentration of 20 μg/ml for *M. tuberculosis,* while the corresponding figure for so-called atypical mycobacteria is more than 65% (KREIS 1970; LUCCHESI 1970). Among the atypical mycobacteria those of Runyon's group I are mostly sensitive, strains from Groups II and III are resistant in more than 20% of the cases, and strains from Group IV are only rarely sensitive. Resistance to CS – which can be detected in isolated cases – is said to be typical for *M. bovis,* strain BCG; wild strains of *M. bovis* on average exhibit greater sensitivity to CS than does *M. tuberculosis* (KREIS 1970).

According to its antibacterial activity CS is largely bacteriostatic, a bactericidal effect being achieved in individual types of pathogens only with extremly high concentrations, 50–100 to more than 1000 times the minimal inhibitory concentrations (COLETSOS et al. 1957, FUST et al. 1958; MEIER 1962; STEENKEN and WOLINSKY 1956).

The efficacy is influenced by the culture and test conditions; the optimal CS activity is found at neutral to slightly acidic pH (6.4–7.0). Higher substance concentrations are necessary at increasingly acid or alkaline pH. For example, four times the amount of CS is needed at pH 5.8 and twice the amount at pH 7.8 (STEENKEN and WOLINSKY 1956). Aqueous stock solutions of CS can be kept at room temperature for 4 weeks (STEENKEN and WOLINSKY 1956). The activity of CS is reduced under the normal culture conditions for mycobacteria at 37 °C in nutrient media such as Kirchner, Sauton, Proskauer-Beck, and Dubos by respectively 39%, 89%, 53%, and 77% (FREERKSEN et al. 1959). In egg medium the loss of activity – especially after the coagulation process – can amount to 90% in comparison with the activity in semi-synthetic media (MEISSNER 1957). For test purposes the Löwenstein-Jensen egg medium has proved successful, provided that care is taken with the pH and the quantity of phosphate buffer, and standardized coagulation times and temperatures are used. Other media, such as Hohn's medium, are less suitable because of their higher alanine content (BÖNICKE and LISBOA 1963). Heating or autoclaving of nutrient media often releases D-alanine, which acts as a D-cycloserine antagonist (HOEPRICH 1963). When egg media containing CS are stored at room temperature there is a loss of activity that has not been observed after 4 weeks of storage in a refrigerator (STEENKEN and WOLINSKY 1956).

D-alanine – an antagonist of CS – is contained in the various nutrient media in various quantities and can thus give rise to corresponding losses of activity. Under certain experimental conditions the antibacterial activity of CS can be eliminated by the addition of D-alanine (BONDI et al. 1957; ZYGMUT 1962, 1963; HAWKINS and MCCLEAN 1966). CS complexes with vitamin B_6 causing activity to be lost (YAMADA et al. 1957). It forms chelates with Cu, Zn, and Co (NEILANDS

1956). Inactivation due to Fe ions, MoO_4, citrate, oxalate, phosphate, etc. is possible (NEUHAUS 1967). Other authors have been unable to observe any loss of the lytic activity of CS against staphylococci due to bonding to Co, Cu, Fe, or Mn ions (SMITH and WEINBERG 1962).

The effect of CS sets in in a delayed fashion; thus, a distinct delayed harmful effect on mycobacteria could only be observed after exposure for 96 h, whereas other antituberculotics such as SM, INH, ETH, EMB, and PZA effected an interruption of growth that persisted for several days after 24 h of in-vitro exposure (DICKINSON 1968). In combination with various antibiotics, CS sometimes exhibits a synergistic potentiation of activity. The test conditions, i.e., the culture conditions and the selection of the test organism are important in this context, as a result of which contradictory findings are possible. When allowed to act on *E. coli* cultures, CS racemate proved to be more effective than the isolated D- or L-form (SMRT et al. 1957; TRIVELLATO and CONCILIO 1958). Combinations of CS with penicillin, bacitracin, oxytetracycline, chlortetracycline, and chloramphenicol acted synergistically on staphylococci and *E. coli*. For example, in the combinations the penicillin concentration could be reduced to $^1/_7$ and the cycloserine concentration to ½, whilst giving the same effects as the correspondingly higher concentrations of the individual active substances (HARRIS et al. 1955). Other authors have described an antagonistic effect of CS in combination with bacteriostatic antibiotics such as chloramphenicol and tetracyclines, provided that the CS has an inhibitory effect on proliferating pathogens (MANTEN et al. 1968). In combination with erythromycin an additive potentiation of activity was found with regard to staphylococci (FUST 1958a).

The combination of CS with INH did not produce any change in the sensitivity to INH when allowed to act upon INH-sensitive and INH-resistant mycobacteria (VIALLIER and CAYRÉ 1956); however, there was a slight potentiation of activity, described as "slight synergism", which did not appear, for example, on combining CS with SM (CUMMINGS et al. 1955). If D-cycloserine is combined with O-carbamyl-D-serine, which has only moderate antibacterial activity, e.g., in the ratio of 90:10 to 50:50, a distinct synergistic effect is obtained (TANAKA and UMEZAWA 1964).

Under the influence of subinhibitory CS concentrations, resistance develops slowly with a stepwise increase (step mutation), the tolerated concentrations being possibly up to more than 50 times the originally effective concentrations (HOWE et al. 1964). Mycobacteria showed a slight loss of sensitivity only after 5 transfers, and after the 11th culture passage the sensitivity had fallen 8 to 16-fold (STEENKEN and WOLINSKY 1956; LUCCHESI 1970).

The resistance that develops in *E. coli* under the influence of subinhibitory concentrations of D-cycloserine has been found to be due to a mutation rate of 10^{-6} to 10^{-7} per passage (CURTISS et al. 1965). This multistep mutation type of resistance development was similarly observed with *Staph. aureus* (HOWE et al. 1964). The mutation rate for *M. tuberculosis* was calculated as 10^{-10} mutants per generation cycle (DAVID 1971).

In the case of *E. coli* which increases its resistance by a factor of 80 after multiple passages, the metabolic transport activity for D-alanine and glycine was found to be reduced by more than 90%, whereas the transport activity for L-alanine was 75% preserved (WARGEL et al. 1971). The original strain was capable of utilizing D- or L-alanine as a source of carbon, while the resistant strain could only metabolize L-alanine. D-cycloserine largely inhibits the metabolism of D-alanine and glycine, whereas L-cycloserine proved to be mainly an inhibitor of the transport of L-alanine (WARGEL et al. 1970).

The disturbance of the alanine metabolism caused by CS leads to a damage of the microbial cell wall. Under the influence of corresponding concentrations and under certain conditions – e.g., proliferation of the microorganism – a bactericidal effect can appear as a result of osmotic dysfunctions (MANTEN et al. 1968; NITTI and TANZI 1957). Under the influence of subinhibitory CS concentrations protoplasts can develop in proliferating cultures – e.g., in staphylococcal cultures (VIRGILIO et al. 1970), *E. coli* cultures (CIAK and HAHN 1959), or in *M. tuberculosis* cultures (HAWKINS and MCCLEAN 1966, RATNAM and CHANDRASEKHAR 1976). After the injection of such spheroplasts of mycobacteria in the guinea pig they remained detectable in the host organism, but hypersensitivity to tuberculin did not develop and no pathological alterations could be detected in the affected organs. Only on reversion of spheroplasts into the bacterial form did pathological changes appear. This correlated with the lifetime of the persistent spheroplasts in the host organism and with their capacity for reversion (RATNAM and CHANDRASEKHAR 1976).

Under specific conditions CS inhibits cell division, while the growth of the pathogens is maintained to a small extent – the result is a formation of filaments with elongation and swelling of the microorganisms (GRULA and GRULA 1965). The sporadically described intensified growth of mycobacteria on nutrient media with cycloserine concentrations that do not inhibit growth (REISS et al. 1960) can be explained in this way.

As a result of its favorable penetration characteristics, CS acts upon mycobacteria stored within the cells; in HeLa cell cultures the damage to the mycobacteria situated outside and inside the cell was the same at equivalent CS concentrations (SHEPHARD 1957).

CS does not exhibit parallel resistance with any commercial antibiotic or chemotherapeutic agent; parallel resistance does appear with terizidone, a condensation product containing 2 molecules of cycloserine.

The results obtained from in-vivo studies allow only a cautious interpretation of the value to be assigned to CS. Because of special conditions, especially regarding the pharmacokinetic behavior with changing metabolic situations in the usual experimental animals, the results of animal studies cannot be used in the same way for grading the efficacy of CS as, for example, in the case of most other antibiotics. The very different serum half-lives in different animal species give an indication of the largely unsuccessful attempts at the treatment of laboratory animals infected with tuberculosis. Thus, the following serum half-lives have been reported after intramuscular injection of CS: mouse 23 min, guinea pig 60 min, rabbit 2.5 h, monkey 7.75 h (CONZELMAN and JONES 1956); in man the half-life is about10 h.

The discrepancy between the in-vitro activity of CS, the in-vivo effect in man, and the lack of activity in small laboratory animals can be further clarified by the

Table 1. Influence of cycloserine on the antituberculotic activity of streptomycin in mice [CUCKLER et al. 1955 (modif.)]

Infection: *M. tuberculosis* H37Rv, induced intravenously.
Therapy: Once a day from the 1st day after the infection until the end of the study, i.e., until 50% of the infected controls had died (about 3 weeks after the infection).
Doses: Streptomycin (0.125, 0.25, 0.50, and 1.0 mg/mouse/day s.c.) and cycloserine (10 mg/mouse/day p.o.) as a combination.
Evaluation: Lung affection index, a value of 0 corresponding to a normal lung and 4 to the score in the infected control group.

Therapeutic regimen	Streptomycin dose (mg/mouse/day)			
	0.125	0.25	0.50	1.00
Streptomycin monotherapy	3.94	3.00	2.94	0.78
Streptomycin + cycloserine (10 mg/mouse/day)	2.42	1.83	0.78	0.22

Cycloserine (10 mg/mouse/day) monotherapy: no significant therapeutic effect.

fact that mouse and guinea pig serum contains D-alanine, a CS antagonist, whereas this is not the case in human serum (HOEPRICH 1965).

According to the efficacy of CS in vitro, CS concentrations 1000 times as high are necessary to produce an effect equivalent to that of INH under otherwise identical conditions (FREERKSEN et al. 1958). This is the reason for the high doses of up to 500 mg/kg needed in animal experiments.

In a therapeutic study on mice infected with tuberculosis, monotherapy with CS exhibited at best a weak effect of statistically questionable significance (CUCKLER et al. 1955; GRUMBACH 1965; STEENKEN and WOLINSKY 1956). Even on administration 4 times a day of high but still tolerable doses of CS, a distinct therapeutic effect could not be discerned in a Tb study on mice (KREIS and FOURNAUD 1965).

In combination therapy a potentiation of the effect of SM could be detected for CS in a study on mice (CUCKLER et al. 1955); see Table 1.

On the basis of the tuberculous lung-affection index, the mouse study revealed the combination of SM and CS to be more than three times as effective as SM alone (CUCKLER et al. 1955). When CS was combined with ETH, no potentiation of the efficacy of the thioamide was observed in a mouse study (GRUMBACH 1965).

In therapeutic studies on guinea pigs infected with tuberculosis no definite therapeutic effect could be demonstrated for CS alone. By using high doses of up to 100 mg/day per guinea pig, it was only possible to prolong the survival time, and the pathomorphological organ findings for the animals treated with CS did not differ essentially from those for the untreated infected controls (GERNEZ-RIEUX and TACQUET 1956; PATNODE et al. 1955a, b; STEENKEN and WOLINSKY 1956); see Table 2.

Table 2. Cycloserine therapy in tuberculous guinea pigs. (Steenken and Wolinsky 1956)

Infection:	*M. tuberculosis* H37Rv, induced intracardially.
Therapy:	Once a day from the 1st week after the infection to the end of the study, i.m.
	The doses listed apply up to and including the 4th week of the study; from 5th week of therapy (LD_{50} in control group) all received uniformly 100 mg/guinea pig/day.
Evaluation:	Survival rate (medians)

Treatment groups	Survival times in days (median and range)
Infected controls	35 (30–44)
Cycloserine 10–15 mg	35 (30–45)
Cycloserine 20–25 mg	31.5 (23–36)
Cycloserine 40–50 mg	41 (29–53)

No distinct therapeutic effect of cycloserine could be detected in rabbits infected with tuberculosis (Gernez-Rieux and Tacquet 1956).

At doses of 100 mg/kg, administered for a treatment period of 50 days a slight effect could be detected in a study on tuberculous monkeys (simian test), although this effect was not equivalent to that achievable with INH doses of 5 mg/kg; the combination of INH with CS proved to be more efficacious than INH on its own (Schmidt 1956).

2. Terizidone (TZ)

As a condensation product, terizidone contains two cycloserine molecules that behave as antibacterially active structural elements, and this explains its largely identical antimicrobial action mechanism and effectiveness (Bonati et al. 1965; Di Perna et al. 1967; Lucchesi et al. 1968; Mariani et al. 1968). The advantages of terizidone over CS appear above all because of its more favorable pharmacokinetic behavior, i.e., its slower elimination evidently results in longer-lasting concentrations of the active substance and thus in better therapeutic results. In rabbits, the spread of a tuberculosis infection induced intraocularly could be prevented by simultaneous therapeutic administration of terizidone in doses of 100 mg/kg/day over an 80-day experimental period (Di Perna et al. 1967).

An intravenous infection of rabbits with *M. bovis* was treated by Nitti et al. (1969) up to 150 days. CS was applicated in doses of 200 mg/kg/d and 400 mg/kg/d, terizidone in doses of equivalent activity. Survival times of the treated animals were significantly prolonged, but there was no significant difference between the various treatment schedules. Macroscopic and microscopic findings at autopsy corroborated the survival data.

Guinea pigs were subcutaneously infected with $^{1}/_{50}$ mg of the H37Rv strain by Di Perna (1969). Oral treatment with 100 mg/kg/d for 60 days beginning on the day of infection was nearly ineffective.

CATENA (1969) infected rabbits intravenously with *M. bovis* and treated the animals for 60 days starting the day after infection. As judged by microscopic findings and by histology, terizidone (200 mg/kg/d) given orally suppressed markedly the infection.

ADÁMEK and TRNKA (1972) determined comparatively the MIC's of CS and terizidone for mycobacteria in several media. On Löwenstein-Jensen egg medium the activity of both compounds was the same except for photochromogenic and scotochromogenic strains, which were more sensitive to terizidone. In liquid Šula medium terizidone was more active than CS against all strains tested. The survival of intravenously infected mice was prolonged a little longer by terizidone than by CS, both drugs given orally in a dose of 200 mg/kg/d.

On the basis of its antibacterial activity and its pharmacokinetic behavior, terizidone – more so than CS – has been put to therapeutic use, apart from tuberculosis, mainly for urinary-tract infections.

3. Concluding Remarks

Because of its antituberculotic activity, which has been confirmed in vitro with a broad action spectrum, and its therapeutic effectiveness in suitable combinations with other antituberculotics, cycloserine is a recognized antituberculotic agent. In view of toxicological problems with tolerance and of its on the whole restricted effective range, cycloserine is used as a reserve agent and is only considered for wider application in the presence of suitable indications. The same holds true for the derivative of cycloserine, terizidone.

References

Adámek L, Trnka L (1972) Comparison of the antituberculotic efficiency of terizidone (Terivalidin, Bracco) and that of D-cycloserine both in vitro and in vivo. Giorn It Mal Tor XXVI:241–247

Barclay WR, Russe H (1955) The in vitro action of cycloserine on *M. tuberculosis*. Am Rev Tuberc 72:236–241

Bönicke R, Lisboa BP (1963) Zur Problematik der Resistenzbestimmung bei D-Cycloserin. Beitr Klin Tuberk 126:212–221

Bonati F, Bertoni L, Rosati G, Zanichelli V (1965) Caratteristiche biologiche ed attività antibatterica del Terizidone. Il Farmaco 20:381–395

Bondi A, Kornblum J, Forte C (1957) Inhibition of antibacterial activity of cycloserine by alpha-alanine. Proc Soc Exp Biol Med 96:270–272

Catena E (1969) Primi rilievi anatomo-istologici sull'attività antitubercolare del Terizidone nel coniglio. Riv Pat Clin Tuberc 42:164–169

Ciak J, Hahn FE (1959) Mechanisms of action of antibiotics. II. Studies on the modes of action of cycloserine and its L-stereo-isomer. Antibiot Chemother (Washington) 9:47–50

Coletsos P, Oriot E, Regel N de (1957) Étude de la sensibilité de *Mycobacterium tuberculosis* à la cycloserine et méthode de titrage in vitro. Ann Inst Pasteur 93:21–29

Conzelman GM Jr, Jones RK (1956) On the physiologic disposition of cycloserine in experimental animals. Am Rev Tub Pulm Dis 74:802–806

Cuckler AC, Frost BM, McClelland L, Solotorovsky M (1955) The antimicrobial evaluation of oxamycin (D-4-amino-3-isoxazolidone) a new broad spectrum antibiotic. Antibiot Chemother (Washington) 5:191–197

Cummings MM, Patnode RA, Hudgins PC (1955) Effects of cycloserine on *Mycobacterium tuberculosis* in vitro. Antibiot Chemother (Washington) 5:198–203

Curtiss R, Charamella LJ, Berg C, Harris PE (1965) Kinetic and genetic analysis of D-cycloserine inhibition and resistance in Escherichia coli. J Bacteriol 90:1238–1250
David HL (1971) Resistance to D-cycloserine in the tubercle bacilli: mutation rate and transport of alanine in parenteral cells and drug-resistant mutants. Appl Microbiology 21:888–892
Dickinson JM (1968) In vitro and in vivo studies to assess the suitability of anti-tuberculous drugs for use in intermittent chemotherapy regimens. Bull Int Union Tuberc XLI:309–315
Di Perna A (1969) Ricerche sperimentali sull'attività antimicobatterica del Terizidone. Riv Pat Clin Tuberc 42:158–163
Di Perna A, Vinciguerra E, Valente S (1967) Effetti de Terizidone sulla tubercolosi sperimentale della camera anteriore dell'occhio dell coniglio. G Ital Mal Tor 21:57–73 Suppl
Freerksen E, Bönicke R, Lisboa B (1958) Über das Verhalten von Cycloserin in vivo. Tuberk Arzt 12:39–49
Freerksen E, Krüger-Thiemer E, Rosenfeld M (1959) Cycloserin. Antibiot Chemother (Basel) 6:303–396
Fust B (1958 a) D-Cycloserin. Medizinische 12:470–478
Fust B (1958 b) Experimentelle Grundlagen zur Wirkung von D-Cycloserin. In: Walter AM (Hrsg) Neue Tuberkulostatika und Tuberkulostatika-Resistenz von Tuberkelbakterien. Thieme, Stuttgart, pp 106–112
Fust B, Böhni E, Pellmont B, Zbinden G, Studer A (1958) Experimentelle Untersuchungen mit D-Cycloserin. Schweiz Z Tuberk 15:129–157
Gernez-Rieux CH, Tacquet A (1956) Action de la cyclosérine sur la tuberculose expérimentale du cobaye et du lapin. Ann Inst Pasteur 91:623–630
Gordon FB, Quan AL (1972) Susceptibility of Chlamydia to antibacterial drugs: test in cell cultures. Antimicrob Agents Chemother 2:242–244
Grula MM, Grula EA (1965) Action of cycloserine on a species of Erwinia with reference to cell division. Can J Microbiol 11:453–455
Grumbach F (1965) Etudes chimiothérapiques sur la tuberculose avancée de la souris. Adv Tuberc Res 14:31–96
Harris DA, Ruger M, Reagan MA, Wolf FJ, Peck RL, Wallick H, Woodruff HB (1955) Discovery, development, and antimicrobial properties of D-4-amino-3-isoxazolidone (oxamycin), a new antibiotic produced by *Streptomyces garyphalus* n.sp. Antibiot Chemother (Washington) 5:183–190
Hawkins JE, McClean VR (1966) Comparative studies of cycloserine inhibition of mycobacteria. Am Rev Respir Dis 93:594–602
Hoeprich PD (1963) Alanine: cycloserine antagonism. III. Quantitative aspects and relations to heating of culture media. J Lab Clin Med 62:657–662
Hoeprich PD (1965) Alanine: cycloserine antagonism. IV. Demonstration of D-alanine in the serum of guinea pigs and mice. J Biol Chem 240:1654–1660
Howe WB, Melson GL, Meredith CH, Morrison JR, Platt MH, Strominger JL (1964) Stepwise development of resistance to D-cycloserine in *Staphylococcus aureus*. J Pharmacol Exp Ther 143:282–285
Kreis B (1970) Resistance of cycloserine. Scand J Respir Dis Suppl 71:266–268
Kreis B, Fournaud S (1965) Les traitements antituberculeux de très courte durée chez la souris II. Résultates. Ann Inst Pasteur 108:117–120
Lucchesi M (1970) Antimicrobial effect of cycloserine. Scand J Respir Dis Suppl 71:13–21
Lucchesi M, Mancini P, Matzen M (1968) Su alcuni aspetti dell' attività antimicobatterica in vitro della cycloserina e del terizidone. Inn Ist Forlanini 28:105–115
Manten A, Klingern B vaan, Voogd CE, Meertens MGP (1968) D-cycloserine as a bactericidal drug. Antagonisms between D-cycloserine and the bacteriostatic antibiotics chloramphenicol and tetracycline. Chemotherapy 13:242–248
Mariani B, Bisetti A, Velluti G (1968) Ricerche sperimentali e clinico-therapeutiche mediante terizidone nella tubercolosi. Minerva Med 59:2445–2458
Meier KE (1962) Beitrag zur Wirksamkeit des D-Cycloserin. Beitr Klin Tuberk 125:222–240

Meissner G (1957) Persönliche Mitteilung: Cycloserin-Stabilität im Ei-Medium. Kolloquium Neue Antituberkulotika Forschungsinstitut Borstel, November 1957
Moulder JW, Novosel DL, Officer JE (1963) Inhibition of the growth of agents of the psittacosis group by D-cycloserine and its specific reversal by D-alanine. J Bacteriol 85:707–710
Nakamura M (1957) Amebicidal action of cycloserine. Experientia 13:29
Neilands JB (1956) Metal and hydrogen-ion binding properties of cycloserine. Arch Biochem Biophys 62:151–162
Neuhaus FC (1967) D-Cycloserine and O-carbamyl-D-serine. In: Gottlieb D, Shaw PD (eds) Antibiotics, vol I: Mechanism of action. Springer, Berlin Heidelberg New York, pp 40–83
Nitti V, Tanzi PL (1957) Sull'attività battericida della cicloserina in vitro. Arch Tisiol Sz Sci 12:42–49
Nitti V, Catena E, Ninni A, Marsico SA (1969) L'attività del terizidone nella tubercolosi sperimentale del coniglio. Arch Tisiol Mal App Resp (Sz Sci) 24:667–698
Patnode RA, Hudgins PC, Cummings MM (1955a) Effect of cycloserine on experimental tuberculosis in guinea pigs. Am Rev Tuberc Pulm Dis 72:117–118
Patnode RA, Hudgins PC, Cummings MM (1955b) Further observation on the effect of cycloserine on tuberculosis in guinea pigs. Am Rev Tuberc Pulm Dis 72:856–858
Ratnam S, Chandrasekhar S (1976) The pathogenicity of spheroplasts of *Mycobacterium tuberculosis*. Am Rev Respir Dis 114:549–554
Reiss J, Townsend SM, Gables C (1960) Cycloserine: Growth enhancement phenomen found during sensitivity studies: clinical implications. J Lab Clin Med 56:607–612
Shepard CC (1957) Use of Hela cells infected with tubercle bacilli for the study of antituberculous drugs. J Bacteriol 73:494–498
Smith JL, Weinberg ED (1962) Mechanisms of antibacterial action of bacitracin. J Gen Microbiol 28:559–569
Smrt J, Beranek J, Sicher J, Skoda J, Hess VF, Sorm F (1957) Synthesis of L-4-amino-isoxazolidone, the unnatural stereoisomer of cycloserine and its antibiotic activity. Experientia 13:291–293
Schmidt LH (1956) Studies on the therapeutic properties of cycloserine. Transact 15th Conf Chemother Tuberc VAAF:353–365
Steenken W Jr, Wolinsky E (1956) Cycloserine: antituberculous activity in vitro and in the experimental animal. Am Rev Tuberc Pulm Dis 73:539–546
Tanaka N, Umezawa H (1964) Synergism of D-4-amino-3-isoxazolidone and O-carbamyl-D-serine. J Antibiotics Ser A 17:8–11
Trivellato E, Concilio C (1958) Stereoisomers of cycloserine. I. Bacteriostatic activity towards some microorganisms. Arch Int Pharmacodyn Ther 117:313–316
Viallier J, Cayré RM (1956) Action bactériostatique sur *Mycobacterium tuberculosis* exercée par l'association cycloserine – isoniazide. Compt Rend Soc Biol Paris 150:1970–1971
Virgilio R, Gonzales C, Munoz N, Cabezon T, Mendoza S (1970) *Staphylococcus aureus* protoplasting induced by D-cycloserine. J Bacteriol 104:1386–1387
Wargel RJ, Shadur CA, Neuhaus FC (1970) Mechanism of D-cycloserine action: transport systems for D-alanine, D-cycloserine, L-alanine, and glycine. J Bacteriol 103:778–788
Wargel RJ, Shadur CA, Neuhaus FC (1971) Mechanism of D-cycloserine action: transport mutants for D-alanine, D-cycloserine, and glycine. J Bacteriol 105:1028–1035
Wilson DE, Williams TW Jr (1966) In vitro susceptibility of nocardia to antimicrobial agents. Antimicrob Agents Chemother 1965:408–411
Yamada K, Sawaki S, Hayami S (1957) Inhibitory effect of cycloserine on some enzymic activities related to vitamin B6. J Vitaminol (Osaka) 3:68–71
Zygmut WA (1962) Reversal of D-cycloserine inhibition of bacterial growth by alanine. J Bacteriol 84:154–156
Zygmut WA (1963) Antagonism of D-cycloserine inhibition of mycobacterial growth by D-alanine. J Bacteriol 85:1217–1220

IX. Thioamides: Ethionamide (ETH), Protionamide (PTH)

H. OTTEN

1. Antimicrobial Activity in Vitro

Ethionamide/protionamide are derivatives of isonicotinic acid. However, although they are structurally similar they are not derivatives of isoniazid. This explains on the one hand their comparable antituberculotic properties and, on the other hand, the major differences between the two substance groups. Ethionamide and protionamide behave in much the same fashion, and thus the data relating chiefly to ethionamide can also be extrapolated to the evaluation of protionamide.

Ethionamide (ETH) is sparingly soluble in water and readily soluble in organic solvents and is bound or degraded as a function of the pH, temperature, and the constituents of the nutrient medium (e.g., heavy metal salts, protein content). The antituberculotically active sulphoxide is formed, which has about the same activity as ETH (BÖNICKE 1965). With increasing alkalization of the solution accelerated inactivation takes place; under the influence of oxidizing agents such as H_2O_2, nitrate or $KMnO_4$ ETH can decompose within minutes (PÜTTER 1964). The details of the degradation vary from one nutrient medium to another, ETH being decreasingly inactivated by the various nutrient media in the following sequence: Dubos, Youmans, 7H9-Middlebrook, and Kirchner. The corresponding sequence for loss of the antituberculotic activity of the sulphoxide is Dubos, 7H9-Middlebrook, Youmans, and Kirchner (GRUNERT et al. 1968). The sulphoxide is less stable than ETH. As a result of faster further degradation in solutions, a state of equilibrium is not reached by a reversion of the sulphoxide to ethionamide (GRUNERT et al. 1968).

In activity determinations the fall in the concentration of ETH in dependence on the nutrient medium, the incubation time, and the starting concentration should be taken into account. Within a few days – the exact time varies from one nutrient medium to the next – a concentration reduction by 30% and sometimes markedly more than 50% sets in, the degradation passing over into an accelerated phase after incubation for about 8 days. The degradation of the sulphoxide is faster, the loss of activity proceeding continuously and independently of the concentration. Concentrations below the detection limit are reached after a few days (GRUNERT et al. 1968). In Löwenstein-Jensen egg medium a loss of activity by as much as 50% is expected after normal coagulation at 85 °C, the bonding to phosphoproteins obviously playing a part in this process (RIST 1960). Important nutrient medium constituents such as ferric chloride, calcium chloride, magnesium citrate, and malachite green have no essential influence on the inactivation processes. By contrast, in a combination of ferric chloride/ammonium chloride/sodium citrate, a distinct fall of the ETH concentration could be induced, so that under certain conditions heavy metal salts can have an inactivating effect (GRUNERT et al. 1968). Addition of protein such as serum or serum albumin to synthetic nutrient media results in increasing inactivation as the concentration of the addition increases. For example, a 10% addition of bovine serum to a Kirchner medium produces a 10-fold reduction of the concentration after a 12-day incubation period compared with a serum-free control (Grunert et al. 1968). ETH is only slightly affected by media containing hydrochloric acid – after 10 days of incubation a fall in the concentration of only about 25% could be found at pH < 2. In the neutral range the loss of activity was between 50% and 70%; at pH 12 (0.05 NaOH) ETH can no longer be detected after incubation for 2 days (Grunert et al. 1968).

The degradation and rearrangement reactions of ETH proceed differently in vitro than in the macro-organism. Evidently there is no conversion into the amide and, moreover, the metabolites detected in vivo with absorption maxima at 315 nm–340 nm are not observed. In most cases a conversion into α-ethylisonicotinic acid or a ring opening is assumed to take place in ETH solutions (Grunert et al. 1968). In microbiological studies no impairment of the results due to conversion of the ETH into the sulphoxide or vice-versa need be expected (Grunert et al. 1968); in ETH/PTH activity tests the inhibitory effects are due to the substance in question.

ETH assays by conventional microbiological and chemical methods yield largely the same value. In addition to the biological detection procedures, such as the vertical diffusion test (Stottmeier et al. 1967), it is predominantly the chemical methods that come into consideration.

Ethylene glycol is suitable as a solvent for ETH/PTH. As far as in-vitro tests are concerned, the intrinsic inhibition due to the corresponding dilution (concentration < 1%) in the test series can be neglected.

The antimicrobial effect of ETH/PTH is confined to mycobacteria; other microorganisms, such as gram-positive and gram-negative bacteria, fungi, viruses, and protozoa are resistant. Besides its good activity against *M. tuberculosis* and *M. bovis,* ETH/PTH sometimes shows good activity against the "atypical mycobacteria". In the event of such infections, therefore, the clinical use of these substances must be based on the evaluation of sensitivity tests. Table 1 shows the minimal inhibitory concentrations.

Table 1. Minimal inhibitory concentrations (MIC) of ethionamide/protionamide (in µg/ml)

	Solid egg medium (e.g. Löwenstein-Jensen)	Semi-synthetic, liquid media, e.g. Dubos, Youmans, sometimes with Tween and serum added
M. tuberculosis	(4–) 8–16 (–32)	ETH: (0.2–) 0.6–0.8–2 (–6) PTH: (0.08–) 0.4–0.8 (–4)
M. bovis	(4–) 8–16–32	(0.5–) 2–4 (–16)
M. kansasii	(4–) 8–32 (–128)	(0.5–) 2–8–32
M. avium	(4–) 16–32–128	(0.5–) 4–16– > 32
Runyon Group I	(4–) 8–16–32 (–128)	(0.5–) 2–8–32 (–128)
Runyon Group II	(8–) 16–32–128	(1–) 4–32–128
Runyon Group III	(4–) 16–32–128	(0.5–) 4–16–128
Runyon Group IV	(8–) 16–32–128	(1–) 4–32–128

References: Bönicke (1965); Hilson (1967); Lefford (1969); Rist (1960); Steenken and Montalbine (1960); Urbancik and Burjanova (1967); Verbist (1966).

With photochromogenic mycobacteria up to 100% sensitivity to thioamides can be expected; the corresponding figure for the scotochromogenic species is up to over 80%. The non-photochromogenic mycobacteria are markedly less sensitive (incidence of sensitivity: about 50%). The fast-growing species are mostly resistant, sensitivity being expected in only about 25% of the cases (GIALDRONI-GRASSI and GRASSI 1966).

Insofar as different effects have been found to exist between the thioamides, PTH can be said to be superior, since it is found to be 1.5 to twice as effective, predominantly in semi-synthetic nutrient media (NOUFFLARD-GUY-LOÉ and BERTEAUX 1962; SCHÜTZ et al. 1969). To what extent PTH has a superior activity in absolute terms, or whether the more favorable in-vitro results are due to its better stability in the various nutrient media, remains an open question.

16 μg/ml is regarded as a critical concentration of the determination of resistance on a Löwenstein-Jensen egg medium.

Time-limited exposure of *M. tuberculosis* to ETH in liquid medium with a concentration of ETH 10 times the MIC (50 μg/ml) delayed resuming of growth after contact only if the exposure exceeded 12 h. After exposure for 24 h an average lag-period of about 7 days was observed which after 96 h of action rose to an average of 11 days. During and after an exposure for 24 h or more the viable count did fall. In the killing kinetics as well as in the duration of the lag-period ETH was very similar to INH at a concentration of 1 μg/ml (DICKINSON and MITCHISON 1966a). This phenomenon of an after-effect with a delayed onset after a limited exposure should be borne in mind in the evaluations of intermittent therapies. After sufficiently long exposure times ETH has a favorable and sustained after-effect on mycobacteria that have remained viable, which are thus more readily accessible to the body's defense mechanisms.

Under sustained activity of 1 μg/ml of ETH in Šula nutrient medium 99% of the microbial units were destroyed within 7 days. On elevation of the ETH concentration to 4 μg/ml the same tuberculocidal effect was achieved within 4 days. A further increase of the concentration to 16 μg/ml did not potentiate the effect during the shorter exposure time of 4 days, although, if allowed to act longer, the higher concentration was found to be more effective. In comparison to this dose- and action-time- dependent intensity of the effect, on interrupted action over a 2-h period per day it was impossible to achieve the same tuberculocidal effect as the one produced by long-term action of 2 μg/ml even by concentrations 5 times as high (KREBS 1967; KREBS and NOACK 1968).

ETH/PTH are primarily bacteriostatic; on elevation of the concentrations by a factor of 5 to 10, the activity becomes bactericidal (RIST 1960); in Tween-albumin nutrient media a tuberculocidal effect is achieved at concentrations 2 to 4 times the MIC (STEENKEN and MONTALBINE 1960). Tuberculocidal concentrations can be reached with doses applicable to animals and man.

The optimal activity is achieved in the slightly acidic pH range (pH 6); in the pH range from 7 to 8 concentrations 3 to 5 times as high are required (NITTI 1959).

Under the influence of subthreshold concentrations of thioamides, resistance rapidly develops, and this can be intensified to high degrees of resistance by culture passages with slowly increasing concentrations. For example, the concentration may rise by 2–3 powers of 10 compared to the original value. The test strain *M. tuberculosis* H37Rv could be trained in thioamide-containing Tween-albumin nutrient media from an initial inhibition level of 3.1 μg/ml to 200 μg/ml after 18 culture passages (STEENKEN and MONTALBINE 1960).

The resistance to ETH "acquired" in the course of therapy is less stable than the primarily existing resistance – it can be made to regress after some 60 culture passages (TSUKAMURA and TSUKAMURA 1967).

As a result of the structural similarity of the side chain $-\mathrm{C}(=\mathrm{S})\mathrm{NH_2}$, parallel resistance appears to various extents with thiosemicarbazone and thiocarlide; cf. Fig. 1 below).

The parallel resistance between thioamides and thiosemicarbazone is largely complete; parallel resistance to thiocarlide corresponds to parallel resistance to thiosemicarbazone (EULE and WERNER 1967). The resistance that develops in the course of thiosemicarbazone therapy automatically means resistance to ETH in 30 to 60 to more than 85% of the cases; however, mycobacteria with a primary resistance to thiosemicarbazone are usually sensitive (EULE and WERNER 1967; LEFFORD 1969; EULE 1965; BARTMANN 1960).

The resistance developing under ETH therapy encompassed resistance to thiosemicarbazone in >80 to 100% of the cases. Simultaneous thiocarlide resistance must also be reckoned with in most cases (EULE and WERNER 1967; SOJKOVÁ et al. 1965; VERBIST 1966).

On the basis of their efficacy and their resistance situation the thioamides are the most effective products in this group of antituberculotics characterized by parallel resistance phenomena. The thioamides are thus the most important compounds for clinical application.

In resistance determinations the aforementioned factors that attenuate the activity in dependence on the culture conditions should be borne in mind. It is found that the proportion method yields more reliable values than the determination of the absolute inhibitory concentrations (URBANCIK and BURJANOVA 1967).

In view of the fact that more than 50% of the activity can be lost within an incubation period lasting a few days, it is sometimes proposed that after a certain time the test cultures should again be treated with ETH/PTH in appropriate quantities (HILSON 1967). At the thioamide concentrations in the culture system

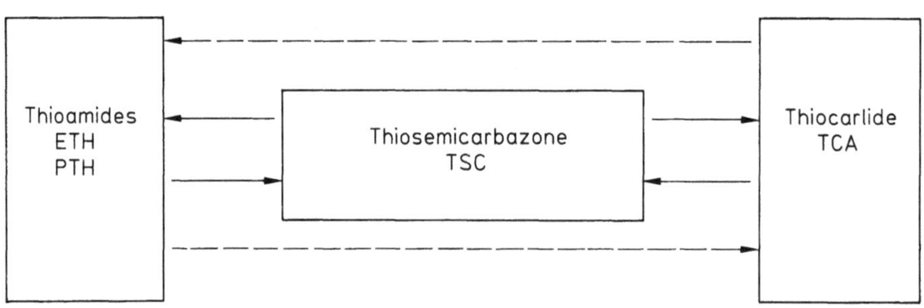

Fig. 1. Resistance relationships – thioamide, thiosemicarbazone, thiocarlide

stabilized in this way, the MIC values obtained in the egg medium are equivalent to those in semi-synthetic media, with values of 1.2 µg/ml to 2.5 µg/ml.

Thioamides penetrate monocytes and behave, for example in monocyte cultures, similarly to INH (RIST 1960). The intracellular penetration capacity explains their high in-vivo activity. According to studies in monocyte cultures, the thioamides act with equal intensity on pathogens localized within and outside the cells (RIST 1960). Mycobacteria are damaged to the same extent in in-vitro systems and in cell cultures (CLINI and GRASSI 1970).

2. Activity of ETH/PTH in Experimental Tuberculosis and Development of Resistance in Vivo

The thioamides exhibit clear therapeutic activity in animal experiments, a dose-effect relationship being found to exist. According to detailed comparative therapeutic studies, above all on mice and guinea pigs, tuberculocidal effects can be demonstrated for the thioamides that are in a specific relationship to those of other antituberculotic agents (WALTER et al. 1960). Daily administration of 10 mg/kg to 15 (to 20) mg/kg is accepted as the threshold-active dose in various animal species and in man (STEENKEN and MONTALBINE 1960; RIST 1960, 1964; GRUMBACH 1961, 1965).

The thioamides are not as effective as INH and RMP. Under certain conditions their effect is superior to that of SM. The remaining antituberculotics are inferior to the thioamides when given in correlating doses (mg/kg) (RIST 1960, 1964; OTTEN 1971; GRUMBACH 1965; DICKINSON and MITCHISON 1966b).

During monotherapy with thioamides resistance develops relatively quickly. In mice treated with ETH (50 mg/kg) from the 14th day after a tuberculous infection, the microbial count decreased in the initial stages of the treatment to as little as 1% of the initial count in the sense of a tuberculocidal effect. After 65 days of therapy – in some cases involving a further reduction of the total microbial counts – ETH-resistant mycobacteria could be detected. In the course of 4 months to 5 months of monotherapy the number of resistant pathogens increased considerably, reaching the size of the originally sensitive population present at the start of treatment (RIST et al. 1958). In combination with INH (5 mg/kg), ETH (50 mg/kg) prevented the development of resistance during 5 months of therapy in mice. The microbial counts fell off permanently, although a residual quantity of 0.001% to 0.01% of the initial values was detectable as sensitive persisters (RIST et al. 1958). The INH-resistance-retarding effect of EHT correlates with the doses of the combination partners used – with rising doses of INH it is possible to reduce the requisite amount of the thioamide. In studies on mice the combinations of 5 mg INH/50 mg ETH per kg, 20 mg INH/25 mg ETH per kg, and 50 mg INH/12.5 mg ETH per kg yielded much the same results, i.e., the INH resistance was equally strongly suppressed in each case (GRUMBACH 1961).

Under the influence of continuous daily therapy for 4 weeks from the time of infection in Tb-infected mice, the survival rate after a treatment-free interval of around 3 weeks, which corresponds to the time it takes for untreated infected controls to die, gives an informative overall picture of the efficacy of the comparatively tested antituberculotics. Table 2 shows the survival rates (in percent) on the

Table 2. Continuous therapy for 4 weeks from the time of infection. (After OTTEN 1971)

Isoniazid	3 mg/kg	97	Ethambutol	100 mg/kg	93
Ethionamide	30 mg/kg	100	Viomycin	100 mg/kg	70
Rifampicin	30 mg/kg	97	Pyrazinamide	100 mg/kg	25
Kanamycin	30 mg/kg	85	Thiocarlide	300 mg/kg	46
Streptomycin	30 mg/kg	75	p-Aminosalicylic acid	1000 mg/kg	10
Thiosemicarbazone	30 mg/kg	20	Infected controls		0

CF_1-Mice, 18–20 g, *M. tuberculosis* H37Rv 10^6–10^7 microbial units i.v., therapy: once a day, 5 times a week; oral administration. Streptomyces antibiotics s.c. Data on survival rate in % on the 50th day after the infection.

50th day after infection with *M. tuberculosis* H37Rv for a number of antituberculotic drugs (OTTEN 1971).

From the values listed in Table 2 it can be seen that ETH has an antituberculotic effect equivalent to that of INH in the Tb-infected mouse at doses 10 times the effective dose of INH (30 : 3 mg/kg). RMP, KM, and SM lie within the same order of magnitude with regard to the intensity of the effect, KM and SM having on the whole a somewhat weaker antituberculotic effect. As far as the other antituberculotic drugs are concerned, a comparable therapeutic result is only achieved with higher doses, e.g., in the case of EMB and VM with 3 times the dose of the ETH.

The efficacy of the antituberculosis agents when administered intermittently is also of therapeutic interest, ETH proving to be highly effective and clearly superior to the other antituberculotics – cf. Table 3 (OTTEN 1971).

When administered intermittently in a simultaneous therapeutic study – i.e., with the treatment started immediately after the infection – ETH displays an activity equivalent to that of INH at a dose 10 times as high (30 :3 mg/kg). Similarly to the case with INH, the therapeutic effect is much the same in groups treated with 1 and 2 treatments per week. When given intermittently in the same doses, ETH is superior to other antituberculosis drugs such as SM and EMB. The high efficacy of ETH can be explained on the one hand by its capacity for intracellular penetration and on the other hand by its beneficial, sustained after-effect, provided that a sufficiently high concentration is allowed to exert its activity on the mycobacteria for a sufficient time.

In a comparison of continuous and intermittent therapy in a Tb-mouse study, different microbial counts were found in the lungs after equivalent total doses. During the first 14 days of the therapy (6×50 mg/kg, 2×150 mg/kg, and 1×300 mg/kg per week) the reduction of the microbial count was more or less the same in all three groups; after 6 and 10 weeks of treatment distinctly lower counts were found in the case of daily administration than in the case of intermittent therapy (KREBS and NOACK 1968).

The doses of the individual drugs in combinations can play a part with regard to toxic effects. In a study on TB-infected mice comparable therapeutic results were achieved with INH and ETH combined in various ratios when the INH fraction was increased and the ETH fraction reduced (GRUMBACH 1961, 1965); see Table 4.

Table 3. Intermittent therapy of tuberculosis in the mouse. (After OTTEN 1971)

			20th	30th	50th	70th	90th day
A	Ethionamide	30 mg/kg	100	100	95	95	45
	Ethambutol	30 mg/kg	100	20	–	–	–
	Streptomycin	30 mg/kg	100	35	20	15	15
	Isoniazid	3 mg/kg	100	100	85	70	50
	Ethionamide	100 mg/kg	100	100	100	100	100
	Ethambutol	100 mg/kg	100	80	80	50	–
	Streptomycin	100 mg/kg	100	95	85	80	55
	Isoniazid	10 mg/kg	100	100	100	100	100
B	Ethionamide	30 mg/kg	100	85	65	60	30
	Ethambutol	30 mg/kg	60	–	–	–	–
	Streptomycin	30 mg/kg	90	30	15	15	–
	Isoniazid	3 mg/kg	100	75	60	30	25
	Ethionamide	100 mg/kg	100	100	100	90	80
	Ethambutol	100 mg/kg	100	50	20	15	–
	Streptomycin	100 mg/kg	95	55	45	35	20
	Isoniazid	10 mg/kg	100	100	100	95	95
	Infected controls		70	1	–	–	–

CF_1-mice; *M. tuberculosis* H37Rv 10^6–10^7 microbial units i.v.
A: Therapy: twice a week = 20 doses over the 10-week period following the infection
B: Therapy: once a week = 10 doses over the 10-week period following the infection
Administration: oral; streptomycin s.c. Data on the survival rates in % on the 20th, 30th, 50th, 70th, and 90th days after the infection.

After 5 months of monotherapy with INH the microbial population was completely resistant to INH. Under the influence of combined therapy with a threshold-active ETH dose (about 12 mg/kg), the resistant fraction was the same although the total microbial count was clearly lower.

In studies on mice a more favorable therapeutic effect was demonstrated for PTH than for ETH in equal doses. The survival times for Tb-infected mice were prolonged under the influence of therapeutically active doses of 20 mg/kg to

Table 4. Effect of therapy with isoniazid and with isoniazid + ethionamide in experimentally induced tuberculosis in mice. (After GRUMBACH 1961, 1965)

	INH 5 mg/kg –	INH 20 mg/kg –	INH 5 mg/kg ETH 12 mg/kg	INH 5 mg/kg ETH 50 mg/kg	INH 20 mg/kg ETH 12 mg/kg	INH 20 mg/kg ETH 25 mg/kg
C:	100%	61%	20%	0.04%	0.08%	0.03%
R:	II–III	III	III	I	II–III	0

Infection: *M. tuberculosis*.
Therapy: 5 months of curative treatment with isoniazid monotherapy or isoniazide-ethionamide combination therapy. Determination of the microbial count in mouse lungs. The microbial count in the group with the highest count (INH 5 mg/kg), which was set to 100% (C) is compared with the counts in the other groups. The degree of resistance (R) to INH is graded from 0 to III.

40 mg/kg. Thus, whereas 50% of the untreated infected controls had died after 17.8 (14.3 to 20.2) days, this time was increased by 8.4 (1.4 to 17.3) days under ETH and by 31.1 (16.1 to 50.7) days under PTH (NOUFFLARD-GUY-LOÉ and BERTEAUX 1962).

In a therapeutic study on guinea pigs infected with tuberculosis ETH yielded a distinct therapeutic effect at doses of 10 mg/kg. After intradermal injection of *M. tuberculosis* (strain H37Rv), the development of ulcerations was dose-dependently delayed or prevented by ETH (RIST 1956; RIST et al. 1958); see Fig. 2.

The protective effect of ETH against tuberculous ulceration is comparable to those of SM and INH, the efficacy at equal doses being about twice that of SM but only about 1/16 that of INH.

After 6 weeks of treatment of guinea pigs in doses of 10 mg/kg to 80 mg/kg per day or every 2nd, 4th, or 8th day, a slow fall in efficacy was observed for ETH with increasing intervals between the doses. According to macroscopic organ findings – especially regarding the spleen – the best results were obtained under the influence of continuous therapy on comparison of the overall quantities of the drug administered. It may be that the weaker effect obtained with longer administration intervals is due to deficient absorption of the higher single doses of ETH. On the basis of an affection index, the values listed in Table 5 were found (DICKINSON 1968).

In a comparative therapeutic study on guinea pigs infected with tuberculosis ETH and PTH proved to be largely equivalent in their effect. Thus, for a survival

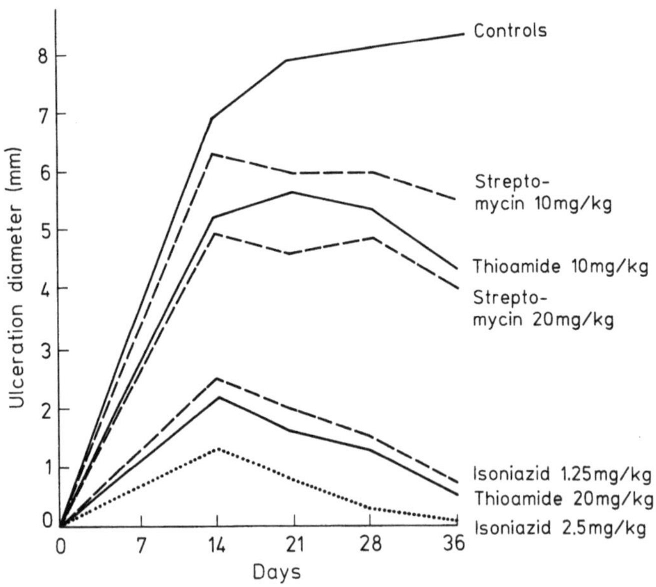

Fig. 2. Comparative effects of ethionamide, streptomycin, and isoniazid on tuberculous skin ulcerations in guinea pigs. [After RIST N et al., Rev. Tuberc. (Paris) 22:278–283 (1958) (modif.)]
Infection: M. tuberculosis H37Rv, 0.05 mg, intradermally
Therapy: daily from the infection for the whole observation period
Evaluation: determination of the diameter of the tuberculous ulcerations

Table 5. Affection index in guinea pigs infected with tuberculosis under ethionamide therapy. (After DICKINSON 1968)

Dose (mg/kg)	Treatment intervals in days during the 6-weeks study period		
	1	4	8
10	0.93	1.03	1.04
20	0.82	0.93	0.94
40	0.68	0.72	0.80

Infected controls: 1.17.

time of 183 (118 to 230) days in the untreated infected control group the corresponding times were 273 days (223 to 306) days in the ETH group and 272 (209 to 341) days in the PTH group (NOUFFLARD-GUY-LOÉ and BERTEAUX 1962).

ETH and PTH were found to be comparable in effect in doses of 20 mg/kg in therapeutic studies on rabbits. The affection index – which is based on the tissue lesions of tuberculosis generalized 40 days after i.v. infection – was 4.3 for the ETH group after 3 months of treatment, compared with 3.4 in the PTH group; the value in the infected control group was 7.7 (SCHMELEV et al. 1971).

Thioamides have favorable distribution characteristics. Thus, the time required for a state of equilibrium to be established regarding the concentrations in the plasma and tissue in rabbits is about 20 min, the corresponding value being e.g. 50 min for INH (HAMILTON et al. 1962). With a half-life of 35 min, a distribution volume of 2.4 litres (in rabbits with a mean body weight of 2.8 kg), and a clearance of 48.3 ml/min. ETH is rapidly distributed over practically the whole organism and is rapidly excreted. The concentrations in the tissues vary largely in the same direction as those in the serum. Within 2 h the serum maxima decreased from about 40 μg/ml after the administration of 20 mg/kg to values below 5 μg/ml, less than 50% being present in the form of free ETH (HAMILTON et al. 1962).

In a study on monkeys with tuberculosis (simian test) a daily ETH dose of 10 mg/kg resulted in a 50% survival rate and was thus equal in effect to an INH dose of 1 mg/kg/day and to an SM dose of 5 mg/kg/day (SCHMIDT 1966). When the evaluation was based on the modification of tissue lesions, especially the lung infiltrations and their elimination and the regional pulmonary lymph nodes, ETH at 10 mg/kg proved to be superior to SM at 5 mg/kg (SCHMIDT 1966).

3. Concluding Remarks

On the basis of their antituberculotic effect both in in-vitro tests and in in-vivo studies on various animal species – mouse, guinea pig, rabbit, and monkey – the thioamides – ethionamide and protionamide – must be classified as reliably effective antituberculotics. The good distribution provides particularly favorable prerequisites for the treatment of generalized tuberculosis. The active doses in the various animal species largely correspond to one another and correlate with the doses determined as effective in man. The possible tuberculocidal and intracellular action – similar to the situation with INH – makes the thioamides particularly effective compared to other antituberculotic agents.

The therapeutic use of the thioamides is encumbered by a relatively high intolerance rate, PTH seeming to be more tolerable, as a result of which drugs belonging to this class of active substance must be graded as highly effective reserve agents in the treatment of tuberculosis.

References

Bartmann K (1960) Kreuzresistenz zwischen α-Äthylthioisonicotinamid (1314 Th) und Thiosemicarbazon (Conteben). Tuberk Arzt 14:525–529

Bönicke R (1965) Vergleichende In-vitro-Untersuchungen zur tuberkulostatischen Wirksamkeit des Aethionamids und seines Sulfoxyds. Beitr Klin Tuberk 132:311–314

Clini V, Grassi L (1970) The action of new antituberculous drugs on intracellular tubercle bacilli. Antibiot Chemother 16:20–26

Dickinson JM (1968) In vitro and in vivo studies to assess the suitability of anti-tuberculous drugs for use in intermittent chemotherapy regimens. Bull Int Union Tuberc XLI:309–315

Dickinson JM, Mitchison DA (1966a) In vitro studies on the choice of drugs for intermittent chemotherapy of tuberculosis. Tubercle 47:370–380

Dickinson JM, Mitchison DA (1966b) Short-term intermittent chemotherapy of experimental tuberculosis in the guinea pig. Tubercle 47:381–393

Eule H (1965) Ethionamid- und Thiosemicarbazon-Kreuzresistenz und ihre Bedeutung für die Klinik. Z Tuberk 123:36–41

Eule H, Werner E (1967) Die Resistenz des Mycobacterium tuberculosis gegen Ethionamid, Thiosemicarbazon und Isoxyl und ihre Beziehung zueinander. Beitr Klin Tuberk 134:247–258

Gialdroni-Grassi G, Grassi C (1966) Chemotherapy of infections caused by atypical mycobacteria. Antimicrobial Agents Chemother 1965:1074–1078

Grumbach F (1961) Le traitement de la tuberculose expérimentale de la souris, par l'association isoniazide-éthionamide à différentes doses. Application des résultats à la posologie clinique. Rev Tuberc (Paris) 25:1365–1385

Grumbach F (1965) Etudes chimiothérapiques sur la tuberculose avancée de la souris. Adv Tuberc Res 14:31–96

Grunert M, Werner E, Iwainsky H, Eule H (1968) Veränderungen des Äthionamides und seines Sulfoxydes in vitro. Beitr Klin Tuberk 138:68–82

Hamilton EJ, Eidus L, Little E (1962) A comparative study in vivo of isoniazid and alpha-ethylthioisonicotinamide. Am Rev Respir Dis 85:407–412

Hilson GRF (1967) Accurate testing of sensitivity to ethionamide. V Congr Chemoth Wien 1967 Vol II/2 541–548

Krebs A (1967) The action of antituberculous drugs. Tuberkuloza 19:328–337

Krebs A, Noack K (1968) Die Wirkungsweise antituberkulöser Medikamente bei kontinuierlicher und intermittierender Anwendung. Jahreskongr Ges Seuchenschutz Leipzig 11.–14. Sept. 1968

Lefford MJ (1969) The ethionamide sensitivity of East African strains of Mycobacterium tuberculosis resistant to thioacetazone. Tubercle 50:7–13

Nitti V (1959) La thioamide dell'acido-α-etilisonicotinico e le sua attività antimicobatterica in vitro. Arch Tisiol 14:819–841

Noufflard-Guy-Loé H, Berteaux S (1962) Etude expérimentale de l'activité antituberculeuse d'un thioamide isonicotinique voisin de l'éthionamide: le 1321 Th (9778 R.P.) Rev Tub Pneumol 26:1204–1215

Otten H (1971) Continuous and intermittent therapy of murine tuberculosis with ethionamide and other antituberculosis drugs. 20th Conf Int Union Tuberc New York Sept 1969 – Symposion: les thioamides. Theraplix-Press Paris 75–79

Pütter J (1964) Photometrische Bestimmung des 2-Äthyl-isothio-nicotinylamid in Organen und Körperflüssigkeiten. Arzneimittelforschung 14:1198–1203
Rist N (1956) Etude expérimentale d'un nouveau médicament antituberculeux, le thioamide de l'acide α-éthylisonicotinique. Atti Soc Lomb Sci Med Biol 11:388–394
Rist N (1960) L'activité antituberculeuse de l'éthionamide (l'alpha-éthyl-thioisonicotinamide ou 1314 Th). Étude expérimentale et clinique. Adv Tuberc Res 10:69–126
Rist N (1964) Die experimentellen Grundlagen der klinischen Anwendung von Ätina bei chronischer Lungentuberkulose. Z Tuberk 122:116–121
Rist N, Grumbach F, Libermann D, Moyeux M, Cals S, Clavel S (1958) Un nouveau médicament antituberculeux actif sur les bacilles isoniazido-résistants: le thioamide de l'acide α-éthylisonicotinique. Etude expérimentale. Rev Tuberc (Paris) 22:278–283
Sojková M, Toušek J, Trnka L (1965) Zur Frage der Kreuzresistenz zwischen Ethionamid, Thiosemikarbazonen und Thioharnstoffderivaten. Praxis Pneumol 19:522–527
Schmelev MA, Korotaev DA, Kozoulitsina TJ (1971) Étude comparative expérimentale et clinique du prothionamide et de l'éthionamide. 20th Conf Int Union Tuberc New York Sept 1969 – Symposion: les thioamides. Theraplix-Press Paris 85–88
Schmidt LH (1966) Studies on the antituberculous activity of ethambutol in monkeys. Ann NY Acad Sci 135:747–758
Schütz I, Bartmann K, Radenbach KL, Siegler W (1969) Vergleich der Verträglichkeit von Prothionamid und Ethionamid im Doppelblindversuch. Beitr Klin Tuberk 140:296–303
Steenken W, Montalbine V (1960) The antituberculous activity of thioamide in vitro and in the experimental animal (mouse and guinea pig). Am Rev Respir Dis 81:761–763
Stottmeier KD, Woodley CL, Kubica GP, Beam RE (1967) A simple biological method for determination of small amounts of tuberculostatic agents in fluids. Bull WHO 37:961–966
Tsukamura M, Tsukamura S (1967) On the instability of ethionamide resistance and on the stability of other drug resistances in tubercle bacilli (five to nine year's in vitro observation). Kekkaku 42:23–27
Urbancik R, Burjanova B (1967) Beitrag zum Problem der Empfindlichkeitsbestimmung von Tuberkelbakterien gegen Äthionamid. Beitr Klin Tuberk 131:339–346
Verbist L (1966) Susceptibility of mycobacteria to 4,4'-diisoamyloxythiocarbanilide. Antimicrobial Agents Chemother 1965:298–305
Walter AM, Otten H, Yamamura Y, Bloch H (1960) Bacterial populations in experimental murine tuberculosis. III. Chemotherapeutic studies. J Infect Dis 107:213–223

X. Kanamycin (KM) and Amikacin

L. Trnka

1. Antimicrobial Spectrum in Vitro

The antimicrobial spectrum of KM is relatively broad. KM acts on most gram-negative cocci and bacteria, including some strains of *Proteus* and *Pseudomonas aeruginosa*. Gram-positives are less sensitive to KM, except for *Staphylococcus aureus, Cornynebacterium diphteriae,* and *Bacillus anthracis.*

In broth dilution tests KM was less active against gram-positive bacteria than other aminoglycoside antibiotics (gentamicin, sisomicin, or tobramycin). *Serratia* strains showed a difference in sensitivity being more susceptible to sisomicin and gentamicin than to tobramycin and kanamycin. Tests with *Mycoplasma* suggest that KM may be slightly less active than sisomicin.

It has been established in several studies that in general KM is less active than the other aminoglycosides (Del Bene and Farrar 1972; Waitz et al. 1972).

2. Antimycobacterial Activity

a) Activity in Artificial Media in Vitro

The results of comparable in-vitro tests are summarized in Table 1. With *M. tuberculosis* strain H37Rv the KM concentration required for complete growth inhibition is determined to some extent by composition of the medium (presence or absence of albumin or serum) and by the duration of the incubation period. The minimal inhibitory concentrations ranged between 0.62 µg/ml and 10 µg/ml, strains of *M. bovis* exhibiting the same susceptibility. The strains of H37Rv resistant to VM or neomycin were not inhibited by 100 µg/ml of KM. Strains of the potentially pathogenic "atypical" species *M. kansasii* (var. luciflava) showed considerable individual variations in their sensitivity to KM in vitro, but the range appeared to be the same as in *M. tuberculosis* strains.

Similar results on the KM sensitivity of mycobacteria in vitro have been reported by YAMAGISAWA and SATO (1957), BROUET et al. (1959), MORELLINI and AVEGNO (1959), and SATO et al. (1960).

YAMADORI (1981 a) used the siliconized slide culture method in Kirchner medium and replaced air by N_2, CO_2, or O_2. Under these unfavorable growth conditions, the effects of antituberculotic drugs in vitro were then found to be dimin-

Table 1. Minimal inhibitory concentrations (MIC) of KM on mycobacteria in vitro

Author	Strain	Medium	MIC µg/ml	Notes
STEENKEN et al. (1958, 1959)	*M. tuberculosis* H37Rv	Proskauer-Beck	5.0	Inoculum 0.1 ml, culture time 15 days
		Proskauer-Beck +10% serum	10.0	
		Dubos-Tween-albumin	2.5	
	H37Rv-VM-R	Proskauer-Beck	>1000	
	H37Rv-Neomycin-R		>1000	
	Photochromogenic PPM[a]		10.0	
PATNODE and HUDGINS (1958)	*M. tuberculosis* H37Rv	Proskauer-Beck	0.62	Inoculum 0.1 ml, culture time 5 weeks
		Proskauer-Beck+0.5% bovine albumin	5.0	
		Proskauer-Beck+5% human serum	5.0	
	M. bovis Ravenel	Proskauer-Beck	0.62	
		Proskauer-Beck+0.5% bovine albumin	0.62	
	BCG	Proskauer-Beck	0.62	
BURJANOVÁ and DORNETZHUBER (1975)	Photochromogenic PPM[a]	Löwenstein-Jensen	10–40	
YAMAMOTO et al. (1975)	*M. tuberculosis* H37Rv	Kirchner semisolid	1.2	
		Dubos-Tween-albumin	0.6	

[a] Potentially pathogenic ("atypical") mycobacteria.

ished; the inhibitory activity of KM was less pronounced than those of SM or RMP, so that uninhibited growth of the bacilli is evidently essential to the action of KM.

α) Factors Affecting the Activity in Vitro. As mentioned above, the addition of 5% human albumin or 0.5% human serum to liquid synthetic Proskauer-Beck medium reduced the inhibitory action of KM on H37Rv strains of *M. tuberculosis*. No such effects have been reported with other media or mycobacteria. It may be assumed that KM is bound to proteins in these media.

The influence of the culture time on the activity of drugs in Löwenstein-Jensen media has been studied in detail by BARTMANN et al. (1966). With KM no end-point in growth was observed within a period of 10 weeks. For practical reasons, therefore, it was recommended to standardize the incubation period, and a period of 4 weeks was proposed. Cultures showing dysgonic growth may be incubated for longer periods. False assessments of sensitivity tests can be avoided if the ratio between the MIC of the patient's strain and the MIC of the standard strain is taken as a basis for the evaluation.

β) Resistance of Bacteria to KM

Development of Resistance in Vitro and its Type: The incidence of mutants naturally resistant to 20 μg/ml of KM in a mycobacterial population previously unexposed to KM was calculated by TSUKAMURA (1977a) as 1 in 10^6–10^8.

According to GROSSET and CANETTI (1962), the median proportions of mutants resistant to the same concentration are 25 in 10^6 after 4 weeks of incubation and 1000 in 10^6 after 6 weeks. In a second experiment, with the same series of 11 strains, the median values were 3 to 4 times as high. While the development of KM resistance in staphylococci was regarded as relatively slow, following the stepwise pattern, its development in mycobacteria was repeatedly evaluated as identical with that of streptomycin resistance – one-step mutation pattern (TSUKAMURA et al. 1960a; ŠIMÁNĚ and KRAUS 1966). YAMADORI (1981b) failed to observe any development of KM resistance, regardless of the duration of the drug's contact with bacilli and of exposure to several kinds of atmospheres producing conditions unfavorable to the growth of tubercle bacilli.

This observation might exclude the possibility suggested by KONDO et al. (1968), that the resistance to KM is caused by the presence of R factors in bacteria.

Primary (initial) resistance to KM has been found in 0.1% of 3598 tested cultures of tubercle bacilli isolated from patients. The critical concentration of KM used for the susceptibility testing was 5.0 μg/ml (KOPANOFF et al. 1978). In potentially pathogenic ("atypical") mycobacteria the prevalence of primary (initial) resistance to KM was higher. 65% of 20 strains of *M. kansasii*, 87% of 23 strains of *M. avium-intracellulare*, and 67% of 12 strains of *M. fortuitum* were evaluated as KM-resistant, using a quantitative proportional test on Löwenstein-Jensen media with a critical proportion of 1% to 20 μg/ml of KM (HEJNÝ 1978).

According to WRIGHT et al. (1958) and ŠIMÁNĚ and KRAUS (1966), secondary (acquired) resistance to KM develops relatively quickly in patients (within 4 months of treatment).

As critical concentrations in susceptibility tests, both for the absolute and the proportion method of testing drug concentrations, either 10 μg/ml or 20 μg/ml KM have been recommended (KUBICA and DYE 1967; HEJNÝ 1978; GÁLVEZ-BRANDON and BARTMANN 1969; CANETTI et al. 1969).

GÁLVEZ-BRANDON and BARTMANN (1969) studied the statistical aspects of the proportion method for testing the drug resistance of tubercle bacilli taking into consideration the size of the inoculum. The random variation in the determination of the proportion of bacterial population capable of growing on a drug-containing medium was investigated with the aid of a mathematical model. For KM some 200 to 1000 viable cells were estimated to constitute an appropriate inoculum.

An expert committee of the WHO (CANETTI et al. 1969) have recommended for sensitivity tests with KM the use of a standard inoculum prepared from the growth on primary diagnostic Löwenstein-Jensen medium. Tests are set up not later than 2 weeks after the slopes have become positive. The tests are performed on Löwenstein-Jensen media.

In the proportion method, mycobacterial populations containing 50% of bacteria growing on media with 10 μg/ml KM or 10% growing on media with 20 μg/ml KM or 1% growing on media with 30 μg/ml KM are regarded as resistant.

KM dependence: No reports dealing with KM dependence have so far been published.

Cross-resistance: "One-way" cross-resistance is known to occur between KM and CM. Mutants resistant to a high concentration of KM which have been selected by KM, are resistant to low concentration of CM. On the other hand, mutants resistant to a low concentration of CM, which have been selected by CM, are susceptible to KM. According to TSUKAMURA (1977b), this phenomenon is based on the fact that quadruply resistant mutants are selected by KM and triply resistant mutants by CM. This stems from the fact that the incidence of triply resistant mutants (resistant to VM, CM, or enviomycin) in the parent H37Rv strains of *M. tuberculosis* is 10^{-5} and that of quadruply resistant mutants is 10^{-7}–10^{-8}.

Similar "one-way" cross-resistance has been described between VM and KM. Several investigators have reported that strains of *M. tuberculosis* which are resistant to VM are also resistant to KM, but that strains resistant to KM maintain their sensitivity to VM (TSUKAMURA 1959a, b; STEENKEN et al. 1958, 1959; TSUKAMURA et al. 1959, 1962).

MCCLATCHY et al. (1977) pointed out, however, that the partial ("one-way") cross-resistance between aminoglycoside antibiotics was variable. A review of the medical histories of 27 patients with tubercle bacilli resistant to KM indicates that cross-resistance occurred with CM and VM, but was unpredictable.

The strain variability in cross-resistance behavior between KM and CM and between KM and VM is probably due to the fact that resistance to these drugs in bacteria might be due to several mechanisms, including a mutational change of the ribosomal targets preventing binding (FUNATSU and WITTMAN 1972), enzymatic inactivation of the drugs by covalent addition of acetyl, adenyl, or phosphoryl groups (BENEVISTE and DAVIES 1973), and impermeability to the drugs (TABER and HALFENGER 1976). TSUKAMURA (1969) has suggested that in mycobacteria mutations to KM resistance might occur at different genetic loci and lead to various degrees of cross-resistance to other similar antibiotics.

The variability in cross-resistance is also reflected in the drug susceptibility studies carried out on cultures of tubercle bacilli isolated from retreated tuberculous patients. According to McClatchy et al. (1977), in these instances cultures resistant to KM were occasionally also found to be resistant to CM and/or to VM, even though the patient had never received either CM or VM. Moreover, KM-resistant tubercle bacilli have been isolated from patients whose medical histories indicated that they had only been treated with either VM or CM.

Cross-resistance between KM and SM – the principal antibiotic of the aminoglycoside group – has been reported by Bartmann (1970) as partial and rare.

Type of Action. For KM a straight line-relationship between the drug concentration and the growth rate of tubercle bacilli has been shown (Tsukamura et al. 1960b; Tsukamura and Mizuno 1980). It has been suggested that KM is primarily bactericidal (Modr et al. 1964), though no direct evidence has yet been presented. Ariji (1971) carried out microscopic examinations of tubercle bacilli exposed to 10 μg/ml of KM. The cytoplasm of these bacilli became coarse and the granular structures of ribosomes were less obvious. Large, homogenous, fairly dense granules, and vacuoles were occasionally observed in the cytoplasm. These morphological changes in the cytoplasm were caused by ribosomal degeneration under the influence of KM. The mesosomes appeared to be poorly organized or fragmented. As shown by the deposition of dense reaction products, enzyme activities of succinic dehydrogenase and cytochrome oxidase were located on the mesosomes in untreated tubercle bacilli, but a remarkable decrease in these activities was found in KM-treated bacilli. Elongated structures were occasionally found in the proximity of large dense granules and vacuoles. These membrane structures were somehow connected with the appearance of large granules and vacuoles.

δ) Effects with Combinations of Antituberculosis Drugs in Vitro. No reports on experiments with combinations of KM and other antituberculotics on tubercle bacilli under "in vitro" conditions have so far appeared.

b) Effect on Mycobacteria in Cell and Tissue Cultures

In a surviving splenic culture KM exerted, similarly to SM, a weak effect on the intracellularly located and a considerable effect on the extracellularly located *M. tuberculosis,* strain H37Rv. A comparative study of the effects produced by the two drugs on the intracellular and extracellular fractions of bacilli in a medium with neutral and acid reactions suggested that the reduced intracellular activity of these antibiotics may be due to the development of an acidic zone around phagocytosed micro-organisms and to the latter's lower physiological activity (Pavlov 1970).

SM like KM, inhibited the growth of tubercle bacilli in monocytes at 10–20 times the inhibitory concentration in vitro. KM at 50 μg/ml and SM at 25 μg/ml showed almost complete growth-inhibiting activity, and the difference between their concentrations was the same as that in vitro (DADDI et al. 1959; IWASAKI 1960).

c) Activity of KM in Experimental Tuberculosis

α) Monotherapy. STEENKEN et al. (1958, 1959) treated guinea pigs infected with *M. tuberculosis* H37Rv with KM given intramuscularly at daily doses of 10 mg/kg–40 mg/kg, obtaining a clear therapeutic effect with 30 mg/kg/day–40 mg/kg/day. The efficacy of this dosage was equivalent to that of 10 mg/kg/day–20 mg/kg/day of SM. Oral doses of KM (25 mg/kg/day–100 mg/kg/day) proved to be ineffective. IWASAKI (1960) used a similar model: guinea pigs were treated for 6 weeks and the effect was evaluated macroscopically. There was a conspicuous difference between KM at daily doses of 40 mg/kg and 60 mg/kg, whereas 20 mg KM/kg/day had much less effect.

The effect of 40 mg KM/kg/day was equal to that of 20 mg SM/kg and a little inferior to oral administration of 4 mg INH/kg. The visceral concentrations of the drug varied in parallel with its blood concentrations, but KM in two divided injections was more effective than in a single injection and INH in three divided doses was also excellent. It was pointed out that the therapeutic effect was due to the long persistence of active blood concentrations.

Using the model of experimental tuberculous meningitis in guinea pigs, TAKAHASHI (1960) estimated that KM was as effective as streptomycin used at half the dosage. To achieve the same antituberculotic effect, KM had to be applied in twice as high doses as SM and in approximately 10 times higher doses than INH (ŠIMÁNĚ and KRAUS 1966).

On the model of guinea pig tuberculosis it has been confirmed that there is no cross-resistance between KM and SM, INH, or PAS, since KM had a favorable influence on infections caused by tubercle bacilli resistant to these three drugs (YAMAGISAWA and KONAI 1958).

β) Combination Therapy. Combination therapy has been studied by STEENKEN et al. (1958, 1959) in tuberculous guinea pigs. KM in daily doses of 5 mg/kg–20 mg/kg was given simultaneously with 5 mg/kg of INH, and the same scale of daily KM doses was administered with 10 mg/kg of SM. Whereas the combination of KM with INH showed a definite antituberculous effect, particularly in cases where higher doses of KM had been used, the effects of combinations of KM with SM were rather doubtful, similar to those after SM monotherapy. It may be concluded that the combination of INH with KM resembles the effects of the combination of INH with SM, particularly in retarding the development of resistance to INH. The combination of SM with KM, however, can not be recommended for clinical use, because the two drugs have the same pattern of toxicity.

Combinations of ETH with SM, KM, VM, and CM were compared by GRUMBACH (1965) in the treatment of advanced tuberculosis in mice. The dose of ETH was 1 mg/mouse and the doses of the other antibiotics 4 mg/mouse. Efficacy was assessed on the basis of viable counts from the organs. The most active combination was ETH + SM followed by ETH + VM, which in turn was clearly superior to ETH + KM. All three combinations were much better than monotherapy with the individual drugs.

3. Antimycobacterial Activity of Amikacin, a Semisynthetic KM Derivative

As shown by YAMAMOTO et al. (1975), SANDERS et al. (1982), and ALLEN et al. (1983), amikacin is highly active in vitro against tubercle bacilli. There is an incomplete cross resistance between amikacin and CM, and complete cross-resistance between amikacin and KM (YAMAMOTO et al. 1975; ALLEN et al. 1983). In murine tuberculosis amikacin was, on a weight basis, more efficient than SM and KM in reducing the viable counts from organs. However, the drug was judged by ALLEN et al. (1983) to have no future in the treatment of human tuberculosis. It cannot be given as an alternative to KM, has no advantages over it, and is more expensive.

4. Concluding Remarks

The activity of KM in vitro is about half of that of SM for extracellular and intracellular tubercle bacilli. In animals, too, the efficacy of KM is half that of SM. In man the effectiveness of KM is likewise clearly inferior to that of SM. Since its lower activity is not compensated by better tolerability, KM ranges among the minor antituberculotics. It is now outdated, but has been used with benefit before the advent of CM, EMB, and RMP in patients harboring SM-resistant bacilli.

References

Allen BW, Mitchison DA, Chan YC, Yew WW, Allan WGL, Girling DJ (1983) Amikacin in the treatment of pulmonary tuberculosis. Tubercle 64:111–118

Ariji F (1971) Electron microscopic studies on tubercle bacilli treated with Kanamycin (in Japanese). Kekkaku 46:53–57

Bartmann K (1970) Discussion remark. Antibiotica et Chemotherapia 16:81–82

Bartmann K, Abel U, Hart R (1966) Die Abhängigkeit des Hemmtiters von der Bebrütungsdauer bei der Bestimmung der Resistenz von M. tuberculosis gegen Antituberkulotika auf Löwenstein-Jensen-Medium. Zentralbl Bakteriol Mikrobiol Hyg (A) 201:538–548

Benveniste R, Davies J (1973) Mechanism of antibiotic resistance in bacteria. Annu Rev Biochem 42:471–493

Brouet G, Marche J, Chevalier J, Liot F, Meur Le G, Bergogne F (1959) Étude expérimentale et clinique de la kanamycine dans l'infection tuberculeuse. Rev Tuberc 23:949–988

Burjanová B, Dornetzhuber V (1975) Empfindlichkeit der Stämme des *M. kansasii* auf verschiedene Antibiotika und Chemotherapeutika in vitro und in vivo. Z Erkr Atmungsorg 142:68–77

Canetti G, Fox W, Khomenko A, Mahler HT, Menon NK, Mitchison DA, Rist N, Šmelev NA (1969) Advances in techniques of testing mycobacterial drug sensitivity, and the use of sensitivity tests in tuberculosis control programmes. Bull WHO 41:21–43

Daddi G, Basilico F, Grassi G (1959) Use of cultures of monocytes for the assessment of activity of antituberculosis drugs (in Italian). G Ital Tuberc 13:123–128

Del Bene VE, Farrar E Jr (1972) Tobramycin: in vitro activity and comparison with kanamycin and gentamycin. Antimicrob Agents Chemother 1:340–342

Funatsu G, Wittman HG (1972) Location of aminoacid replacements in protein S12 isolated from Escherichia coli mutants resistant to streptomycin. J Mol Biol 68:547–556

Gálvez-Brandon J, Bartmann K (1969) Statistical aspects of the proportion method for determining the drug resistance of tubercle bacilli. Scand J Respir Dis 50:1–18

Grosset J, Canetti G (1962) Teneur des souches sauvages de *Mycobacterium tuberculosis* en variants résistants aux antibiotiques mineurs. Ann Inst Pasteur 103:163–184

Grumbach F (1965) Etudes chimiothérapiques sur la tuberculose avancée de la souris. Adv Tuberc Res 14:31–96
Hejný J (1978) Mycobacteriological aspects of the treatment of mycobacterioses. I. In vitro studies (in Czech.). Stud pneumol phtiseol cechoslovac 38:579–583
Iwasaki T (1960) Experimental pathologic study on the effects of kanamycin on tuberculosis. Ann Rep Jap Soc Tuberc No 5:27–50
Kondo S, Akanishi M, Utahara R, Maeda K, Umezawa H (1968) Isolation of kanamycin and paromamine inactivated by E. coli carrying R factor. J Antibiot 21 A:22–29
Kopanoff DE, Kilburn JO, Glassroth JL, Snider DE Jr, Farer LS, Good RC (1978) A continuing survey of tuberculosis primary drug resistance in the United States: March 1975 to November 1977. Am Rev Respir Dis 118:835–843
Kubica GP, Dye WE (1967) Laboratory methods for clinical and public health mycobacteriology. Public Health Service Publications Nr 1547. US Govt Printing Office
McClatchy JK, Kanes W, Davidson PT, Moulding TS (1977) Cross-resistance in *M. tuberculosis* to kanamycin, capreomycin and viomycin. Tubercle 58:29–34
Modr Z, Heřmanský M, Vlček V (1964) Antibiotics and their pharmaceutical products (in Czech.). Avicenum Prague
Morellini M, Avegno P (1959) Antimicrobial activity of kanamycin both in vitro and in vivo (in Italian). Ann Inst Forlanini 19:195–201
Patnode RA, Hudgins PC (1958) Effect of kanamycin on Mycobacterium tuberculosis in vitro. Am Rev Tuberc Pulm Dis 78:138–139
Pavlov EP (1970) Several factors influencing the activity of streptomycin, kanamycin and isoniazid in intracellularly located tubercle bacilli (in Russian). Probl Tuberk 48, issue 9:72–76
Sanders WE Jr, Hartwig C, Schneider N, Cacciatore R, Valdez H (1982) Activity of amikacin against Mycobacteria *in vitro* and in murine tuberculosis. Tubercle 63:201–208
Sato N, Murohashi T, Yanagisawa K (1960) Antimycobacterial activity of kanamycin derivates in vitro and in vivo. J Antibiot 13 A:177–179
Šimáně Z, Kraus P (1966) Antituberculous drugs (in Czech) Spofa, Prague
Steenken W Jr, Montalbine V, Thurston JR (1958) The antituberculosis activity of kanamycin in vitro and in the experimental animal (guinea pig). Ann NY Acad Sci 76:103–110
Steenken W Jr, Montalbine V, Thurston JR (1959) The antituberculous activity of kanamycin in vitro and in the experimental animal (guinea pig). Am Rev Tuberc Pulm Dis 79:66–71
Taber H, Halfenger GM (1976) Multiple-aminoglycoside-resistant mutants of *Bacillus subtilis* deficient in accumulation of kanamycin. Antimicrob Agents Chemother 9:251–259
Takahashi H (1960) Experimental tuberculosis meningitis in guinea pigs. 4. Effect of the administration of kanamycin (in Japanese). Kekkaku 35:216–218
Tsukamura M (1959 a) One-way cross resistance of *Mycobacterium avium* between kanamycin and viomycin. Jpn J gen Microb 34:268–273
Tsukamura M (1959 b) Further studies on the one-way cross resistance in *Mycobacterium tuberculosis* with special reference to streptomycin resistance, kanamycin resistance and viomycin resistance. Jpn J gen Microb 34:275–281
Tsukamura M (1969) Cross-resistance relatonships between capreomycin, kanamycin, and viomycin resistances in tubercle bacilli from patients. Am Rev Respir Dis 99:780–782
Tsukamura M (1977 a) Cross-resistance of tubercle bacilli (a review II) (in Japanese). Kekkaku 52:47–49
Tsukamura M (1977 b) Cross-resistance of tubercle bacilli (a review III) (in Japanese) Kekkaku 52:171–175
Tsukamura M, Noda Y, Yamamoto M (1959) Studies on the kanamycin resistance in *Mycobacterium tuberculosis*. V. Sensitivity of kanamycin-resistant mutants to various antituberculosis drugs and mutation frequency to various drug resistance in kanamycin-resistant mutants. J Antib 12 A:323–324
Tsukamura M, Noda Y, Hayashi M, Torii F (1960 a) Studies on the kanamycin-resistance in Mycobacterium tuberculosis. I. J Antib 13 A:70–73

Tsukamura M, Noda Y, Torii F (1960b) Relationship between antibacterial action of kanamycin and growth phase of *Mycobacterium avium*. J Antib 13A:406–409
Tsukamura M, Yamamoto M, Haashi M, Noda Y, Torii F (1962) Further studies on cross resistance in Mycobacterium tuberculosis, with special reference to streptomycin-, kanamycin-, and viomycin resistance. Am Rev Respir Dis 85:427–431
Tsukamura M, Mizuno S (1980) A comparative study on the relationship between the growth rate of tubercle bacilli and the concentration of antituberculous agents (in Japanese). Kekkaku 55:365–370
Waitz JA, Moss EL Jr, Drube CG, Weinstein MJ (1972) Comparative activity of sisomicin, gentamicin, kanamycin, and tobramycin. Antimicrob Agents Chemother 2:431–437
Wright KW, Renzetti AD, Lunn J, Bunn PA (1958) Observations on the use of kanamycin in patients in a tuberculosis hospital. Ann NY Acad Sci 76:157–165
Yamadori H (1981a) In vitro effects of several kinds of gas exposure on the antimicrobial activities of antituberculous agents. II. Bactericidal effects (in Japanese). Kekkaku 56:465–470
Yamadori H (1981b) In vitro effects of several kinds of gas exposure on the antimicrobial activities of antituberculous agents. III. The development of drug resistance (in Japanese). Kekkaku 56:521–524
Yamagisawa K, Sato N (1957) Studies on kanamycin, a new antibiotic against tubercle bacilli. I. Effect on virulent tubercle bacilli in vitro and in mice. J Antib 10A:233–242
Yamagisawa K, Konai K (1958) Studies on kanamycin. IV. Effect of kanamycin on experimental tuberculosis of guinea pigs infected with the strain resistant to various drugs. Jpn J Bact 13:95–103
Yamamoto K, Sakurai H, Inoue I, Yamagami K (1975) Experimental studies on the antituberculous effect of BB-K8 (in Japanese). Kekkaku 50:235–239

XI. Thiocarlide (DATC)

L. Trnka

DATC, a member of the large series of diaryl thioureas, synthesized by Buu-Hoi and Xuong (1953), is used exclusively by the oral route. When it is given parenterally, its absorption is insufficient owing to its poor solubility in water.

The protein affinity of DATC may influence its activity in the host organism. On the other hand, the binding of DATC to albumin enhances its solubility, and this might augment the concentration of DATC in the blood, though it could also limit the amount taken up by the tissues. This could account for the observations reported by Tacquet et al. (1963) and by Meissner and Meissner (1970) on ^{35}S-labelled DATC.

1. Antimicrobial Spectrum in Vitro

The inhibitory activity of DATC on organisms other than mycobacteria has not so far been reported.

2. Antimycobacterial Activity

a) Activity in Artificial Media in Vitro

Viallier et al. (1962) used Youmans' liquid medium with bovine serum and found an MIC of 2 µg/ml–10 µg/ml for 85% of 46 strains of *M. tuberculosis;* 45 of 47 strains of atypical mycobacteria had an MIC of 7.5 µg/ml or higher.

LUCCHESI (1963) observed that in Dubos liquid medium with Tween 80, but without albumin the growth of *M. tuberculosis* was inhibited by a concentration of 1.0 μg/DATC/ml to 5.0 μg/DATC/ml, the growth of *M. bovis* strains by concentrations of 0.1 μg/ml to 0.5 μg/ml, and the same concentrations were needed to inhibit the growth of photochromogenic strains of mycobacteria.

The other species of mycobacteria were inhibited only by much higher DATC concentrations.

Using 0.5% albumin in liquid media, EIDUS and HAMILTON (1964) observed that two-thirds of 92 strains isolated from patients were inhibited by 0.5 μg/DATC/ml, 85% by 1.0 μg/ml, and 98% by 2 μg/ml. These results are in agreement with the findings of URBANCIK and TRNKA (1963), TRNKA et al. (1963 a, b, c), ŠIMÁNĚ et al. (1966), and TACQUET et al. (1963, 1970).

The effect of albumin on the minimal inhibitory concentration of DATC has been demonstrated by EIDUS and HAMILTON (1964). In a medium containing 0.5% of albumin the minimal inhibitory concentration of DATC for *M. bovis* BCG was 0.4 μg/ml, while 4.0 μg/ml was necessary in a medium containing 4% albumin.

VIRTANEN (1963) and MUZIKRAVIĆ (1970) tested DATC incorporated into Tarshis' blood agar. The MIC for a small inoculum of otherwise sensitive strains was 4 μg/ml.

In tests on the susceptibility of tubercle bacilli to DATC on Löwenstein-Jensen solid media, higher minimal inhibitory concentrations (10 μg/ml to 40 μg/ml) were found by URBANCIK and TRNKA (1963). The results were subsequently confirmed by EIDUS and HAMILTON (1964), who considered that the relative insensitivity of tubercle bacilli to DATC on egg media was due mainly to protein binding, precipitation and sedimentation of DATC during the coagulation procedure (particularly at high DATC concentrations), and partial deterioration due to the coagulation temperature. Variations in this temperature can cause variations in the DATC activity in individual batches of the medium.

Using the absolute concentration method, VERBIST (1966) reported a MIC of 100 μg/ml for 97% of strains isolated from 591 patients never treated before with DATC. KUBALA and KUBALA (1970) observed a median MIC of 30.35 μg/ml on Löwenstein-Jensen medium, whereas in liquid Šula medium the median MIC was 1.12 μg/ml.

Low DATC concentrations are thus necessary to inhibit the growth of *M. tuberculosis*, *M. bovis*, and photochromogenic strains of tubercle bacilli in liquid media with or without a small amount of albumin. The addition of larger amounts of protein reduces the antimycobacterial activity of the drug. This has also been reported by FAVEZ et al. (1963), GUBLER and FRIEDRICH (1965), and MEISSNER and STOTTMEIER (1965).

α) Factors Affecting the Activity in Vitro. Many factors are capable of influencing the antimycobacterial activity of DATC in vitro. Some of them have already been mentioned, concerning the effects of the albumin concentration or the effects of egg proteins in solid Löwenstein-Jensen media.

According to TACQUET et al. (1963), a number of other factors can influence the results of tests of the susceptibility to DATC. These include the Tween 80 content, the pH, and the storage temperature of the medium. Storage of DATC for 1 week at 37 °C decreases the bacteriostatic activity of the drug by a factor of 10.

β) Resistance of Tubercle Bacilli to DATC

Development of Resistance in Vitro and in Vivo and Its Type: From a comparison of the incubation periods and the minimal inhibitory concentrations observed in in-vitro tests it may be assumed that the development of DATC resistance is rather slow and that it follows the multistep pattern. This assumption is supported by the results of animal experiments (TRNKA et al. 1963a, b; TACQUET et al. 1959).

The appearance of initial resistance to DATC was mentioned by MEISSNER (1965), but because of the cross-resistance with thiosemicarbazones it was difficult to establish its prevalence. MEISSNER (1965) noted initial resistance to thiosemicarbazones (1 μg TSC/ml to 10 μg TSC/ml) in 3.5% of 314 German children treated during 1961–1963 and in 1.9% of 1429 adults who came under observation during 1956–1963.

The development of secondary DATC resistance during treatment of patients was also mentioned by MEISSNER (1965). EMERSON et al. (1969) observed an at least fourfold increase in the resistance ratio in 6 out of 17 patients treated daily with 8 g DATC. However, the numbers of patients ever treated with DATC, particularly in monotherapy, are very small.

The criteria for the determination of sensitivity or resistance of cultured tubercle bacilli to DATC were therefore not generally agreed but selected individually. MEISSNER (1965) used Löwenstein-Jensen media. DATC in polyethylene glycol was added at concentrations of 50 μg/ml to 1000 μg/ml, and the results were evaluated by the resistance ratio method. A ratio of 2:1 was regarded as indicating resistance.

In their experimental work with animal models, URBANCIK and TRNKA (1963) used growth on Löwenstein-Jensen media containing 80 μg/DATC/ml as the criterion of resistance.

DATC Dependence: DATC dependence is not mentioned in any of the available papers.

Cross-Resistance of DATC: No cross-resistance with other antituberculotic drugs has been found, except with thiosemicarbazones.

The cross-resistance between DATC and thiosemicarbazones was reported by MUROHASHI and YANAGISWA (1963), TRNKA et al. (1963 a, b), and MEISSNER (1965). The latter author observed resistance to DATC in 93% of 54 strains resistant to 1 μg TSC/ml–10 μg TSC/ml. SOJKOVÁ et al. (1965) observed cross-resistance between DATC and thiosemicarbazones in a thiosemicarbazone-resistant strain of *M. tuberculosis* (H37Rv), and MUZIKRAVIĆ (1970) in all strains made resistant in vitro to either DATC or TSC.

Possible cross-resistance between DATC and ETH (EULE and WERNER 1967) was intensively studied. URBANCIK and TRNKA (1963) suggested that it might be strain-dependent. SOJKOVÁ et al. (1965) found that tubercle bacilli which had become resistant to ETH (410 strains) were still sensitive to DATC. VERBIST (1970) observed cross-resistance in 7 out of 18 strains with secondary resistance to ETH, but none in 5 strains with initial resistance to ETH.

No definite opinion is possible, since the emergence of additional resistant strains soon stopped because the two drugs were no longer widely used.

γ) Type of Action. DICKINSON and MITCHISON (1966) observed a negligible fall in the viable counts of tubercle bacilli exposed for up to 4 days to 10 μg DATC/ml in liquid Dubos medium. Growth started again immediately after removal of the drug. The results strongly suggest a purely bacteriostatic action.

δ) Effects in Combination with Other Antituberculotic Drugs in Vitro. At the time of the discovery of DATC few investigations were done on combined chemotherapy in vitro, and the drug combination were tested largely in animal models. No reports are available on the effects of combinations of DATC with other antimycobacterial drugs in vitro.

b) Effects on Mycobacteria in Cell and Tissue Cultures

No reports have so far appeared on the intracellular activity of DATC. Like other thioureas and thiocompounds it may act predominantly extracellularly, since its accumulation in the host cells in sufficient concentrations might be rather difficult.

c) Activity of DATC in Experimental Tuberculosis

α) Monotherapy. The activity of DATC in vivo has been tested in various animal models, including guinea pigs, mice, and rabbits. Experiments on guinea pigs disclosed the antimycobacterial activity of DATC in skin lesions. LUCCHESI (1963) and URBANCIK et al. (1964) used the method of intracutaneous infection induced by virulent tubercle bacilli, described in detail by URBANCIK et al. (1963). DATC at a daily oral dose of 50 mg/kg–100 mg/kg prevented the development of skin lesions and caused their regression if given to animals with already developed lesions. The effect was superior to those of PAS, VM, and TSC, but inferior to those of INH and SM.

Rabbits were used by FREERKSEN and ROSENFELD (1962, 1963), by FREERKSEN (1963), and by URBANCÍK et al. (1964). The criteria adopted were the mortality of the infected animals and X-ray changes of lung lesions produced by intravenous infection and their pathomorphological assessment. DATC at 100 mg/kg/day or 200 mg/kg/day seemed to be superior to PAS (500 mg/kg) or ETH (50 mg/kg). FREERKSEN (1963) was enthusiastic, concluding that DATC and ETH completely cured miliary tuberculosis of rabbits after administration for 6 weeks. There were supposedly no radiological differences between the results obtained with DATC and INH (5 mg/kg).

More detailed information was obtained in mouse models used by CROWLE et al. (1963), FREERKSEN (1963), MUROHASHI and YANAGISAWA (1963), TRNKA et al. (1963 a–c), and URBANCIK and TRNKA (1963). In all these experiments the mice were infected intravenously and the treatment was started either immediately after the infection or at the time of already developed tuberculosis. The effects were assessed by estimating the mortality (survival time), changes in the weight of the treated animals, and by counting of cultivable tubercle bacilli in organs from sacrificed animals.

According to MUROHASHI and YANAGISAWA (1963), 5 mg INH/kg and 50 mg ETH/kg were equivalent to 50 mg DATC/kg. In contrast to this, FREERKSEN (1963) concluded that DATC at a daily dose of 100 mg/kg was evidently less effective than INH at 5 mg/kg or SM at 50 mg/kg, but superior to PAS at 500 mg/kg. This was also confirmed by other authors.

β) Combination Therapy. Using combinations of DATC with either INH (5 mg/kg) or ETH (50 mg/kg), TRNKA et al. (1963 a–c) estimated that DATC contributes to the activity of INH to the same extent as ETH. GRUMBACH (1965) treated mice with advanced tuberculosis with 25 mg/kg/day of INH + 100 mg/kg, 200 mg/kg, or 400 mg/kg/day of DATC. The results were no better than those obtained with INH + TSC. ROSENFELD (1970) compared INH + DATC with INH + PAS in intravenously infected rabbits. As measured by the survival time, INH + PAS was superior to INH + DATC during the first 8 weeks. In long-term treatment over 5 months the combination of ETH + DATC was more effective than ETH + PAS.

3. Concluding Remarks

The activity of DATC in vitro depends largely on the experimental conditions. Its efficacy in experimental animals was equal to that of ETH in some models, while in others it was no better than that of TSC of PAS; in no case was it of the same order as that of INH or SM. From the body of the experimental evidence some investigators felt justified in proposing clinical trials with the view to replacing the poorly tolerated PAS by DATC in combination with other leading drugs like INH to prevent secondary resistance. Controlled clinical trials have shown, however, that DATC did not live up to its promise.

References

Buu-Hoï NP, Xuong ND (1953) Sur les composés tuberculostatiques du groupe de la thiourée et leur mécanisme d' action. C R Acad Sci (Paris) 237:498–500
Crowle AJ, Mitchell RS, Petty TL (1963) The efectiveness of a thiocarbanilide (Isoxyl) as a therapeutic drug in mouse tuberculosis. Am Rev Resp Dis 88:716–717
Dickinson JM, Mitchison DA (1966) In vitro studies on the choice of drugs for intermittent chemotherapy of tuberculosis. Tubercle 47:370–380
Eidus L, Hamilton EJ (1964) In vitro tests with 4,4'-diisoamyloxythiocarbanilide. Am Rev Resp Dis 90:258–260
Emerson PA, Lacey BW, Breach MR (1969) A bacteriological study of thiocarlide monotherapy. Tubercle (Lond) 50:273–279
Eule H, Werner E (1967) Die Resistenz des M. tuberculosis gegen Ethionamid, Thiosemicarbazon und Isoxyl und ihre Beziehungen zueinander. Beitr Klin Tuberk 134:247–258
Favez G, Vulliemoz P, Breaud P (1963) Tuberculostatic properties of 4,4'-diisoamyloxythiocarbanilide (Isoxyl) (in German). Schweiz Med Wochenschr 93:1208–1210
Freerksen E (1963) Experimental experiences with 4,4'-diisoamyloxythiocarbanilide (Isoxyl). Acta Tub Pneumol Belg 54:12–34
Freerksen E, Rosenfeld M (1962) Experimentelle Therapie mit 4,4'-Diisoamyloxythiocarbanilid. Arzneimittelforsch 12:280–282
Freerksen E, Rosenfeld M (1963) Zur experimentellen Wertermittlung des Tuberkulostaticum Isoxyl. Beitr Klin Tuberk 127:386–397

Gubler HV, Friedrich T (1965) Sensitivity testing of tubercle bacilli to Diisoamyloxythiocarbanilid (in German). Schweiz Med Wochenschr 95:1691–1693
Grumbach F (1965) Etudes chimiothérapiques sur la tuberculose avancée de la souris. Adv Tuberc Res 14:31–96
Kubala E, Kubala J (1970) Discussion remark. Antibiotica et Chemotherapia 16:196–198
Lucchesi M (1963) Recherches expérimentales sur le 4,4'-diisoamyloxythiocarbanilide (Isoxyl). Acta Tub Pneumol Belg 54:42–58
Meissner G (1965) Häufigkeit der Resistenz für Conteben und deren Bedeutung für das Auftreten der Resistenz für Isoxyl (4,4'-Diisoamyloxythiocarbanilid) bei Tuberkelbakterien. Prax Pneumol 19:387–395
Meissner G, Stottmeier D (1965) Die Empfindlichkeit der Mycobakterien für 4,4'-Diisoamyloxythiocarbanilid (Isoxyl) und ihre Bestimmung auf Löwenstein-Jensen Nährböden. Beitr Klin Tuberk 130:289–295
Meissner G, Meissner J (1970) Untersuchungen an Kaninchen über Resorption und Verteilung von ^{35}S–^{3}H markiertem 4,4'-Disisoamyloxythiocarbanilid (Thiocarlid). Nuklearmedizin Suppl 8:177–182
Murohashi I, .Yanagisawa I (1963) Experimental study on Isoxyl (Disoxyl). Acta Tub Pneumol Belg 54:35–41
Muzikravić T (1970) Chemoresistance to Isoxyl. Antibiotica et Chemotherapia 16:177–181
Rosenfeld M (1970) Discussion remark. Antibiotica et Chemotherapia 16:201
Šimáně Z, Kraus P, Krausová E (1966) Antituberculotic drugs (in Czech.). Spofa, Prague pp 112
Sojková M, Toušek J, Trnka L (1965) Zur Frage der Kreuzresistenz zwischen Ethionamid, Thiosemicarbazonen und Thioharnstoffderivaten. Prax Pneumol 19:522–527
Tacquet A, Gernez-Rieux C, Macquet V, Buu-Hoï NP, Xuong ND (1959) Étude in vitro et in vivo de l'activité antituberculeuse de la 4,4'-diisoamyloxythiocarbanilide. Ann Inst Pasteur Lille 10:43–50
Tacquet A, Guillaume J, Macquet V (1963) Etude expérimentale du métabolisme de la 4,4'-diisoamyloxythiocarbanilide marquée au soufre radioactif. Acta Tub Pneumol Belg 54:59–65
Tacquet A, Devulder B, Tison F, Martin JC (1970) Activité de l'Isoxyl sur Mycobacterium kansasii: etudes *in vitro* et chez le cobaye pneumoconiotique. Antib Chemother 16:160–176
Trnka L, Urbancik R, Polenská H (1963a) Antimicrobial activity of isoxyl (4,4'-diisoamyloxythiocarbanilide) in vitro and in vivo (in Czech.). Rozhl Tub 23:147–151
Trnka L, Urbancik R, Polenská H (1963b) Antimykobakterielle Aktivität von Isoxyl. I. In Vitro- und Mäuseversuche. Path Microb 26:817–833
Trnka L, Urbancik R, Polenská H (1963c) Experimental results in animals with new antituberculous drugs (in Roumanian). Ftisiologia (Bucuresti) 12:215–216
Urbancik R, Trnka L (1963) Report on the antimicrobial activity of Isoxyl on M. tuberculosis "in vitro" and "in vivo". Acta Tub Pneum Belg 54:66–86
Urbancik R, Trnka L, Polenská H (1963) The suitability of intracutaneous infection in guinea pigs induced by virulent tubercle bacilli for the use in chemotherapeutic trials. Experientia 19:23
Urbancik R, Trnka L, Kruml J, Polenská H (1964) Antimykobakterielle Aktivität von Isoxyl. II. Versuche an Meerschweinchen und Kaninchen. Path Microb 27:79–87
Verbist L (1966) Susceptibility of mycobacteria to 4,4'-diisoamyloxythiocarbanilide. Antimicrobial Agents Chemother 1965:298–305
Verbist L (1970) Discussion remark. Antibiotica et Chemotherapia 16:190–192
Viallier J, Cayré RM, Lanéry R (1962) Activité bactériostatique exercée *in vitro*, sur les Mycobactéries par la 4,4'-diisoamyloxythiocarbanilide. CR Soc Biol 156:854–856
Virtanen S (1963) Determination of the sensitivity of Mycobacteria to Isoxyl *in vitro*. Ann Med exp Fenn 41:430
Wagner WH, Winkelmann E (1969) Tuberkulostatisch wirksame N,N'-Diarylthioharnstoffe, 2. Mitteilung. Arzneimittelforsch 19:719–730
Winkelmann E, Wagner WH, Hilmer H (1969) Tuberkulostatisch wirksame N,N'-Diarylthioharnstoffe, 1. Mitteilung. Arzneimittelforsch 19:543–558

XII. Capreomycin (CM)

H. OTTEN

1. Antimicrobial Activity in Vitro

Because of its good solubility in water, CM is suitable for in-vitro studies in all kinds of media – solid, semi-solid, and liquid. For activity tests it is best to use the fairly standardizable, semi-synthetic media such as Kirchner, Proskauer-Beck, Dubos, Middlebrook 7H10, Youmans, etc. For special test purposes it is sometimes useful to add Tween 80 (e.g., 0.05%) or agar (e.g., 0.2%–1.5%) to these media. Protein-rich media, e.g., ones to which serum has been added or egg media such as Löwenstein-Jensen, require higher substance concentrations – sometimes up to more than 10 times the minimal inhibitory concentrations (MIC) determined in semisynthetic media. In addition to the serial dilution test, plate or tube diffusion tests, e.g., with *M. butyricum* as the test microorganism, or turbidimetric determinations with *Klebsiella pneumoniae* are suitable for activity testing (STARK et al. 1963).

The effect of CM is evidently diminished by bonding to egg protein (BLACK et al. 1964). To what extent other inactivations are caused by nutrient media constituents is unknown. Since the inhibitory effect is influenced by the amount of the test microorganism added to the nutrient medium, standardized inocula should be used in comparative tests. A culture medium (Löwenstein-Jensen) to which CM has been added can be stored for more than 8 weeks at +4 °C without loss of activity. In the event of prolonged incubation at 37 °C the activity does fall off, which should be borne in mind when using extremely slow-growing Tb strains for a resistance evaluation (SCHRÖDER and HENSEL 1970).

In the form of a standard solution – e.g., for test purposes – aqueous solutions of CM are largely stable when stored in a refrigerator (4 °C). It is expedient to subject such solutions to sterile filtration through membrane filters.

The action spectrum of CM covers above all mycobacteria and in addition a large proportion of the Nocardia strains isolated from patients' material. The MIC's determined for gram-positive and gram-negative micro-organisms are largely above 100 µg/ml, so that CM has no clinical significance for infections with these pathogens. Table 1 gives a guide to the intensity and range of CM activity. The MIC values have been taken from various reports and the values are thus based on various experimental techniques, which should be borne in mind in comparative evaluations (SUTTON et al. 1966; BLOOM 1970; HAVEL and ŠIMONOVA 1970; LUCCHESI 1970; STARK et al. 1963; BLACK et al. 1964; WILSON and WILLIAMS 1966).

On egg medium wild strains of *M. tuberculosis* are largely expected to be sensitive, with MIC's of up to 16 µg/ml. SM-resistant strains are sensitive to CM. In addition, "atypical" mycobacteria of Runyon groups I, II, and IV isolated from patients' material prove sensitive in more than 60% of the cases; strains from Runyon's group III – especially *M. avium* – are only sensitive to CM in around 40% of the cases (HAVEL and ŠIMONOVA 1970; KUBALA and KUBALA 1970). According to other authors, different sensitivity data are obtained for individual mycobacterial species, *M. bovis* strains being sensitive in only about 60%

Table 1. Antimicrobial action spectrum of capreomycin. Minimum inhibitory concentrations in μg/ml

Gram-positive bacteria		
Enterococci		(64–) 250–1000
Staphylococcus aureus		(1–) 16–64 (–500)
Streptococcus pneumoniae		250–1000
Streptococcus pyogenes		(32–) 128–500 (–1000)
Streptococcus viridans		(32–) 128–256
Mycobacterium tuberculosis	in egg medium	(2–) 8–16 (–32– >64)
	in liquid medium	(0,5–) 1–4 (–8–32)
Mycobacterium bovis		(4–) 8–16 (–64)
Runyon Group I	Photochromogenic Mycobacteria	(1–) 8–16–32
Runyon Group II	Scotochromogenic Mycobacteria	(<2–8–) 16–32 (–64)
Runyon Group III	Non-chromogenic Mycobacteria	(2–8–) 16–64 (–128– >128)
Runyon Group IV	Fast-growing Mycobacteria	(<2–4) 8–32 (–64– >128)
Nocardiae		16–32– >128
Gram-negative bacteria		
Escherichia coli		(8–) 32–128–500
Enterobacter aerogenes		16– >128
Klebsiellae		16–32– >128
Pasteurella multocida		128
Proteus vulgaris		128–1000
Proteus mirabilis		250–1000– >1000
Proteus rettgeri		16– >32
Pseudomonas aeruginosa		>500
Salmonellae		64– >256
Shigellae		16– >128

of the cases, *M. kansasii* in only about 30%, and *M. avium* being largely resistant. Likewise, fast-growing mycobacteria are mostly resistant, though some strains may be highly sensitive (LUCCHESI 1970). From this it can be seen that in each individual case only a sensitivity test can give a true picture of the situation.

The type of antituberculotic activity exerted by capreomycin is variously described: mostly it is said to be bacteriostatic (GUNELLA 1965; COLETSOS and ORIOT 1964a, b); if a special experimental technique is used a tuberculocidal effect can be observed. To kill 99.9% of the bacterial population a concentration 4 to 8 times that of SM is necessary (STARK et al. 1963).

In monocyte cultures CM is found to exert comparable activity on Mycobacteria to that observed with conventional culture techniques (CLINI and GRASSI 1970).

In subculture techniques the development of resistance can be rapidly induced at subinhibitory concentrations, although in comparison with SM about twice the number of passages is necessary; for example, the degree of resistance is 2000 and 8000 times the initial value after 12 and 21 subcultures (SUTTON et al. 1966).

The effect of combinations of CM with other antituberculotics is variously assessed: according to in-vitro experiments, combinations with INH, SM, PAS, or

VM do not lead to a synergistic potentiation of the effect (SUTTON et al. 1966). Other authors report intensification of the activity in combinations with SM (COLETSOS and ORIOT 1964a). According to animal studies, CM can be observed to potentiate activity when used in combinations with other antituberculosis drugs (SUTTON et al. 1966).

In the case of *M. tuberculosis* on egg medium a primary resistance rate of 100 mutants in 10^6 culturable units has been determined at CM concentrations of 20 µg/ml. From this it emerges with regard to resistance evaluation that a test strain with 1% of resistant mutants should be regarded as resistant, and if the proportion of resistant mutants is 5%, the resistance can be regarded as certain (RIST and GRUMBACH 1965).

Because of the similarity in their chemical structures, largely complete parallel resistance exists between CM and VM, i.e., the resistance determined by CM gives rise to VM resistance and vice-versa (RIST and GRUMBACH 1965; ALGEORGE and PETRE 1970; VERBIST 1970). Other authors have been unable to confirm the existence of complete parallel resistance between CM and VM, and some exclude this possibility (STARK et al. 1963; HERR et al. 1962; COLETSOS and ORIOT 1964a, b).

Partial parallel resistance exists between CM and KM. CM is included in the resistance relationships between KM and VM owing to partial parallel resistance: the resistance determined by CM gives rise to complete VM resistance, but only in some cases to KM resistance as well. In the case of KM resistance determined by KM with parallel CM resistance, on the other hand, it does not necessarily follow that VM resistance will also appear (RIST and GRUMBACH 1965).

Figure 1 illustrates the relationships of parallel resistance between CM, VM, and KM. SM has also been included. There is no parallel resistance with other antituberculotic agents and antibiotics, with the exception of neomycin.

The incidence of parallel resistance between capreomycin, viomycin, and kanamycin depends on the selecting antibiotic, as can be seen from Table 2, which is based on the data reported by RIST and GRUMBACH (1965).

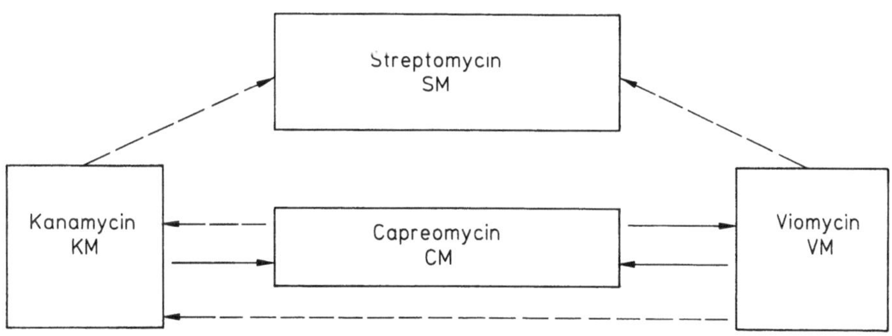

Fig. 1. Parallel resistance between capreomycin and other antituberculotics

Table 2

Resistance selected by	Incidence of parallel resistance (after RIST and GRUMBACH, 1965)	
Capreomycin	Viomycin 100%	Kanamycin 54% (28% slightly, 26% highly resistant)
Viomycin	Capreomycin 100%	Kanamycin 36%
Kanamycin	Capreomycin 64%	Viomycin 40%

2. Activity of CM in Experimental Tuberculosis and Development of Resistance in Vivo

CM is active in experimental tuberculosis in various animal species (SUTTON et al. 1966; RIST and GRUMBACH 1965; GUNELLA 1965). Since after oral administration active capreomycin is absorbed little or not at all, parenteral administration is the only route that can be considered, intramuscular or subcutaneous injection being the method of choice. After intravenous injection a halflife of about 1 h is determined in the dog, up to 80% of the dose being excreted within 6 h of an injection of 10 mg/kg (WELLES et al. 1966).

a) Chemotherapeutic Activity in Infections in the Mouse

In staphylococcal infections an ED_{50} of 155 mg/kg is obtained for two subcutaneous injections, the requisite dose in streptococcal infections being 58 mg/kg. In pneumococcal infections no effect could be achieved with doses higher than 800 mg/kg (SUTTON et al. 1966).

Klebsiella infections could be favorably influenced by two dosages with an ED_{50} of 30 mg/kg; in other infections, due to gram-negatives such as *Proteus* or *E. coli,* the ED_{50} values are over 160 mg/kg to 240 mg/kg, whereas a similar effect was achieved in *Salmonella* infections only after 5 doses of 115 mg/kg. Infections due to *Pseudomonas aeruginosa* remain unaffected even at high doses (SUTTON et al. 1966).

Since these high doses of more than 100 mg/kg are within the toxic range on repeated medication, according to orienting animal experiments in the mouse, CM cannot be considered as an agent for the treatment of infections caused by banal gram-positive and gram-negative pathogens, for which many more effective antibiotics and chemotherapeutics are available.

More favorable therapeutic results were achieved in tuberculosis infections in the mouse (Table 3), the effect of CM proving stronger than that of VM but not equal to those of KM and SM (RIST and GRUMBACH 1965). In infections with SM-resistant mycobacteria CM to be proved fully effective, and its activity in *M. bovis* infections is comparable to that in *M. tuberculosis* infections (SUTTON et al. 1966). *M. kansasii* infections can evidently be more beneficially influenced by CM than by SM (SUTTON et al. 1966).

Combinations of CM with antituberculotics such as SM, INH, and PAS have given a better effect on *M. tuberculosis* infections – especially in the case of combinations with PAS – than the individual agents (SUTTON et al. 1966).

Table 3. Tabulated synopsis of the antimycobacterial activity of capreomycin in infections in the mouse. Mortality rate (%) during therapy in mycobacterial infections

M. tuberculosis infections. Therapy from 13th day after infection	Day after infection: 23.	Day after infection: 100.
Infected controls	100	
Streptomycin 200 mg/kg	0	0
Capreomycin 200 mg/kg	25	50
Capreomycin 400 mg/kg	17	25
Viomycin 200 mg/kg	67	84

M. tuberculosis infection

Infected controls	Streptomycin		Capreomycin	
	250 mg/kg	5 mg/kg	250 mg/kg	5 mg/kg
80	0	60	12	83

M. tuberculosis-SM-resistant infection

Infected controls	Streptomycin		Capreomycin	
	250 mg/kg	50 mg/kg	250 mg/kg	50 mg/kg
57	60	50	0	39

M. bovis infection

Infected controls	Capreomycin 500 mg/kg
80	0

Mycobacterial affection index (necrotic foci and pathogen counts in the lungs and, in some cases: kidneys, in relation to the findings in the infected control group taken as 100%) under the influence of therapy

M. tuberculosis infection

		Combination therapy	
Infected controls	100		
Capreomycin 500 mg/kg	34		
Streptomycin 250 mg/kg	31	CM 500 + SM 250	31
Isoniazid 2 mg/kg	10	CM 500 + INH 2	7
p-Aminosalicyclic acid 112 mg/kg	38	CM 500 + PAS 112	21

M. kansasii infection

Infected controls 100

Capreomycin		Streptomycin	
500 mg/kg	250 mg/kg	500 mg/kg	250 mg/kg
36	52	80	84

M. lepraemurium infection

Leprosy index (organ lesions) after 3-months of therapy	Infected controls	Capreomycin 500 mg/kg	Streptomycin 100 mg/kg
	100	38–46	56

References: Rist and Grumbach (1965); Sutton et al. (1966); Chang (1965).

Various reports are available on the development of resistance to CM in the course of the treatment. On the one hand no reduction of sensitivity was observed after 9 weeks of treatment with daily doses of 500 mg/kg (Sutton et al. 1966), while resistance has been observed to develop after 3 months of therapy with 200 mg/kg (Grumbach 1965). The latter observation is frequently confirmed in clinical practice, where resistance can develop within a treatment period of 2 months to 3 months in accordance with the "fall and rise" phenomenon (Rist and Grumbach 1965).

CM has proved to be effective in experimentally induced leprosy due to *M. leprae* and *M. lepraemurium* (Shepard 1964; Gaugas 1967; Chang 1965).

CM is effective in tuberculous infections in guinea pigs, daily doses of 20 mg/kg to 40 mg/kg to 80 mg/kg giving a clear protective effect (Gunella 1965; Nakamura et al. 1964).

3. Concluding Remarks

According to the experimental investigations, CM has proved to be predominantly antituberculotic in its activity. CM is only used to a limited extent in clinical practice, especially in patients with SM-resistant tubercle bacilli, because of its restricted potency and the possibility of oto – and nephrotoxic side effects. For this reason only a small number of animal experimental studies in particular have been published, and most of these relate to the mouse.

As can be seen from the table, even when high doses of up to 200 mg/kg or more are given it is impossible to bring about a reliable protective effect in mycobacterial infections in the mouse.

In accordance with its in-vivo and in-vitro efficacy CM is classified as a 2nd-series antituberculotic.

References

Algeorge G, Petre A (1970) Some experimental aspects of cross-resistance between capreomycin and viomycin. Antibiot Chemother 16:32–35

Black HR, Griffith RS, Brickler JF (1964) Preliminary laboratory studies with capreomycin. Antimicrob Agents Chemother 1963:522–529

Bloom C (1970) Capreomycin laboratory studies. Antibiot Chemother 16:1–9

Chang YT (1965) Effects of capreomycin, ethambutol, vadrine, neovadrine, tapazole, griseofulvin and five long-acting sulfonamides in murine leprosy. Antimicrob Agents Chemother 1964:777–782

Clini V, Grassi C (1970) The action of new antituberculous drugs on intracellular tubercle bacilli. Antibiot Chemother 16:20–26

Coletsos PJ, Oriot E (1964a) Action de la capréomycine sur *Mycobacterium tuberculosis* en milieux de culture liquides, seule ou associée à la streptomycine, à l'INH et au PAS Ann Inst Pasteur 107:215–231

Coletsos PJ, Oriot E (1964b) Etude de l'activité antibacillaire in vitro de la capréomycine. Rev Tuberc (Paris) 28:413–432

Gaugas JM (1967) Antimicrobial therapy of experimental human leprosy (Myco. leprae) infection in the mouse foot pad. Lepr Rev 38:225–230

Grumbach F (1965) Etudes chimiothérapiques sur la tuberculose avancée de la souris. Adv Tuberc Res 14:31–96

Gunella G (1965) Microbiological, histological and clinical results following the use of capreomycin. Symposium on capreomycin held by Royal Society of Medicine London 15th Jan 1965, Eli Lilly and Comp Press 51–55

Havel A, Šimonova S (1970) The effect of capreomycin on "atypical" and avian mycobacterial strains in vitro. Antibiot Chemother 16:17–19
Herr EB Jr, Sutton WB, Stark WM (1962) Chemical and biological studies of capreomycin. Trans 21th Res Conf Pulm Dis VAAF:367–369
Kubala E, Kubala J (1970) Experimental and clinical evaluation of the tuberculostatics – discussion on capreomycin. Antibiot Chemother 16:75–77
Lucchesi M (1970) The antimicrobial activity of capreomycin. Antibiot Chemother 16:27–31
Morse WC, Sproat EF, Arrington CW, Hawkins JA (1966) M. tuberculosis *in vitro* susceptibility and serum level experiences with capreomycin. Ann NY Acad Sci 135:983–988
Nakamura RM, Kanai K, Murohashi T (1964) Effectiveness of capreomycin against experimental tuberculosis of mice and guinea pigs. Kekkaku 39:161–165
Rist N, Grumbach F (1965) Antituberculous activity of capreomycin in vitro and in mice and cross-resistance against capreomycin, viomycin and kanamycin in in vitro and clinical studies. Symposium on capreomycin held by Royal Society of Medicine London 15th Jan 1965, Eli Lilly and Comp Press 19–25
Shepard CC (1964) Capreomycin: activity against experimental infection with Mycobacterium leprae. Science 146:403–404
Sutton WB, Gordee RS, Wick WE (1966) In vitro and in vivo laboratory studies on the antituberculous activity of capreomycin. Ann NY Acad Sci 135:947–959
Schröder KH, Hensel I (1970) The determination of resistance of M. tuberculosis to capreomycin. Antibiot Chemother 16:69–72
Stark WM, Higgens CE, Wolfe RN, Hoehn MM, McGuire JM (1963) Capreomycin, a new antimycobacterial agent produced by *Streptomyces capreolus* sp. n. Antimicrob Agents Chemother 1962:596–606
Verbist L (1970) Experimental and clinical evaluation of the tuberculostatics – discussion on capreomycin. Antibiot Chemother 16:73–75
Welles JS, Harris PN, Small RM, Worth HM, Anderson RC (1966) The toxicity of capreomycin in laboratory animals. Ann NY Acad Sci 135:960–973
Wilson DE, Williams TW Jr (1966) In vitro susceptibility of *Nocardia* to antimicrobial agents. Antimicrob Agents Chemother 1965:408–411

XIII. Ethambutol (EMB)

H. Otten

EMB was tracked down as an antituberculotically active racemate among a large number of ethylenediamines; the dextro-isomer is used for therapeutic purposes, in the form of EMB hydrochloride (Shepherd et al. 1966; Thomas et al. 1961).

1. Antimicrobial Activity in Vitro

In vitro the d-isomer is some 200 times as antituberculotically effective as the l-form (Wilkinson et al. 1961). A white, crystalline substance, EMB is readily soluble in water and, because of its thermal stability, well suited for test purposes. In conventional nutrient media the antituberculotic activity of EMB remains intact over a 7-week culture period at an incubation temperature of 37 °C (Mostardini et al. 1968). In some of the test strains the MIC can be slightly elevated compared with the initial value after 10 weeks of incubation; in a Löwenstein-Jensen egg medium EMB remains fully active when stored in a refrigerator – at 4 °C – for 6 weeks, although in the event of longer storage a slight loss of activity must be reckoned with (Schröder and Hensel 1970).

The antimicrobial activity of EMB is restricted to Mycobacteria and various Nocardia species; other microorganisms, such as gram-positive and gram-negative strains, fungi, viruses, and protozoa, are resistant to EMB.

The antituberculotic effect remains largely consistent over a broad spectrum of mycobacteria, including the so-called atypical species. The minimal inhibitory concentrations – in μg/ml nutrient medium – are as follows:

M. tuberculosis	
in liquid, semi-synthetic media as Dubos, Youmans, Sauton, Middlebrook 7H10 and others, sometimes with Tween added	(0.1–) 0.5–1 (–2)
in Löwenstein-Jensen egg media Egg yolk agar (Herrold) and others	(0.1–) 0.5–1–2 (–4– >8)
M. bovis	(0.5–) 1–2 (– >4)
M. avium	(0.5–) 1–4 (–8)
M. kansasii	(0.5–) 1–2–4
Runyon Group I	(0.5–) 1–2–4 (–8– >16)
Runyon Group II	(1–) 2–4–8 (– >16)
Runyon Group III	(0.2–) 1–4–8 (–16)
Runyon Group IV	(1–) 2–8–16– >16
Nocardia	(1–) 8–32–128

References: GIALDRONI-GRASSI and GRASSI (1966); BÖNICKE (1962); KARLSON (1961b); LUTZ and BERGER (1962); LUCCHESI and MANCINI (1970); SCHRÖDER and HENSEL (1970); KUBALA and KUBALA (1970).

Individual mycobacterial species (e.g., *M. borstelense, M. friedmanii*) consistently exhibit high resistance to EMB, and as a result this has been proposed as a typing characteristic (PORTAELS and PATTYN 1970).

Pathogenic mycobacteria of Group II (scotochromogenic) and Group III (non-photochromogenic) are resistant to EMB (on Ogawa egg medium at concentrations of 5 μg/ml), whereas non-pathogenic mycobacteria from these groups are EMB-sensitive (TSUKAMURA 1970).

Among the so-called atypical mycobacteria, individual species display different sensitivities so that the sensitivity ranges to be assigned to the individual Runyon groups can only serve as a guide. In practice a sensitivity test is necessary in each individual case.

EMB diffuses into mycobacteria, in concentrations proportional to those in the nutrient medium. As a result of intramycobacterial binding, the concentrations in the bacterium can be up to twice those in the medium (FORBES et al. 1966).

EMB acts upon proliferating mycobacteria, the inhibitory effect setting in after a latent phase. Under the influence of optimal concentrations the growth phase can remain unaffected for up to about 24 h (KUCK et al. 1963). EMB diffuses rapidly into mycobacteria, the concentration reached after 2 h of exposure corresponding to that determined after 96 h (KUCK et al. 1963). However, raising the concentration does not result in a faster onset of action; the inhibition of mycobacteria under the influence of EMB depends on the exposure time and not so much on the concentration (BEGGS and JENNE 1970).

Dormant pathogens are virtually unaffected by ethambutol, even though high intracellular concentrations are obtained as a result of its diffusion capacity (FORBES et al. 1962).

If the exposure is short, the damage induced by EMB is reversible. After a lag phase, prolonged in proportion to the damage incurred, the mycobacteria begin to proliferate again (FORBES et al. 1966):

The uptake of EMB by mycobacteria is increasingly inhibited by increasing ionization in the medium. Thus, in demineralized water mycobacteria can take up 10 times (or more) the amount of EMB taken up in NaCl or KCl solutions or in Na or K phosphate buffers (FORBES et al. 1966).

Various polyamines such as spermidine, spermine, putrescin, cadaverine as well as magnesium inhibit the effect of EMB. In cultures the effect of EMB can be eliminated if such substances are added (FORBES et al. 1962; FORBES et al. 1966; REUTGEN and IWAINSKY 1970). Vitamins such as nicotinamide, aneurine, p-aminobenzoic acid, and pantothenic acid, and purines, pyrimidines, and various amino acids added to cultures have no influence on the effect of EMB (BÖNICKE 1962; FORBES et al. 1966).

Under the influence of EMB mycobacteria lose their resistance to acids. The effect sets in after a delay while metabolic processes are in progress, since the reduction of the acid resistance only reaches its maximum after 2 days to 4 days and can be prevented on simultaneous exposure to fast-acting antituberculotics such as SM (GRUMBACH 1966).

On continued exposure to EMB concentrations of the order of the MIC a progressive reduction of the microbial count is observed. Short-term single or even repeated exposures to high concentrations, e.g., of 5 µg/ml, have a weaker inhibitory effect than continuous exposures to lower concentrations, e.g., of 1 µg/ml. If the intervals between the intermittent exposures are too long, e.g., 2 h of exposure to EMB concentrations of 5 µg/ml every 3 days, no inhibition is produced (KREBS and NOACK 1968). The activity – especially on intermittent exposure – is variously described, which to some extent may be due to the methods used, e.g., to the use of different media. Thus, on the one hand, a tuberculocidal effect is reported for concentrations of up to 10 µg/ml (LUTZ and BERGER 1962), whilst on the other hand proliferation was observed immediately after short-term exposures of 2 h to 6 h to 10 µg/ml. When the contact period was prolonged to 24 h a delay of renewed growth by about 2.5 days was found. Only during a contact of 96 h the viable count did fall (to below 1%) and the delay of renewed growth extended to 4.5 days (DICKINSON 1968).

The development of resistance to EMB is of the one-step type, primarily resistant mutants possibly occurring among *M. tuberculosis* and *M. bovis* strains at the rate of $1:10^5$ (TSUKAMURA 1965). However, the development of resistance in vitro and in vivo is delayed – even after very many culture passages the resistance value, once reached (and it is rarely more than 10 times the initial value), does not undergo any further essential change (BÖNICKE 1962; GRUMBACH 1966; KARLSON 1961 b; SCHMIDT et al. 1962; SCHMIDT 1966; TSUKAMURA 1965). Once acquired the resistance is largely stable (TSUKAMURA and TSUKAMURA 1967; LUCCHESI and MANCINI 1970).

Under clinical conditions, in an observation series of 278 patients before EMB therapy 9.4% of the *M. tuberculosis* strains were still exhibiting growth at 4 µg/ml

(Löwenstein-Jensen egg medium), the corresponding figures after 3 months and after 6 months of therapy being respectively 13.6% and 43%. At a concentration of 8 μg/ml, losses of sensitivity only occurred for the first time after 3 months of treatment (in 12.3% of the cases), this figure increasing to 17.7% of the isolates after a further 3 months (LUCCHESI and MANCINI 1970).

Under the influence of monotherapy with EMB (~15 mg/kg), EMB-resistant tubercle bacilli could be isolated in 17% of the patients after 2 months of treatment, in 37% of the cases after 4 months, and in 58% of the cases after 6 months. The MIC was 5 μg/ml, although high resistance to 10 μg/ml was found only in 5% of the isolates (DONOMAE and YAMAMOTO 1966). Other authors fail to confirm a similarly high loss of sensitivity under EMB therapy (TACQUET et al. 1970; PYLE 1966).

EMB does not display parallel resistance with other antituberculotics; in combination therapy, especially with *M. tuberculosis* and *M. bovis*, a potentiation of the effect is more marked than with the "atypical" mycobacteria, this potentiation of the effect being sometimes described as synergism (GUPTA 1964; GRUMBACH 1966; LAL and ROBSON 1963; SCHMIDT 1962; TACQUET and TISON 1963).

Tests on the sensitivity of mycobacteria to EMB can also be carried out by the vertical diffusion test. In conventional arrangements in test-tubes inhibition zones of 37 mm are reached with concentrations on the borderline of effectiveness (KALICH 1969).

In monocyte cultures ethambutol acts with the same intensity as in conventional culture media (CLINI and GRASSI 1970). LISS (1982) has shown that human alveolar macrophages obtained by bronchial lavage accumulate EMB to a level 7 times higher than the extracellular drug concentration of 5 μg/ml. After 5 days of incubation of infected macrophages in medium containing 5 μg/ml EMB electron microscopy revealed tubercle bacilli within phagosomes exhibiting membrane swelling and various stages of bacteriolysis, whereas the bacilli in the control were quite normal. The viable count of bacilli had decreased to about 10%. INH (0.5 μg/ml) reduced the count to 1%, INH + EMB to less than 1%. Using human monocyte-derived macrophages CROWLE et al. (1985) also observed a marked reduction of viable counts: 80%–90% of intracellular bacilli were killed within 7 days when 5 μg/ml EMB were added immediately after infection; 1 μg/ml EMB prevented multiplication. Addition of the drug 2 days after infection resulted in an even higher killing rate than immediate application.

2. Activity of EMB in Experimental Tuberculosis and Development of Resistance in Vivo

EMB has proved to be a reliably active antituberculotic in experimental tuberculosis induced in animals with various mycobacterial species. After oral administration EMB is absorbed at much the same high speed in various animal species and is excreted largely – more than 90% – with the urine, some 10% in metabolized form.

At therapeutic EMB doses concentrations of 0.6 μg/ml to 2 μg/ml to 5 μg/ml are reached in the blood of various animal species, thus covering the sensitivity range of the majority of mycobacteria (BUYSKE et al. 1966; SCHMIDT 1966).

EMB is therapeutically effective in experimental tuberculosis in the mouse with therapy commencing from the time of infection and involving daily s. c. administration of doses from 12 mg/kg. At doses 4 times this threshold active dose (50 mg/kg) a complete protective effect can be achieved in the course of the therapy, i.e., a 100% survival rate. As the dose is increased further to 30 times the original level (1500 mg/kg), the acutely toxic concentrations are reached (THOMAS et al. 1961).

If the therapy is started 4 days after the infection with EMB doses of 50 mg/kg, the effect is equivalent to that of INH therapy with 1 mg/kg, the INH: EMB dose ratio being about 1 : 50. If the start of the treatment is delayed (8th day after the infection) a complete protective effect can only be achieved by increasing the dose to 100 mg/kg–200 mg/kg. A while after the end of treatment reactivation takes place in dose-dependent fashion with an increasing mortality rate over time (FREERKSEN and ROSENFELD 1962).

When treatment of mice began simultaneously with infection by *M. tuberculosis*, EMB doses of 50 mg/kg administered orally or subcutaneously exhibited respectively half and $^{1}/_{20}$ of the equivalent activity of ETH and INH. In the therapeutic study (treatment started from the 14th day after the infection), the mortality rate was 62% for EMB doses of 50 mg/kg as compared with 0% in the groups treated with 5 mg/kg of INH or 50 mg/kg of ETH (GRUMBACH 1966). After 6 months of curative therapy with EMB doses of 100 mg/kg, EMB-resistant mycobacteria could be detected in 50% of the surviving animals. Resistance developed slowly, and as it did so it was characterized by relatively slight losses of sensitivity. Nevertheless it was impossible to suppress a reactivation of the tuberculous process (GRUMBACH 1966). Combined therapy with EMB + INH or EMB + ETH proved to be highly effective, the EMB suppressing the development of resistance to INH and ETH (GRUMBACH 1966). In intermittent therapy the effect of twice-weekly EMB doses of 100 mg/kg, measured by the survival rate, corresponded to about $^{2}/_{3}$ of the effect of an INH dose of 3 mg/kg and to about 50% of the effect of an ETH dose of 30 mg/kg. SM doses of 30 mg/kg were equivalent to only about 30% of the effect of EMB, but at SM doses of 100 mg/kg its effect was about 1 ½ times as strong as that of EMB. After a single weekly ad-

Table 1. Dose-effect relationship of antituberculotic agents in a simultaneous continuous therapy study in mice with experimental tuberculosis (OTTEN 1971)

	mg/kg	Surviving %		mg/kg	Surviving %
Infected controls	–	0	Streptomycin	30	85
Ethambutol	30	68	Thiosemicarbazone	30	25
Isoniazid	3	97	Viomycin	100	90
Ethionamide	10	53	Pyrazinamide	100	30
Kanamycin	10	40	Thiocarlide	100	48
Rifampicin	10	50	p-Aminosalicylic acid	1000	45

Infection: *M. tuberculosis* (H37Rv). Therapy: once a day from the 1st to the 28th day after infection – total of 20 times. Survival rate: given as % on the 40th day after infection

ministration of EMB (100 mg/kg) only a trace of the effect remained discernible, being more or less equivalent to the effect of 30 mg/kg of SM, half as strong as the effect of 3 mg/kg of INH, and 25% as strong as the effect of 30 mg/kg of ETH (OTTEN 1971).

Table 1 gives a synopsis of the dose-effect relationships for active doses of the antituberculotic agents in a simultaneous therapy study on mice infected with *M. tuberculosis*.

Under the influence of therapeutically active doses of EMB in experimental Tb infection of the cornea in the albino mouse, immune reactions were fully effective without secondary infections occurring. On the other hand, the more effective therapy with corresponding doses of INH or combinations of INH and EMB suppressed the development of immunobiological defense reactions (LAL and ROBSON 1963).

In experimental tuberculosis in the mouse with atypical mycobacteria, e.g. *M. kansasii*, EMB exerts an effect comparable to that in *M. tuberculosis* infections (TACQUET and TISON 1963).

In a therapeutic study on guinea pigs infected with tuberculosis, oral EMB doses of 100 mg/kg produced a marked curative effect. In 50% of the animals autopsy revealed only minor lesions, whereas all the infected and untreated animals had very severe organ tuberculosis leading to death (LUTZ and BERGER 1962). The combination of INH (0.2 mg/guinea pig/day) and EMB (25 mg/guinea pig/day), administered daily for 60 days after the infection is more effective than the individual components and is comparable to therapy with 100 mg of EMB/guinea pig/day (KARLSON 1962). The therapeutic effect of EMB after subcutaneous administration is reported as being greater. In the course of the therapy only moderately pronounced organ tuberculosis developed in 60% of the subcutaneously treated group, whereas in the orally treated group the same number of severe organ tuberculoses developed as in the controls, some of which led to death (KARLSON 1961 a).

According to histomorphological studies, EMB has a favorable effect on specific focus reactions in experimental guinea pig tuberculosis: cellular absorption is promoted, epitheloid cell tubercles begin to regress, formation of lympho-reticulocytic follicles is stimulated, and the fibrillar delimitation of tuberculous tissue damage is favored (DIACONIȚĂ 1971).

In experimental tuberculosis in rabbits treated from the 10th to the 30th day after the infection with doses of 50 mg/kg to 100 mg/kg the therapeutic efficacy of EMB more or less corresponds to that brought about by PAS doses of 300 mg/kg to 500 mg/kg (FREERKSEN and ROSENFELD 1962).

In experimental tuberculosis in monkeys (rhesus monkeys or Simia) EMB exhibits dose-dependent activity in the course of continuous therapy with doses of 12.5 mg/kg to 100 mg/kg. The optimal still tolerable EMB dose remains inferior to an INH dose of 10 mg/kg with regard to efficacy. The combination of EMB and INH doses with borderline activity is therapeutically more effective than the administration of the individual components; as a partner in a combination, EMB is superior to PAS in conventional therapeutic schemes (SCHMIDT 1966).

In experimental leprosy in the mouse following an infection with *M. lepraemurium* EMB has an effect comparable with that of 4,4′-diaminodiphenylsulphone (DDS) (CHANG 1964). By contrast, in infections with *M. leprae* EMB was not found to have any effect in the mouse model (SHEPARD and CHANG 1964).

3. Concluding Remarks

The antimicrobial activity of EMB, which is confined almost exclusively to mycobacteria, covers the majority of the mycobacteria with the same relative degree of activity both in in-vitro experiments and in experimental mycobacterioses in animals. The development of ethambutol resistance is relatively rare compared with other highly active antituberculotics. The acquired resistance is restricted in most cases to only a slight loss of sensitivity and is largely stable.

There is no parallel resistance with other known antituberculotics, and therefore, in view of its different action mechanism, EMB is regarded as an ideal substance for use in combination therapies.

References

Beggs WH, Jenne JW (1970) Growth inhibition of *Mycobacterium tuberculosis* after single-pulsed exposures to streptomycin, ethambutol, and rifampin. Infect Immun 2:479–483

Bönicke R (1962) In vitro-Untersuchungen über die tuberkulostatische Aktivität von Dextro-2,2′-(Äthylendiimino)-di-1-Butanol (Dadibutol). Beitr Klin Tuberk 126:108–117

Buyske DA, Sterling W, Peets E (1966) Pharmacological and biochemical studies on ethambutol in laboratory animals. Ann NY Acad Sci 135:715–725

Chang YT (1965) Effects of capreomycin, ethambutol, vadrine, neovadrine, tapazole, griseofulvin and five long-acting sulfonamides in murine leprosy. Antimicrob Agents Chemother 1964:777–782

Clini V, Grassi C (1970) The action of new antituberculous drugs on intracellular tubercle bacilli. Antibiot Chemother 16:20–26

Crowle AJ, Sbarbaro JA, Judson FN, May MH (1985) The effect of ethambutol on tubercle bacilli within cultured human macrophages. Am Rev Respir Dis 132:742–745

Diaconiţă G (1971) Die Dynamik der experimentellen tuberkulösen Entzündung des Meerschweinchens unter Einwirkung der Ethambutol-Therapie. Pneumonologie 144:69–81

Dickinson JM (1968) In vitro and in vivo studies to assess the suitability of anti-tuberculous drugs for use in intermittent chemotherapy regimens. Bull Int Union Tuberc XLI:309–315

Donomae J, Yamamoto K (1966) Clinical evaluation of ethambutol in pulmonary tuberculosis. Ann NY Acad Sci 135:849–881

Forbes M, Kuck NA, Peets EA (1962) Mode of action of ethambutol. J Bacteriol 84:1099–1103

Forbes M, Peets EA, Kuck NA (1966) Effect of ethambutol on mycobacteria. Ann NY Acad Sci 135:726–731

Freerksen E, Rosenfeld M (1962) Dextro-2,2′-(Aethylendiimino)-di-1 butanol-dihydrochlorid in der experimentellen Tuberkulose-Therapie. Arzneimittelforsch 12:359–360

Gialdroni-Grassi G, Grassi C (1966) Chemotherapy of infections caused by atypical mycobacteria. Antimicrob Agents Chemother 1965:1074–1078

Grumbach F (1966) Activité antituberculeux chez la souris de l'éthambutol (dextro-2,2′-éthylènediimino-di-1-butanol) en association avec d'isoniazide ou l'éthionamide. Ann Inst Pasteur 110:69–85

Gupta SK (1964) Combined effect of d-2,2′-(ethylenediimino)-di-1-butanol (ethambutol) with other tuberculostatic agents against different strains of mycobacteria. Indian J Exp Biol 2:81–85

Kalich R (1969) Sensibilitätsprüfung von Mykobakterien gegenüber Ethambutol mit dem Vertikaldiffusionstest. Z Erkr Atmungsorgane 131:107–111

Karlson AG (1961 a) Therapeutic effect of ethambutol (dextro-2-2′-(ethylenediimino)di-1-butanol) on experimental tuberculosis in guinea pigs. Am Rev Respir Dis 84:902–904

Karlson AG (1961 b) The in vitro activity of ethambutol (dextro-2,2′-(ethylenediimino)di-1-butanol) against tubercle bacilli and other microorganisms. Am Rev Respir Dis 84:905–906

Karlson AG (1962) The combined use of ethambutol (dextro-2,2′-(ethylenediimino)-di-1-butanol) and isoniazid in experimental tuberculosis of guinea pigs. Am Rev Respir Dis 86:439–441

Krebs A, Noack K (1968) Die Wirkungsweise antituberkulöser Medikamente bei kontinuierlicher und intermitterender Anwendung. Jahreskongr Ges für Seuchenschutz Leipzig 11.–14.9.1968

Kubala E, Kubala J (1970) Experimental and clinical evaluation of the tuberculostatics. Antibiot Chemother 16:75–77

Kuck NA, Peets EA, Forbes M (1963) Mode of action of ethambutol on Mycobacterium tuberculosis strain H37Rv. Am Rev Respir Dis 87:905–906

Lal HM, Robson JM (1963) Ethambutol in experimental murine tuberculosis. Relation of effectiveness of antimicrobial drugs to immunity. Am Rev Respir Dis 87:870–876

Liss RH (1982) Bactericidal activity of ethambutol against extracellular *Mycobacterium tuberculosis* and bacilli phagocytized by human alveolar macrophages. S Afr Med J 62:15–19

Lucchesi M, Mancini P (1970) The anti-mycobacterial activity of ethambutol. Antibiot Chemother 16:230–238

Lutz A, Berger MA (1962) Données expérimentales sur l'action antituberculeuse in vitro et in vivo du d-2,2′-(éthylènediimino)-di-1-butanol. Ann Inst Pasteur 103:216–221

Mostardini G, Saletti M, Barnabe R (1968) Stability of d-2,2′-(ethylenediimino)di-1-butanol (ethambutol) in I.U.T.M. medium. Quad Sclav Diagn Clin Lab 4:515–519

Otten H (1971) Continuous and intermittent therapy of murine tuberculosis with ethionamide and other antituberculosis drugs. 20th Conf Int Union Tuberc New York Sept 1969 – Symposium: les thioamides. Theraplix-Press Paris: 75–79

Portaels F, Pattyn SR (1970) Resistance to ethambutol as an aid to the identification of *Mycobacterium friedmannii* (abscessus) and *M. borstelense*. J Med Microbiol 3:674–676

Pyle MM (1966) Ethambutol in the retreatment and primary treatment of tuberculosis: a four year clinical investigation. Ann NY Acad Sci 135:835–845

Reutgen H, Iwainsky H (1970) Wirkungsmechanismus des Ethambutol. Z Erkr Atmungsorgane 133:457–459

Schmidt LH (1966) Studies on the antituberculous activity of ethambutol in monkeys. Ann NY Acad Sci 135:747–758

Schmidt LH, Lang J, Good RC, Hoffman R (1962) Experimental studies on the toxicity and antituberculosis activity of ethambutol. Trans 21th Conf Pulm Dis VAAF: 355–366

Schröder KH, Hensel I (1970) Determination of resistance of M. tuberculosis to ethambutol. Antibiot Chemother 16:302–304

Shepard CC, Chang YT (1964) Activity of antituberculosis drugs against Mycobacterium leprae. Studies with experimental infection of mouse footpads. Int J Lepr 32:260–271

Shepherd RG, Baughn CO, Cantrall ML, Goodstein B, Thomas JP, Wilkinson RG (1966) Structure activity studies leading to ethambutol, a new type of antituberculous compound. Ann NY Acad Sci 135:686–710

Tacquet A, Tison F (1963) Activité in vitro et in vivo du dextro 2-2′ (éthylènediimino)di-1-butanol, utilisé seul ou en association sur les mycobactéries atypiques. Rev Tuberc (Paris) 27:431–443

Tacquet A, Devulder B, Pochart E (1970) L'èthambutol dans le traitement de la tuberculose pulmonaire. Antibiot Chemother 16:257–277

Thomas JP, Baughn CO, Wilkinson RG, Shepherd RG (1961) A new synthetic compound with antituberculous activity in mice: ethambutol (dextro-2,2′-(ethylenediimino)-di-1-butanol). Am Rev Respir Dis 83:891–893

Tsukamura M (1965) Resistance pattern of Mycobacterium tuberculosis and Mycobacterium bovis to ethambutol. Act Tuberc Scand 46:89–92
Tsukamura M (1970) Differentiation between pathogenic and nonpathogenic mycobacteria of group II and group III by susceptibility to ethambutol. Kekkaku 45:237–240
Tsukamura M, Tsukamura S (1967) On the instability of ethionamide resistance and on the stability of other drug resistance in tubercle bacilli (five to nine year's in vitro observation). Kekkaku 42:23–27
Wilkinson RG, Shepherd RG, Thomas JP, Baughn CO (1961) Stereospecificity in a new type of synthetic antituberculous agent. J Am Chem Soc 83:2212–2213

XIV. Rifampicin (RMP)

L. TRNKA

RMP, also appearing under the names of rifampin, rifamycin AMP, and rifaldazine in the literature, is a semisynthetic antibiotic belonging to the family of rifamycins. In 1957 a strain of *Streptomyces mediterranei* was isolated from a soil sample collected at a pine arboretum near St. Raphael, France. The strain, receiving a collection number ME/83, was cultured in shake-flasks and the fermentation broth showed the presence of at least five forms of an antibiotic which was called "rifamycin" (MARGALITH and BERETTA 1960).

Only the B form of rifamycin was produced in the presence of diethylbarbituric acid, and this was readily oxidized to rifamycin O, which underwent hydrolysis with loss of glycolic acid and the formation of rifamycin S. The reduction product of rifamycin S, namely rifamycin SV, was active against gram-positive bacteria, including *Mycobacterium tuberculosis,* but required parenteral administration.

The subsequent synthesis of 3-formylrifamycin SV paved the way for the development of derivatives. An aldehyde group introduced in position 3 and an N,N-disubstituted hydrazone formed with 1-methyl-4-aminopiperazine resulted in the RMP molecule which had the special advantage of better absorption after oral administration (SEYDEL 1970).

The biological properties of the rifamycins were first described in 1966 by SENSI et al., who also reported the results of a detailed investigation of RMP. In 1967, ARIOLI et al., PALLANZA et al., and FURESZ et al., in a series of three interrelated reports, presented extensive results of their laboratory studies and preliminary clinical observations and gave the pharmacokinetic parameters of RMP.

1. Antimicrobial Spectrum in Vitro

In vitro RMP is highly active against a wide range of pathogenic bacteria, including strains that often present problems in antimicrobial therapy. The minimal inhibitory concentrations of RMP (in µg/ml) for collection strains in liquid media were as follows: *Staphylococcus aureus* 0.002 µg/ml–0.005 µg/ml, *Streptococcus haemolyticus* 0.02 µg/ml–0.05 µg/ml, *Streptococcus faecalis* 0.01 µg/ml–0.5 µg/ml, *Diplococcus pneumoniae* 0.01 µg/ml, *Clostridium perfringens* 0.002 µg/ml, *Bacillus anthracis* 0.01 µg/ml, *Haemophilus influenzae* 0.02 µg/ml, *Neisseria gonorrhoeae* 0.02 µg/ml, *Pseudomonas aeruginosa* 10 µg/ml, *Escherichia coli* 1 µg/ml–

10 μg/ml, *Klebsiella pneumoniae* 5 μg/ml–10 μg/ml and *Brucella* 1 μg/ml–2 μg/ml (MANTEN and VAN WIJNGAARDEN 1969; FURESZ 1970; WHITE and LANCINI 1971).

RMP is generally more active than cephaloridine, cephalothin, lincomycin, and gentamicin on gram-positive micro-organisms, while its activity on gram-negatives is comparable with that of cephaloridine and cephalothin.

In a cell culture system (L cells and Hela cells) RMP considerably inhibited the intracellular multiplication of *Shigella flexneri* and enteropathogenic *Escherichia coli*. Its intracellular action was more pronounced than that of kanamycin and streptomycin, which could be in part attributed to the fact that RMP penetrated the cells more easily than the other two (OSADA et al. 1972). In contrast, PESANTI (1980) estimated that RMP was no more active than penicillin on *Staphylococcus aureus*, which was ingested by normal mouse peritoneal macrophages in vitro.

No activity of RMP against fungi *(Nocardia asteroides, Candida albicans, Trichophyton mentagrophytes)* was found by FURESZ (1970). Amphotericin B, however, stimulated the antifungal effects of RMP, probably by increasing the penetration of this drug through the fungal cytoplasmic membrane (MEDOFF et al. 1972).

RMP is active against some of the oncogenic viruses and appears to be one of the few known drugs that can block viral growth without damaging host cells (Editorial 1969).

2. Antimycobacterial Activity

a) Activity in Artificial Media in Vitro

The minimal inhibitory concentrations of RMP against various species of mycobacteria, as summarized from papers with complete documentation, are given in Table 1.

Most of the papers were published in 1968–1970. The results indicate that strains of *M. tuberculosis*, regardless of whether they are of laboratory origin (H37Rv or H37Ra) or isolated from tuberculous patients (so-called wild strains) are highly sensitive to RMP. The MIC values on solid agar media with Tween ranged between 0.005 μg/ml and 1.0 μg/ml. The corresponding values in liquid media were in the same range, as has also been confirmed by HOBBY (1972) who tested more than 1000 strains isolated in 1968–1970. The MIC values on egg media (Löwenstein-Jensen, Ogawa, or IUAT) were, however, higher, ranging between 2.5 μg/ml and 10 μg/ml of RMP per ml of the medium. The reasons for this difference will be discussed below.

The general sensitivity of *M. tuberculosis* for RMP has also been reported by ATLAS and TURCK (1968), WOZNIAK et al. (1969), BABA and AZUMA (1971), and WOODLEY et al. (1972).

Strains of *M. bovis* have the same sensitivity to RMP, or are even slightly more sensitive than *M. tuberculosis* strains. All of the 16 strains tested by CLARK and WALLACE (1967) were inhibited by 0.25 μg/ml RMP.

Mycobacterial species of potential pathogenicity (atypical mycobacteria) exhibit variable sensitivity to RMP, which is not absolutely consistent with the

Table 1. Minimal inhibitory concentrations (MIC) of RMP for various species (strains) of mycobacteria

Author	Mycobacteria	MIC (μg/ml)	Medium	Comments
CLARK and WALLACE (1967)	*M. tuberculosis* H37Rv	0.06	Dubos Albumin-Tween liquid (DAT)	2 Weeks of culture
		0.12–0.25		3
	M. tuberculosis 15 wild strains	0.06–0.5		2
	M. bovis	0.06–0.12		2
	16 strains	0.06–0.25		3
	M. avium	>4		2
	22 strains	>4		3
	Photochromogenic	0.12–>4		2
	25 strains	0.25–>4		3
	Scotochromogenic	0.06–>4		2
	3 strains	0.25–>4		3
GRUMBACH (1967)	*M. tuberculosis* H37Rv	10	Löwenstein-Jensen solid	RMP before coagulation
VERBIST and GYSELEN (1968)	*M. tuberculosis* 500 wild strains	2.5–5	Löwenstein-Jensen solid	
HOBBY et al. (1969a)	*M. tuberculosis* H37Rv	0.045–0.9	DAT liquid	1.68×10^2 cells/inoculum
HOBBY et al. (1969b)	*M. tuberculosis* wild	0.06	7H10 solid with OADC enrichment	
	M. tuberculosis wild	0.018	DAT liquid	
	M. tuberculosis wild	0.168	Albumin liquid without Tween	
HUSSELS and SCHÜTZ (1968)	*M. tuberculosis* wild	5	Löwenstein-Jensen solid	
KAWAMORI (1969)	*M. tuberculosis* 14 wild strains	0.1–0.25	DAT liquid	
	M. tuberculosis 14 wild strains	0.1–0.25	Kirchner semisolid with albumin	
LORIAN and FINLAND (1969)	*M. tuberculosis* 20 wild strains	0.05–0.2	7H9 solid without Tween	7×10^5–7×10^8 cells/inoculum
	M. tuberculosis 20 wild strains	0.005–0.02	7H9 solid with Tween	
	Photochromogenic 5 strains	0.1–0.3	7H9 solid with Tween	
	Photochromogenic 5 strains	0.1–0.3	7H9 solid without Tween	
	Photochromogenic 5 strains	0.3–2.5	7H10 solid	

Table 1 (continued)

Author	Mycobacteria	MIC (μg/ml)	Medium	Comments
	Scotochromogenic 2 strains	0.3	7H9 solid without Tween	
		0.25	7H9 solid with Tween	
		1.25	7H10 solid	
	Non-chromogenic 8 strains	0.02–20	7H9 solid without Tween	
	Non-chromogenic 8 strains	0.02–20	7H9 solid with Tween	
	Non-chromogenic 8 strains	1–20	7H10 solid	
	Rapid growers 4 strains	0.3–20	7H9 solid without Tween	
	Rapid growers 4 strains	0.7–20	7H9 solid with Tween	
	Rapid growers 4 strains	1–20	7H10 solid	
MCCLATCHY et al. (1969)	*M. tuberculosis* wild	0.1–0.5	7H11 solid	3 Weeks 5% CO_2
	M. kansasii 6 strains	0.1–0.5	7H11 solid	
	Scotochromogenic	0.1–20	7H11 solid	
	Non-chromogenic	2–20	7H11 solid	
	Rapid growers	20		
TACQUET et al. (1969)	*M. tuberculosis* H37Rv	10	Löwenstein-Jensen solid	
	M. tuberculosis H37Ra	10	Löwenstein-Jensen solid	
	M. bovis Ravenel	0.5	Löwenstein-Jensen solid	
GRUMBACH (1970)	*M. tuberculosis* H37Rv	0.1	DAT liquid	
	M. tuberculosis H37Rv	0.5	Youmans liquid	
	M. tuberculosis H37Rv	5	Löwenstein-Jensen solid	
LUCCHESI and MANCHINI (1970)	*M. tuberculosis* 55 wild strains	0.05–0.5	Dubos liquid with Tween without albumin	
	Photochromogenic	5	Dubos liquid with Tween without albumin	
	Scotochromogenic 28 strains	5–50	Dubos liquid with Tween without albumin	
	Non-chromogenic 13 strains	5–50	Dubos liquid with Tween without albumin	
	Rapid growers	50	Dubos liquid with Tween without albumin	
NAITO et al. (1970)	*M. tuberculosis*	0.05	Kirchner liquid with 10% serum	Inoculum 0.01 mg 7 days
	Photochromogenic 8 strains	0.1	Kirchner liquid with 10% serum	
	Scotochromogenic 6 strains	0.1	Kirchner liquid with 10% serum	

Table 1 (continued)

Author	Mycobacteria	MIC (μg/ml)	Medium	Comments
	Non-chromogenic 48 strains	0.006	Kirchner liquid with 10% serum	
NITTI (1970, 1972)	*M. tuberculosis* H37Rv	1–5	Ogawa egg solid	
	M. tuberculosis H37Rv	0.2	Dubos albumin without Tween liquid	
	M. tuberculosis 16 wild strains	0.1–0.5	Dubos albumin without Tween liquid	
	Photochromogenic 9 strains	0.1–0.5	Dubos albumin without Tween liquid	
	Scotochromogenic 8 strains	0.05–1	Dubos albumin without Tween liquid	
	Non-chromogenic 5 strains	0.1–5	Dubos albumin without Tween liquid	
	Rapid growers	10–100	Dubos albumin without Tween liquid	
	Rapid growers	>100	Dubos albumin without Tween liquid	
TOYOHARA (1971)	*M. tuberculosis* H37Rv	0.05 0.2–0.5 10–20	Dubos liquid Kirchner semisolid agar Ogawa 1% solid	
DENIS-BOTTIN (1972)	*M. tuberculosis* wild	25–40	Löwenstein-Jensen solid	
SAITO et al. (1972)	*M. kansasii* 6 strains	0.05–0.5	DAT liquid	
	M. marinum 7 strains	0.05–0.1	DAT liquid	
BYALIK and KLIMENKO (1973, 1976)	*M. tuberculosis* H37Rv	1	Proskauer-Beck liquid	
	M. bovis	1	Proskauer-Beck liquid	
HOBBY et al. (1974)	*M. tuberculosis* wild	1	7H10 solid	
BABA and AZUMA (1976)	*M. tuberculosis* wild 1 779 strains	10	Ogawa egg solid	
KUZE et al. (1977)	*M. kansasii*	0.001–0.1	DAT liquid	Inoculum 0.01 mg

Runyon grouping of these mycobacteria. It is generally agreed that *M. kansasii* and most photochromogenic species are RMP sensitive. This characteristic feature has been confirmed not only by the authors listed in Table 1, but also by TANZIL et al. (1972), SHIMOIDE (1977), HEJNÝ (1978), and YATES and COLLINS (1981).

The last-mentioned authors used the modal resistance method and were able to confirm that all 130 strains of the *M. avium/intracellulare* complex were resistant to RMP. The relative resistance of these strains, as well as that of the group of non-chromogenic mycobacteria, has been confirmed by CLARK and WALLACE (1967), LORIAN and FINLAND (1969), and MCCLATCHY et al. (1969). Most of these strains were not inhibited by 2 µg/ml to 20 µg/ml RMP. RYNEARSON et al. (1971) observed that domed opaque colonies of the non-chromogens were more susceptible to RMP than the translucent colonies of the same strains.

The sensitivity of other potentially pathogenic mycobacteria varies from strain to strain and is hardly species-dependent.

The growth of *M. lepraemurium* was also suppressed by RMP, as observed by RIGHTSEL et al. (1978) by the diffusion chamber technique.

α) Factors Affecting the Activity in Vitro. The data presented in Table 1 show that the activity of RMP is influenced by the type of the medium. The activity was higher in Dubos Tween-albumin medium and lower in egg media. This has been confirmed by KARLSON (1970), who compared egg-yolk agar, Middlebrook-Cohn 7H10 agar, and a Proskauer-Beck liquid medium containing 5% of serum in RMP mycobacterial sensitivity tests.

When RMP was incorporated in egg medium, such as Löwenstein-Jensen, before inspissation there was an approximately 90% loss of activity. Only 11%–20% of the RMP activity was lost on boiling or autoclaving in aqueous solutions. Therefore, like SM, RMP seems to be inactivated by the egg-yolk phospholipids (STOTTMEIER et al. 1969).

The same authors found that the stability of RMP in aqueous solutions is similar to that of aqueous solutions of dihydrostreptomycin sulphate. Both drugs lose less than 10% of their antituberculous potency if stored for up to 3 months at −20 °C.

The influence of the inoculum size and the presence of bovine serum in the culture medium was studied by NAITO et al. (1970) in Kirchner's liquid medium. With an inoculum size of 0.1 mg the MIC was 0.25 µg/ml, while with the smaller inoculum of 0.001 mg the MIC decreased down to 0.025 µg/ml. An increase in the serum content did not reduce the activity of RMP.

β) Resistance of Tubercle Bacilli to RMP

Development of Resistance in Vitro and Its Type: The classical experiments of GRUMBACH and RIST (1967), revealed that RMP concentrations of 0.25 µg/ml or 0.5 µg/ml in Dubos Tween albumin media caused not only inhibitory effects but also, after 21 days of culture, selected RMP-resistant bacilli. Identical results were reported by HOBBY and LENERT (1970) with concentration of 0.9 µg/ml RMP/ml in a liquid medium.

These data indicate that under the influence of some RMP concentrations, a population of tubercle bacilli characterized by its resistance to a given RMP concentration can develop. The in-vitro results are consistent with those observed in experimental animals and in patients (e.g., DAVIDSON and WAGGONER 1976). It is likely that mutation/selection mechanisms are responsible for this development.

The fluctuation test designed by LURIA and DELBRÜCK shows that tubercle bacilli mutate to RMP resistance spontaneously and at random. A low mutation

Table 2. Proportion of RMP-resistant mutants in populations of *M. tuberculosis* (H37Rv) as found on Löwenstein-Jensen media

Author	RMP (μg/ml)						
	2.5	5.0	10.0	20.0	40.0	80.0	500.0
Grumbach and Rist (1967)	25%	2%	0.7%		3×10^{-7}	3×10^{-7}	10^{-8}
Verbist and Gyselen (1968)	10^{-3}	10^{-6}	10^{-7}	10^{-8}	2×10^{-8}		
Rist (1969)	25%	2%	10^{-3}	10^{-6}	3×10^{-7}		10^{-8}
Grumbach (1970)			10^{-3}	10^{-6}	3×10^{-7}		10^{-8}
Le Lirzin and Djurovic (1971)		2×10^{-5}	10^{-8}				

rate, calculated to be 3.32×10^{-9} to 7.53×10^{-10} mutations per bacterium per generation was estimated by David (1970), who analyzed the increase in the proportion of mutants with time in growing populations of tubercle bacilli. Spontaneous resistant mutants appear according to a single-step pattern – no intermediate or transient forms have ever been detected (Tsukamura 1972a).

The mutation rate determines the proportion of spontaneous (primary) resistant mutants in a population of tubercle bacilli never exposed to RMP. On the other hand, the proportion of primary resistant mutants is an important factor determining the outcome of selection under the influence of RMP. The higher this proportion, the sooner a resistant population will develop by multiplication of selected resistant mutants.

The proportion of RMP-resistant mutants has therefore been studied ever since the discovery of the bactericidal activity of RMP. Two groups of authors used serial dilution plating on solid media, a relevant method in this respect. The results reported in the various papers are presented in Table 2.

The data indicate that the proportion of primary RMP-resistant mutants in a population of tubercle bacilli, strain H37Rv is low in comparison with proportions of mutants with primary resistance to other antituberculosis drugs, including INH. At a concentration of 20 μg RMP/ml only one mycobacterial cell in a population of 10^6–10^8 will survive and can give rise to a resistant population. It was found that in tuberculous cavities the population of tubercle bacilli amounts to 10^6–10^8 bacilli. The in-vitro results have subsequently been found to have valid implications for clinical chemotherapy.

It is evident from the data summarized in Table 2 that in a population of tubercle bacilli primary mutants to various RMP concentrations are present in different proportions; generally speaking those resistant to lower concentrations are present in greater numbers. Under a selection pressure of a given RMP concentration a population develops with a higher proportion of resistant bacterial units, but still heterogeneous enough.

The estimation of a critical concentration for defining RMP resistance is therefore important for practical reasons. The critical concentration must be determined by considering the distribution of the degree of resistance in previously untreated tuberculous patients and by considering resistance-development patterns. The critical concentrations should be higher than the upper limit of distribution of the resistance degrees in previously untreated patients, and should be selective for low-resistance mutants.

CANETTI et al. (1969) defined in this way criteria applicable in the proportion method of resistance testing. As the criteria of resistance the authors adopted 10% of bacterial units growing in the presence of 20 µg RMP/ml or 1% of those growing in the presence of 40 µg RMP/ml on Löwenstein-Jensen media. NITTI (1972) proposed a lower resistance level: 10% growing at 10 µg RMP/ml or 1% growing at 20 µg RMP/ml on egg media. TSUKAMURA (1972b) recommended growth in the presence of 25 µg RMP/ml as the critical concentration on Ogawa egg medium. The differences in these proposed critical concentrations are not substantial.

In principle, bacteriological methods of resistance testing using solid egg media and either the absolute or the proportion method are generally accepted and used. The other methods of laboratory testing of RMP resistance, such as the use of ^{32}P-incorporation test (REUTGEN 1972; 1973) or the use of CO_2 from radiolabelled substrate (SNIDER et al. 1981) should only be mentioned, since they are not in general use.

With the absolute or the proportion method of sensitivity tests the incidence of RMP-resistant populations of tubercle bacilli was estimated in tuberculous patients not previously treated with RMP (primary or initial RMP resistance). DENIS-BOTTIN (1972) estimated the incidence of strains with primary resistance to RMP as less than 5% for all isolated strains of *M. tuberculosis,* as 36% for *M. bovis* strains, and as about 50% for isolated strains of potential pathogenic mycobacteria (atypical mycobacteria).

In a cooperative study carried out in the Federal German Republic in 1972 to 1975, HUSSELS (1977) found the incidence of primary RMP resistance to be very low (0.1%). Similar results were reported from the United States (between 1975 and 1977 only 0.3%, KOPANOFF et al. 1978), from Poland (JANOWIEC et al. 1979), from the Soviet Union (BIBIK 1972), and from other countries. It can thus be concluded that primary resistance to RMP was low, and since that time no alarming reports have so far been published.

Features of Resistant Populations: It was suggested by TSUKAMURA (1972a) that a resistant population of tubercle bacilli might have phenotypic characteristics different from those of a "sensitive" population, i.e., one containing only spontaneous primary mutants in negligible numbers. MANTEN et al. (1969), several authors cited by BINDA et al. (1971), and OHSATO and SHIZUMI (1972) have reported a reduced virulence of RMP-resistant strains. SCHRÖDER and KOPERSKA (1972), however, did not find any correlation between RMP resistance and the decrease in virulence or loss of catalase-activity, as is known for INH-resistant populations. HUI et al. (1977) emphasized the importance of changes in the permeability barrier in RMP-resistant cells, since the DNA-dependent RNA polymerase isolated from an RMP-resistant population of tubercle bacilli was found to be susceptible to RMP.

Cross-resistance: No cross-resistance has been reported to exist between RMP and all other antituberculosis drugs, (except rifamycins), both in vitro and in animal models, and this was borne out by clinical experience. The observation of SIDDIQI et al. (1981) that all 55 strains isolated by them in Indonesia and resistant to RMP were also resistant to INH, while many strains resistant to INH were found to be susceptible to RMP, has not been confirmed by other authors. It cannot be excluded that the observed resistance was secondary, appearing after unchecked administration of RMP.

γ) Type of Action. The fact that RMP exerts a bactericidal effect was pointed out already in the early studies. GRUMBACH and RIST (1967) estimated that by using a concentration of 1 μg RMP/ml on Dubos Tween albumin medium (which corresponds to a concentration of 500 μg/ml on Löwenstein Jensen medium) sterilization of the test tubes was accomplished after 21 days of culture. With RMP concentrations of 0.25 μg/ml or 0.5 μg/ml, the bactericidal effect needed more time and a few resistant mutants appeared.

HOBBY and LENERT (1972) performed in-vitro experiments in which the numbers of viable cell units per ml of medium were determined at various times during the incubation of tubercle bacilli with 1 μg/ml of RMP, EMB, or INH. A rapid reduction in the number of viable cell units was noted with RMP and INH, but not with EMB. After 21 days of incubation, however, the number of viable cell units demonstrable in the INH-containing medium had risen while the number in the RMP-containing medium remained undetectable. RMP appeared, therefore, to be at least as bactericidal as INH, and more active in this respect than EMB.

DICKINSON et al. (1977) analyzed the bactericidal activity of RMP in in-vitro experiments in which log-phase cultures of tubercle bacilli in liquid media were exposed to drug concentrations in the range likely to occur in serum during treatment of patients. The bactericidal activity was measured by the reduction in the viable counts at 4 days and 7 days. The mean reduction in the number of colony-forming units during the first 4 days of exposure increased with increasing drug concentration. The reduction for RMP was about the same as that for INH. The same relative ratings for the bactericidal activity were obtained by comparing the reduction in counts during the first 7 days of incubation. The difference between the bactericidal activities of RMP and INH was again not significant, but significant differences were found between the activities of these two drugs and the activity of SM on the one hand and of EMB on the other.

BYALIK and KLIMENKO (1976) studied the bactericidal effect of RMP against different strains of tubercle bacilli in a liquid synthetic Proskauer-Beck medium. A complete bactericidal effect was achieved with a concentration of 5 μg RMP/ml and 7 days to 9 days of exposure or with a concentration of 40 μg RMP/ml and 5 days to 7 days of exposure. Lower concentrations and shorter exposures produced only a partial bactericidal effect.

JENNE and BEGGS (1973) analyzed the effect of the RMP concentration and estimated that RMP is ultimately bactericidal but can be considered to pass from a bacteriostatic to a bactericidal action as its concentration is increased during continued drug exposure. An example of this is the transition from bacteriostatic to bactericidal action on *M. tuberculosis* strain H37Rv as the RMP concentration in the broth culture is increased from 0.005 μg/ml to 5.0 μg/ml.

The concentration of the drug is one factor determining its effect on microbial cells; another is the duration of the exposure. It has been postulated that the drug effect is related to the total exposure, i.e., to the product of time (exposure period) and concentration, and much effort was made to clarify this relationship in the case of RMP. DICKINSON et al. (1972) estimated that, within the concentration range of 0.0625 μg/ml to 4 μg/ml, the effect was proportional to the product [concentration]$^{0.378}$ × exposure period. JENNE and BEGGS (1973) were rather sceptical about the validity of this proportionality.

From these studies, however, one important factor has emerged, and that is the "after-effect" (inhibition of growth after the drug has been removed from the medium), which occurs in experiments using transient periods (pulses) of drug exposure.

DICKINSON and MITCHISON (1970) and MITCHISON (1971) showed that 0.2 μg RMP/ml was more bactericidal in the first 24 h of exposure than 1.0 μg INH/ml, and that there was a lag before the growth recommenced after exposure for about 2 h. The lag period after exposure to RMP was shorter than that after exposure to other bactericidal drugs. This estimation was utilized in the formulation of the specific RMP activity, as will be mentioned below.

The existence of a lag time before recommencement of growth has been confirmed by TOYOHARA (1971), who used the DICKINSON's method of culture in membrane filter holders.

Correlating the bactericidal activity of RMP with its peak serum levels, GROSSET (1978b) stated that RMP, and INH have the lowest minimal inhibitory concentrations for tubercle bacilli. As the peak serum levels of these drugs are high, the ratio of the serum levels to the MIC is some 50–100 for both of these drugs. From these data it can be predicted that both drugs could exert a strong bactericidal activity on tubercle bacilli in vivo.

A third factor that might influence the activity of RMP in vitro is the functional state of the microbial population, as has been suggested by GULEVSKAYA and MILOVANOVA (1977), KANAI and KONDO (1979), and by DOLZHANSKY (1982). In-vitro experiments with streptomycin-dependent strains of tubercle bacilli have confirmed that RMP is effective on multiplying and to a certain degree upon resting tubercle bacilli.

The functional state of cultured tubercle bacilli can be altered by changes in the pH of the medium or by changes in the environment of the culture media. According to GROSSET (1981), at a neutral pH of the medium RMP has the same activity as INH on actively growing tubercle bacilli. Tubercle bacilli growing in vitro at neutral pH may be compared to a large population of tubercle bacilli growing actively in tuberculous cavities. GROSSET (1978b) pointed out further that RMP also exerts its bactericidal activity in bacilli with a reduced multiplying activity at an acid pH, and it is the only known drug that also acts in this way on bacilli with a reduced multiplying activity at a neutral pH.

DICKINSON and MITCHISON (1981) achieved a uniform slowing down of the growth rate of tubercle bacilli by replacing air by another gas, and by lowering the pH of the culture medium or the incubation temperature. This uniform slowing down caused a reduction in bactericidal activity that was similar for RMP and for INH. However, when the cultures had been held dormant at 8 °C and then allowed to metabolize briefly by increasing the temperature for 1 h or 6 h per day, RMP seemed to be more bactericidal than INH. The explanation for the greater bactericidal activity of RMP under these conditions comes from earlier experiments carried out by these authors with pulsed exposure to the drug, as already mentioned. The results thus confirmed and refined GROSSET's findings. The population of tubercle bacilli within tuberculous lesions is not homogenous. It consists of actively multiplying bacilli, of bacilli that are truly dormant and occasionaly dying, and of a fraction that is dormant but sometimes metabolizes actively for short periods (DICKINSON and MITCHISON 1981). It was postulated that RMP exerts an effect not only on actively multiplying bacilli (like INH and other drugs), but specifically on the last mentioned fraction, which is considered responsible for many of the relapses occurring after the termination of chemotherapy (DICKINSON and MITCHISON 1976).

δ) Effects in Combination with Other Antituberculosis Drugs in Vitro. Initial experiments with RMP in combination with other antituberculosis drugs were reported in 1970 by HOBBY and LENERT, who used the conventional microbiological technique for counting microbial populations in vitro.

RMP alone in a concentration equivalent to 0.9 μg/ml reduced the number of viable cell units of tubercle bacilli (H37Rv) from 1.7×10^6 to 8.5×10^1 after 10 days of incubation in Tween albumin liquid medium. After 21 days of incubation, however the population had risen again to 1.5×10^5 viable cell units and the strain was now fully resistant to RMP. The addition of low, subinhibitory, concentrations of INH (0.05 μg/ml), EMB (0.5 μg/ml), SM (0.1 μg/ml), or PAS (1.0 μg/ml) to the above-mentioned concentration of RMP was capable of preventing to some degree the secondary increase in the number of tubercle bacilli after 21 days of incubation, but it failed to prevent the emergence of RMP-resistant organisms.

In subsequent experiments the same concentration of RMP was combined with higher, (but still subinhibitory) concentrations of other antituberculosis drugs. INH in a concentration of 0.1 μg/ml or 0.2 μg/ml, SM at 0.2 μg/ml or 0.3 μg/ml, PAS at 2 μg/ml or 5 μg/ml, and EMB at 0.1 μg/ml or 0.5 μg/ml were used. These selected concentrations are not far below the minimal inhibitory levels. As a result, all combinations produced sterilization of the cultures and prevented the emergence of resistant cells. It may thus be concluded that the antimycobacterial action of RMP may be enhanced, and the emergence of RMP-resistant cells prevented, by the addition of just subinhibitory amount of INH, SM, PAS, or EMB (HOBBY 1972).

Further experiments (HOBBY and LENERT 1972) yielded results indicating, on the other hand, that subinhibitory amounts of RMP may increase the effectiveness of low concentrations of SM or INH and may prevent the emergence of SM- or INH-resistant cells. However, RMP failed to prevent the emergence of EMB-resistant microbial cells. There have been numerous papers on attempts to observe synergism, addition, or antagonism of combinations of RMP with other antituberculotics in vitro.

Using a cross-dilution method, NAITO et al. (1970) found that RMP exerted some degree of synergism in combination with SM or PAS, TSC, VM, and INH and particularly with EMB. No antagonism was demonstrable with the selected drug combinations and concentrations.

JANOWIEC et al. (1977) used the serial dilution test tube method with Youmans medium containing 10% of calf serum and evaluated the action of RMP with INH and PAS as synergistic. In contrast to this, DICKINSON and MITCHISON (1976) making serial viable counts on tubercle bacilli exposed in vitro to RMP 0.2 μg/ml, INH 1.0 μg/ml, or EMB in a concentration of 10 μg/ml in a Tween albumin liquid medium, failed to see any bactericidal synergism between RMP and INH or any influence of EMB on the bactericidal activity of INH and RMP.

In subsequent experiments DICKINSON et al. (1977) used tubercle bacilli in the log phase grown in Tween-albumin liquid media and exposed them to combinations of RMP with other drugs in concentrations in the range likely to be achieved in the serum during treatment of patients. The bactericidal activity of the drugs was measured by the decrease in viable counts after 4 days and 7 days. Bactericidal synergism was found for the combination of RMP (0.11 μg/ml–1.0 μg/ml) and SM (1.0 μg/ml to 4.0 μg/ml), indifference for the combination of RMP and INH (0.2 μg/ml to 5.0 μg/ml), and antagonism for RMP and EMB (2.0 μg/ml to 8.0 μg/ml).

Using quantitative plate counting on solid media TRNKA et al. (1974) and TRNKA and ŠTAFLOVÁ (1974) studied the action of RMP with other drugs in relation to the concentration. The effect of drug-resistant mutants was excluded. The results indicate that RMP and EMB act synergistically in a wide range of concentrations and proportions both drugs participating equally in the increased effectiveness of a given combination. The increased interaction in associations of RMP with other drugs is limited to certain concentrations particularly those of RMP.

Summarizing the factors affecting the activity of RMP in vitro, the enhancing effect of some substances cannot be disregarded. Thus, HAVEL and ROSENFELD (1975) found in in-vitro experiments that the activity of RMP was enhanced by the addition of 4,4-diaminodiphenyl sulphone (DDS) which, given alone, was ineffective. The degree of enhancement depended on the DDS concentration. A reduction in RMP concentration could be compensated by increasing the dose of DDS; for example, 4 μg/ml of RMP combined with 4 μg/ml of DDS was equivalent in antimycobacterial activity to a combination of 2 μg/ml of RMP and 16 μg/ml of DDS.

b) Effects on Mycobacteria in Cell and Tissue Cultures

In cultures of isolated monocytes infected with *M. tuberculosis* which mimic infected macrophages in vivo the activity of RMP was similar to that of INH. PZA had a higher activity, whereas SM had no activity at all at concentrations achieved in patients (GROSSET 1981). According to STOICA (1972), the effective intracellular concentrations of RMP are between 0.2 μg/ml to 1.0 μg/ml, which was confirmed by PAVLOV et al. (1974). A killing effect of RMP on intracellular tubercle bacilli has been demonstrated by CARLONE et al. (1985).

The effective concentrations of RMP are somewhat higher than those estimated by CLINI and GRASSI (1970), who reported that RMP was active on tubercle bacilli at about the same concentrations in monocyte cultures and in artificial culture media. The MIC in Dubos medium was 0.2 μg RMP/ml, whereas that in monocyte cultures was 0.5 μg RMP/ml.

Comparing the intracellular activity of RMP with those of penicillin and gentamicin, SOLBERG and HELLUM (1978) found the former to be more pronounced, indicating a greater penetration of RMP into phagocyte vacuoles.

The mode of the intracellular activity of RMP has been studied in a series of investigations. In leucocytes the concentration of RMP exceeded that in the supernatant by a factor of 2 (MANDELL 1973), and this was confirmed with the aid of velocity gradient centrifugation by PROKESCH and HAND (1982). A higher concentration was achieved after 2 h of incubation. The activity of this higher concentration of RMP could be potentiated by the low intraphagolysosomal pH and other phagolysosomal bacteriostatic factors that affect particularly phagocytosed staphylococci and other extracellular parasites (LAM et al. 1983). A higher intracellular than extracellular concentration has been found by ACOCELLA et al. (1985). An accumulation of lipid-soluble RMP may also occur in alveolar macrophages. HAND et al. (1985) estimated that RMP was present in several times higher concentrations in the alveolar macrophages of smokers than in the extracellular environment. The increased uptake was attributed to some structural and functional alterations induced by smoking.

c) Activity of RMP in Experimental Tuberculosis and Development of Resistance in Vivo

α) *Monotherapy, Continuous Treatment*

In mice: Experimental tuberculosis in mice has been used most often in the study of RMP activity. The methodological aspects of this work, if clearly indicated in the papers reviewed, have been summarized in Table 3.

Table 3 shows that a wide variety of mouse strains was used, and the natural resistance to tuberculous infection may vary considerably between strains, even if the mice are comparatively little susceptible to tuberculous infections.

The majority of authors used the laboratory strain H37Rv and the intravenous route of infection; certain other strains not comparable in their virulence and pathogenicity in mice with the strain H37Rv have also been used. About one-half of the experiments were of the curative type (treatment being started when the infection was established, i.e., after 10 days to 14 days), and the remaining ones were of the preventive type (treatment started a few days after the challenge). The challenging doses varied considerably.

Relative uniformity was achieved in the methods of evaluation. Whereas the first experiments were based on the evaluation of survival time, later there was an almost complete change-over to following the dynamics of the mycobacterial population in lung and spleen homogenates in the course of treatment.

Differences in methodology make it necessary to evaluate individual studies, and care must be taken with any generalizations.

Table 3. Methodological aspects of experimental murine tuberculosis used in reviewed papers dealing with RMP activity

Author	Strain of mice	Challenge	Starting day of RMP treatment	Evaluation criteria
HOBBY and LENERT (1968)	Swiss white	*M. tuberculosis* H37Rv i.v.	3	Survival time, % survival
HOBBY and LENERT (1969b)	Swiss white	*M. tuberculosis* H37Rv i.v.	3	Mean survival time at 42 days
VERBIST (1968)	Inbred Gif-TB	*M. tuberculosis* Middelburg 217, 0.15 mg, i.v.	10	Counts of viable bacilli in lungs and spleens
VERBIST (1969)	Inbred Gif-TB	*M. tuberculosis* Middelburg 217, 0.1 mg, i.v.	8 (11)	Mean survival time Mean counts of viable bacilli in lungs and spleens
VERBIST (1970)	Inbred Gif-TB	*M. tuberculosis* Middelburg 217, 0.1 mg, i.v.	8 (11)	Mean survival time Mean counts of viable bacilli in lungs and spleens
GRUMBACH and RIST (1967)	ML white	*M. tuberculosis* H37Rv 0.1 mg, 2×10^6, i.v.	1 (14)	Viable counts in lungs and spleens
BATTEN (1968)	Schneider	*M. tuberculosis* ICI, 10^6, i.v.	21	Viable counts in lungs and spleens
BATTEN (1969)	Schneider	*M. tuberculosis* ICI, 10^6, i.v.	21	Viable counts in lungs and spleens
BATTEN (1970)	Schneider	*M. tuberculosis* ICI, 10^6, i.v.	21	Viable counts in lungs and spleens
GRUMBACH et al. (1969)	Conventional	*M. tuberculosis* H37Rv 10^6 i.v.	14	Viable counts in lungs and spleens
HAVEL et al. (1970)	White H	*M. tuberculosis* H37Rv, i.v.	2 (10)	Viable counts in lungs and spleens
NAITO et al. (1970)		*M. tuberculosis* 0.07 mg, i.v.	7	Viable counts in lungs and spleens
SUZUKI (1971)		*M. tuberculosis* Schacht strain INH- and SM-R i.v.		Body weight, survival rate, viable counts in lungs and spleens
KRADOLFER and SCHNELL (1971)	MF_2 mice	*M. bovis* Ravenel i.v.	11	Viable counts in lungs and spleens, cumulalative-frequency distribution curve
KONDO and KANAI (1977a)	Conventional	*M. bovis* Ravenel	1	Counts of viable bacilli in lungs and spleens
SOSNOWSKI and TOMASZKIECZ (1973)	Balb c	*M. tuberculosis* H37Rv, i.v., 10^7	14	Counts of viable bacilli in lungs and spleens

Table 3 (continued)

Author	Strain of mice	Challenge	Starting day of RMP treatment	Evaluation criteria
GROSSET et al. (1978)	MLA	*M. tuberculosis* H37Rv, 3×10^6, i.v.	11	Counts of viable bacilli in lungs and spleens
TOYOHARA (1969)	Conventional	*M. tuberculosis* Kurowo strain, i.v.	15	Counts of viable bacilli in lungs and spleens
KUZE et al. (1979)	Conventional	*M. intracellulare* TMC strain 1469 i.v.	10	Counts of viable bacilli in lungs and spleens

Papers dealing with the antimycobacterial activity of rifamycin SV in murine tuberculosis, such as those of TSUKAMURA et al. (1963) and SPITZY (1963), were in the late "sixties" replaced by ones in which the activity of a new rifamycin derivate, namely RMP, was analyzed in vivo. In these papers some findings were reported which later contributed to the formulation of the modern principles of antituberculosis chemotherapy.

The pioneering work was done in 1967 by GRUMBACH and RIST, who found that the minimal orally active dose of RMP in a mouse model was 20 times lower than that of subcutaneously injected rifamycin SV.

From the very start the experiments were aimed more at the basic problems of RMP activity. Reports referring to the efficacy of RMP against *M. intracellulare* (KUZE et al. 1979), *M. kansasii* (BURJANOVÁ and DORNETZHUBER 1975), or other species of tubercle bacilli in vivo (YOSHIDA 1970) are rather exceptional.

The curative type of treatment of mice with acute advanced tuberculosis (high bacterial loading in the lungs) using RMP at daily doses of 25 mg/kg or 50 mg/kg resulted in negativity of about 50% of lung homogenates after 3 months of daily administration. RMP at a daily dose of 5 mg/kg was rather ineffective (GRUMBACH and RIST 1967).

In a model of less advanced tuberculosis used by BATTEN (1968), a daily dose of 40 mg RMP/kg led to completely negative cultures already after 3 weeks of treatment. 20 mg RMP/kg produced a considerable fall in the viable count compared to the controls.

The dose-dependent effects of RMP were studied in greater detail by VERBIST and GYSELEN in 1968 and by VERBIST in 1968. It was found that the bactericidal effect of RMP became manifest quickly and was strongly dose-dependent. In the lungs the mean number of viable units dropped from 10^8, to 10^3, 10^1, and 10^0 with RMP at doses of 5 mg/kg to 40 mg/kg. With INH the effect was slower and a dose-effect relationship was hardly discernible in the 10th week of treatment.

It was also found that after 3 weeks of daily treatment there was no difference in the mean survival time between RMP given at 5 mg/kg and INH given at the same dose. Using more sensitive criteria (viable counts) and longer administration times, VERBIST (1969) and HAVEL et al. (1970) confirmed the finding of HOBBY and LENERT (1968) that an RMP dose of 10 mg/kg was equivalent to a daily INH dose of 5 mg/kg.

The sterilizing activity of RMP was studied by culturing the organs for a certain time after the end of the treatment. VERBIST (1969) reported that the secondary increase in the number of viable tubercle bacilli after discontinuation of treatment was slower in the group treated with RMP at higher doses (20 mg/kg or 40 mg/kg) than in the low-dosage groups (5 mg/kg to 10 mg/kg) or in the groups treated with INH regardless of the dosage. TOYOHARA (1979) observed that the percentage of bacteriological relapses was dependent on the duration of RMP administration: 60% after 8 weeks, 40% after 3 months of monotherapy, and zero after 6 months of daily administration.

In chronic murine tuberculosis KRADOLFER (1970) and KRADOLFER and SCHNELL (1971) estimated that after 4 months of daily administration of RMP at a daily dose of 40 mg/kg, the majority of the mice were not bacteriologically sterile despite the apparent negativity achieved during the treatment, since viable tubercle bacilli were again found in the mice after a recovery period of 50 days–100 days. A similar phenomenon has been observed in less advanced tuberculosis by BATTEN (1968).

The other aspect of the administration of RMP in monotherapy is the emergence of RMP resistance. Analysing previous experiments, GRUMBACH (1969) found that after 4 months populations homogeneously resistant to high RMP concentrations appeared in the lungs of mice that had not become negative by that time (50%).

With the various monotherapy regimens implemented by VERBIST (1970), 29%–40% of the positive cultures isolated from the lungs and the spleens displayed some degree of RMP resistance, especially after several months of therapy. There was no statistical difference in the incidence of RMP-resistant strains between daily and intermittent application of the drug.

In guinea pigs: In the work on RMP guinea pigs have been used considerably less often than mice as a model of experimental tuberculosis. The purpose of the experiments was more variable.

In the first reports NITTI et al. (1967); NITTI and NINNI (1969) used disseminated tuberculosis in guinea pigs to study the protective and therapeutic activity of RMP. The activity was assessed by the extent of macroscopic lesions according to the schemes proposed by FELDMAN. Later the authors used also the cutanous ulcer technique developed by RUBBO and PIERSON.

It was estimated that 20 mg RMP/kg/day exerted a complete protective effect and a definite, even if only partial, curative effect. The action was dose-dependent, with an optimum at 40 mg/kg/day. A further increase in the dosage, while appreciably accelerating the regression of the local lesions, did not significantly affect the final result of the treatment. The type of action was regarded as predominantly bactericidal with a typical resolution of focal lesions and cellular and exudative reactions reflecting allergic responses to the products released by rapid and intensive bacterial lysis. The effectiveness of 20 mg–40 mg RMP/kg both in the preventive and the curative type of administration was later confirmed by LUCCHESI and MANCINI (1970) in similarly designed experiments.

The results reported by TOYOHARA (1970) were consistent with the above. Similar doses were used successfully in the prevention of the development of lesions in infected guinea pigs by ALGEORGE et al. (1971). UVAROVA et al. (1976) applied RMP in a daily dose of 30 mg/kg 3 weeks after subcutaneous infection of guinea pigs with a low infectious dose (0.0001 mg) for 5 months. High therapeutic activity was achieved with this dosage, particularly in the first 3 months of therapy. However, the authors pointed out that, despite prolonged treatment with high doses of RMP, tissue sterilization could not be achieved, thus observing the same phenomenon as had been seen in experimental murine tuberculosis.

SHINIBEROV (1979) observed that RMP at the above-mentioned dose, administered orally, led to an inhibition of proliferative blast-cell transformation in the spleen and lymph nodes of the treated animals and to some other changes indicating its immunosuppressive effect in the host (AOYAGI et al. 1979; ROOK 1973; KRAMER and BERGMANN 1976; TRNKA et al. 1977).

The results were consistent with the earlier observations of ESKENAZY et al. (1971) dealing with immunomorphological features of the action of RMP and with ones of ALGEORGE and RUDESCU (1973) who studied tuberculin hypersensitivity and the humoral antibody response. BELLASHENE and FORSGREN (1980) confirmed the immunosuppressive effect by the split-heart allograft technique.

WESTFAL et al. (1974) studied the pathomorphology of lesions in tuberculous guinea pigs treated with RMP. Extensive cell vacuolation was seen in the liver. Cytolysis was taking place in some cells in the lobules. There were no inflammatory infiltrations, nor any proliferation of the connective tissues. Extensive vacuolation in the hepatic parenchyma indicates damage of the liver cells provoked by high doses of RMP.

In rabbits: KREBS (1969) reported on the experiments of BLASI et al. from 1967. RMP at a daily dose of 15 mg/kg prevented the development of tuberculosis and exerted bactericidal activity in a curative type of treatment of corneal infection. ROSENFELD (1970) investigated the inhibitory serum activity of rabbit serum after administration of 10 mg RMP/kg, 5 mg INH/kg, 20 mg SM/kg, or 25 mg EMB/kg. The serum activity after taking RMP was greater during a period of 1 h to 23 h than after the administration of the other drugs.

β) Monotherapy, Intermittent Treatment

In mice: VERBIST noticed already in 1969 that a single high dose of RMP (100 mg/kg) administered once a week was more effective in reducing the number of culturable bacilli in mice than the same dose divided into daily portions.

SUZUKI demonstrated in 1971 that a single weekly dose of 20 mg RMP/kg was more effective than a daily dose of 5 mg or 10 mg in twice-weekly regimens. RMP at a dose of 20 mg/kg given once was almost as effective as when it was given in two divided doses. The once-weekly regimen of 10 mg RMP/kg was inferior to that of 5 mg/kg given daily, but superior to that of 5 mg/kg 2 or 3 times a week. These experiments have been confirmed by KONDO and KANAI (1977a, b, 1978).

The suitability of RMP for intermittent administration is in part due to its long half-life, especially in mice. Effective blood levels are maintained for a longer time than with other antituberculotics (KRADOLFER 1968; VERBIST 1969; TOYOHARA and IWASAKI 1971).

In guinea pigs: The experiments in guinea pigs contributed considerably to the formulation of the principles of modern tuberculosis chemotherapy. DICKINSON and MITCHISON (1970) treated guinea pigs with established tuberculosis (3 weeks after the infection) for 6 weeks with RMP at doses of 2.5 mg/kg to 80 mg/kg. At each mean daily dosage level groups were given the doses at intervals of 1 day, 2 days, 4 days, or 8 days. Their response to the treatment was then assessed on the basis of macroscopic lesions in the organs and viable counts in the spleen.

The efficacy of the treatment increased with increasing interval between successive doses. The benefit derived from high doses of RMP given intermittently may in part be due to the disproportionately high peak serum concentrations and the prolonged excretion of large doses.

TOYOHARA (1970) stated that intermittent administration of 60 mg RMP/kg twice a week or of a dose of 120 mg RMP/kg once a week had about the same effect as continuous treatment.

These findings suggested that RMP may be particularly suitable for intermittent administration in man, provided that the increase in the size of the individual doses would not provoke serious toxicity.

γ) Combination Therapy

In mice: The experiments with RMP monotherapy in mice can be summed up as follows: The effect of RMP depends on the tubercle bacilli loading of the tissues. The smaller the loading, the faster and more permanent is the negativation. These effects can be achieved either with daily or with intermittent administration of RMP. Finally, no definite sterilization was achieved by RMP monotherapy in the murine models used. Bacterial relapses were usually caused by RMP-resistant populations arising in consequence of selection effects.

This led naturally to studies of combinations of RMP with other antituberculosis drugs. Two aspects were followed very intensively: the bactericidal effect and the prevention of emergence of resistance.

The first drug examined in combination with RMP was INH, the leading antituberculotic at that time. In an already cited paper, GRUMBACH and RIST (1967) demonstrated the apparent negativation of all animals after 3 months of treatment with RMP and INH, both at a daily dose of 25 mg/kg. In 1968 VERBIST and GYSELEN reported that the addition of a low dose of INH (2 mg/kg) to 10 mg RMP/kg was able to prevent the emergence of RMP resistance for the period of drug administration. In very similar experiments, GRUMBACH (1969) found that after 3 months of treatment with 25 mg RMP/kg + 5 mg INH/kg tubercle bacilli retained their sensitivity to RMP. After 6 months all animals were negative. With combinations of the same doses of RMP and INH (25 mg/kg) the bactericidal effect achieved was more pronounced then that after RMP monotherapy, and the small populations of tubercle bacilli cultured from lung homogenates after 3 months or 4 months of the treatment were RMP-sensitive.

In later papers, GRUMBACH et al. (1970) and GRUMBACH (1975a, b) estimated that discontinuation of the treatment after 6 months was followed by bacteriological relapses in about 20% of the animals within next 6 months. After 12 months of treatment no relapses occurred in the subsequent 6 months, but the tissues of the treated animals had not been sterilized, since cortisone treatment provoked again the appearance of bacteriological relapses; the tubercle bacilli retained their sensitivity to RMP.

In chronic murine tuberculosis treated with 40 mg RMP/kg + 25 mg INH/kg KRADOLFER and SCHNELL (1971) confirmed the high bactericidal activity of this combination. GROSSET (1978a) noticed that no drug in combination with RMP was capable of making mice completely culture-negative after 4–6 months of treatment.

The combinations of RMP with other antituberculotics were consequently less effective, despite the fact that after a short treatment period (3 weeks) the mean survival times with combinations of RMP (10 mg/kg) with INH (5 mg/kg), EMB (15 mg/kg), or SM (100 mg/kg) were practically identical (HOBBY et al. 1969b). This means that some time is needed before the differences between the various drug combinations become manifest.

SM (250 mg/kg) combined with RMP (40 mg/kg) was not more effective than RMP monotherapy (KRADOLFER and SCHNELL 1971). Addition of SM to the combination of RMP + INH did not have any clear-cut benefit at the end of 5 months of treatment in the experiments of GRUMBACH et al. (1969), despite the fact that the reduction in the bacterial counts was faster at the beginning of treatment.

EMB was regarded as an effective combination partner for RMP, next to INH, by GRUMBACH et al. (1969). SOSNOWSKI and TOMASZKIEWICZ (1973) and FREERKSEN and ROSENFELD (1976) used a very low dose of EMB for potentiation (5 mg/kg–20 mg/kg), whereas other authors used 100 mg/kg–200 mg/kg (KOZULICINA and PETROV 1976; KONDO and KANAI 1977b).

In contrast, KRADOLFER and SCHNELL (1971) and GROSSET (1978a) estimated that EMB at the doses used in the experiments contributed little to the effectiveness of RMP, since only 75% of the treated animals were culture-negative after 6 months of the treatment and the remaining ones harbored RMP-resistant tubercle bacilli.

It is evident that, on the basis of up-to date evaluation criteria, addition of EMB to RMP cannot accelerate the negativation rate or the sterilizing effect, nor can it prevent the appearance of resistant populations. This is true even if EMB is used as a third drug in combination of RMP + INH, as reported by MABUCHI (1982) for murine tuberculosis.

ETH combined with RMP was also unable to prevent the emergence of RMP resistance (GRUMBACH 1969).

PZA is known to be highly effective in murine tuberculosis as already mentioned. According to GROSSET (1978a), in combination with INH, PZA can be considered as one of the main drugs in short-course chemotherapy of experimental murine tuberculosis. However, its addition (150 mg/kg) to a combination of RMP (10 mg/kg) and INH (25 mg/kg) for another 3 months did not contribute to the sterilizing effect or to the rate of negativation (GROSSET et al. 1980; GROSSET 1981). When PZA is added to INH + RMP in the initial phase of treatment for 2 months the sterilizing effect is improved from 65.5% to 89.3% with statistical significance (GROSSET et al. 1983). KM (40 mg/kg), CM (40 mg/kg), and VM (40 mg/kg) were combined with RMP by SUZUKI (1971). According to this author, better effects than with corresponding monotherapies were observed, but it is not clear whether they actually improved on the effect of RMP monotherapy.

From the above experiments it may be concluded that not one of the combinations studied was superior to RMP+INH in respect to the rate of negativation and the prevention of RMP resistance. Therefore, this combination was mainly used for studying two other aspects of tuberculosis chemotherapy.

The first aspect concerns intermittency. GRUMBACH et al. (1969) showed that the combination of RMP+INH given twice a week was only slightly inferior to the same combination administered daily. The difference consisted in 80% of negative spleen cultures instead of 100%, and resistance to INH (but not to RMP) developed in one animal.

The once-weekly regimen proved to be considerably inferior. After 6 months the combination of RMP and INH led to culture negativity of only 33% of the lungs and 44% of the spleens.

The second question of tuberculosis chemotherapy studied in experimental models of murine tuberculosis was whether the addition of RMP to a good regime for a short period would have a lasting benefit.

GRUMBACH et al. (1969) used the combination of INH+SM. RMP was added during the first month. The results were assessed at 4 months. The combination of INH+SM given for 4 months daily or intermittently produced results characterized by inability to achieve tissue negativity. The residual populations were of the order of 10^2 to 10^3. If RMP was added for 1 month, the results were surprisingly good. Some of the animals were negativized, and the residual populations were very low, of the order of 10^1. These results came far closer to those of the regimens comprising RMP for the entire duration of treatment.

There was clear-cut evidence that the addition of RMP for only 1 month had produced a benefit which was still demonstrable as late as 3 months after withdrawal of the drug. Further experiments by GROSSET et al. (1978a) confirmed that, in terms of bacteriological relapses, the best results can be achieved if the RMP can be administered for as long as possible, particularly if its combination with INH is used instead of INH monotherapy in the second phase of two-phase chemotherapy.

In guinea pigs: INH at daily doses of 4 mg/kg combined with 40 mg RMP/kg produced a strong bactericidal effect during 42 days of treatment, as was discovered by NITTI and NINNI (1969) by counting viable bacterial units in the spleens of guinea pigs sacrificed after various times. The effects were definitely better than those of a combination of INH and SM (40 mg/kg i.m.).

On the other hand, SM at the dose indicated above combined with RMP produced bactericidal effects which were better than those of RMP monotherapy and equal to those obtained with the combination of INH and SM.

Finally, EMB (100 mg/kg/day) combined with RMP did not appreciably increase the bactericidal activity of RMP (NITTI and NINNI 1969).

A basic contribution to the formulation of the principles of modern tuberculosis chemotherapy was made by DICKINSON and MITCHISON (1976a, b) and was based on guinea pig studies. The methods were similar to those described earlier; the animals were treated for 11 weeks, RMP was given at a dose of 30 mg/kg, INH at 8 mg/kg, and EMB at 45 mg/kg. The drugs were administered alone or in various combinations. The extent of the tuberculosis was scored and the spleens were cultured from groups killed at intervals of up to 7.5 months after the end of chemotherapy. It was estimated that the regimens containing RMP were no more bactericidal than the corresponding regimens without RMP. However, in the RMP-containing regimens bacteriological relapses were delayed for at least 2 months. It was concluded that RMP may act selectively on a small fraction of the bacterial population, and that it may be unnecessary to prescribe it for long periods in short-course chemotherapy in man.

The results in the guinea pig model led to same conclusions as had been derived from the already described in-vitro studies. The fraction of tubercle bacilli growing in vivo that is inhibited specifically by RMP may consist of persistent tubercle bacilli with spurts of metabolizing activity. The sterilizing activity of RMP in the guinea pig model was regarded as equivalent to that of INH and superior to those of other antituberculosis drugs. In contrast, in the experimental model of murine tuberculosis the sterilizing activity of RMP or INH was equal to that of PZA. In this respect this group of drugs was superior to other antituberculosis drugs (BARTMANN et al. 1985).

3. Concluding Remarks

The minimal inhibitory concentrations of RMP for *M. tuberculosis* and *M. bovis* in vitro are as low as those of INH and therefore better than those of the other 12 antituberculotics. In contrast to INH, RMP is active against many "atypical" mycobacteria. Like INH, RMP is growth-dependently bactericidal on extracellularly and intracellularly located bacilli. The killing rate of RMP is the same as that of INH, but the effect sets in more quickly with RMP. There is no cross-resistance with the other antituberculotics. The proportion of primarily resistant mutants in wild strains is very low, in contrast to the situation with INH. In experimental animals RMP is as active as INH, but it kills more or less resting bacilli in mice better than INH. A combination of RMP with INH is more active than either drug alone. Apart from INH, certain other antituberculotics when given in combination in appropriate dosage are able to prevent the development of secondary bacterial resistance to RMP, but except for PZA, they do not contribute appreciably to the sterilization effect. RMP is well suited for intermittent treatment. In regimens characterized by treatment in phases, RMP can be used in the initial intensive as well as in the continuation phase. Together with INH, RMP constitutes the back-bone of modern short-course regimens for the treatment of human tuberculosis, which have to be applied for 6 months–9 months. In many respects the activity of RMP must be judged as equal to that of INH, while being superior in other respects which have a bearing on clinical application and have been indicated above.

References

Acocella G, Carlone NA, Cuffini AM, Cavallo G (1985) The penetration of rifampicin, pyrazinamide, and pyrazinoic acid into mouse macrophages. Am Rev Respir Dis 132:1268–1273

Algeorge G, Sibilla A, Rudesco D, Stoian M (1971) Recherches sur l'action protectrice de la rifampicine en administration intermittente dans la tuberculose expérimentale du cobaye. Ftiziologia (Bucuresti) 20 Suppl:69–74

Algeorge G, Rudescu D (1973) Rifampicin effect on tuberculin hypersensitivity and humoral antibody response in tuberculous guinea pigs. Z Immun Forsch 144:459–466

Aoyagi T, Izumi T, Toyohara M, Kawai T, Shima K, Umeda H (1979) Immunological, pharmacological and dynamic action of rifampicin (in Japanese). Kekkaku 54:573–582

Arioli V, Pallanza R, Furesz S, Carniti G (1967) Rifampicin: a new rifamycin. I. Bacteriological studies. Arzneimittelforsch 17:523–527

Atlas E, Turck M (1968) Laboratory and clinical evaluation of rifampicin. Am J Med Sci 256:247–254

Baba H, Azuma Y (1976) The clinical significance of the critical drug concentration of rifampicin. Report I. Studies on the MIC of rifampicin to tubercle bacilli isolated from the rifampicin untreated patients using 1% Ogawa medium (in Japanese). Kekkaku 51:1–5

Bartmann K, Radenbach KL, Zierski M (1985) Wandlungen in den Auffassungen und der Durchführung der antituberkulösen Chemotherapie. Eine Übersicht mit praktischen Schlußfolgerungen. Prax Klin Pneumol 39:397–420

Batten J (1968) Experimental chemotherapy of tuberculosis. Brit Med J 3:75–82

Batten J (1969) Rifampicin in treatment of experimental tuberculosis in mice. Tubercle 50:294–298

Batten J (1970) Rifampicin in the treatment of experimental tuberculosis in mice: sterilization of tubercle bacilli in the tissues. Tubercle 51:95–99

Bellahsene A, Forsgren A (1980) Effect of rifampicin on the immune response in mice. Infect Immun 27:15–20

Bibik HF (1972) Frequency and clinical importance of primary drug resistance of Mycobacterium tuberculosis in patients with pulmonary tuberculosis (in Russian). Probl Tuberk 50, issue 8, 20–25

Binda G, Domenichini E, Gottardi A, Orlandi B, Ortelli E, Pacini B, Fowst G (1971) Rifampicin, a general review. Arzneimittelforsch 21:1907–1977

Burjanová B, Dornetzhuber VL (1975) Empfindlichkeit der Stämme des M. kansasii auf verschiedene Antibiotika und Chemotherapeutika in vitro und in vivo. Z Erkr Atmungsorgane 142:68–77

Byalik IB, Klimenko MT (1973) Effect of rifampicin and ethambutol on Mycobacterium tuberculosis in vitro (in Russian). Probl Tuberk 51 issue 2:56–61

Byalik IB, Klimenko MT (1976) Bactericidal action of rifampicin (in Russian). Probl Tuberk 54 issue 9:74–80

Canetti G, Le Lirzin M, Porven G, Rist N, Grumbach F (1968) Some comparative aspects of rifampicin and isoniazid. Tubercle 49:367–376

Canetti G, Fox W, Khomenko A, Mahler HT, Menon NK, Mitchison DA, Rist N, Šmelev NA (1969) Advances in techniques of testing mycobacterial drug sensitivity, and the use of sensitivity tests in tuberculosis control programmes. Bull WHO 41:21–43

Carlone NA, Acocella G, Cuffini AM, Forno-Pizzoglio M (1985) Killing of macrophage-ingested mycobacteria by rifampicin, pyrazinamide, and pyrazinoic acid alone and in combination. Am Rev Respir Dis 132:1274–1277

Clark J, Wallace A (1967) The susceptibility of mycobacteria to rifamide and rifampicin. Tubercle 48:144–148

Clini V, Grassi C (1970) The action of new antituberculous drugs on intracellular tubercle bacilli. Antibiot Chemother 16:20–26

David HL (1970) Probability distribution of drug-resistant mutants in unselected populations of *Mycobacterium tuberculosis*. Appl Microb 20:810–814

Davidson PT, Waggoner R (1976) Acquired resistance to rifampicin by Mycobacterium kansasii. Tubercle 57:271–273

Denis-Bottin C (1972) Activité „in vitro“ de la rifampicine sur des souches de mycobactéries tuberculeuses et atypiques. Act Tub Pneum Belg 63:127–139

Dickinson JM, Mitchison DA (1970) Suitability of rifampicin for intermittent administration in the treatment of tuberculosis. Tubercle 51:82–94

Dickinson JM, Jackett PS, Mitchison DA (1972) The effect of pulsed exposures to rifampin on the uptake of uridine-^{14}C by *Mycobacterium tuberculosis*. Amer Rev Resp Dis 105:519–527

Dickinson JM, Mitchison DA (1976a) Bactericidal activity *in vitro* and in the guinea-pig of isoniazid, rifampicin and ethambutol. Tubercle 57:251–258
Dickinson JM, Mitchison DA (1976b) Experimental investigations of bacteriological mechanisms in short course chemotherapy. Bull Int Union Tuberc 51:79–86
Dickinson JM, Aber VR, Mitchison DA (1977) Bactericidal activity of streptomycin, isoniazid, rifampin, ethambutol and pyrazinamide alone and in combination against *Mycobacterium tuberculosis*. Am Rev Resp Dis 116:627–635
Dickinson JM, Mitchison DA (1981) Experimental models to explain the high sterilizing activity of rifampin in the chemotherapy of tuberculosis. Am Rev Resp Dis 123:367–371
Dolzhansky VM (1982) Conditions favourable for rifampicin activity and development of resistance in vitro (in Russian). Probl Tuberk 60 issue 3:59–62
Dutt AK, Stead WW (1982) Present chemotherapy of tuberculosis. J Inf Dis 146:698–704
Editorial (1969) Rifampicin and viruses. Brit Med J 2:588–589
Eskenazy A, Diaconitza G, Ionesco J (1971) Enzymatic et immunomorphological features of rifampicine action in experimental tuberculosis (in French). Ftiziologia (Bucuresti) 20 Suppl:85–90
Freerksen E, Rosenfeld M (1976) Fortschritte in der Tuberkulosebehandlung. Prax Pneumol 30:489–502
Fujiwara H, Negoro S, Tsuyuguchi, Kishimoto S (1976) Immunosuppressive effect of rifampicin (in Japanese). Kekkaku 51:47–53
Furesz S (1970) Chemical and biological properties of rifampicin. Antibiot Chemother 16:316–351
Furesz S, Scotti R, Pallanza R, Mapelli E (1967) Rifampicin: a new rifamycin. III. Absorption, distribution and elimination in man. Arzneimittelforsch 17:534–537
Grosset J (1978a) The sterilizing value of rifampicin and pyrazinamide in experimental short course chemotherapy. Tubercle 59:287–297
Grosset J (1978b) Experimental data on short-course chemotherapy. Bull Int Union Tuberc 53:265–267
Grosset J (1981) Studies in short-course chemotherapy for tuberculosis. Basis for short-course chemotherapy. Chest 80:710–720
Grosset J, Grumbach F, Rist N (1978) La rôle de la rifampicine dans la phase ultime du traitement de la tuberculose murine expérimentale. Rev Fr Mal Resp 6:515–520
Grosset J, Truffot C, Boval C, Fermanian J (1980) Efficacité stérilisante de l'isoniazide et du pyrazinamide en association avec la rifampicine dans la tuberculose expérimentale de la souris. Rev Fr Mal Resp 8:31–32
Grosset J, Truffot-Pernot C, Bismuth R, Lecoeur H (1983) Recent results of chemotherapy in experimental tuberculosis of the mouse. Bull Int Union Tuberc 58:90–96
Grumbach F (1969) Experimental "in vivo" studies of new antituberculosis drugs: capreomycin, ethambutol, rifampicin. Tubercle 50 Suppl:12–22
Grumbach F (1970) L'activité de la rifampicine sur la tuberculose expérimentale de la souris. Développement de la résistance à la rifampicine. Effets thérapeutiques des associations de différents médicaments à la rifampicine. Antib Chemother 16:392–405
Grumbach F (1975a) La durée optimale de l'antibiothérapie par l'association isoniazide + rifampicine dans la tuberculose expérimentale de la souris. Étude de la phase post-thérapeutique. Épreuve de la cortisone. Rev Fr Mal Resp 3:625–634
Grumbach F (1975b) Traitement de la tuberculose de la souris par l'association isoniazide-rifampicine. Essais de l'adjonction de traitements courts pendant la période post-thérapeutique pour éviter la reviviscence bacillaire. Rev Fr Mal Resp 3:1027–1036
Grumbach F, Rist N (1967) Activité antituberculeuse expérimentale de la rifampicine, dérivé de la rifamycine SV. Rev Tub Pneumol 31:749–762
Grumbach F, Canetti G, Le Lirzin M (1969) Rifampicin in daily and intermittent treatment of experimental murine tuberculosis, with emphasis on late results. Tubercle 50:280–293
Grumbach F, Canetti G, Le Lirzin M (1970) Caractère durable de la stérilisation de la tuberculose expérimentale de la souris par l'association rifampicine-isoniazide. Épreuve de la cortisone. Rev Tuberc Pneumol 34:312–319

Gulevskaya SA, Milovanova EV (1977) The action of isoniazid and rifampicin on viability and the ultrastructure of Mycobacterium tuberculosis (in Russian). Probl Tuberk 55 issue 5:67–73
Hand WL, Boozer RM, King-Thompson NL (1985) Antibiotic uptake by alveolar macrophages of smokers. Antimicrob Agents Chemother 27:42–45
Havel A, Adámek L, Šimonová S (1970) Rifampicin in experimental investigations on mice. Antibiot Chemother 16:406–415
Havel A, Rosenfeld M (1975) Potenzierung der Wirkung von Rifampicin und Ethionamid durch das gegen M. tuberculosis unwirksame 4,4-Diamino-Diphenylsulfon (DDS) in vitro. Prax Pneumol 29:453–458
Hejný J (1978) Mycobacteriological aspects of the treatment of mycobacterioses. I. In vitro studies (in Czech.). Stud pneumol phtiseol cechoslovac 38:579–583
Hobby GL (1972) Summation of experimental studies on the action of rifampin. Chest 61:550–554
Hobby GL, Lenert TF (1968) The antimycobacterial activity of rifampin. Am Rev Resp Dis 97:713–714
Hobby GL, Lenert TF, Maier-Engallena J (1969 a) *In vitro* activity of rifampin against the H37Rv strain of *Mycobacterium tuberculosis*. Am Rev Resp Dis 99:453–456
Hobby GL, Lenert TF, Maier-Engallena J (1969 b) Experimental observations on the antimycobacterial activity of rifampin. Proc Soc exp Biol Med 131:323–326
Hobby GL, Lenert TF (1970) The action of rifampin alone and in combination with other antituberculous drugs. Am Rev Resp Dis 102:462–465
Hobby GL, Lenert TF (1972) Observations on the action of rifampin and ethambutol alone and in combination with other antituberculous drugs. Am Rev Resp Dis 105:292–295
Hobby GL, Johnson PM, Boytar-Papirnyik V (1974) Primary drug resistance: a continuing study of drug resistance in tuberculosis in a veteran population within the United States. X. September 1970 to September 1973. Am Rev Resp Dis 110:95–100
Hui J, Gordon N, Kajioka R (1977) Permeability barrier to rifampin in mycobacteria. Antimicrob Agents Chemother 11:773–779
Hussels H, Schütz I (1968) Rifampicin-Hemmtiter bei Tuberkulosebakterien-Wildstämmen und Rifampicin-Serumkonzentrationen bei Tuberkulosekranken. Beitr Klin Tuberk 140:304–312
Hussels H (1977) Die Häufigkeit der primären Resistenz von Tuberkelbakterien in der Bundesrepublik Deutschland einschließlich Berlin (West) im Beobachtungszeitraum 1972 bis 1975. Prax Pneumol 31:664–670
Janowiec M, Zwolska-Kwiek Z, Wisniewska A, Wroblewska H (1977) Interaction of antituberculous drugs. I. Combined action of rifampicin, nicotinic acid hydrazide, streptomycin and para-aminosalicylic acid on growth of strains of tubercle bacilli (in Polish). Pneum Pol 45:425–430
Janowiec M, Zwolska-Kwiek Z, Bek E (1979) Drug resistance in newly discovered untreated tuberculosis patients in Poland, 1974–1977. Tubercle 60:233–237
Jenne JW, Beggs WH (1973) Correlation of in vitro and in vivo kinetics with clinical use of isoniazid, ethambutol and rifampin. Am Rev Resp Dis 107:1013–1021
Kanai K, Kondo E (1979) Bactericidal effect of rifampicin on resting tubercle bacilli in vitro (in Japanese). Kekkaku 54:89–92
Karlson AG (1970) Comparison of three mediums for rifampin-susceptibility tests of mycobacteria. Am Rev Resp Dis 101:765–767
Kawamori Y (1969) Antituberculous activity of rifampicin. Progress in Antimicrobial and Anticancer Chemotherapy. Proc 6th Intern Congr Chemother, Tokyo, August 10–15 1969. Vol 1. University Park Press, Baltimore, pp 1206–1208
Kondo E, Kanai K (1977 a) Experimental studies on the effective regimens of antituberculous drugs in the treatment of tuberculosis. I. Intermittent drug administration with single or combined drugs (in Japanese). Kekkaku 52:339–343
Kondo E, Kanai K (1977b) Experimental studies on the effective regimens of antituberculous drugs in the treatment of tuberculosis. II. Long-term chemotherapy in mice by daily and intermittent administration with changing drug combination (in Japanese). Kekkaku 52:373–376
Kondo E, Kanai K (1978) Comparative studies on therapeutic effect of rifampicin and isoniazid on experimental mouse tuberculosis (in Japanese). Kekkaku 53:261–264

Kopanoff DE, Kilburn JO, Glassroth JL, Snider DE, Farer LS, Good RC (1978) A continuing survey of tuberculosis primary drug resistance in the United States: March 1975 to November 1977. A United States Public Health Service Cooperative Study. Am Rev Resp Dis 118:835–842

Kozulicina TI, Petrov IV (1976) Experimental study of the intermittent use of rifampicin and ethambutol (in Russian). Probl Tuberk 54 issue 5:72–74

Kradolfer F (1968) Relationship between chemotherapeutic activity and blood concentration of rifampicin in murine tuberculosis. Amer Rev Resp Dis 98:104–106

Kradolfer F (1970) Rifampicin, isoniazid, ethambutol, ethionamide and streptomycin in murine tuberculosis: comparative chemotherapeutical studies. Antibiot Chemother 16:352–360

Kradolfer F, Schnell R (1970) Incidence of resistant pulmonary tuberculosis in relation to initial bacterial load. Rifampicin and INH in experimental tuberculosis. Chemotherapy 15:242–249

Kradolfer F, Schnell R (1971) The combination of rifampicin and other antituberculous agents in chronic murine tuberculosis. Chemotherapy 16:173–182

Kramer H, Bergmann KC (1976) Zum Einfluß von Rifampicin auf die Lymphozytentransformation. Z Erkr Atmungsorgane 144:163–167

Krebs A (1969) Experimentelle Chemotherapie der Tuberkulose. Z Erkr Atmungsorgane 130:417–448

Kuze F, Naito Y, Takeda S, Maekawa N (1977) Sensitivities of atypical mycobacteria to various drugs. IV. Sensitivities of atypical mycobacteria originally isolated in the USA to antituberculous drugs in triple combinations (in Japanese). Kekkaku 52:505–513

Kuze F, Lee Y, Maekawa N, Suzuki Y (1979) A study on experimental mycobacterioses provoked by atypical mycobacteria. 2. Combined antituberculous chemotherapy against conventional mice infected intravenously with Mycobacterium intracellulare (in Japanese). Kekkaku 54:453–460

Lam C, Mathison GE (1985) Effect of low intraphagolysosomal pH on antimicrobial activity of antibiotics against ingested staphylococci. J Med Microbiol 16:309–316

Le Cam M, Madec Y, Bernard S (1971) Comportement métabolique de *Mycobacterium tuberculosis,* souche H37 RA sous l'action de la rifampicine. Éléments de comparaison avec l'isoniazide. Ann Inst Pasteur 120:186–195

Le Lirzin M, Djurovic V (1971) Étude sur milieu de Loewenstein-Jensen de la composition des souches sauvages de *Mycobacterium tuberculosis* en variants résistant à la rifampicine et en variants résistant à l'éthambutol. Ann Inst Pasteur 120:531–548

Lorian V, Finland M (1969) In vitro effect of rifampin on mycobacteria. Appl Microb 17:202–207

Lucchesi M, Mancini P (1970) Antimycobacterial activity of rifampicin. Antibiot Chemother 16:431–443

Mabuchi H (1982) Studies on the intensification of chemotherapeutic regimens in experimental tuberculosis (in Japanese). Kekkaku 57:73–79

Mandell GL (1973) Interaction of intraleukocytic bacteria and antibiotics. J Clin Inv 52:1673–1679

Manten A, Van Wijngaarden LJ (1969) Development of drug resistance to rifampicin. Chemotherapy 14:93–100

Margalith P, Beretta G (1960) Rifamycin XI. Taxonomic study on Streptomyces mediterranei nova species. Mycopath Mycol Appl 13:321–325

McClatchy JK, Waggoner RF, Lester W (1969) In vitro susceptibility of mycobacteria to rifampin. Am Rev Resp Dis 100:234–236

Medoff G, Kobayashi GS, Kwan CN, Schlessinger D, Venkov P (1972) Potentiation of rifampicin and 5-fluorocytosine as antifugal antibiotics by amphotericin B. Proc Nat Acad Sci USA 69:196–199

Mitchison DA (1971) The principles of intermittent chemotherapy (in Czech.). Stud Pneumol Phtiseol Cechoslovac 31:288–296

Naito M, Maekawa N, Tsukuma S, Nakanishi M (1970) Studies on a new antituberculous antibiotic rifampicin. Progress in Antimicrobial and Anticancer chemotherapy. Proc 6th Intern Congr Chemother Tokyo, August 10–15, 1969, Vol I. University Park Press, Baltimore, pp 1058–1061

Nitti V (1970) Experimental and clinical studies on the antituberculous activity of rifampicin alone or combined with other drugs. Antibiot Chemother 16:444–470
Nitti V (1972) Antituberculous activity of rifampicin. Report of studies performed and in progress (1966–1971). Chest 61:589–598
Nitti V, Catena E, Ninni A, Di Filippo A (1967) Activity of rifampicin in experimental tuberculosis of the guinea pig. Chemotherapia 12:369–400
Nitti V, Ninni A (1969) In vivo bactericidal activity of rifampicin in combination with other antimycobacterial agents. Chemotherapy 14:356–365
Ohsato T, Shizumi H (1972) Virulence of rifampicin-resistant tubercle bacilli for experimental animals (preliminary report) (in Japanese). Kekkaku 47:129–134
Osada Y, Nakajo M, Une T, Ogawa H, Oshima Y (1972) Application of cell culture in studying antibacterial activity of rifampicin to Shigella and enteropathogenic Escherichia coli. Japan J Microbiol 16:525–533
Pallanza R, Arioli V, Furesz S, Bolzoni G (1967) Rifampicin: a new rifamycin. II. Laboratory studies on the antituberculous activity and preliminary clinical observations. Arzneimittelforsch 17:529–534
Pavlov EP, Tušov EG, Kotljarov LM (1974) The action of rifampicin on intracellular tubercle bacilli (in Russian). Probl Tuberk 52 issue 12:64–67
Pesanti EL (1980) Protection of staphylococci ingested by macrophages from the bactericidal action of rifampin. Antimicrob Agents Chemother 18:208–209
Prokesch RC, Hand WL (1982) Antibiotic entry into human polymorphonuclear leukocytes. Antimicrob Agents Chemother 21:373–380
Reutgen H (1972) Ein neues Verfahren zur Bestimmung der Rifampicin-Resistenz bei Mycobacterium tuberculosis. Acta Biol Med Germ 28:395–409
Reutgen H (1973) Zur Resistenzbestimmung von Mycobacterium tuberculosis gegenüber INH, Streptomyzin, PAS, Äthionamid, Ethambutol und Rifampicin mittels ^{32}P-Inkorporations-Test. Acta Biol Med Germ 30:309–316
Rightsel WA, Sawyers MF, Peters JH (1978) Comparative effects of sulfones and rifampin on growth of *Mycobacterium lepraemurium* in macrophage diffusion chamber cultures. Antimicrob Agents Chemother 13:509–513
Rist N (1969) La résistance du bacille tuberculeux à la rifampicine. Rev Tuberc Pneumol (Symposium Rifadine) 33:33–38
Rook GAW (1973) Is the macrophage the site of the immunosuppressive action of rifampicin? Tubercle 54:291–295
Rosenfeld M (1970) Rifampicin, Myambutol, Isoxyl and capreomycin as combination partners in animal experiments. Antibiot Chemother 16:501–515
Rynearson TK, Shronts JS, Wolinsky E (1971) Rifampin: in vitro effect on atypical mycobacteria. Am Rev Resp Dis 104:272–274
Saito H, Yamamoto S, Yamura T (1972) Susceptibility of Runyon group I mycobacteria to rifampicin. Hir J Med Sci 21:35–40
Schröder KH, Koperska C (1972) Rifampicin-Resistenz und Virulenz von M. tuberculosis für Meerschweinchen. I. Mitteilung. Zbl Bakt Hyg, I. Abt Orig A 219:112–113
Sensi P, Maggi N, Füresz S, Maffii G (1967) Chemical modification of biological properties of rifamycins. Antimicrob Agents Chemother 1966:699–714
Seydel JK (1970) Physico-chemical studies on rifampicin. Antibiot Chemother 16:380–391
Shimoide H (1977) The disease due to *Mycobacterium kansasii* in Japan (in Japanese). Kekkaku 52:577–585
Shiniberov VA (1979) Effect of rifampicin on the nonspecific reactivity and natural resistance of tuberculosis guinea pigs (in Russian). Probl Tuberk 57, issue 1, 50–54
Siddiqi SH, Aziz A, Reggiardo Z, Middlebrook G (1981) Resistance to rifampicin and isoniazid in strains of *Mycobacterium tuberculosis*. J Clin Pathol 34:927–929
Snider DE Jr, Good RC, Kilburn JO, Laskowski LF Jr, Lusk RH, Marr JJ, Reggiardo Z, Middlebrook G (1981) Rapid drug-susceptibility testing of *Mycobacterium tuberculosis*. Am Rev Resp Dis 123:402–406
Solberg CO, Hellum KB (1978) Protection of phagocytosed bacteria against antimicrobial agents. Scand J Infect Dis Suppl 14:246–250

Sosnowski W, Tomaszkiewicz L (1973) Bacteriological results of the treatment of mice tuberculosis by rifampicin and ethambutol administered daily or intermittently (in Polish). Gruzlica 41:214–224
Spitzy KH (1963) Position of Rifamycine in the antibacterial chemotherapy (in German). Chemotherapie 7:317–320
Stoica E (1972) L'action de l'éthambutol (EMB) et de la rifampicine (RFM) sur les mycobactéries phagocytées par la macrophage alvéolaire. Acta Tuberc Pneumol Belg 63:501–509
Stottmeier KD, Kubica GP, Woodley CD (1969) Antimycobacterial activity of rifampin under in vitro and simulated in vivo conditions. Appl Microbiol 17:861–865
Suzuki T (1971) Experimental studies on intermittent use of rifampicin alone or combined with other secondary antituberculous drugs (in Japanese). Kekkaku 46:153–164
Tacquet A, Devulder B, Martin JC, Daniel H, Le Bouffant L (1969) Activité antimycobactérienne de la rifampicine. Etudes „in vitro" et „in vivo". Rev Tuberc Pneumol (Symposium Rifadine) 33:61–80
Tanzil HOK, Chatim A, Rachim A, Judanarso D (1972) "In vitro" action of rifampicin on typical and atypical mycobacteria. Acta Tuberc Pneumol Belg 63:140–147
Toyohara M (1970) Antituberculous activity of rifampicin for the experimental tuberculosis of guinea pigs (in Japanese). Kekkaku 45:375–378
Toyohara M (1971) An experimental study on the antituberculous activity of rifampicin (in Japanese). Kekkaku 46:211–216
Toyohara M (1979) Experimental model of the short-course chemotherapy (in Japanese). Kekkaku 54:369–374
Toyohara M, Iwasaki T (1971) Antituberculous activity of rifampicin for experimental tuberculosis of mice (in Japanese). Kekkaku 46:19–22
Trnka L, Štaflová S (1974) Experimental principles on the use of rifampicin in the intermittent chemotherapy of tuberculosis. Ain Shams Med J 25 (Suppl):157–159
Trnka L, Mison P, Staflova S (1974) Interaction aspects of antimycobacterial drugs in the chemotherapy of tuberculosis. II. The role of rifampicin and other drugs in the dependent or independent action of drug associations *in vitro*. Chemotherapy 20:82–91
Trnka L, Škvor J, Mišoň P (1977) The effect of antituberculotics on in vitro lymphocyte transformation (in Czech.). Stud pneumol phtiseol cechoslovac 37:233–238
Tsukamura M (1972a) The pattern of resistance development to rifampicin in Mycobacterium tuberculosis. Tubercle 53:111–117
Tsukamura M (1972b) Critical concentration for definition of rifampicin resistance of tubercle bacilli (in Japanese). Kekkaku 47:113–119
Tsukamura M, Imazu S, Tsukamura S (1963) Alcune osservazioni sul meccanismo di azione della rifamicina SV. Ann Inst Carlo Forlanini 23:40–50
Tsukamura M, Imazu S, Tsukamura S (1963) Combined effect of Rifamycin SV with other antituberculosis drugs: experiments in mice. Chemotherapia 7:470–477
Uvarova OA, Kozulitsyna TI, Korotaev GA (1976) Features specific for the action of rifampicin on experimental tuberculosis (in Russian). Probl Tuberk 54 issue 1:65–70
Verbist L (1968) Étude expérimentale de l'activité de la rifampicine in vitro et in vivo. Taux sanguins. Rev Tuberc Pneumol 33 bis :59–60
Verbist L (1969) Rifampicin activity "in vitro" and in established tuberculosis in mice. Acta Tub Pneumol Belg 60:397–412
Verbist L (1970) Experimental base of intermittent chemotherapy. Pneumonology Suppl 1970 Neue Wege der Tuberkulosetherapie:31–37
Verbist L, Gyselen A (1968) Antituberculous activity of rifampin *in vitro* and *in vivo* and the concentrations attained in human blood. Am Rev Resp Dis 98:923–932
Westfal I, Zengteler G, Szymaczek-Meyer L (1974) Microscopic changes in the liver in experimental tuberculosis of guinea pigs treated with rifampicin (in Polish). Gruzlica 42:879–885
White RJ, Lancini G (1971) Uptake and binding of ^{3}H-rifampicin by Escherichia coli and Staphylococcus aureus. Biochim Biophys Acta 240:429–434
Woodley CHL, Kilburn JO, David HL, Silcox VA (1972) Susceptibility of mycobacteria to rifampin. Antimicrob Agents Chemother 2:245–249

Wozniak S, Tomaszkiewicz L, Zierski M (1969) Tuberculostatic activity of rifampicin (rifampin) in vitro (in Polish). Gruzlica 37:983–989
Yamadori H (1971) In vitro effects of several kinds of gas exposure on the antimicrobial activities of antituberculous agents. Chapter I. Bacteriostatic effects (in Japanese). Kekkaku 46:429–433
Yates MD, Collins CH (1981) Sensitivity of opportunistic mycobacteria to rifampicin and ethambutol. Tubercle 62:117–121
Yoshida F (1970) Experimental therapy with rifampicin. Antibiot Chemother 16:416–423

CHAPTER 3

Experimental Evaluation of Chemoprophylaxis and Preventive Treatment in Animals

H. H. KLEEBERG

A. Definitions

The word prophylaxis is derived from the Greek phulaxis, which means "a guarding". Properly speaking it should be applied only when speaking of diseases where infection can be prevented. However, in tuberculosis control we use the term BCG prophylaxis, although the bacillus Calmette-Guerin cannot prevent the tubercle bacillus from settling in a non-infected host: it can only prevent the further spread of infection. The terms primary chemoprophylaxis and secondary chemoprophylaxis have therefore been introduced, the first meaning protection from infection and the second prevention of the progression of infection to disease. In the control of tuberculosis the use of drugs on non-infected persons with the aim of preventing clinical disease or the spread of infection is practised widely. The terms chemoprevention, preventive therapy and chemoprotection are sometimes used instead of secondary prophylaxis. The U.S. Committee on Therapy used the term infection prophylaxis for primary prophylaxis, and disease prophylaxis for secondary prophylaxis.

B. Objectives of Laboratory Experiments

Soon after the discovery of the antimycobacterial effect of isoniazid (INH), experiments with chemoprophylaxis and preventive treatment were done on a number of animal species in several countries and institutions as it was essential to have experimental evidence of the biological efficacy of the drug. DOMAGK et al. (1952), FUST et al. (1952), and GRUNBERG and SCHNITZER (1952) were the first to work in this field. AVELLINI (1953) and BADIALI (1954) published the findings of their experiments with cattle. In 1955, BARTMANN began publishing a series on his experiments with guinea pigs and in 1956, SCHMIDT reported his experiments with primates (SCHMIDT 1956). Numerous publications appeared during the fifties and sixties and were reviewed by DEBRÉ et al. (1959), LAMBERT (1959), OMODEI-ZORINI (1963), SPIESS (1963), DEBORAH SYMPOSIUM (1959), LUCCHESI et al. (1957; 1958; 1959; 1960; 1961), BARTMANN (1960), KLEEBERG (1966) and BARTMANN et al. (1971). Experimental data exist on subjects such as choice of drug, choice of animal species, correct dosing schedule, limitations of prophylaxis, attainable and required levels of *in vivo* drug concentrations, limits of reliability, frequency of side effects, effect of exposure and susceptibility, duration of dosing, drug administration routes, interference with immune response, effect on tuberculin reaction and failure rate, adverse reactions, the question of drug resistance, the possibility of eradicating the microbial population and combining immune prophylaxis with chemoprophylaxis. Questions were posed: would INH prevent the spread of tubercle bacilli? Would it prevent generalization of lesions? Would it reduce the bacterial population to a minimum? How specific was it, and how toxic? Could it be taken over long periods? Would it provide protection for the period of administration or would protection last beyond that time? Would it simply retard the progress of the disease or would it only prevent complications?

C. Results of Animal Experiments

It is fortunate that tubercle bacilli, and in particular *Mycobacterium tuberculosis* and *M. bovis,* have such a wide host spectrum among mammals. Many different animal species, including the larger domestic animals, could be utilized in the study of chemoprophylaxis. Seldom before had drug prophylaxis of any kind been studied so thoroughly prior to its widespread use on man. Large-scale trials were done on guinea pigs, monkeys and cattle, but a great many mice and rabbits were also used. However, the multiplicity of experimental designs and methods used makes it difficult both to evaluate and to compare the experimental results. The number of infective organisms varied widely and so did their virulence. Many different routes of infection and many different drug dosages were used, and the criteria for evaluation differed, as did the duration of observation.

Experiments to prevent the fixation of tubercle bacilli in tissues should be so devised that infection is similar to natural infection. It can be brought about by means of animal feed, inhalation or injection. It is relatively easy in such experiments to show the ineffectiveness of a substance or a certain dose, but it is difficult to prove complete protection or that all organisms have been destroyed. It is not enough to show that death or disease has been prevented, as latent infection with tubercle bacilli is known to last for very long periods and several conditions must be fulfilled before complete protection of the host is proved. Tests must be done with small numbers of highly virulent organisms, so that the animal's susceptibility remains high.

The first reports by FERREBEE and PALMER (1956) showed that large numbers of organisms produced a degree of resistance to infection in the host, as did untreated infections. If survival is to be tested then experiments must continue for 6 months to 9 months after cessation of drug treatment so that late relapses can be detected. If animals are sacrificed early, cultures must be made so as to show that the tissues are free of tubercle bacilli. A few important and well-controlled prophylactic experiments will be discussed.

I. Experiments with Monkeys

Monkeys are the most susceptible of the mammals and they can be used to test any drugs active against tuberculosis. SCHMIDT (1956) was the first to expose animals to natural infection. He exposed 51 noninfected animals to 127 tuberculous ones and treated all of them for 10 weeks with a low dose of INH (5 mg/kg) and then for a further 42 weeks with 20 mg/kg. Exposure and treatment were stopped at the same time. Half of the prophylactically treated animals developed tuberculin allergy and tuberculosis. In his second series SCHMIDT (1959) used a single intratracheal injection of about 750 tubercle bacilli and treated the infected animals for 16 weeks–24 weeks. All of them remained tuberculin negative throughout the one-year follow-up period. Bacteriologically no bacilli could be shown to have survived. His trials indicate that prophylaxis must be given not only during exposure but for a few months following it if multiplication of the organisms is to be inhibited. An infection which takes place towards the end of the exposure time will not be wiped out by INH.

II. Experiments with Guinea Pigs

A convincing experiment on 209 guinea pigs was done in Denver (COHN et al. 1962). The animals were infected by aerosol inhalation in such a way that the lung surfaces of each of the 42 control animals showed 35 tubercles–50 tubercles after 3 weeks. The other 167 animals were treated with INH subcutaneously, the dose being 14 mg/kg for 10 days. One-seventh (i.e., 24) of the treated animals converted to tuberculin positive, and 6 months–12 months later tuberculosis was diagnosed. Infection was successfully prevented in the remaining 6/7ths (i.e., 143) animals.

BARTMANN et al. (1955; 1956; 1957 a–c; 1958 a–c; 1959 a) undertook extensive therapy and prophylaxis experiments on guinea pigs which included intermittent INH administration. In his prophylactic experiments medication was started simultaneously with infection, and the infective dose was similar to that in natural infection. After the subcutaneous infection of guinea pigs with 2–25 organisms of a highly virulent strain all the controls developed generalized tuberculosis. The INH dose was 5 mg/kg–10 mg/kg and was injected subcutaneously every third or fourth day. After 4 months' treatment 50% of the animals were free of organisms, and after 8 months 75% were free of them. When the same dose was given daily for 4 months after infection to animals which had received 33 viable units, 95% (19 of 20) animals remained tuberculin negative. Nine months later none of the animals used in the experiment showed histological signs of tuberculosis and all cultures were negative.

Some of the classical work by BJERKEDAL and PALMER (1962, 1964) deals with primary INH prophylaxis. In their first experiment on 1188 guinea pigs the lowest challenge dose administered was 130 viable units, which infected 85% of the 72 control animals. INH was given in the drinking water at 4 mg/kg for periods of 10 weeks, 18 weeks, 26 weeks. The level of INH in the blood was too low to be measurable. Between 88% and 100% of the treated guinea pigs did not become diseased. Repeated negative tuberculin reactions were seen as proof of the eradication of tubercle bacilli and this disease-free state lasted for as long as 20 weeks after treatment had ended. The group whose treatment period was the longest, i.e., 26 weeks, did not fare any better than the group treated for only 16 weeks. The same authors later tested the antimicrobial effect of a daily dose of 10 mg/kg INH administered in two different ways: all at once in a single daily injection, and in multiple small doses in drinking water. This experiment was performed on 1620 guinea pigs and lasted for 133 weeks. The minimum infective dose given was an inoculum of 380 viable bacillary units. INH was given to the group receiving this inoculum for only 8 weeks and successfully prevented infection in 60% to 70% of the animals. This can be considered true chemoprophylaxis. The intention had been to give INH for just long enough to eradicate the infection in about half of the animals. The study proved that the degree of tuberculin sensitivity generated by the challenge is less in animals given a single daily dose than in those given multiple smaller doses. Both methods of administration were equally effective in preventing virulent bacilli from causing tuberculous disease for as long as the drug was being given. Dosages producing high peak levels had the same antimicrobial effect as those producing a low constant tissue concentration of INH.

III. Experiments with Cattle

Investigations into tuberculosis chemoprophylaxis in cattle have been reported from many countries. Italian veterinarians in Perugia (BADIALI 1954; BADIALI and BARACCIA 1959; BADIALI and DE MAJO 1962; MORETTI and PEDINI 1953; ROSATI and TINI 1955; ROSATI and BADIALI 1959, 1960) were the first to experiment with prophylactic INH and natural exposure. The first pilot trials were done with small numbers of animals observed for short periods. These workers employed 10 mg/kg INH intramuscularly and 4 mg/kg subcutaneously. Tuberculin reactions remained negative in the 8 protected cattle, while 7 of the 9 control calves became tuberculous. CASTELLANI et al. (1959) kept 15 calves in a highly infectious environment, and treated 10 of them with 10 mg/kg initially and later with 5 mg/kg. The protected calves' reactions to tuberculin tests were negative and the animals were free of any bacteriologically detectable tubercle bacilli 2 months after the commencement of the trial.

In the USSR ANDRUSCHENKO (1962) experimented on 108 cattle which were given 5.0 mg/kg to 7.5 mg/kg INH per os. Tuberculin tests disclosed that only 2 of the animals became infected. The Dairy Research Institute in Kiel (SEELEMANN et al. 1957a, b, 1958) showed that 10 mg/kg of an INH derivative given daily or every second day could protect calves which were either exposed in the stable or infected per os. Of the 14 control animals in 2 trials 8 became tuberculin positive while 22 of the 24 treated animals remained tuberculin negative. In another series 34 calves were exposed during an 8-month period and given 4.5 mg of the drug; 18 of 19 animals given INH prophylaxis during the first 4 weeks of life remained tuberculin negative, the exception being a congenitally-infected calf. Three of 15 animals whose prophylaxis began 6 weeks–12 weeks after birth became infected. In Prague (KUBIN et al. 1959) calves were intravenously infected with 10 mg of virulent *M. bovis* and treated with 15 mg/kg–20 mg/kg per os 3 times weekly. No tuberculous lesions could be found in animals given INH for 2 months, but the controls showed generalized TB. Veterinarians in Poland (SPRYSZAK 1961, 1964) undertook 2 INH prophylaxis trials. They infected 25 calves intravenously with 5 mg of *M. bovis* and fed them milk containing tubercle bacilli. Twenty calves were given 15 mg/kg INH for 4 months, after which the tuberculin reactions of 17 of them were negative, one was positive and 2 suspicious. In another experiment 30 calves were fed tuberculous milk and 18 of them were treated with 20 mg/

kg INH every second day. All the treated animals afterwards reacted negatively to tuberculin. This experiment formed the basis of an attempt to control TB in a herd varying in size from 150 to 350 head of cattle. The 88 tuberculous cattle in the herd were gradually replaced by newborn purchased calves which were given 20 mg/kg in their milk. After 2½ years the herd was declared free of TB.

Tuberculosis was eradicated from an infected herd of 800 cattle in Peru within 5 years by means of INH prophylaxis and gradual replacement (SEIFERT 1962). Clean young stock were not segregated from tuberculous cows. The INH derivative was given in milk to 300 suckling heifer calves at the rate of 500 mg per animal per day during the first 6 months of life. The calves were then separated from the cows. An equal number of bull calves were not treated and many became infected, yet all but 3 of the treated animals remained tuberculin negative.

My investigation spanned the years 1958 to 1969 (KLEEBERG 1959, 1966, 1967a, b; Kleeberg and Worthington 1963; Kleeberg et al. 1966), and was part of a large-scale countrywide trial to determine the usefulness of INH in the control of cattle tuberculosis.

Calves were infected artificially per os and by means of air droplets, and were treated with 10 mg/kg per day per os. The untreated controls developed lesions but the INH-treated calves did not. However, the protection conferred by the drug was limited to the period of administration. When INH was discontinued and the source of infection removed simultaneously, tubercle bacilli survived and were detected in normal or enlarged lymph nodes. To determine the duration of continuous prophylaxis necessary to sterilize calves infected with *M. bovis*, each of 16 calves was given 0.4 mg per os of virulent *M. bovis*. The calves were treated for varying lengths of time beginning on the day of infection. After an observation period of 2 months–3 months during which tuberculin tests were done at monthly intervals, all calves were sacrificed and investigated bacteriologically (Table 1).

Table 1. Sterilisation of bovine TB infection by continuous chemoprophylaxis

Experimental animals	Infection	Isoniazid	Tuberculin	Reaction	Trial period	Pathology	Bacteriology
No. of calves	Live *mycobact. bovis* per os over 10 days	Dosing of 10 mg/kg daily	Skin fold measurement mean increase at		Days	Grossly visible lesions	Culturing of lymph node material
			2 months	End of trial			
2	4 mg	Nil	17 mm	17 mm	65	TB in L. nodes	2 × positive
2	4 mg	1 week	9 mm	1 mm	110	None	1 × positive 1 × negative
4	4 mg	1 month	7.5 mm	2 mm	140	None	1 × positive 3 × negative
4	4 mg	2 months	6.5 mm	0 mm	170	None	4 × negative
4	4 mg	3 months	5.5 mm	0 mm	170	None	4 × negative

It was shown that one month of treatment was not sufficient to rid all the animals of tubercle bacilli, but 2 months or 3 months' treatment resulted in the elimination of viable tubercle bacilli. All the animals had reacted positively to tuberculin 1 month–2 months after challenge, thus proving established infection. In the animals under prophylaxis the reactions gradually decreased in size and were negative after 5 months. However, bacillary isolation was possible from some calves which had been treated for 16 days–40 days and showed a weak reaction just before slaughter.

The effect of chemoprophylaxis on the dissemination of bovine tuberculosis was studied in 17 herds containing 1670 TB-free cattle and 1198 tuberculous cattle. The field trials were done in the South African provinces of Transvaal and Natal. Farmers administered INH powder in cattle feed at 10 mg/kg once daily. Only in 4 of the 17 herds were tuberculous cattle segregated. The tuberculous stock ceased to be infective within a period of 2 months. Cattle which had reacted either negatively or suspiciously to the initial tuberculin test were re-tested 2 months–3 months later. Most of the 73 cattle which reacted positively to the re-test were believed to have been recently infected and to have been in the pre-allergic phase at the time of the first test (Table 2).

Eight of the cows which had reacted negatively or doubtfully to the first test but positively to the second were seen at slaughter to have chronic lesions or generalized tuberculosis. The initial tuberculin test must have exerted a reminder-like influence on specifically committed lymphocytes and the skin test became positive for the re-test 2 months later. Most of the new reactors were considered to have been previously infected. Even if all of the 76 new reactors are counted as failures,

Table 2. Arrest of disease transmission by chemoprophylaxis; isoniazid dosed per os at 10 mg/kg bodyweight once daily

Herd code	Infectious pool No. pos. cattle	Exposed clean stock No. neg. cattle	Period of INH dosing (in months)	New positive reactors at first retest	Further ractors during 2 years of control
St	79	50	8	1	0
Ha	66	7	9	2	0
Th	26	34	5	0	0
Ri	68	66	8	13	0
We	157	160	2	6	1
Vi	134	35	3	1	0
Ho	86	66	5	2	0
vdW	56	26	2	0	0
Gr	61	108	2½	7	1
El	54	79	2	1	0
Bre	14	66	2	4	0
Fr	34	30	2	0	1
Co	34	66	2	7	0
Cr	42	260	2	4	0
Sc	69	100	2	15	0
Wo	161	314	2	5	0
Swan	57	203	2	5	0

95% protection was nevertheless achieved. As a result of this demonstration the method has been used successfully in South Africa for many years.

D. Discussion of Experimental Data

Before conclusions can be drawn the factors which have influenced the data obtained in the experiments discussed should be examined. There are three variables in these experiments: the host organism, the parasite and the drug. As far as the host is concerned, all the workers quoted here used fully susceptible non-infected, i.e., tuberculin negative, animals. Guinea pigs and calves can be considered to be highly susceptible and are therefore very suitable species. In all trials in which the tuberculin reaction's conversion to positive is employed as the criterion for infection and its negativity as the criterion for protection, accurate judgement is possible. The tuberculin test is a reliable biological test and elicits the most consistent reaction of a host to invading tubercle bacilli. Delayed hypersensitivity to tuberculin is readily demonstrated in cattle and guinea pigs but less so in man (BJERKEDAL and PALMER 1964; KLEEBERG 1966). Trials which ended with negative reactions to tuberculin after a long period of control have special significance. In experiments in which animals given INH did not become tuberculin positive, the test proved that infection had not taken place.

The majority of investigators allowed enough time for the surviving latent tubercle bacilli to create tuberculin allergy. In most investigations bacteriological examination of the exposed tissues was undertaken. A short-coming of the early work with cattle was that conclusions were drawn from relatively small trials conducted over short periods with insufficient numbers of cattle. This resulted in the unwarranted condemnation of INH prophylaxis for cattle.

I. Technique of Infection

In most cases virulent tubercle bacilli were used and the controls showed generalized tuberculosis. Where 130 bacilli per guinea pig were used, which infected less than 100% of the controls, one wonders whether they were all viable or infective. Attenuated strains would have given wrong, but more favorable, results. As far as mode of infection is concerned, fortunately in several of the trials in cattle, monkeys and guinea pigs natural infection, or the aerogenic route, was used. This enhanced the practical value of the experimentation. In cattle, infection per os can be regarded as infection by one of the natural routes. In guinea pigs subcutaneous and aerogenic infection with the same amounts of viable units can be regarded as equally effective.

II. Infective Dose

The experiments so far considered were all done using natural infection or minimal artificial infection, since large numbers of viable organisms would have influenced the result both positively and negatively. In chemoprophylaxis both natural and acquired immunity must be taken into consideration. The infective dose can be so great that it may cause the animals to develop specific immunity, which would help to combat the infective agent. This undesirable condition can arise when large numbers of tubercle bacilli are injected parenterally. The dying organisms and their breakdown products can be immunogenic even when multiplication has been inhibited by the drug. Large numbers of bacilli can cause abscess formation and necrosis and these can result in host conditions unfavorable for drug action against the bacilli. Non-proliferating bacilli are not killed by the drug. A large bacterial mass would be likely to contain bacilli with stagnant metabolism, or dormant bacilli, which would not be influenced by the drug. After discontinuation of INH, relapses would occur. In practice, however, primary prophylaxis is used in exposed, non-infected individuals.

III. Animal Species Differences

In my opinion the ox is naturally more resistant to *M. bovis* than man is to *M. tuberculosis*, and the monkey and the guinea pig are more susceptible to these two organisms than man is. TB in monkeys, for example, can be prevented in only half of the animals if the infection and treatment end at the same time (SCHMIDT 1956). INH given intermittently to guinea pigs over many months was not able to eradicate infection. A low dose of INH provided throughout the day in the drinking water was also not able to cure the animals in 10 days, or even in 30 days, but continued dosing for 2 months–4 months did cure them (BARTMANN 1962a; COHN et al. 1962).

Investigations in cattle have shown that good protection is provided by dosages between 5 mg/kg and 10 mg/kg, although peak serum levels following such dosages are much lower in cattle than in man.

It would be interesting to ascertain whether an individual animal in which an infection has been successfully overcome by either chemoprophylaxis or chemoprevention has a higher degree of immunity than a fully susceptible tuberculosis-free individual. Several studies with laboratory animals in which the immunity from a treated infection was measured have been reported (BARTMANN et al. 1958a, 1959b; BARTMANN 1962a; CANETTI et al. 1958; JANKOV 1960). It was found that strong immunity developed in guinea pigs when a substantial infective dose had been treated. Weak immunity, or none at all, was detected after a small infective dose had been treated.

Two Italian experiments with cattle contradict the findings of South African field trials. BADIALI and DE MAJO (1962) and ROSATI and BADIALI (1960) concluded after trials with 7 and 6 calves respectively, that the resistance acquired by the animals was equal to that conferred by BCG vaccination and that it lasted for at least 6 months. KLEEBERG (1966) reported studies done on a herd of 80 cattle, consisting of 37 tuberculous cows that had been treated with INH and rendered almost tuberculin negative and 43 disease-free cattle. Infectious cattle were accidentally introduced into this herd and within six months 200 newly-infected cases which reacted strongly to tuberculin were detected. Half of these had been previously treated stock and the other half non-infected, non-treated stock. Thus no enhancement of resistance could be seen and there were strong indications that successful chemoprophylaxis leaves the individual animal fully susceptible.

IV. The Drug as Factor

Only INH is discussed here as none of the other anti-TB drugs has its advantages. Its effectiveness is superior to that of any other drug, it is cheaper, easier to administer and has few adverse effects. Other drugs used in preventive treatment will be discussed below, but the few chemoprophylactic experiments done with them will not be reviewed.

The effectiveness of INH was not affected by the administration route. This observation holds true for all the animal species investigated. INH was shown to diffuse easily and to be distributed quickly in all organs, regardless of the administration route (BARTMANN and FREISE 1963; KLEEBERG 1966; BARTMANN 1960; VIVIEN and GROSSET 1961) (Table 3).

For a long time it was questioned whether continuous moderate blood levels or daily high peaks were the better indicator of greater therapeutic value. In the sixties short high peaks were considered to be preferable. It is now known that the effectiveness of INH is related to the total exposure of the body to the drug. Total exposure is defined as the product of concentration and duration of exposure.

Reviewing the work of BJERKEDAL and PALMER and COHN et al., CANETTI (1966) wondered whether a high dose of INH might make it possible to shorten the duration of chemoprophylaxis which otherwise requires a full year. BARTMANN and BLISSE (1967) therefore infected guinea pigs with about 50 viable units of inoculum each and then treated them for 2 weeks, 4 weeks, and 8 weeks using 10 mg/kg, 25 mg/kg and 50 mg/kg. Treatment was started the day after infection and the drug was administered subcutaneously 6 times weekly. Two weeks' treatment resulted in 30%–53% protection and 4 weeks' treatment in 84%–100% protection. It was not possible to compensate for shorter treatment periods by increasing the dose. Eight weeks of INH at 10 mg/kg protected all of 20 guinea pigs from infection, while 4 weeks at 50 mg/kg did not (84% protection). It appears that even the higher doses are not bactericidal. These findings confirm those of BJERKEDAL and PALMER (1964) who infected guinea pigs with 4400 viable units and treated the animals for 20 weeks with 4 mg/kg, 16 mg/kg and 20 mg/kg daily. Understandably the 4 mg/kg dose was less effective than the other doses, but 30 mg/kg did not prove to be superior to 16 mg/kg. The 30 mg/kg dose protected 78% and the 16 mg/kg dose 67%. The difference was not significant. In guinea

Table 3. Isoniazid serum and tissue levels in four mammalian species – Determined microbiologically

Species	INH dosis (mg/kg)	Time interval (h)	Serum level (mcg/ml)	Lung level	Spleen level	Authors
Man	5	1	5.0	4.5	–	BARTMANN and FREISE
Guinea pig	10	1	5.3	2.2	2.8	BARTMANN and FREISE
Mouse	5	1	2.5	0.9	1.0	BARTMANN and FREISE
Cattle	20	3	1.8	1.7	1.5	KLEEBERG

pigs intermittent INH medication was found to be less protective than daily dosing (BARTMANN 1960). Surprisingly, varying dosage regimens all produced the same high degree of protection in cattle, in which 5 mg/kg INH did not cause blood levels to exceed 0.7 mcg/ml. Protection was nevertheless provided. It should be mentioned that the dosages shown in Table 3 are relatively non-toxic in all species studied.

Several investigators proved that the protective value of INH ceases the moment treatment is discontinued. In man INH must therefore be given continuously as long as infection persists. It would thus be of little use to start chemoprophylaxis without at the same time implementing other measures against the source of infection.

Tubercle bacilli which survive the short period of prophylaxis, or which enter the body shortly before the end of prophylaxis, can cause tuberculous infection, making it necessary to continue treatment. The duration of treatment depends on the natural resistance of the species. In cattle it has been shown that treatment should continue for 2 months, and in monkeys and guinea pigs for 2 months–3 months. In man, 2 months' treatment after exposure has ended should be sufficient providing dormant bacilli and exogenous sources of infection are absent. The experimental data obtained on animals can be used as guidelines for the use of INH in man, because a dose of 5 mg/kg causes similar blood peaks in man to those produced by a dose of 10 mg/kg in guinea pigs and a dose of 30 mg/kg in cattle. The only difference is that certain individuals inactivate INH more rapidly than others, and a rapid inactivator would not reach the desired peak of 1 mcg/ml. It would thus be wrong to give 5 mg/kg chemoprophylactic INH in divided doses.

A number of facts that have a bearing on human treatment have emerged from experimental chemoprophylaxis. The drug of choice is isoniazid, which consistently prevents natural infection and eliminates artificially introduced tubercle bacilli when treatment is started simultaneously with infection and is continued for an adequate period. With a sufficiently high drug level protection is absolute. INH chemoprophylaxis can thus be superior to the separation of the infectious source from the exposed person and it can also be superior to BCG prophylaxis.

Under average conditions of natural exposure to infection INH prophylaxis can prevent tuberculin allergy. Delayed type sensitivity normally develops after high infective doses but disappears gradually as dosing continues. Tubercle bacilli can survive short periods of drug exposure, and it is necessary to continue dosing for 2 months after the last exposure. A certain degree of acquired immunity can develop in animals that have been subjected to both exposure and treatment, but this is of short duration.

The results of experiments on animals can be utilized as a basis for decisions on the treatment of man as INH has been shown to be successful even against the unfavorable combination of heavy exposure, high virulence and low host resistance. The following conclusions can be drawn. No treatment regimen has been found which simultaneously protects against infection and allows immunity to be acquired. Primary chemoprophylaxis is most useful when heavy exposure of short duration has occurred. The rate of failure in man would be very small if the problem of default in pill-taking could be overcome. INH-resistant mutants have not been shown to develop while minimal infections are being treated. In the natural conditions of human infection the numbers of bacilli actually entering the body are so small that the chances of resistant mutants being selected are infinitesimal.

E. Preventive Treatment in Animals

Most of the early animal experiments with antituberculosis drugs were done on artificially infected animals. Laboratory animals were injected with large numbers of tubercle bacilli and treatment was started either immediately or when tuberculosis had established itself. Many of these studies were designed to test preventive treatment and our present knowledge of antituberculosis drugs is based on their findings. Terms such as disease prophylaxis, relapse prophylaxis, generalization prophylaxis, secondary prophylaxis and chemoprevention are used in the literature, but none of these is either as suitable or as explicit as the term preventive treatment.

The reasons for using INH in most of the studies under review are manifold. It possesses most of the qualifications that an effective antituberculosis drug should have. Depending on the concentration at which it is used its action is tuberculocidal or tuberculostatic and its toxicity is low. It is selective and does not interfere with beneficial microbes in the alimentary tract. Its ability to diffuse into diseased tissue is superior to that of any other anti-TB drug. It is highly soluble in water and is easily absorbed in the alimentary canal. It readily enters all body fluids and structures and permeates cell membranes, and none of the constituents of necrotic tissue are antagonistic to it. It is easily administered and is thus suitable for long-term treatment. It is only mildly allergenic, if at all, and is minimally neutralized by body protein.

As regards work with guinea pigs the following workers contributed important data which will be summarized below: DOMAGK et al. (1952); FUST et al. (1952); HEILMEYER (1952); UEHLINGER et al. (1952); KARLSON and FELDMAN (1953); HUMBERT (1954); VELTMAN (1955a, b); BARTMANN et al. (1955, 1956, 1958b); FEREBEE and PALMER (1956); SHER et al. (1957); NASTA et al. (1957, 1960); PEIZER et al. (1957); LUCCHESI and SPINA (1957–1961); PALMER (1959); SPIESS (1959); BARTMANN (1960); BJERKEDAL and PALMER (1962); and PALMER et al. (1956). Some of the studies are extremely well-controlled demonstrations of effective INH therapy.

The aims and achievements of the early studies of preventive chemotherapy differed widely. Some workers attempted to achieve biological cure, some the elimination of all bacilli, and some the localization of tuberculosis, i.e., the prevention of hematogenous and lymphatogenous spread. The question of the most effective dose and the possibility of intermittent administration had still to be investigated. Most of the studies involved artificial primary infection followed by early treatment with INH. In judging this work it was sometimes difficult to separate preventive treatment from pure therapy. Two main questions arose out of the interpretation of the experimental data: what did the author set out to achieve, and what tuberculous condition did he treat?

As had been the case with work done on primary prophylaxis, results were found to differ according to animal species, type and virulence of inoculum, inoculation route, size of dose, frequency of its administration and duration of treatment. Studies of long duration which allowed for long-term observation after stoppage of treatment were more valuable than those of short duration.

I. Experiments with Guinea Pigs

Most of the experiments were done by inoculating large quantities of inoculum, i.e., 100000 and more tubercle bacilli, into each animal. The intraperitoneal, subcutaneous and intramuscular routes were all used for infection, and treatment was started either simultaneously with the infection or after an interval of up to a month. The doses of INH varied from 5 mg/kg to 50 mg/kg and the period of administration varied from 3 months to 12 months. The drug was usually given continuously, but in some trials it was given intermittently. The results range from complete failure to complete cure and they seem to depend more on the virulence of the strain used for infection than on the drug as such.

As already explained, the treatment of massive infection is conducive to the development of immunity, and this immunity can inhibit or even prevent reactivation of disease. The lower the virulence of the bacilli which survive the first therapy, the stronger the effect. In these studies the interaction of the tubercle bacilli and the natural resistance, now enhanced by acquired resistance, rather than the chemotherapeutic effect of the INH, were being examined. Good studies are those in which fully virulent test strains are used, the follow-up periods are sufficiently long and the search for surviving organisms is intensive. The elimination of all bacilli from the guinea pig was usually not achieved, even with long-continued therapy, but during preventive treatment tuberculosis could not establish itself, and hematogenous spread was prevented.

II. Experimental Studies with Mice

When the therapeutic effect of drugs on experimental infections in mice is studied, the results are expressed as the prevention of either death or lesions, or the prolongation of life, or the eradication of infecting microorganisms as shown by culturing the tissue of the mice. The last is probably the most valuable.

Murine tuberculosis lends itself very well to the experimental approach. Methods of studying experimental chemotherapy in mice are given in detail by GRUMBACH (1965). Her experimental model of advanced tuberculosis in mice can be regarded as a suitable model for human pulmonary tuberculosis. With this technique therapeutic treatment starts 14 days after infection (GRUMBACH 1962; 1965; GRUMBACH et al. 1967; GRUMBACH 1969; GRUMBACH et al. 1969; CANETTI and GROSSET 1958; GRUNBERG and SCHNITZER 1952; JESPERSEN and RASMUSSEN 1955; LAMBERT 1959; MCCUNE et al. 1957; TAI et al. 1961). The excellent therapeutic effect of a combination of INH and streptomycin in experimental murine TB was shown by HOBBY et al. (1953). MCCUNE et al. (1957) determined the fate of *M. tuberculosis* in mouse tissue by means of the microbial enumeration technique. This showed the persistence of drug-susceptible tubercle bacilli despite prolonged antimicrobial therapy.

Animal experiments with intermittent chemotherapy were already being done in 1960 (Bartmann). The success of both continuous and intermittent treatment with INH and SM in murine TB was compared.

Two-phase treatment, which is now so popular in the treatment of man, was introduced by GRUMBACH as early as 1962. In her treatment of experimental murine tuberculosis she used different combinations of INH and SM in the 3-month initial phase and INH alone in the 9-month second phase. She showed that the results of only 3 months' treatment with the INH and SM combination were as good as those obtained with a continuous 12-month double regimen. A large dose of INH yielded results more rapidly than a small one. Combined treatment yielded results more rapidly when SM was given daily than when it was given every second day. She also showed that 6 month treatment was insufficient. When therapy was stopped at 6 months the bacterial population recurred and lesions developed. The recurrence of bacterial populations was observed even after the best initial treatment. The results of her work led Canetti to recommend that on theoretical grounds initial treatment of a tuberculous infection should begin with a high-quality combination, i.e., large doses of INH and SM daily. Five years later GRUMBACH et al. (1967) admitted that long-lasting sterilization of severe murine tuberculosis was not possible with INH and SM. Viable bacilli were seen to reappear in all animals.

When rifampicin (RMP) was added to regimens containing INH they showed efficacy not previously seen. GRUMBACH (1969) reported the sterilization of the lung and spleen in 100% of animals treated for only 4 months with 25 mg/kg INH. In this combination 5 mg/kg RMP was found to be insufficient. Sterilization was also achieved in all the mice treated with 25 mg/kg RMP and 5 mg/kg INH when treatment lasted for 6 months.

Adopting an experimental model similar to that employed by Grumbach, KRADOLFER (1970) compared the bactericidal effect of RMP with that of INH and that of SM. He determined that the minimum dose required to elicit a chemotherapeutic effect was 5.6 mg/kg RMP and as little as 3 mg/kg INH. Larger doses of RMP prolonged the survival of the infected mice to a greater extent than did his maximum dose of INH. The effect of RMP could be enhanced by administering the drug in combination with a second antituberculosis drug instead of administering it alone. No surviving bacilli could be detected on culture.

GRUMBACH et al. (1969) compared the efficacy of two combinations, RMP plus INH and RMP plus ethambutol, which were administered daily, twice weekly and once weekly for 6 months. In both the daily and the intermittent regimens RMP plus INH was found to be the more effective combination.

Animal experimentation showed the way to two-phase treatment. A regimen consisting of an initial one-month daily phase followed by a continuation phase in which RMP and INH were given intermittently was almost as effective as regimens in which treatment was given daily throughout. The addition of SM to the regimen INH plus RMP did not appear to be beneficial, but the addition of RMP to the regimen INH plus SM for only one month produced long-lasting and beneficial effects. This was the first indication that the addition of another drug to a preventive regimen for a short period might well enhance that regimen's effectiveness (GRUMBACH 1965).

RMP acts differently in mice and guinea pigs. In guinea pigs 40 mg/kg RMP daily, given per os, is as effective as 4 mg/kg INH daily when judged by the number of bacilli surviving in the spleen (NITTI 1967). By contrast, several other authors found RMP to be as effective as INH at similar doses in the mouse. RMP's low efficacy in the guinea pig is due to the animal's serum level which is 10 to 20 times lower than man's and the mouse's. In intracardially infected guinea pigs the combination of INH and RMP was found to be superior to monotherapy with either of these two drugs. These experiments confirm the sterilizing action of a combination of the two drugs.

In the course of the international tuberculosis conference in Mexico in 1975 experimental investigations using murine tuberculosis were reviewed by DICKINSON and MITCHISON (1976). The evidence suggested that the two drugs pyrazinamide (PZA) and RMP could make important contributions to modern short-course treatment regimens. Established disease in mice was treated with single drugs and with combinations of drugs which included INH, and two distinct phases were detectable: a bactericidal phase lasting 20 days to 30 days, and a sterilization phase. A few positive spleen cultures were obtained when INH and SM were given, but when the companion drug to INH was PZA, sterilization occurred. When the mice were allowed to survive after 3 months of treatment with INH and PZA, about two-thirds eventually relapsed. However, relapse did not occur when treatment had been given for 6 months. Experiments at the Pasteur Institute showed that the contribution made by SM to the sterilizing activity of a regimen was very small. Murine tuberculosis studies proved that although most drugs enhanced the early bactericidal phase, only RMP and PZA are capable of specific sterilizing action. The sterilization phase is most effective when the combination contains INH. It was also established that the sterilizing activities of PZA and RMP are not evinced in an *in vitro* situation. Since PZA is active only at an acid pH it was possible to show that the efficacy of PZA as a sterilizing drug in the second phase of treatment is due to its ability to act on small numbers of slowly-metabolizing persistent organisms found in acid intracellular sites.

In the late seventies a murine tuberculosis treatment model was convincingly used in Paris by Grosset, who published several papers (GROSSET 1978a, b). Today clinicians are not satisfied with the bactericidal action of drugs (best observed in an actively growing bacillary population) but expect a treatment regimen to have a sterilizing effect on the total population so as to prevent relapse after cessation of treatment. It was shown that RMP was the only drug which acted equally well on both rapidly multiplying and dormant bacilli. Only INH can, when combined with RMP, render the mouse totally culture-negative after 4 months–6 months of treatment. The administration of RMP for a short time seems to improve the final results of standard therapy. It was also shown that no relapses occur in mouse tuberculosis after 9 months of treatment with the INH plus RMP regimen. The evidence obtained from murine tuberculosis studies has greatly strengthened the case for the short-course treatment of man. Workers agree that it is very difficult to cure tuberculosis in mice because the spleen cannot easily be cleared of tubercle bacilli which are located intracellularly in these animals.

Much of the information obtained from mouse studies can be applied to man. It has been shown that in man, as in the mouse, the results obtained after 6 months of treatment with INH and RMP are as good as those obtained after 18 months of treatment with INH and SM. The usefulness of experimental animal models has thus been proved.

The effect of INH on experimental tuberculosis in *Macacca mulatta* was investigated by CLARKE and SCHMIDT (1969). The monkeys were inoculated intratracheally, 15 were treated with 10 mg/kg daily and 10 were untreated controls. To determine the development of hypersensitivity and bacterial shedding, the animals were tuberculin tested every 48 hours and a tracheal washing was done every 3 days. Three-quarters of the animals on INH became tuberculin hypersensitive but after 20 days of INH, only one animal still reacted. All but 2 anergic animals in the control group were tuberculin positive by the 16th day. On the 11th day all the monkeys were excreting bacilli, but by the 17th day only 13% were still excreting. Three animals excreted *M. tuberculosis* for the remainder of the study. On the basis of the data they accumulated in the course of this study the authors feel that INH should not be administered prophylactically to primates which have not completed a 16-day quarantine period. This interval will permit identification and removal of any tuberculin reactors. Apparently INH can affect the development of hypersensitivity without preventing the excretion of organisms. In Rhesus monkeys the prophylactic use of INH involves the risk of masking the disease.

A number of zoos use INH prophylaxis. The drug is commonly administered prophylactically to colonies of primates, particularly in the USA. Experience with ruminants, carnivores and marsupials was reported by FRANKE (1964), HAUSER (1963), HEYMANN (1959), and TEUSCHER (1956). A local epizootic of TB in a small laboratory colony of baboons was controlled with 40 mg/kg–80 mg/kg INH in daily doses. Prophylactic treatment was considered to be justified in the control of the disease in this colony, so as to save animals needed for short-term experiments (ALLGOOD and PRICE 1971).

III. Mink and Rabbits

The Russian KHAIKIN (1970) infected 60 minks by mouth and treated half of them with 10 mg/kg INH for 75 days. Guinea pig inoculation disclosed no tubercle bacilli in any of the treated mink, but bacilli were found in 83% of the controls. However, in two field trials in which animals exposed to infection were treated with 7.5 mg/kg INH, only a few remained free of tuberculosis.

Reactivation was seen in 41% of rabbits treated with INH for 4 months and in 25% of those treated with the drug for 12 months (FREERKSEN 1956, 1957a, b, 1959; KUBIN et al. 1959).

IV. Intermittent Treatment

Studies of the treatment of experimental guinea pig tuberculosis with intermittent doses of INH were done by DICKINSON et al. (1973). They inoculated the animals intramuscularly with 1 mg inoculum. Treatment was initiated 3 weeks after infection using dosages of 1 mg/kg, 2 mg/kg and 4 mg/kg administered at intervals ranging from one day to 14 days. The response was assessed on the basis of macroscopic disease and viable counts. The efficacy of treatment remained constant when the intervals between doses were increased from one day to 4 days, but decreased considerably when the intervals were longer. When the size of the dose was increased, 20 mg/kg–30 mg/kg INH gave the best response. Higher dosages did not improve response. Doses given twice weekly were more effective than those given at 7-day intervals, and those given at 10-day intervals were even less effective.

V. Preventive Treatment in Cattle

Investigations involving cattle present a more favorable picture. Experiments were done on large numbers of animals with naturally occurring tuberculosis, employing long periods of control. In West Germany calves were treated with 10 mg/kg of an INH derivative 3 months–4 months after natural infection. After 10 months of treatment no viable organisms could be found (SEELEMANN et al. 1957a, b, 1958). SPRYSZAK (1961) infected 55 calves intravenously and treated 38 with INH. The animals were sacrificed shortly afterwards, and also those sacrificed 2 months later, were all found to be free of lesions, while the control animals showed severe disease.

KUBIN et al. (1959) in Czechoslovakia also used calves, which they infected intravenously with 10 mg of a *Mycobacterium bovis* strain and then treated per os 3 times weekly with 10 mg/kg–15 mg/kg INH. Cultures made from the organs of calves sacrificed immediately after therapy were negative, as were those from calves sacrificed after an interval of 4 months. Several reports published in Italian scientific journals between 1953 and 1958 were reviewed by KLEEBERG (1966). The Italian workers studied the curative effect of INH therapy in advanced cattle tuberculosis and often used low dosages for short periods. They concluded that INH was effective in controlling disease but not in freeing lesions of tubercle bacilli.

NAI and PERINI (1960) later showed that preventive treatment of postprimary tuberculosis was effective, and created a continuous state of tuberculin negativity. They treated 413 positive reactors with 5 mg/kg–10 mg/kg for 3 months–12 months, either per os or subcutaneously, and 73% became tuberculin negative. For 6 months 42 of these animals were in continuous contact with 271 tuberculosis-free cattle. None of the treated animals which had previously reacted re-converted to positive, nor did any of the control animals.

In the years 1958–1968 preventive chemotherapy in cattle was tested in field trials in South Africa. These trials involved 30 herds, numbering on average 240 cattle each. Of the total of 7000 cattle, 30% were tuberculous. The symptomatology, tuberculin sensitivity, pathology, bacteriology (including drug resistance), pharmacology and epizootiology of bovine tuberculosis under treatment were described by KLEEBERG (1959, 1966, 1967a, b), and KLEEBERG et al. (1963, 1966). The tuberculous cattle received INH continuously for periods of 7 months–11 months and the noninfected cattle were segregated but used as indicators of further spread. The method of administration was per os, usually in the rations.

Tuberculin-testing the whole herd and repeating the test after 2 months enabled all infected animals to be identified and branded, and their treatment to begin immediately. All cattle having clinically or bacteriologically recognizable advanced tuberculosis were eliminated.

In some of the herds INH prophylaxis was used in the noninfected cattle for the first 2 months and in others the noninfected cattle were segregated for the first 2 months. Subsequent post mortem examination revealed that at the start of the investigation 55% of the cattle had localized disease, 20% were moderately diseased and 25% were in an advanced state of disease. All positive reactors were treated with INH daily, mostly at 10 mg/kg but in some herds at 20 mg/kg and 25 mg/kg. Tuberculin tests were done quarterly or every six months, mainly to check for new infection among the controls. The follow-up period was between 2 years and 6 years. Autopsies were performed on 209 tuberculous cattle at the Onderstepoort Institute and special emphasis was placed on bacteriological examination since the aim of the investigation was the elimination of all live tubercle bacilli from as many cattle as possible. About 400 organs from treated cattle were investigated, more than 1000 guinea pigs were injected with suspicious material and 4000 cultures were made.

Table 4 gives the results of all the bacteriological tests done on tuberculous and suspicious material. Treatment lasting 2 months–3 months resulted in bacteriological cure of 58% of the cattle, and the same applied when treatment had lasted 4 months–6 months, but 80% of cattle treated for 7 months–11 months were completely cured. These results correlate well with those obtained on live cattle in the field, on which loss of tuberculin reactivity was observed 2 years after therapy. The most striking observation was a rapid decrease in tuberculin allergy in most of the INH-treated cattle. After 6 months 28% of the cattle tuberculin positive at the start of treatment no longer reacted to 7000 units of PPD. One year after cessation of therapy 70% of the cattle which had previously reacted posi-

Table 4. Preventive isoniazid treatment in tuberculous cattle. Summary of bacteriological and biological test restults in relation to duration of treatment

Category of tubercle bacilli isolated	Period of INH treatment at farm			
	2–3 months	4–6 months	7–8 months	9–11 months
No. cattle with virulent *M. bovis*	6	2	2	1
No. cattle with INH resistant, attenuated *M. bovis* only	4	8	18	10
No. cattle with visible, but not cultivable *M. bovis* only	3	7	21	12
No. cattle fully sterilised plus cases without lesions	11	5	51	31
Evaluation as to cure				
No. of former tuberculous organs examined	50	50	190	93
No. of cattle examined	24	22	92	54
Percentage cured in bacteriological sense	58%	55%	78%	80%
Percentage reactivation possible	30%	11%	3%	3.5%

tively became negative reactors, and 1½ years later 90% of them had become nonreactors.

To save time and work and to improve the cure rate, a two-phase high-dose treatment was instituted, consisting of a daily dose of 20 mg/kg–25 mg/kg for 4 months followed by an intermittent regimen of 30 mg/kg twice weekly for 3 months. This resulted in a still more rapid decline in tuberculin allergy. Three months after the start of treatment, 55% of the previous reactors were negative to PPD. Cattle which after therapy were negative twice in an interval of 6 months were cured, and no relapses occurred. Only 5 of 157 cattle (3%) harbored virulent *M. bovis* after regular treatment for 7 months or more. These 5 had previously been in an advanced stage of disease. The high cure rate (79%) can be ascribed partly to the very low virulence of INH-resistant *M. bovis* which was demonstrated by infecting 9 different species of mammals intravenously with 17 strains of this organism.

Dissemination of the disease in the treated tuberculous herds was monitored by means of regular tuberculin testing. When all the infected cattle in a herd were treated, dissemination was halted within 2 months (Table 5). New outbreaks occurred in 3 of the 30 herds because of poor farm management, a lack of veterinary control and overlooking a case of tuberculous mastitis at the start of therapy. Arrest of further spread of the disease can be readily explained by the pathological findings. Autopsy showed that all tuberculous lesions were well encapsulated within 3 months, that open cavities were empty and that diseased lung tissue had collapsed and was fibrotic. In 38 herds in which the epizootic had been studied for 2 years–5 years, 3% of the new positive reactors were found among noninfected animals after treatment had been completed. Two months after the start of therapy dissemination was halted in all herds. In the following 18 months only 1.3% were found to be new reactors. In the 3 years–5 years that followed no new cases were found, although 5%–25% of the cattle in these herds had been tuberculous and had received treatment.

Brazilian veterinarians have been able to confirm the sterilizing effect of INH treatment (LANGENEGGER et al. 1981). In a herd of 210 cattle tuberculin testing revealed 149 reactors and infection with *M. bovis* was confirmed. INH was given by mouth at 25 mg/kg per day, initially for 60 consecutive days, and then another

Table 5. Transmission of bovine tuberculosis after a course of preventive and curative INH treatment

Disease transmission according to tuberculin test results	Situation at start of treatment			Number of new reactors			
	No. herds	TB free cattle	Tuberculous cattle	1st year	2nd year	3rd year	4th–5th year
No spread	16	1705	891	0	0	0	0
Few new cases	11	2554	894	15	26	7	7
Full new outbreaks	3	563	358	0	0	59	19

60 doses were given at the rate of 3 per week. Post mortem and bacteriological examinations were carried out on 28 animals whose causes of death were unrelated. *M. bovis* could not be cultured from any of the 28, but lesions were found in some, and guinea pig inoculation had negative results. Tuberculin tests showed that by the end of the observation period the mean reaction had dropped from 7.5 mm to 1.5 mm. Therapeutic efficacy was estimated to be 93%.

INH chemoprophylaxis was used in many herds in the Ukraine (Didovets et al. 1978). After whole herds had been tuberculin tested and positive reactors had been killed, INH was given in daily doses ranging from 200 mg for calves aged 2 months to 500 mg for heifers. The drug was given in colostrum, milk or drinking water. Treatment was instituted immediately on detection of tuberculous infection and normally lasted for 2 months, followed by a further 2 months of treatment the next autumn or spring. After one year restrictions in half of the herds undergoing treatment could be lifted.

It can be concluded that both lymphatogenous and hematogenous dissemination can be prevented if the host is subjected to preventive treatment with an adequate dosage of INH. No manifest tuberculosis will then develop, apart from the original inoculation focus or the natural primary lesions. The organisms which do spread are apparently eliminated by the host. Mammalian species differ in their ability to overcome massive infection with virulent organisms under cover of preventive treatment. A short course of prophylactic treatment may not be curative. Cattle, by virtue of their high natural resistance to INH-resistant *M. bovis*, are exceptionally suitable for therapy with INH alone. Preventive treatment will cure most bovine tuberculosis cases, and treated animals will usually revert to tuberculin negative. A combination of INH and RMP used at the beginning of preventive treatment may have bactericidal action and may be superior to INH alone.

F. Immunological Questions of Chemoprophylaxis and Vaccine Prophylaxis

It is understandable that many investigators questioned whether chemoprophylaxis and preventive treatment would interfere with the natural defence mechanism and immunity against tuberculosis. It is important to know how both natural and acquired resistance, whether created by artificial or natural infection, will function once the bacilli have been killed by INH. Many workers have compared BCG vaccination with chemoprophylaxis, and some have investigated a combination of the two in the hope of achieving greater protection. It must be stressed that INH acts against the microorganisms only, while BCG influences the host by affording it greater protection against the spread of infection. The drug acts immediately, but only for as long as it is being taken, while BCG acts only after 5 weeks or 6 weeks. In man BCG continues to protect for several years. Some authors consider the immune response aroused by BCG or by a primary TB complex to be too valuable to impede with medical treatment.

It has already been said that an individual undergoing preventive treatment of a minimal infection is not protected against subsequent infection. However, prophylactic treatment of an infection brought about by a large quantity of inoculum was found to give rise to immunity. This occurred in the experiments in which there was an interval between treatment and superinfection, and also in those in which superinfection followed immediately after the start of treatment (BARTMANN et al. 1959b; BARTMANN 1962a, b; BLOCH and SEGAL 1955; BRETEY and CANETTI 1957; JANKOV 1960).

Seven studies of guinea pigs and mice deal with the protection against superinfection afforded by the chemotherapeutic treatment of a primary infection and compare the treated animals with untreated controls (DEBRÉ et al. 1959; EBINA 1959; LAMBERT 1960; LUCCHESI and SPINA 1957–1961; SPIESS 1961; TOYOHARA et al. 1959; SERI and BALOGH 1962). It was shown that the immunizing effect of BCG is suppressed if INH is administered at the same time. However, the protection afforded by BCG is maintained in principle if the treatment is started 6 weeks after BCG vaccination (SPIESS 1961). Other experiments confirm that INH given shortly after infection will influence the development of immunity, whether that immunity is induced by BCG or by virulent tubercle bacilli. If treatment is started 4 weeks–8 weeks after vaccination, immunity is not suppressed either in mice or in guinea pigs. However, when virulent organisms were used in guinea pigs, the development of immunity was slightly suppressed because INH either killed the organisms or inhibited their multiplication.

Comparisons were made in both cattle and guinea pigs between the degrees of immunity created by BCG and by a tuberculosis infection which had been cured by INH treatment (BADIALI and BARACACCIA 1959; NASTA et al. 1960; ROSATI and BADIALI 1960). The degrees of immunity were found to be similar. It was shown that as long as 2 years after a therapeutically treated group of guinea pigs had been cured and had become tuberculin negative, resistance to reinfection had increased (SPIESS 1961).

To summarize, protection against superinfection will develop after preventive treatment provided the treatment is not started too soon after infection. This protection will be moderate and will last for quite some time – at least six months if therapy is started 6 weeks–8 weeks after infection and if the tubercle bacilli are not very invasive. Long treatment can eliminate the survivors completely (GRUMBACH 1962). This can be expected to prevent further immunogenic stimulation, and the question arises whether complete eradication of the bacterial population and the host's consequently diminished immune response are preferable to partial eradication coupled with continued immunity or protection. In man the answer will depend on the general epidemiological situation, i.e., on the likelihood of his exposure to infection in the future.

Combination of Chemoprophylaxis and Immune Prophylaxis

Investigations in which vaccination was done with normal INH-sensitive BCG will be discussed first. Experiments were done on mice by JESPERSEN and RASMUSSEN (1955), on guinea pigs by KIKUTH and POTHMANN (1959) and NASTA et al. (1960), on monkeys by SCHMIDT (1959) and on rabbits by FREERKSEN (1957a). Vaccination before virulent infection, which was then treated with INH, generally improved survival rates or other parameters of the disease. Rabbits which were first vaccinated and then treated with 20 mg/kg INH, for example, lived longer than those which were either only vaccinated or only treated. Similarly, BCG vaccination during INH prophylaxis inhibited the course of tuberculosis (JANKOV 1960; MENEMENLI and ERASLAN 1959). However, LUCCHESI and SPINA (1960) observed an adverse effect when they combined BCG and INH. Vaccination after non-sterilizing treatment always tended to be protective (LUCCHESI and SPINA 1960; NASTA et al. 1960). Because the tuberculostatic effect of INH prevents the BCG organisms from multiplying, vaccination must be done either before INH treatment is begun or after it has ceased.

INH-Resistant BCG

When it had become clear that the effect of vaccination with normal BCG was poor when it coincided with INH treatment, the development of INH-resistant BCG was proposed (CANETTI 1955). The factors that influence protection by BCG vaccination are known to be the dose, the route of vaccination, the viable count, the stability, the dispersion and, most of all, the virulence of the strain. Effective immunization depends on the ability of BCG to persist in lymphatic tissue. When *M. tuberculosis, M. bovis* or BCG become fully INH-resistant and catalase negative they are almost avirulent in most of the species investigated. Consequently the problem was: would INH-resistant BCG organisms be able to multiply effectively in the host, thus giving sufficient protection? Several authors have observed that large doses of INH-resistant BCG are able to produce good immunity (BRETEY and CANETTI 1957; MEDORO et al. 1960; SCHAEFER et al. 1957). However, doses as large as those administered to animals cannot be administered to man. It has been shown by others that INH-resistant BCG at the usual concentrations produced less immunity in the guinea pig than INH-sensitive BCG did (BARTMANN 1960; CANETTI et al. 1958; NAGATA 1959). In the early sixties GAINSFORD and GRIFFITH (1961); UNGAR et al. (1961) claimed that a different kind of INH-resistant BCG vaccine gave rise to an allergy in both animals and man which was as strong as that caused by classical BCG vaccine. However, according to many experts allergenic potency is not identical to immunizing potency. Immunizing effect is correlated to the ability of a vaccine to sustain high tuberculin hypersensitivity. I infected cattle with INH-resistant *M. bovis* which gave rise to tuberculin allergy, but 6 months–12 months later all the cattle had become tuberculin negative, something that would not have happened had INH-sensitive *M. bovis* been used. The evidence leads one to conclude that INH-resistant BCG vaccine does not afford as much protection against infection as does the normal INH-sensitive BCG vaccine.

References

Allgood MA, Price GT (1971) Isoniazid therapy of tuberculosis in baboons. Primates 12:81–90

Andruschenko VV (1962) Chimioprofilaktyka tuberkul'ozu tvaryn. Socialist Tvaryunyctvo Kyiv 34:57

Avellini G (1953) Compartamento del sangue periferico in bovini affetti da tuberculosi e trattati con idrazide dell'acido isonicotinico. Clin Vet (Milano) 76:361–381

Badiali L (1954) L'idrazide dell'acido isonicotinico nella bovina, esperimento di profilassi tuberculosi. Vet Ital 5:7–18
Badiali L, Baraccia E (1959) La chemioprofilassi nella tuberculosi bovina. Prime prove pratiche di risanamento. Vet Ital 10:292
Badiali L, De Majo F (1962) Ulteriori ricerche sulla chimioprofilassi isoniazidica della tuberculosi bovina. Rev Tuberc Mal App Resp 10:3–30
Bartmann K (1959) Isoniazid prophylaxis in exposed or minimally infected animals. Bull Int Union Tuberc 29:214–226
Bartmann K (1960a) Die experimentellen Grundlagen der Chemoprophylaxe der Tuberkulose mit Isonicotinsäurehydrazid (INH). Adv Tuberc Res 10:127–215
Bartmann K (1960b) Weitere Untersuchungen über das Vaccinationsvermögen INH-resistenter BCG-Stämme. Beitr Klin Tuberk 123:132–138
Bartmann K (1962a) Die Prophylaxe der Tuberkulose durch BCG and Isoniazid, einzeln und in Kombination, bei Tier und Mensch. Tuberk Arzt 16:329–357
Bartmann K (1962b) Formen und Indikationen der Chemoprophylaxe der Tuberkulose mit Isoniazid. Tuberk Arzt 16:136–147
Bartmann K, Blisse A (1967) Kurzfristige, primäre INH-Prophylaxe mit hohen Dosen bei minimal infizierten Meerschweinchen. Beitr Klin Tuberk 135:351–356
Bartmann K, Freise G (1963) Mikrobiologisch bestimmte INH-Konzentrationen im Gewebe von Tier und Mensch. Beitr Klin Tuberk 127:546–560
Bartmann K, Millberger H (1959) Das Vaccinationsvermögen INH-resistenter BCG-Stämme bei Meerschweinchen. Beitr Klin Tuberk 119:536–546
Bartmann K, Kleeberg HH, Spiess H (1971) Chemoprophylaxe und präventive Chemotherapie gegen Tuberkulose. In: Meissner G, Schmiedel A, Nelles A (Hrsg) Mykobakterien und mykobakterielle Krankheiten, Teil VIII. VEB Fischer, Jena, pp 277–311
Bartmann K, Villnow J, Schwarz CH (1955) Tierexperimentelle Untersuchungen zu einer intermittierenden Chemotherapie und -prophylaxe der Tuberkulose. I. Der Erfolg intermittierender Gaben von 10 mg INH je Kilogramm Körpergewicht im Simultanversuch an Meerschweinchen. Beitr Klin Tuberk 115:79–86
Bartmann K, Villnow J, Schwarz CH (1956) Tierexperimentelle Untersuchungen zu einer intermittierenden Chemotherapie und -prophylaxe der Tuberkulose. II. Der Erfolg zweimal wöchentlich verabfolgter Gaben von INH in verschiedener Dosierung beim Simultanversuch an Meerschweinchen. Beitr Klin Tuberk 115:269–275
Bartmann K, Villnow J, Schwarz CH (1957a) Tierexperimentelle Untersuchungen zu einer intermittierenden Chemotherapie und -prophylaxe der Tuberkulose. III. Prophylaktische Versuche mit INH an massiv infizierten Meerschweinchen. Beitr Klin Tuberk 116:471–478
Bartmann K, Villnow J, Schwarz CH (1957b) Tierexperimentelle Untersuchungen zu einer intermittierenden Chemotherapie und -prophylaxe der Tuberkulose. IV. Prophylaktische Versuche mit INH bei einer Minimalinfektion von Meerschweinchen. Beitr Klin Tuberk 116:687–698
Bartmann K, Villnow J, Schwarz CH (1957c) Tierexperimentelle Untersuchungen zu einer intermittierenden Chemotherapie und -prophylaxe der Tuberkulose. V. Virulenz- und Resistenzprüfungen von Kulturen aus Gewebe INH-behandelter Meerschweinchen. Beitr Klin Tuberk 117:344–349
Bartmann K, Villnow J, Schwarz CH (1958a) Tierexperimentelle Untersuchungen zu einer intermittierenden Chemotherapie und -prophylaxe der Tuberkulose. VI. Die Infektionsimmunität von Meerschweinchen bei einer prophylaktisch mit INH behandelten Tuberkulose. Beitr Klin Tuberk 118:87–101
Bartmann K, Villnow J, Schwarz CH (1958b) Tierexperimentelle Untersuchungen zu einer intermittierenden Chemotherapie und -prophylaxe der Tuberkulose. VII. Der Erfolg kontinuierlicher und intermittierender Gaben von INH und der Tripelkombination INH, Streptomycin, PAS im therapeutischen Versuch an Meerschweinchen. Beitr Klin Tuberk 118:297–313
Bartmann K, Villnow J, Schwarz CH (1958c) Tierexperimentelle Untersuchungen zu einer intermittierenden Chemotherapie und -prophylaxe der Tuberkulose. VIII. Der Bakteriengehalt des Gewebes minimal infizierter Meerschweinchen während der INH Prophylaxe. Beitr Klin Tuberk 119:75–84

Bartmann K, Villnow J, Schwarz CH (1959a) Tierexperimentelle Untersuchungen zu einer intermittierenden Chemotherapie und -prophylaxe der Tuberkulose. IX. Versuche an Meerschweinchen zur Prophylaxe einer Minimalinfektion mit kontinuierlichen und intermittierender INH-Gaben. Beitr Klin Tuberk 121:460–465
Bartmann K, Villnow J, Schwarz CH (1959b) Acquired resistance and isoniazid medication. Am Rev Tuberc 79:97–101
Bjerkedal T, Palmer CE (1962) Effect of isoniazid prophylaxis in experimental tuberculosis in guinea pigs. Am J Hyg 76:89–123
Bjerkedal T, Palmer CE (1964) Effects of different concentrations of isoniazid on tubercle bacilli in guinea pigs. Acta Tuberc Scand 45:179–204
Bloch H, Segal W (1955) Viability and multiplication of vaccines in immunization against tuberculosis. Am Rev Tuberc 71:228–248
Bretey J, Canetti G (1957) Vaccination par BCG normal et BCG isoniazido-résistant en présence et en absence d'un traitement par l'isoniazide. Ann Inst Pasteur 92:441–450
Canetti G (1955) Une méthode de prophylaxie antituberculeuse associant la vaccination et la chimioprévention. Vaccination par le BCG isoniazido-résistant et administration d'isoniazide jusq' à apparition de la résistance spécifique vaccinale. Rev Tuberc (Paris) 19:1392–1395
Canetti G (1966) Wege zur Ausrottung der Tuberkulose. Prax Pneumol 19:602–610
Canetti G, Grosset J (1958) L'influence du taux maximum d'INH libre du sérum sur la structure des souches isoniazido-résistantes apparaissant au cours de l'INH-thérapie. Rev Tuberc (Paris) 22:778–805
Canetti G, Bretey J, Saenz A, Grosset J (1958) Effet d'un traitement précoce par l'isoniazide sur l'immunité engendrée chez un cobaye par une dose de BCG standard faible. Ann Inst Past 95:262–271
Castellani G, D'Esposito C, Zacchi B (1959) Quimioprofilaxis de la tuberculosis. Proc XVIth Int Vet Congr (Madrid) 2:699–700
Clarke GL, Schmidt JP (1969) Effect of prophylactic isoniazid on early developing experimental tuberculosis in *Macaca Mulatta*. Am Rev Respir Dis 100:224–227
Cohn ML, Davis CL, Middlebrook G (1962) Chemoprophylaxis with isoniazid against aerogenic tuberculous infection in the guinea pig. Am Rev Respir Dis 86:95–97
Deborah Symposium (1959) Chemoprophylaxis of tuberculosis. Am Rev Respir Dis 80:1–139
Debré R, Noufflard H, Foussereau S (1959) "Chimioprophylaxie" par l'isoniazide et immunité antituberculeuse. Contribution à l'étude expérimentale. Rev Fr Étud Clin et Biol 4:32–39
Dickinson JM, Aber VR, Mitchison DA (1973) Studies on the treatment of experimental tuberculosis of the guinea pig with intermittent doses of isoniazid. Tubercle 54:211–224
Dickinson JM, Mitchison DA (1976) Experimental investigations of bacteriological mechanisms in short course chemotherapy. Bull Int Union Tuberc 51:79–86
Didovets SR, Rotov VI, Chenurov KP (1978) Chemoprophylaxis of tuberculosis in cattle (using isoniazid). Veterinariya (Moscow, USSR) 10:50–57
Domagk G, Offe HA, Siefken W (1952) Weiterentwicklung der Chemotherapie der Tuberkulose. Beitr Klin Tuberk 107:325–337
Ebina A (1959) Multiplication and antituberculosis immunity in mice by vaccination with BCG. Sci Rep Res Inst Tohoku Univ 8:455–467
Ferebee SH, Palmer CE (1956) Prevention of experimental tuberculosis with isoniazid. Am Rev Tuberc 73:1–18
Franke R (1964) Erfahrungen mit INH-Dauertherapie zur Tuberkulose-Prophylaxe. T Diergeneesk 89 (Suppl):176–180
Freerksen E (1956) Resistenz, Immunität, Allergie bei der Tuberkulose. Klin Wochenschr 34:881–887
Freerksen E (1957a) Angeborene und erworbene Widerstandskraft bei der Tuberkulose. Tuberk Arzt 11:65–75
Freerksen E (1957b) Discussion remarks. Bull Int Union Tuberc 27:220–221, 245–247
Fust B, Studer A, Böhni E (1952) Experimentelle Erfahrungen mit dem Antituberkulotikum „Rimifon". Schweiz Z Tuberk 9:226–242

Gainsford W, Griffiths MI (1961) A freeze-dried vaccine from isoniazid-resistant BCG. Brit Med J 1:1500–1501
Grosset J (1978a) The sterilising value of rifampicin and pyrazinamide in experimental short course chemotherapy. Tubercle 59:287–297
Grosset J (1978b) Short course chemotherapy in experimental tuberculosis. Selected Papers 18:5–31
Grumbach F (1962) Treatment of experimental murine tuberculosis with different combinations of isoniazid/streptomycin followed by isoniazid alone. Am Rev Respir Dis 86:211–215
Grumbach F (1965) Etudes chimiothérapiques de la tuberculose avancée de la souris. Adv Tuberc Res 14:31–96
Grumbach F (1969) Experimental "in vivo" studies of new antituberculous drugs: capreomycin, ethambutol, rifampicin. Tubercle 50 (Suppl):12–21
Grumbach F, Canetti G, Grosset J (1964) Further experiments on long-term chemotherapy of advanced murine tuberculosis, with emphasis on intermittent regimens. Tubercle 45:125–135
Grumbach F, Canetti G, Grosset J, Le Lirzin M (1967) Late results of long-term, intermittent chemotherapy of advanced murine tuberculosis. Limits of the murine model. Tubercle 48:11–26
Grumbach F, Canetti G, Le Lirzin M (1969) Rifampicin in daily and intermittent treatment of experimental murine tuberculosis, with emphasis on late results. Tubercle 50:280–293
Grunberg E, Schnitzer RJ (1952) Studies on the activity of hydrazine derivates of isonicotinic acid on the experimental tuberculosis of mice. Quart Bull Sea View Hosp 13:3–11
Hauser H (1963) Beitrag zur Tuberkulose-Morphologie bei Zoo-Ruminaten nach Rimifon-Behandlung. Schweiz Arch Tierheilkd 105:655–662
Heilmeyer L (1952) Vorläufiger Bericht über Isonikotinsäurehydrazid (Rimifon, Neoteben) aufgrund experimenteller und klinischer Untersuchungen. Münch Med Wochenschr 94:1303–1308
Heymann H (1959) Use of isoniazid in zoo animals. Kleintierpraxis 4:123
Hobby GL, Lenert TF, Rivoire ZC, Donikian M, Pikula D (1953) In vitro and in vivo activity of streptomycin and isoniazid singly and in combination. Am Rev Tuberc 67:808–827
Humbert R (1954) Biologische Heilung experimenteller Tuberkulose durch Isoniazid? Z Ges Exp Med 124:355–370
Jankov M (1960) Immunization with BCG during the course of chemoprophylactic and chemotherapeutic treatment of guinea pigs infected with virulent tubercle bacilli. Bull Int Union Tuberc 30:123–132
Jespersen A, Rasmussen KN (1955) Comparative studies on the effect of dihydrostreptomycin and isoniazid on immunised and non-immunised red mice following intravenous challenge with bovine tubercle bacilli. Acta Pathol Microbiol Scand 36:548–557
Karlson AG, Feldman WH (1953) Effective therapeutic doses of isoniazid for experimental tuberculosis of guinea pigs. Am Rev Tuberc 68:75–81
Kikuth W, Pothmann FJ (1959) Zur Kombination von INH-Prophylaxe und BCG-Schutzimpfung. Dtsch Med Wochenschr 81:360–364
Khaikin B YA (1970) Chemoprophylaxis of tuberculosis in mink using isoniazid. Krolik Vod Zverovod 3:30
Kleeberg HH (1959) The treatment of tuberculosis in man and animals with isoniazid. J S Afr Vet Med Assoc 30:69–73
Kleeberg HH (1966) Chemotherapy and chemoprophylaxis of tuberculosis in cattle. Adv Tuberc Res 15:189–269
Kleeberg HH (1967a) The use of chemotherapeutic agents in animal tuberculosis. Veterinarian (London) 4:197–211
Kleeberg HH (1967b) Die Chemotherapie als neues Mittel zur Tilgung der Rindertuberkulose. Vet Med Nachr 2/3:223–239
Kleeberg HH, Worthington RW (1963) A modern approach to the control of bovine tuberculosis. J S Afr Vet Med Assoc 34:383–391

Kleeberg HH, Nixon RC, Worthington RW (1966) Evaluation of isoniazid in the field control of bovine tuberculosis. J S Afr Vet Med Assoc 37:219–228
Kradolfer F (1970) Rifampicin, isoniazid, ethambutol, ethionamide and streptomycin in murine tuberculosis. Antibiot Chemother 16:352–360
Kubin M, Zavadilová Z, Freslová A (1959) Chemoprofylaxe pokusné tuberkulózy hydrazidem Kys. isonikotinové. Vet Med (Praha) 32:577–586
Lambert HP (1959) The chemoprophylaxis of tuberculosis. Am Rev Respir Dis 80:648–658
Lambert HP (1960) The influence of chemoprophylaxis on immunity in experimental tuberculosis. Am Rev Respir Dis 82:619–626
Langenegger J, Langenegger CH, De Oliveira J (1981) Tratamento da tuberculosa bovina con isoniazida. Pesquisa Veterinaria Brasileira 1:1–6
Lucchesi M, Spina G (1957) Basi sperimentali de la chemioprofilassi antitubercolare mediante isoniazide. Nota I: Riv Ital Tuberc 5:320–336
Lucchesi M, Spina G (1958) Basi sperimentali de la chemioprofilassi antitubercolare mediante isoniazide. Nota II: Riv Ital Tuberc 6:103–130
Lucchesi M, Spina G (1959) Basi sperimentali de la chemioprofilassi antitubercolare mediante isoniazide. Nota III: Riv Ital Tuberc 6:131–147
Lucchesi M, Spina G (1960) Bases expérimentales de la chimioprophylaxie antituberculeuse par l'isoniazide. Bull Int Union Tuberc 30, 133–148
Lucchesi M, Spina G (1961) Basi sperimentali de la chemioprofilassi antitubercolare mediante isoniazide. Nota IV: Riv Tuberc App Resp 9:42–56
McCune R, Lee SH, Deuschle K, McDermott W (1957) Ineffectiveness of isoniazid in modifying the phenomenon of microbial persistence. Am Rev Tuberc 76:1106–1109
Medoro GA, Rause G, Termine A (1960) Esperienze di chemio-vaccinoprofilassi con isoniazide e BCG INH-resistente. Lotta C Tuberc 20:383–387
Menemenli N, Eraslan A (1959) A pilot study on preventive and prophylactic effects of isoniazid in contact children. Bull Int Union Tuberc 29:259–266
Moretti P, Pedini B (1953) Sulla attivatà preventiva antitubercolare nel vitello dell'idrazide dell'acido isonicotinico. Nuova Vet 28:315–322
Nagata S (1958) Kekkaku 33:699–702
Nagata S (1959) Kekkaku 34:7–10, 552–555
Nai DD, Perini G (1960) Ulteriori osservazioni sulla negativizzazione allergica dei bovini tuberculino-positivi trattati con isoniazide. Atti Soc Ital Sci Vet 14:612–616
Nasta M, Algeorge G, Arhiri M, Negulescu VL (1957) Recherches sur la chimioprophylaxie de la tuberculose expérimentale du cobaye. Rev Tuberc (Paris) 21:1013–1017
Nasta M, Algeorge G, Arhiri M (1960) Bases expérimentales de la chimioprophylaxie de la tuberculose. Bull Int Union Tuberc 30 No 2–3:149–156
Nasta M, Arhiri M, Algeorge G (1960) Evolutia tuberculozei de suprainfectie la cobaii tuberculosi supusi chimioprofilaxei si chimioterapiei. Probl Tuberc (Bucureşti) 1:185–195
Nitti V (1967) Activity of rifampicin in experimental tuberculosis of the guinea pig. Chemotherapia 12:369–400
Omodei-Zorini A (1963) La chemioprofilassi antitubercolare mediante isoniazide in campo umano e bovine. Ann Ist Forlanini 23 (Suppl):227–423
Omodei-Zorini A (1963) Further developments in human and bovine antituberculosis chemoprophylaxis with isoniazid in Italy. Dis Chest 43:131–141
Palmer CE (1959) The effect of isoniazid on experimental tuberculosis in the guinea pig. Bull Int Union Tuberc 29:273–275
Palmer CE, Ferebee SH, Hopwood L (1956) Studies on the prevention of experimental tuberculosis with isoniazid. II. Effects of different dosage regimens. Am Rev Tuberc 74:917–939
Peizer LR, Chaves AD, Widelock D (1957) The effects of early isoniazid treatment in experimental guinea-pig tuberculosis. Am Rev Tuberc 76:732–751
Rosati T, Tini R (1955) Sull'andamento della reazione in bovini naturalmente infetti e trattati con idrazide dell'acido isonicotinico. Vet Ital 6:895–905
Rosati T, Badiali L (1959) La chemioprofilassi della tuberculosi bovina mediante isoniazide. Riv Tuberc App Respir 7:207–227

Rosati T, Badiali L (1960) Investigations on antituberculous chemoprophylaxis and comparative tests with BCG vaccination. Am Rev Respir Dis 82:577–578
Schaefer WB, Cohn ML, Middlebrook G (1957) Comparative study of the vaccinating properties of BCG and its isoniazid-resistant mutant in guinea pigs. Am Rev Tuberc 75:656–658
Schmidt LH (1956) Some observations on the utility of simian pulmonary tuberculosis in defining the therapeutic potentialities of isoniazid. Am Rev Tuberc 74 Suppl: 138–153
Schmidt LH (1959) Observations on the utility of isoniazid in the prophylaxis of experimental tuberculosis. Bull Int Union Tuberc 29:276–284
Seelemann M, Buschkiel H, Rackow HG (1957a) Chemoprophylaktische Versuche bei Rindertuberkulose. 1. Mittlg. Zbl Vet Med 4:80–93
Seelemann M, Buschkiel H, Rackow HG (1957b) Chemoprophylaktische Versuche bei Rindertuberkulose. 2. Mittlg. Zbl Vet Med 4:101–118
Seelemann M, Buschkiel H, Rackow HG (1958) Chemoprophylaktische Versuche bei Rindertuberkulose. 3. Mittlg. Zbl Vet Med 5:609–628
Seifert H (1962) "Chemoprophylaxe" zur Verhütung von Infektionskrankheiten bei Rindern. Vet Med Nachr 4:207
Seri I, Balogh Z (1962) Zur Frage der tuberkulösen Superinfektion, II. Mitteilung. Tuberk Arzt 16:677–682
Sher BC, Czaja ZG, Takimura Y, Popper H (1957) The course of experimental tuberculosis inhibited by isoniazid. Am Rev Tuberc 75:295–302
Spiess H (1959) Chemoprophylaxe und präventive Chemotherapie gegen die Tuberkulose. Dtsch Med Wochenschr 84:1410–1415
Spiess H (1961) Zur Kombination von Impf- und Chemoprophylaxe der Tuberkulose. Dtsch Med Wochenschr 86:2162–2163
Spiess H (1963) Tuberkulose. Chemo- und Impfprophylaxe. Hdb Kinderheilk 5:807–834
Spryszak A (1961) Control of bovine tuberculosis with reference to chemoprophylaxis in calves. Bull Off Int Epizoot 56:954–958
Spryszak A (1964) An accelerated restoration to health of a tuberculous herd by the preventive application of isoniazid. Bull Vet Inst Pulawy 8:44–48
Tai FH, Jen TM, Chu BY, Han SH (1961) Isoniazid prophylaxis of tuberculous infection in mice. Am Rev Respir Dis 83:711–717
Teuscher E (1956) Zur Känguruhtuberkulose. Thesis, Zürich
Toyohara MA, Kidoh YO, Bayashi O (1959) Studies on the effect of isoniazid upon the antituberculous immunity induced by BCG vaccination. Tubercle 40:184–191
Uehlinger E, Siebenmann R, Frei H (1952) Erste Erfahrungen mit Rimifon „Roche" bei experimenteller Meerschweinchentuberkulose. Schweiz Med Wochenschr 33:335–338
Ungar J, Thomas V, Muggleton PW (1961) Freeze-dried BCG vaccine from an isoniazid resistant strain. Brit Med J 1:1498–1500
Veltman T (1955) Experimentelle Untersuchungen zur Chemotherapie der Tuberkulose. 1. Mittlg. Zbl Bkt I Orig 163:177–209
Veltman T (1955a) Experimentelle Untersuchungen zur Chemotherapie der Tuberkulose. 2. Mittlg. Zbl Bkt I Orig 163:210–218
Veltman T (1955b) Experimentelle Untersuchungen zur Chemotherapie der Tuberkulose. 3. Mittlg. Zbl Bkt I Orig 163:484–504
Vivien JN, Grosset J (1961) Le taux d'isoniazide actif dans le sérum sanguin. Adv Tuberc Res 11:45–110

CHAPTER 4

Experimental and Clinical Activity of Antituberculosis Drugs and Other Antimicrobial Agents Against Mycobacteria Other than Tubercle Bacilli, Except *M. Leprae*

K. BARTMANN

A. Introduction

Besides *M. tuberculosis, M. bovis,* and the intermediate *M. africanum,* which give rise to "typical" tuberculosis, many other mycobacteria can be pathogenic, especially if the local or systemic resistance mechanisms are impaired. To distinguish this group from the typical causative agents, their members are often called "atypical", but this is a misleading term because most of these bacteria can now be assigned to well-defined groups and species. As shown in Table 1, the groups are classified on the basis of certain characteristics, such as generation time, pigment production, and pathogenicity. The grouping in Table 1 originally devised by RUNYON (1959), should not be considered a mandatory taxonomic scheme. For example, other authors place *M. ulcerans* and *M. xenopi* in Group III (SELKON 1969; KUBICA et al. 1975). Lepra is a clinically distinct entity and it is therefore not usually dealt with under the heading of mycobacterioses. We too shall follow this convention. For the remaining mycobacteria that do not belong to the *M. tuberculosis* complex there is no accepted common designation. Therefore, we shall use the descriptive term "Mycobacteria other than tubercle bacilli", abbreviated to "MOTT bacilli" or to MOTT. For surveys of the bacteriology, epidemiology, clinical features, and treatment of diseases caused by the MOTT bacilli, the reader is referred to FORSCHBACH (1975, in German), and to WOLINSKY (1979, in English). A comprehensive review (in German) is presented in Part VII of "Mykobakterien und mykobakterielle Krankheiten" edited by MEISSNER and SCHMIEDEL (1970). Monographs have been published in English by WEISZFEILER (1973) and by CHAPMAN (1977). A review specially devoted to experimental and clinical chemotherapy was published in English by BURJANOVÁ and URBANCIK (1970).

The reader may also consult the section on "antimycobacterial activity" of each antituberculosis drug in Chapter 2.

The experimental and clinical evaluation of diseases caused by MOTT is beset with many difficulties. In the earlier publications the microorganisms were often not identified to the species that have since been defined, but only to the group. However, pathogenicity and drug sensitivity may differ widely between different members of a given group. In this review, therefore, attention will be focussed on

Table 1. Currently accepted species of Mycobacterium. (After GOOD 1979)

Group	RUNYON group No.	Strictly or potentially pathogenic	Rarely or never pathogenic
Slowly growing or "nonculturable", strictly pathogenic		*M. tuberculosis* *M. bovis* *M. africanum* *M. ulcerans* *M. leprae*	
Photochromogens	I	*M. kansasii* *M. marinum* *M. simiae* *M. asiaticum*	
Scotochromogens	II	*M. scrofulaceum* *M. szulgai* *M. xenopi*	*M. gordonae* *M. flavescens*
Nonphotochromogens	III	*M. avium* *M. intracellulare* *M. malmoense* *M. haemophilum*	*M. terrae* *M. triviale* *M. nonchromogenicum*
Rapidly growing	IV	*M. fortuitum* *M. chelonei*	*M. vaccae* *M. smegmatis* *M. phlei* *M. parafortuitum* *M. neoaurum* *M. thermoresistible* *M. chitae* *M. gadium* *M. gilvum* *M. duvalii* *M. aurum*
Pathogenic in animals		*M. lepraemurium* *M. microti* *M. paratuberculosis* *M. farcinogenes* *M. senegalense*	

those papers in which the species of the micro-organism in question is either mentioned or can be reliably assumed.

Although susceptibility studies with MOTT present no problems from a technical point of view, the results can be compared only for one and the same technique. Since the proportion method is the most widely used and seems to give the most reproducible results, those studies are preferred for a review that make use of this technique. Furthermore, the number of strains should not be less than 5–10 per species. For the rapidly growing Mycobacteria of Group IV, the standardized techniques used for non-acid fast microorganisms such as staphylococci or enterobacteriaceae, are often applied. Publications in which the clinical outcome is correlated with in-vitro susceptibility are considered only if the drug concentrations in the sensitivity tests were spaced in such a way that different degrees of intermediate sensitivity could be distinguished, because this is the most critical range for the correlation of treatment results and in-vitro data. Another problem is the interpretation of the sensitivity tests. For *M. tuberculosis* the classification of strains as sensitive or resistant is based on careful correlations between the results of treatment and in-vitro tests. No precise information is available for the MOTT bacilli. Most authors use the same criteria as for true tuberculosis, but it may well be that – because of the lower pathogenicity of MOTT – these criteria are too rigid and that partial inhibition of multiplication of the whole population or complete inhibition of a fraction of the population at a particular drug concentration would be more useful for predictive purposes than the criteria used for *M. tuberculosis*. For further discussion see HOBBY et al. (1967). In the tables showing the prevalence of sensitivity and resistance that we present below, we have used the criteria adopted for *M. tuberculosis,* but we use these terms merely as a descriptive shortcut and not in a prognostic sense. If the data are allocated to the classes S (sensitive) or R (resistant), this means that at least 90% of the strains have the respective characteristic.

Although in-vivo models for some species do exist, the selection of the best parameters for their evaluation and the significance of these models is open to many questions.

Controlled therapeutic studies in human subjects are lacking, because the number of patients is limited and because – in the assumed presence of tuberculosis – a more or less effective treatment has usually already been implemented for some time before the true causative agent is detected. Furthermore, the criteria used for the evaluation of the clinical course are not as uniform as in tuberculosis, and their prognostic relevance is less certain. For example, in tuberculosis, bacteriology proved to be the most sensitive indicator of the value of chemotherapy. Nevertheless, it is questionable whether in pulmonary infections due to the *M. intracellulare-avium* complex the aim should be to stop the excretion of bacilli at the price of severe adverse reactions, because the patient is not a source of infection, the symptoms and signs are often mild, and the disease may remain stable for years despite continual excretion of bacilli (ROSENZWEIG 1979). For the evaluation of treatment, therefore, we have applied (besides the "hard core" criteria i.e., disappearance of the excretion of bacilli and relapse), criteria that imply more subjective elements, such as improvement (mainly roentgenologically) or inactivity of the disease (inactivity as defined by the older standards of the American National Tuberculosis Association).

In spite of all these difficulties, much has been learned about the proper management of patients infected by MOTT. If investigators from one and the same group have reported several times on the same patient population, then only the latest reports are considered as well as those dealing with particular aspects. In addition to the abbreviations used in other parts of this book, we use DDS for diaminodiphenyl sulphone, the drug widely applied in lepra infections.

The different species belonging to MOTT will be dealt with in the order of grouping according to Table 1.

As treatment with antituberculosis drugs is ineffective against some species of MOTT, brief mention will be made of the activity of other antimicrobials.

B. Possible Reasons for the Lower Sensitivity of MOTT to many Antituberculotics Compared to *M. tuberculosis*

Various possible mechanisms to explain the relatively low susceptibility of MOTT to many antituberculotics have been discussed by DAVID (1981), who arrived at the conclusion that the assumption of high incidence of spontaneous mutations or drug-resistance factors is not supported by the available data. The most likely explanation is a permeability barrier, due either to a special structure or function at the level of the cytoplasmic membrane or to the fact that the drugs are prevented from reaching the cytoplasmic membrane at the outer layers of the cell wall. The concept of a permeability barrier is supported by the following facts: The RNA-polymerase isolated from a strain of *M. intracellulare* that exhibited natural resistance to RMP was susceptible to RMP (HUI et al. 1977). MIZUGUCHI et al. (1983) found that the resistance of *M. intracellulare,* strain 103, to the aminoglycosides and peptide antituberculotics was not due to enzymatic inactivation of the drugs. The ribosomes were found to be sensitive to the antibiotics. The level of resistance in this and other strains could be markedly reduced by adding Tween 80 to the medium. An analogous observation was made by HUI et al. (1977) with RMP. Both groups of researchers assumed that Tween enhanced permeability. It has been shown by many authors (for references see MIZUGUCHI et al. 1983) that in the *M. avium* complex a change in appearance of the colors from the translucent to the opaque type is accompanied by an increased sensitivity to several antituberculosis drugs, increased growth rate, and loss of virulence. RASTOGI et al. (1981) have shown by comparative ultrastructural studies that the bacteria of the translucent-colony type have an outer polysaccharide cell wall layer which is not found in the bacilli of the opaque colonies. Since MIZUGUCHI et al. (1981) have found that translucent cells bear two plasmids, whereas opaque cells bear only one, it may be argued that the production of the outer polysaccharide layer is under the control of a plasmid.

C. Efficacy of Antituberculosis Drugs and Other Antimicrobial Agents Against the Various MOTT Species

I. Group I. Photochromogenic Mycobacteria

1. *M. Kansasii* (Yellow Bacillus, *M. Luciflavum*)

In man, *M. kansasii* causes mainly pulmonary disease, followed in frequency by cervical adenitis. Lesions at other extrapulmonary sites have been observed in rare instances. If untreated, the pulmonary disease runs a slowly progressive course over the years without any significant symptoms in the majority of cases (GOLDMAN 1968; JOHANSON and NICHOLSON 1969; FRANCIS et al. 1975).

a) Activity of Antituberculosis Drugs in Vitro

The publications on the in-vitro activity of antituberculosis drugs have been compiled in Table 2. It can be seen at once that, despite differences in technique, all

Table 2. Prevalence of sensitivity and resistance to antituberculosis drugs in *M. kansasii*. Relative prevalence of sensitivity (*S*) and resistance (*R*). The authors are coded numerically (see list below)

	S	S>R	S≃R	R>S	R
PAS		21		12, 13	1–4, 6, 8, 9, 17, 18, 22, 23, 25, 27
SM		12, 19, 21, 22, 23, 26	18	2, 4, 6, 8, 13, 25	1, 9, 17, 20, 27
TSC	1, 9, 17	13, 25			
PZA				5	1, 9, 13, 18, 25, 27
INH				2, 12, 19, 21, 22, 23	1, 4, 6, 8, 9, 13, 17, 18, 25, 26, 27
TC					27
VM	21, 23	18, 22, 25		3, 4, 6, 8, 9, 13	
CS	1, 9, 17, 21, 23	4, 6, 8, 13, 18, 22, 25			
ETH	6, 8, 9, 13, 21, 23, 25	12, 22			
KM		18, 21		9, 25	6, 8, 13, 20
DATC	7, 9, 13, 17, 25				
CM	21	14		11, 15, 25	6, 8
EMB	17, 18, 21, 24, 25	9, 19, 26, 27		11, 13, 23	
RMP	10, 15–19, 21, 22, 24, 26	11, 23, 25, 27			

[1] Wolinsky et al. (1957)
[2] Lester et al. (1958)
[3] Urbančik (1959)
[4] Lewis et al. (1959)
[5] Stottmeier (1964)
[6] Wichelhausen and Robinson (1965)
[7] Tacquet et al. (1966)
[8] Hobby et al. (1967)
[9] Burjanová and Urbančík (1967)
[10] McClatchy et al. (1969)
[11] Schröder et al. (1969)
[12] Johanson and Nicholson (1969)
[13] Meissner (1970)
[14] Havel and Šimonová (1970)
[15] Molavi and Weinstein (1971a)
[16] Rynearson et al. (1972)
[17] Schröder (1973)
[18] Burjanová and Dornetzhuber (1975)
[19] Harris et al. (1975)
[20] Martin-Luengo et al. (1978)
[21] Jakschik (1979)
[22] Kuze et al. (1981)
[23] Kim et al. (1981)
[24] Yates and Collins (1981)
[25] Hejný (1982)
[26] Ahn et al. (1983)
[27] De Kantor et al. (1985)

authors agree that the large majority of strains is sensitive to RMP, EMB, ETH, TSC, DATC and CS, and resistant to PAS and PZA.

Furthermore, *M. kansasii* must be classified as mainly resistant against INH and SM if the criteria valid for *M. tuberculosis* are applied. However, many strains show only a partial resistance to both drugs. As regards VM, KM and CM, the results vary, probably for technical reasons. Taking all the respective investigations together, more strains are resistant than sensitive to these three drugs. Combinations of INH with SM and/or EMB at various concentrations were investigated by TSANG et al. (1978), who showed that the INH + EMB combination reduces the amount of growth more than it could be expected from additive action of the two drugs. For INH + SM the interaction was suggestive of a superadditive effect, but this was not statistically significant. KUZE et al. (1981) tested various triple combinations at a fractional concentration of 0.2 mg/l, which by itself was ineffective except for RMP in a small percentage of strains. Combinations without RMP, i.e., INH + SM + PAS or EMB and INH + EMB + KM inhibited 40%–70% of the strains. All 13 strains were inhibited by triple combinations of RMP + ETH + VM or RMP + EMB + KM. The authors recommend therefore that the *M. kansasii* infections be treated with triple combinations including RMP, one of the aminoglycosides, and either EMB or ETH.

b) Activity of Other Antimicrobial Agents in Vitro

M. kansasii was found to be sensitive to the following drugs: DDS (PATTYN and VAN ERMENGEM 1968, BURJANOVÁ and DORNETZHUBER 1975; DE KANTOR et al. 1985), clofazimine (BURJANOVÁ AND DORNETZHUBER 1975), sulphonamides (HEJNÝ 1982; DEMOULIN et al. 1982; DE KANTOR et al. 1985), erythromycin (MOLAVI and WEINSTEIN 1971 b; HEJNÝ 1982), lincomycin (HEJNÝ 1982), and perhaps minocycline (TSUKAMURA 1980a, b). DE KANTOR et al. (1985) reported for the majority of strains sensitivity to erythromycin, but resistance to lincomycin. SALFINGER and KAFADER (1986) observed inhibition of 3 strains tested by the new quinolone Ro 23-6240 at a concentration of 0.5 mg/l.

The species is resistant to penicillin (ROGUL et al. 1957), cephalosporins (SANDERS et al. 1980; GARCIA-RODRÍGUEZ and MARTIN-LUENGO 1980; SAKURAI 1983), chloramphenicol (WOLINSKY et al. 1957; GUY and CHAPMAN 1961), oleandomycin (BURJANOVÁ and DORNETZHUBER 1975), spiramycin (DE KANTOR et al. 1985) and the aminoglycosides: gentamicin, sisomicin, tobramycin, dibekacin and amikacin (BURJANOVÁ and DORNETZHUBER 1975; GANGADHARAM and CANDLER 1977a; MARTIN-LUENGO et al. 1978; HEJNÝ 1982). SANDERS et al. (1982) and DE KANTOR et al. (1985) found nearly half of their strains sensitive to amikacin.

Most of the strains are resistant to tetracycline and oxytetracycline (WOLINSKY et al. 1957; ROGUL et al. 1957; GUY and CHAPMAN 1961; HEJNÝ 1982; DE KANTOR et al. 1985).

In vitro, 2 mg/l of ciprofloxacin were found to inhibit about 50% of the strains, whereas the MIC of norfloxacin was in the range of 8 µg/ml to >16 µg/ml (GAY et al. 1984). According to the results obtained with a few strains, the quinolone Ro 23-6240 has a MIC of 0.5 mg/l (SALFINGER and KAFADER 1986). HEIFETS and ISEMAN (1985) found *M. kansasii* sensitive to ansamycin, a spiro-piperidyl rifamycin, to the same degree as to RMP.

c) Activity of Antituberculosis Drugs and some Other Antimicrobial Agents in Animals

Only a few years after human MOTT infections had become evident, animal models were developed to study their chemotherapy in vivo. In 1958, STEENKEN et al. reported in detail their studies with four strains of *M. kansasii* on mice infected intravenously. Treatment was started immediately and was continued for

31 days. The daily doses of the drugs were as follows: CS 200 mg/kg, SM 125 mg/kg, both applied parenterally. The other drugs were mixed in with the diet so as to give 200 mg/kg/day (INH) and 500 mg/kg/day (TSC, thiocarbanilide, and thiocarbanidin). Efficacy was evaluated by the survival time and by the scores allotted to macroscopic lesions in lungs and kidneys. CS and TSC were found to be ineffective. SM and thiocarbanilide had a limited effect on 2 strains. INH and thiocarbanidin were judged to be fair in 1 strain and good in 2. Infections due to one strain proved to be refractory to all the drugs tested.

MAYER et al. (1958) infected mice intravenously. Several strains of *M. kansasii* were used in a comparison with *M. tuberculosis* (strain H37Rv). Treatment for 30 days was started immediately after the infection. Besides various thiocarbanilide derivatives the following drugs were applied daily: SM and VM 150 mg/kg s.c., INH 0.1% in the feed, and PAS 1% in the feed. The efficacy criteria were scores of gross pathological involvement of the lungs and the kidneys and the survival time. SM and VM prolonged the survival time and reduced the extent of kidney lesions but not of lung lesions. INH had in addition a favorable influence on the lung disease. The results differed to some extent among the 6 strains used, but all pointed in the same direction.

WOLINSKY (1959) infected mice intravenously and started the treatment 18 days later, continuing for a further 35 days. The daily doses in mg/kg were as follows: SM 250 s.c.; mixed with the feed: INH 200, CS 1500, TSC 500, DDS 150 (later 100) and sulphadiazine 2000. The same doses were applied in combined treatment. The evaluation criteria were survival, macroscopic lung and kidney involvement, development of spinning disease, bacteriaemia, bacteriuria, and the numbers of colony-forming units (CFU) in the lungs, spleen, liver, kidneys, and brain. CS and sulphadiazine were very slightly effective. A weak effect was noted for TSC and DDS. The best activity was displayed by INH and SM. In combination with INH, neither CS, DDS, TSC, nor sulphadiazine was additive or synergistic. INH + SM seemed to be slightly more effective than either drug alone.

KARLSON (1959) tried DDS in mice, 200 mg/kg/day being given with the feed to intravenously-infected mice for 20 days reckoning from the day of the infection. Judging from the histology, there was a slight effect.

HEDGECOCK and BLUMENTHAL (1965) started treatment a few days before the infection of mice by the intravenous route. The daily doses per kg were as follows: SM 125 mg/kg i.m., INH 120 mg/kg, and PAS from 600 mg/kg to 2400 mg/kg, both drugs mixed with the feed. The results were evaluated by the volume and macroscopic appearance of the livers and spleens, histopathology and CFU's in the various organs. The treatment lasted for 28 days–32 days. PAS was either ineffective or actually aggravated the disease, SM had a definite but limited activity. INH reduced effectively the viable counts of a strain that was partially sensitive, but had no effect on a strain resistant to 5 mg/l INH.

SAKAMOTO and GODA (1966) found good effectiveness of 50 mg EMB/kg per day, on the basis of the survival time and the macroscopic changes.

BURJANOVÁ AND URBANCÍK (1967) tested several drugs in intravenously-infected mice, oral treatment for 30 days being started 10 days after the infection. INH, PAS, TSC, and PZA were ineffective or aggravating. DATC in a daily dose of 200 mg/kg suppressed the bacterial multiplication. This was also reported by BURJANOVÁ and DORNETZHUBER in 1967.

In 1967, GERNEZ-RIEUX et al. summarized their experiments on dust-exposed and then intravenously-infected guinea pigs. Treatment was started either immediately or 30 days after the infection, with daily doses of 10 mg/kg INH, 20 mg/kg ETH, 50 mg/kg EMB, all given subcutaneously, and thiocarbanilide, 300 mg/kg per os. Evaluation was by the radiological index, lesion index, and the number of CFU per lung. ETH and EMB were slightly superior to INH. The combination of INH + ETH was no better than ETH alone.

In 1968 ROSENFELD presented a review of her experiments on intravenously-infected mice. Treatment for short periods was always started a few days after the infection and was evaluated by mortality curves. Under these conditions the following survival rates in % were found after about 10 months (daily doses in mg/kg in brackets): 45 for ETH (50) and DATC (100), 30 for SM (50), 20 for EMB (100), 5 for INH (10), and 0 for CS (500), TSC (100), and DDS (50). However, CS, TSC, and DDS prolonged the median survival time. The results with combined treatment which confirm the in-vitro data for multiple drug combinations are of great interest. The survival rates with 100 mg/kg/day DATC were markedly improved by the addition of 3 or 4 other drugs in low doses. 90%–100% of the animals survived after 3 months on combinations of daily 100 mg/kg DATC + 20 mg/kg SM + 20 mg/kg ETH + 10 mg/kg INH or 100 mg/kg DATC + 20 mg/kg SM + 10 mg/kg ETH + 20 mg/kg sulphamethoxypyrazine + 20 mg/kg demethylchlortetracycline.

OLITZKY et al. (1968) infected mice intraperitoneally. Treatment was started 50 days later with subtoxic doses by the subcutaneous route for about 2½ weeks, and was evaluated by histopathology and quantitative cultures from organs. Streptovaricin C in a dose of 250 mg/kg/day had a marked effect. Some activity was reported for bluensomycin, spectinomycin, lincomycin, and kanamycin.

The activity of DATC in dust-exposed guinea pigs was tested by TACQUET et al. (1970). 150 mg/day were given to each animal. The results were judged by the mortality rate, body weight, tuberculin allergy, radiological, anatomical and histological indices, and by the counts of culturable bacilli from the lungs. It was concluded that DATC was more effective than INH, ETH, and EMB, tested in earlier experiments. Therapy was started immediately or 30 days after the infection and lasted for 30 days or 60 days.

Using a similar experimental design to that adopted by ROSENFELD (1968), YOSHIDA (1970) studied the efficacy of RMP alone and in various combinations. Taking the survival time as the criterion, RMP showed a clear dose-response correlation for the doses tested (5 mg/kg to 50 mg/kg). In monotherapy, the survival time after 110 days was highest (65%) with RMP 50 mg/kg, followed by 20 mg/kg RMP (55%), 100 mg/kg DATC (40%), 10 mg/kg RMP (30%), and 5 mg/kg RMP (0%). In the same experiment a combination of daily 100 mg/kg DATC + 5 mg/kg INH + 10 mg/kg ETH + 20 mg/kg SM was the most effective treatment giving a survival rate of 80%. Further studies showed that double combinations of 10 mg/kg RMP per day with 100 mg/kg DATC, 20 mg/kg CS, 5 mg/kg INH, 20 mg/kg SM, 25 mg/kg EMB, 10 mg/kg ETH, or 20 mg/kg sulphamethoxypyrazine did not reach the activity of 20 mg/kg RMP alone, except for the combination with SM.

In the review by BURJANOVÁ and URBANCIK (1970) some unpublished experiments by BURJANOVÁ are mentioned that demonstrate a limited activity of EMB and a good activity of clofazimine.

SHRONTS et al. (1971) carried out a series of experiments on intravenously-infected mice. As measured by viable counts from the kidneys, a clear dose-response relationship was found for RMP applied with the feed in doses of 10 mg/kg/day, 20 mg/kg/day, 40 mg/kg/day and 100 mg/kg/day. In an experiment with start of the treatment 10 days after the infection the animals were treated for 49 days with INH 25 mg/kg or RMP 25 mg/kg, 125 mg/kg EMB, or 25 mg/kg INH + 25 mg/kg RMP. Treatment with RMP or EMB reduced the mortality, whilst INH alone did not. Viable counts from the kidneys were not influenced by INH or EMB, but were slightly reduced by RMP. The combination of RMP + INH was obviously not more effective. In a third experiment higher doses were given for 45 days. RMP in a dose of 40 mg/kg/day clearly reduced the viable counts in the kidneys. This effect was surpassed by the combination of 40 mg/kg RMP with 250 mg/kg INH and 40 mg/kg RMP + 250 mg/kg INH + 125 mg/kg ETH, all drugs being mixed in with the feed. However, the activity of 100 mg/kg RMP alone was higher than that of the combinations. The best effects were achieved with the combination of 40 mg/kg RMP + 125 mg/kg SM; addition of INH gave no improvement.

The most extensive experiments on single drugs and their combinations were published by BURJANOVÁ and DORNETZHUBER (1975). Treatment of the intravenously-infected mice was started 10 days after the infection for 30 days and was evaluated by viable counts from the lungs as the main criterion. All orally applicable drugs were mixed in with the feed. The daily doses calculated in mg/kg were as follows: INH 12, ETH 60, TSC 120, PAS 600, PZA 120, RMP 30 and 120, EMB 180, SM 60, KM 180, VM 180, CM 30, and clofazimine 12. INH was combined with a number of these drugs and also with DATC (100 mg/kg). No protective effect was observed for INH, PAS, ETH, TSC, CM, for combinations of INH + ETH or PZA or TSC, or for combinations of ETH with DATC and ETH + DATC + PZA. A weak activity was noted for SM, VM, and KM, a good one for RMP, EMB, and clofazimine. Addition of INH or SM to RMP did not improve the results. RMP + DATC or EMB were marginally better than RMP alone. The activity of RMP + DATC was excellent, but was still surpassed by RMP + DATC + EMB.

The results of all the animal experiments outlined above are categorized in Table 3. Like the in-vitro data, they favor multiple drug regimens. To what extent they are actually indicative for the therapy of human infections remains an open question, and this mainly for two reasons. In the first place, long-term treatment has not been carried out, as in experiments with *M. tuberculosis*, and secondly, one of the most effective drugs, namely DATC, has only a weak activity on *M. tuberculosis* in human patients despite its effectiveness in vitro and in smaller laboratory animals against the microorganism.

d) Treatment of *M. Kansasii* Infections in Man

In cervical adenitis chemotherapy is only an adjunct to surgical intervention (for a review see LINCOLN and GILBERT 1972). This topic is therefore excluded from

Table 3. Classification of the activity of drugs and regimens in animal experiments with *M. kansasii*

Drugs	Activity		
	Zero or very weak	Weak to moderate	Good or better
Antituberculotics	PAS TSC CS PZA	INH EMB SM VM KM	DACT RMP Combinations: RMP+DACT RMP+DACT+EMB RMP+SM DACT+ETH+SM+sulphonamide or INH
Other antimicrobial drugs	Sulphadiazine DDS	Bluensomycin Lincomycin	Streptovaricin C Clofazimine

further discussion, which deals mainly with pulmonary disease. In most of these cases, the first diagnosis is tuberculosis, and treatment is therefore started with antituberculotics. Consequently, the earlier reports deal mainly with the effect of the classical drugs used in combination: INH + PAS and/or SM. Later EMB and RMP were added, replaced PAS and sometimes SM.

The results achieved over the years are condensed in Table 4. The efficacy of all those regimens that did not include RMP was considerably lower in infections due to *M. kansasii* than in those due to *M. tuberculosis*. This is reflected by the relatively low conversion rates even after two years of treatment – despite persistent sensitivity of the bacilli, by the very low rates of cavity closure, the high proportions of patients with active status at 12 months or 24 months, and the large percentages of surgical interventions. The main reason for the unsatisfactory effectiveness of these regimens is certainly the partial or complete resistance to INH, SM, and PAS. It was shown by JOHANSON and NICHOLSON (1969) that the sputum conversion, cavity closure, rate of return to work, and the rate of relapses were all better, with statistical significance, if at least half of the bacterial population had been inhibited by 1 mg INH/l. PEZZIA et al. (1981) did not find any correlation between susceptibility to INH and the conversion rate, but they compared the rates after a duration of treatment at which the maximum of conversions had obviously nearly been reached. Comparisons at earlier dates might have revealed differences, as AHN et al. (1981) have observed in their patients (cf. Fig. 2 of their paper). After 3 months of therapy about 35% of the patients were still positive if the bulk of the bacterial population was resistant to 1 mg INH/l. In contrast, only 7% or 8% were still positive if at least a part of the bacteria was sensitive to this concentration. After 6 months the difference became much smaller: about 15% vs. 4%. For streptomycin, JOHANSON and NICHOLSON (1969) did not observe any correlation between the sputum conversion and the degree of susceptibility, but the number of patients treated by this drug was rather small and the duration of treatment was in many cases less than 2 months. PEZZIA et al. (1981) found that

Table 4. Clinical efficacy of antituberculosis drugs in pulmonary infections due to *M. kansasii*

Authors	No. of patients[1]	Medical treatment	Improved on X-ray %	Sputum conversion %	Cavity closure %	Still active %	Relapse %	With surgery %
WOOD et al. (1956)	17	INH + SM and/or PAS	44			20		35
LESTER et al. (1958)	49	INH + SM and/or PAS		24 (12)[2]; 88 (24) + S[3]		12 (24)		33
JENKINS et al. (1960)	61	INH + SM and/or PAS, additional drugs in 61%		60 (12); 66 (24)	25,5 (24)	15	8	54
KASS and DYE (1962)	12	ETH + VM		92				42
PFUETZE et al. (1965)	152	INH + SM and/or PAS, additional drugs in 18%		81			<10	37,5
ZVETINA (1965)	15	INH + SM or PAS		58 (12); 33 (24)		47 (12–24)	14	20
KETTEL (1965)	12	INH + SM or PAS	70	33 (12)	0 (12)			0
ZVETINA (1966)	122	INH + SM or PAS, additional drugs in 43%	51	72 (12) + S	18 (24)	35 (24) + S	10 + S	20
JOHANSON and NICHOLSON (1969)	91	Various combinations, mostly INH, SM, ETH	90	85 (≧12)	64.5 (≧12)	≧27 (≧12)	13 (≧12)	25
RAUSCHER et al. (1974)	33	INH + SM + PAS in 70%, EMB in 51%, ETH in 30%, PZA and RMP in 10%		84 (15)			0	12
HARRIS et al. (1975)	35	INH + SM + EMB, in some pat. additional drugs, but no RMP		74 (18)			0	2
DAVIDSON (1976b)	27	INH + SM + RMP, in some pat. additional drugs		100 (18) + S			1, 5 (58) + S	12
AHN et al. (1981)	256	INH + EMB(+SM) + RMP		100 (4)			0 (+RMP) 7 (−RMP)	3
PEZZIA et al. (1981)	158	INH + 1 other drug ($n = 63$) INH + 2 other drugs ($n = 63$) Regimens incl. RMP ($n = 32$)		78 (6) 85 (6) 93 (6)			12	31

Table 4 (continued)

Authors	No. of pa- tients[1]	Medical treatment	Im- proved on X-ray %	Sputum con- %	Cavity closure %	Still active %	Relapse %	With surgery %
BENJAMIN and SPAGNOLO (1982)	20	All RMP, most + INH + EMB		100 (7)			0 (1–24)	
AHN et al. (1983)	40[4]	INH + RMP + EMB for 12 m; + SM twice weekly for 3 m		100 (3)			2,5 (31)	0
BANKS et al. (1983b)	33	RMP + EMB in 21 pat.; + a third drug in 12		100	80 (≧12)		0 (66)	
GONZÁLES-MONTANER et al. (1983)	13	RMP + EMB (+ other?)		90 (2)				

1, number eligible for evaluation; 2, in brackets: months of treatment; 3, + *S:* operated patients included; 4, all cases cooperative initial treatment patients.

high degrees of SM resistance had an adverse influence on the sputum conversion. Whereas ETH did not contribute to the clinical efficacy of chemotherapy according to JOHANSON and NICHOLSON (1969), EMB was a step forward expressed mainly by a reduction in the incidence of surgery. A truly dramatic improvement was achieved with the introduction of RMP, first reported by DAVIDSON et al. (1972) with the short statement of 12 successes in 13 patients treated with RMP in combination with other drugs. The effectiveness of RMP in the initial treatment and repeated treatment of a larger number of patients was clearly shown by HARRIS et al. (1975), AHN et al. (1981), and PEZZIA et al. (1981). In the series of HARRIS et al. (1975) 85% converted without RMP on the initial treatment and 62% on repeated treatment; with regimens including RMP 100% became negative on first and repeated treatment. PEZZIA et al. (1981) observed sputum conversion after 6 months on regimens without RMP in 81.5% of the cases and in 93% with RMP. In consequence of the improved efficacy of treatment provided by EMB and RMP, the degree of INH sensitivity of the bacilli no longer influenced the conversion rate (HARRIS et al. 1975; AHN et al. 1981). The high activity of RMP is further reflected by the development of secondary resistance not only on monotherapy (DAVIDSON and WAGGONER 1976) but also during combined treatment (PEZZIA et al. 1981). This emphasizes the necessity of combined therapy. AHN et al. (1981) analyzed the time required for conversion by treatment with RMP in various combinations. Their data are shown in Table 5. It will be evident that RMP + INH in combination with EMB are more active than in combination with SM or with other drugs. The quadruple regimen consisting of RMP + INH + EMB + SM seems to be a little superior to the triple regimens. Sputum conversion could be obtained in *M. kansasii* infections with practically the same speed as in *M. tuberculosis* infections. SCHRAUFNAGEL et al. (1984), however, observed even with RMP containing regimens, a slower bacteriological and radiological improvement in patients with *M. kansasii* infection. Data on long-term results and on the optimal duration of treatment are rare. For these reasons, an Adhoc Committee of the American Thoracic Society (BAILEY et al. 1983) still recommended a treatment duration of 18 months to 24 months. But in the same year, AHN et al. (1983) showed that a triple drug regimen consisting of INH + RMP +

Table 5. Time required for the conversion of sputum from positive to negative after treatment with rifampicin in combination with various drugs for infections due to *Mycobacterium kansasii*. (After AHN et al. 1981)

Drugs	Initial treatment		Repeated treatment	
	No. of patients	Average no. of weeks to conversion	No. of patients	Average no. of weeks to conversion
RMP+INH+EMB+SM	52	6,5	10	7,3
RMP+INH+EMB	25	6,9	5	8,5
RMP+INH+SM	5	7,5	4	8,5
Other RMP combinations	10	7,3	4	8,0
Total	92		23	

EMB for 12 months intensified in the first 3 months by SM twice weekly, produced sputum conversion in all 40 cooperative patients treated for the first time, with a relapse rate of 2.5% during an average follow up period of 31 months. In the compromised host infected with *M. kansasii* treatment is even more difficult. It may be successful (FRASER et al. 1975) or it may fail (MCGEADY and MURPHEY 1981). Here too regimens including RMP offer a better chance of survival than regimens without RMP (MCGEADY and MURPHEY 1981).

2. *M. Marinum (M. Balnei)*

M. marinum was first isolated from human patients in 1949 on the occasion of an epidemic outbreak of skin disease (HERLITZ et al. 1951). The contaminated water of a municipal swimming pool was traced as the source of the infection. Later, reports came in from different parts of the world. Infections occurred when superficial lesions came into contact with contaminated water from swimming pools, fish tanks, ocean beaches, lakes, and rivers. The lesions are usually confined to the skin – due to the low temperature optimum of *M. marinum* – but may also spread to deeper structures of the legs. Spontaneous healing occurs after 3 months to 3 years, but cases have been reported in which the lesions had persisted for decades (KELLY 1976).

a) Activity of Antituberculosis Drugs in Vitro

Resistance to INH, PAS, and TSC and moderate sensitivity to SM was noted by the first reporters and confirmed in all subsequent papers. Most strains of the species are sensitive to RMP, EMB, CS, KM, ansamycin and – quite unusually – for PZA, moderately sensitive to VM (RYNEARSON et al. 1971; SCHRÖDER 1973; VAN DYKE and LAKE 1975; SILCOX and DAVID 1971; YATES and COLLINS 1981; HEIFETS and ISEMAN 1985). The majority of strains is sensitive to the tetracyclines; there are no clear differences in activity between tetracycline, doxycycline, and minocycline (TORRES et al. 1978; TSUKAMURA 1980a, b; SANDERS and WOLINSKY 1980; WALLACE et al. 1981 b; STONE et al. 1983).

b) Activity of Other Antimicrobial Agents in Vitro

For cephradine more strains were found to be sensitive than resistant, but for the other cephalosporins like cefazolin or cefoxitin the strains were resistant (GARCIA-RODRÍGUEZ and MARTIN-LUENGO 1980). HAAS et al. (1982) reported sensitivity to cefoxitin as well as to cephaloridine, cephalexin and cefuroxime. Their strains were highly resistant to cefamandole and cefazolin. The species is resistant to the aminoglycosides gentamicin, sisomicin, tobramycin, and dibekacin, but sensitive to amikacin (MARTIN-LUENGO et al. 1978; SANDERS and WOLINSKY 1980; WALLACE et al. 1981 b; HAAS et al. 1982).

The majority of strains was reported as resistant to erythromycin (SANDERS and WOLINSKY 1980). Regarding cotrimoxazole, many authors observed sensitivity (FLOWERS 1970; BLACK and EYKYN 1977; STONE et al. 1983). EVEN-PAZ et al. (1976), however, judged their strains to be resistant, as did SANDERS and WOLINSKY (1980). According to WALLACE et al. (1981 b) *M. marinum* is sensitive to the sulfamethoxazole component but resistant to trimethoprim. DEMOULIN et al. (1982) found most strains sensitive to sulfonamides. One strain of *M. marinum* was tested against clofazimine and found to be sensitive in vitro and in vivo (BANERJEE and HOLMES 1976). Two strains tested were sensitive to the new quinolone Ro 23-6240 (SALFINGER and KAFADER 1986).

c) Activity of Antituberculosis Drugs and Other Antimicrobial Agents in Animals

The appropriate model is the footpad infection in mice. LEACH and FENNER (1954) treated mice i.p. with about 75 mg/kg/day of SM, either from the day of the infection or beginning when early foot lesions were present, or at an advanced stage. The lesions could be favorably influenced by both early and delayed treatment.

PATTYN and ROYACKERS (1965) treated footpad-infected mice for 48 days from the day after the infection. The following drugs were administered with the diet: INH (0.02%), CS (0.2%), DDS (0.1%), and PAS (0.6%). SM (about 150 mg/kg) was injected s.c. 6 times a week. Lesions developed in all the animals treated with INH, PAS, and CS and in none treated with SM or DDS.

BANERJEE and HOLMES 1976, evaluated the therapeutic effect on the basis of viable counts from homogenized footpads. The drugs, RMP and clofazimine, were given with the feed from the day of the infection. RMP produced a certain bactericidal effect at the level of 0.03% in the diet, yielding serum concentrations of 7 mg/l–12 mg/l. Clofazimine needed a level of 0.1% in the diet in order to show an effect, which was assessed by the authors as small.

d) Treatment of M. *Marinum* Infections in Man

Over the last decade a number of papers have been published on the chemotherapy of human infections with and without additional surgery. Good effects have been obtained with EMB, in most cases combined with RMP, and with a combination of ETH + CS (WOLINSKY et al. 1972; WILLIAMS and RIORDAN 1973; VAN DYKE and LAKE 1975; BAILEY et al. 1982; RAZ et al. 1984). Tetracyclines have been used successfully either in the form of tetracycline, 1 g/day–2 g/day (KIM 1974; IZUMI et al. 1977) or as minocycline 0.2 g/day (LORIA 1976; LOCKSHIN 1977; CONTORER and JONES 1979). The lesions reacted promptly and healed within weeks or a few months. The same results were obtained with cotrimoxazole (BARROW and HEWITT 1971; TURNER et al. 1975; KELLY 1976; BLACK and EYKYN 1977; HUGH and COLEMAN 1981). Cotrimoxazole seems at the present time to be the treatment of choice. More chronic and/or extended cases may need prolonged treatment with RMP + EMB up to one year (HUGH and COLEMAN 1981; RAZ et al. 1984). Erythromycin and lincomycin did not give satisfactory results in a few cases treated (CORTEZ and PANKEY 1973; WILLIAMS and RIORDAN 1973).

3. *M. Simiae*

In 1965 KARASSEVA et al. reported the isolation of two new species, *M. simiae* and *M. asiaticum*, from monkeys. VALDIVIA and SUAREZ (1971) in Cuba described the isolation of a new species of mycobacteria, called *M. habana*, from patients with pulmonary disease. Later it was shown that *M. simiae* and *M. habana* are in fact identical (MEISSNER and SCHRÖDER 1975; WEISZFEILER and KARCZAG 1976). Meanwhile, patients with pulmonary disease due to *M. simiae* have been encountered outside Cuba (BOISVERT 1974; BELL et al. 1983). The information on drug sensitivity is scarce. In vitro, the strains were resistant to INH, SM, PAS, EMB, and RMP and probably sensitive to CS (PATTYN and DOMMISSE 1973; WEISZFEILER et al. 1981; BELL et al. 1983). The species seems to be resistant also to ansamycin (HEIFETS and ISEMAN 1985). In patients, combinations containing INH, SM, EMB and RMP proved to be ineffective (BELL et al. 1983).

4. *M. Asiaticum*

M. asiaticum was isolated for the first time from humans by BLACKLOCK et al. (1983) in Australia. Three patients were considered to have chronic secondary colonization of areas of damaged or poorly draining lung tissue. Two patients had progressive pulmonary cavitary disease with repeated isolation of *M. asiaticum*. Susceptibility studies by the resistance ratio method revealed that the five strains were sensitive to CS and ETH but resistant to INH, PAS, RMP and TSC. They differed in sensitivity to SM, EMB and CM. Treatment with antituberculosis drugs was given in both patients with progressive disease but could not be evaluated because bad cooperation made the results unreliable.

II. Group II. Scotochromogenic Mycobacteria

1. Introductory Remarks

Group II comprises the slowly growing mycobacteria that produce pigments when growing in the dark. In human pathology they are mostly found in superficial lymphadenitis. Cases of pulmonary disease have been described, and very few with disseminated diseases including osteomyelitis and meningitis (LINCOLN and GILBERT 1972). The group was differentiated into species mainly after 1965. The older literature deals only with the group as a whole. We therefore present the data separately first for the group and then for the various species. Epidemiological investigations have shown that the scotochromogenic species responsible for lymphadenitis is *M. scrofulaceum*. The species *M. xenopi* and *M. szulgai* have been found as causative agents of pulmonary disease, besides a few cases due to *M. scrofulaceum*. Except under unusual conditions, *M. gordonae* is apathogenic. One case of cavitary lung disease caused by *M. flavescens* has been reported (CASIMIR et al. 1982). *M. scrofulaceum* is considered by some investigators as a member of the *M. avium* complex, because pigmentation is a variable characteristic, but the biochemical reactions, surface antigens, and the drug sensitivity pattern are similar. The broader complex has been called *M. avium-intracellulare-scrofulaceum* (MAIS) complex.

2. Publications on Group II Without Identification of the Species

a) Activity of Antituberculosis Drugs in Vitro

The publications have been compiled in Table 6. Strains of the group are resistant to INH, PAS, and PZA. More strains are resistant than are sensitive to SM,

Table 6. Prevalence of sensitivity and resistance to antituberculosis drugs in scotochromogenic strains tested as a group. Relative prevalence of sensitivity (*S*) and resistance (*R*). The authors are coded numerically (see list below)

Drug	S	S>R	S≃R	R>S	R
INH					1, 3–10, 11, 13, 14
SM	2	7, 9		4–6, 8, 11, 13, 14	1, 3
PAS				6	1–4, 7–11, 14
RMP			12		
EMB				11, 13	
ETH		6, 8, 9, 13, 14		10	
TSC		9		6, 7	1, 5, 11
DACT					
CS	1	4, 6, 9, 11, 13, 14			3, 8
VM		11	1	4–6, 8, 13, 14	3
KM		5, 8, 9, 11			
CM		15			
PZA					1

[1] Wolinsky et al. (1957)
[2] Rogul et al. (1957)
[3] Urbančik (1959)
[4] Lewis et al. (1959)
[5] Virtanen (1961)
[6] Carruthers and Edwards (1965)
[7] Mulder-de Jong (1964)
[8] Wichelhausen and Robinson (1965)
[9] Yamamoto et al. (1967)
[10] Pattyn et al. (1968)
[11] Meissner (1968)
[12] McClatchy et al. (1969)
[13] Edwards (1969)
[14] Burjanová (1970)
[15] Havel and Šimonová (1970)

EMB, TSC, and VM. About 50% are sensitive to RMP. Sensitivity is found for ETH, CS, KM, and CM.

b) Activity of Other Antimicrobial Agents in Vitro

The data are not really representative, because some publications deal only with a few strains. Sensitivity to DDS has been reported by Pattyn and van Ermengem (1968). More strains were sensitive than were resistant to erythromycin (Virtanen 1961; Yamamoto et al. 1967) and sulphonamides (Lewis et al. 1959; Virtanen 1961). Yamamoto et al. (1967), however, reported a preponderance of resistance to sulphisoxazole. Resistance pre-dominated for chloramphenicol, tetracyclines (Lewis et al. 1959; Virtanen 1961; Yamamoto et al. 1967), oleandomycin (Lewis et al. 1959; Virtanen 1961), and penicillin (Rogul et al. 1957). The group was found to be resistant to lincomycin (Olitzki et al. 1967).

c) Activity of Drugs in Animal Experiments

There is only one report by Sakamoto and Goda (1966). The authors tried EMB without any success (cited from Burjanová and Urbancik 1970).

d) Treatment of Group II Infections in Man

Therapy of adenitis is not considered, because the treatment is mainly surgical. Lewis et al. (1959) reported on 14 cases with pulmonary disease. 11 were made inactive by INH + PAS, sometimes also with SM and/or other drugs.

Wolinsky (1963) observed 4 patients with cavitary lung disease. One was treated by SM + PAS, the others by INH + SM (+ PAS in 2 cases). All failed to close the cavity and required surgery. Relapses occurred in 2 of them after 2 years. The other 2 patients were well after 4 years and 5 years.

Pulmonary disease was treated in 7 cases by Carruthers and Edwards (1965). 5 were treated with INH, SM and/or PAS: 4 became negative on culture, one patient required additional antituberculotics, and the last also surgery. All improved on X-rays.

The largest series, comprising 22 patients, was reported by Yamamoto et al. (1967). In 10 surgical measures were applied. The type of the antituberculosis treatment is not specified. After 6 months 45% were negative on culture and 32% had improved on X-rays. 12 patients (7 of them operated) had a follow-up of 3 years. 9 patients were considered as cured and 3 as improved. The authors also observed 4 cases of meningitis: all 4 were cured.

3. Infections by *M. Flavescens*

Chronic cavitary lung infection was observed by Casimir et al. (1982) in a patient with melanoma. The organisms were sensitive to RMP. Triple drug treatment with INH + RMP + EMB improved symptoms and led to sputum conversion by culture.

Table 7. Prevalence of sensitivity and resistance to antituberculosis drugs in *M. gordonae* and *M. scrofulaeceum*. Relative prevalence of sensitivity (*S*) and resistance (*R*). The authors are coded numerically (see list below)

Drug	Sensitivity pattern of	
	M. gordonae	M. scrofulaceum
PAS	R > S (9); R (4)	R (1, 4, 8, 10, 11)
SM	S > R (9); R (8)	S (1); S > R (10); S ≃ R (11); R (8)
TSC	R (8)	S (8); R > S (1)
PZA	R (3)	R (11)
INH	R (4, 8, 9)	R (1, 4, 8, 11)
VM	S ≃ R (9)	S > R (1, 10)
CS	S > R (9)	S (8); S > R (1); S ≃ R (10)
ETH	S > R (9)	S ≃ R (10)
KM	S ≃ R (9)	S > R (10)
DACT	–	–
CM	S ≃ R (9)	R (5)
EMB	S (2); S > R (9); R (8)	S (10); R > S (5, 11)
RMP	S (7); S > R (6, 9)	S (10); S > R (7); S ≃ R (5, 6, 11)

[1] Manten (1959)
[2] Tacquet and Tison (1963)
[3] Stottmeier (1964)
[4] Kestle et al. (1967)
[5] Schröder et al. (1969)
[6] Rynearson et al. (1971)
[7] Molavi and Weinstein (1971a)
[8] Schröder (1973)
[9] Jakschik (1979)
[10] Kuze et al. (1981)
[11] De Kantor et al. (1985)

4. Infections by *M. Gordonae*

(previously *M. aquae*, "tap water" bacillus)

a) Activity of Antituberculosis Drugs in Vitro

The sensitivity pattern is described in Table 7. The rifampicin derivative ansamycin has an activity equal to RMP (HEIFETS and ISEMAN 1985).

b) Activity of Other Antimicrobial Agents in Vitro

The strains seem fairly sensitive to minocycline (TSUKAMURA 1980). For erythromycin, more are sensitive than are resistant (MOLAVI and WEINSTEIN 1971 b).

c) Treatment of *M. Gordonae* Infections in Man

Too few cases have been reported for any conclusions to be drawn. A case of chronic olecranon bursitis was described by LORBER and SUH (1983). The man was treated with INH + RMP to which the organisms were judged as sensitive. After one year the elbow had healed with a small scar.

5. Infections by *M. Scrofulaceum* (Formerly *M. Marianum, M. Paraffinicum*)

a) Activity of Antituberculosis Drugs in Vitro

The data have been compiled in Table 7. Comparison of the sensitivity patterns for the whole group and for *M. gordonae* and *M. scrofulaceum* (see Tables 6 and 7) does not disclose any differences that would exceed technical variations. From the sensitivity tests one could expect the best results for both species after treatment with regimens including RMP, CS, ETH, KM, and VM.

b) Activity of Other Antituberculosis Agents in Vitro

The majority of strains is sensitive to sulfonamides, and all were so to DDS (DEMOULIN et al. 1982; DE KANTOR et al. 1985). The species is resistant against clofazimine according to DE KANTOR et al. 1985, but sensitive according to DAMLE et al. 1978. A varying percentage is sensitive to erythromycin (GUY and CHAPMAN 1961; MOLAVI and WEINSTEIN 1971 b; DE KANTOR et al. 1985). For minocycline the sensitivity is somewhat lower than that of *M. tuberculosis* (TSUKAMURA 1980 a, b). To tetracycline most strains were resistant (GUY and CHAPMAN 1961; DE KANTOR et al. 1985), as they were to the aminoclycosides (GANGADHARAM and CANDLER 1977 a; MARTIN-LUENGO et al. 1978; DE KANTOR et al. 1985) and to cephalosporins (GARCIA-RODRÍGUEZ and MARTIN-LUENGO 1980; DE KANTOR et al. 1985). SAKURAI (1983), however, observed a good activity of several compounds like cephalothin or cefazolin. The new quinolone Ro 23-6240 had a MIC of 0.5 mg/l (SALFINGER and KAFADER 1986).

c) Activity of Drugs in Animal Experiments

Nothing known.

d) Treatment of *M. Scrofulaceum* Infections in Man

Except for reports on isolated cases in immunocompromised hosts (e.g., McNUTT and FUDENBERG 1971), no information is available on the chemotherapy of pulmonary or disseminated diseases due to this species. As has already been pointed out, chemotherapy in superficial lymphadenitis is disappointing. Cures were obtained by antituberculosis drug regimens with or without incision in 1 of 29 children, infected by Group-II or Group-III organisms, but in over 90% by excision, a percentage not improved by the additional drug therapy (McKELLAR 1976).

6. Infections due to *M. Szulgai*

DAVIDSON (1976a) has reviewed all 13 cases known that have been caused by this scotochromogenic species; 10 had a pulmonary disease, 2 olecranon bursitis, and 1 cervical adenitis. In vitro, using *M. tuberculosis* as the reference, the strains are resistant to INH, PAS, CS, and TSC and/or moderately sensitive to SM, CM, VM, RMP, EMB, and ETH (MARKS et al. 1972; SCHAEFER et al. 1973). YATES and COLLINS (1981), however, found two of two strains highly resistant to RMP and EMB. About a third of the strains investigated by DEMOULIN et al. (1982) were sensitive to sulphonamides. HAAS et al. (1982) tested 3 strains and found them sensitive to some cephalosporins, especially to cefoxitin, and to amikacin. According to DAVIDSON (1976a), the best treatment appears to be a three-drug regimen consisting of RMP + INH + EMB. The parenteral drugs (SM, CM, or VM) should be used as a fourth or substitute drug. An additional case in Australia was described by POCZA (1981). The patient, an alcoholic and heavy smoker, had pulmonary cavitary disease. Response to treatment with RMP + INH + EMB and temporarily + PTH or CM was poor, probably because of irregular drug taking.

7. Infections due to *M. Xenopi* (Formerly *M. Littorale, M. Xenopei*)

This microorganism, with a temperature optimum of about 43 °C, is grouped by some authors among the non-chromogenic Group III because the pigment production starts late. Pulmonary infections caused in man by this opportunist mycobacterium were first described by MARKS and SCHWABACHER in 1965. Nosocomial pulmonary infections related to the hospital water system were reported by COSTRINI et al. (1981).

a) Activity of Antituberculosis Drugs and Other Antimicrobial Agents in Vitro

Among the MOTT this species is relatively sensitive to antituberculotics. The strains are usually sensitive to CS and CM. In larger series, most of the strains were sensitive to SM, EMB, ETH and KM; more were sensitive than were resistant to PAS, RMP, ansamycin and VM. At least 50% were inhibited by 0.2 mg/l INH, i.e., they were fully sensitive (MEISSNER 1970; JAKSCHIK 1979). *M. xenopi* seems to be resistant to TSC and PZA (ENGBAEK et al. 1967), DDS (PATTYN and VAN ERMENGEM 1968) and cephalosporins (GARCIA-RODRÍGUEZ and MARTIN-LUENGO 1980), but sensitive to various aminoglycosides and related compounds like sisomicin, tobramycin, and amikacin (MARTIN-LUENGO et al. 1978). About two third of the strains tested by DEMOULIN et al. (1982) were sensitive to sulphonamides. The new quinolone Ro 23-6240 had a MIC of 0.5 mg/l (SALFINGER and KAFADER 1986).

b) Treatment of *M. Xenopi* Infections in Man

In human clinical practice the outcome is not predictable, and not clearly related to the chemotherapy applied, even if treatment is guided by the results of sensitivity tests (ENGBAEK et al. 1967; MEISSNER et al. 1970; THIBIER et al. 1970; MCDONALD et al. 1971; ELSTON and DUFFY 1973; TELLIS et al. 1977; COSTRINI et al. 1981; BOGAERTS et al. 1982; SMITH and CITRON 1983; BANKS et al. 1984). Development of secondary resistance has been observed (MCDONALD et al. 1971). Multiple drug regimens are therefore recommended, for a period of 18 months–24 months (SMITH and CITRON 1983). The best regimen appeared to be INH + RMP + either SM or EMB (BANKS et al. 1984). But failure and relapse rates were high. Only 23% of patients were considered as cured by chemotherapy alone. Since several patients were cured by resection the authors suggest that operation might be part of first line treatment.

III. Group III

1. *M. Avium* Complex (Including *M. Avium* and *M. Intracellulare*, Formerly also "Battey-Bacillus")

a) Introductory Remarks

The species *M. avium and M. intracellulare* cannot be separated by common laboratory procedures. They are separable by serological typing, pathogenicity tests in animals, and skin sensitins. In most papers the two species have not been differentiated. Unless the species has been explicitly stated, our data refer to the complex. Besides superficial lymphadenitis and rare disseminated disease which occurs mainly in immunocompromised patients, these organisms can cause chronic, indolent, often cavitary pulmonary disease, especially in persons with a reduced local or systemic resistance. If untreated, the disease usually deteriorates (HUNTER et al. 1981), and a comparison of the treatment results in *M. kansasii* and *M. avium* complex infections shows that both early and late results are worse in infections due to *M. avium* complex. As has already been mentioned in Section B, strains of the *M. avium* complex produce two types of cells with different drug sensitivity. According to MOULDING (1978), most of the available evidence suggests that the most sensitive opaque forms do not occur in vivo and, consequently, that their relative drug susceptibility has nothing to do with therapeutic success. However, Moulding was able to show that in vitro subinhibitory concentrations of RMP, EMB, and ETH produced a morphological shift in the direction of the opaque forms. This would constitute an example of sensitization and could in part explain the effectiveness of chemotherapy despite drug resistance. Another technique that has been discussed for "resensitisation" by GLASSER (1978) is additional application of dimethyl sulphoxide (DMSO). Several authors have found that in vitro DMSO can reduce the resistance to antituberculotics in *M. tubercu-*

losis and also in strains of the *M. avium* complex (NASH and STEINGRUBE 1982). The concentrations of DMSO tried were 5% and 2.5%. As 1% of DMSO already has a growth-retarding effect, it must be questioned whether the reduced MIC in the presence of 2.5% or 5% DMSO is not simply an expression of the intrinsic bacteriostatic activity of this substance instead of an amplifying mechanism, e.g., by increasing the permeability barrier to drugs as in the case of Tween 80.

b) Activity of Antituberculosis Drugs in Vitro

The data are presented in Table 8, which shows in comparison to Table 2 that the *M. avium* complex is more resistant to all antituberculosis drugs than is *M. kansasii*. The difference is slight for PAS and PZA, a little larger for SM, VM, KM, CM, and INH, and marked for RMP, EMB, ETH, TSC, DATC, and CS.

Table 8. Prevalence of sensitivity and resistance to antituberculosis drugs in the *M. avium* complex. Relative prevalence of sensitivity (*S*) and resistance (*R*). The authors are coded numerically (see list below)

Drug	S	S < R	S ≃ R	R > S	R
PAS				14	1–7, 9, 12, 13, 18–23, 25, 26
SM			7	1–4, 6, 8, 12, 14, 22	5, 12, 13, 18, 19, 20, 21, 23, 25, 26
TSC				4, 7, 14, 23, 25	2, 3, 5, 12, 13, 18, 26
PZA					1, 13, 21, 23, 25
INH					1–8, 9, 12, 13, 18–23, 25, 26
KM		2, 3, 22		6, 19, 20, 25	8, 13, 21
CS	1, 18, 25	5, 7, 20, 23	12	6, 8, 13, 19, 21, 22	26
ETH	7	12		6, 8, 13, 14, 19–23, 25	5
VM				5, 6, 20, 22	8, 13, 19, 25
DATC				25	13
CM				15, 20	6, 8, 10, 19, 21, 23–26
EMB				12, 19, 20, 22, 25	10, 13, 18, 21, 23–24, 26
RMP		17, 22		16, 20, 21	10, 11, 18, 19, 23–26

[1] WOLINSKY et al. (1957)
[2] LEWIS et al. (1960)
[3] VIRTANEN (1961)
[4] MULDER DE JONG (1964)
[5] CARRUTHERS and EDWARDS (1965)
[6] WICHELHAUSEN and ROBINSON (1965)
[7] YAMAMOTO et al. (1967)
[8] HOBBY et al. (1967)
[9] KESTLE et al. (1967)
[10] SCHRÖDER et al. (1969)
[11] MC CLATCHY et al. (1969)
[12] EDWARDS (1969)
[13] MEISSNER (1970)
[14] BURJANOVÁ (1970)
[15] HAVEL and ŠIMONOVÁ (1970)
[16] RYNEARSON et al. (1971)
[17] MOLAVI and WEINSTEIN (1971a)
[18] SCHRÖDER (1973)
[19] DUTT and STEAD (1979)
[20] JAKSCHIK (1979)
[21] DAVIDSON (1981)
[22] KUZE et al. (1981)
[23] ENGBAEK et al. (1981)
[24] YATES and COLLINS (1981)
[25] HEJNÝ (1982)
[26] GREENE et al. (1982)

Some reports on the testing of drug combinations have been published. STOTTMEIER et al. (1968) used an in-vitro model simulating the serum pharmacokinetics. These authors studied combinations of INH, erythromycin, oxacillin, and methenamine. Two-drug combinations delayed growth, three-drug combinations maintained the numbers of bacilli at the original level. Bactericidal effects were obtained only by triple-drug combinations with concentrations above the therapeutic levels. The best results were obtained by continuous exposure to triple-drug combinations even in low concentrations, which had a marked bactericidal efficacy.

KUZE et al. (1981) tested 13 strains of *M. intracellulare*. The effectiveness of various triple-drug combinations (each drug in a final concentration of 0.2 mg/l) was compared to the activity of the single drugs. Under the experimental conditions chosen, the lowest MIC for 50% of the microorganisms (MIC_{50}) was that of RMP, being surpassed only by the combinations of RMP + ETH + VM and RMP + EMB + KM. With regard to the MIC_{100}, all the combinations tested were better than any single drug. The order of decreasing activity was RMP + ETH + VM = RMP + EMB + KM > INH + RMP + EMB = INH + SM + EMB > INH + RMP + CS = INH + EMB + KM > INH + SM + PAS > INH + ETH + KM.

HEIFETS (1982) investigated 3 strains of *M. intracellulare* by a technique adjusted to statistical treatment by the combined use of probit analysis and isobologram methods. The clearest results were obtained by plotting the bacteriostatic concentrations for 75% of the bacterial population with their confidence limits on the isobolograms. The drugs investigated were RMP, SM, EMB, and ETH. The double combinations RMP + EMB, RMP + SM, EMB + SM, and EMB + ETH showed little or no synergistic effect, in contrast to the combinations of ETH + RMP and ETH + SM. Of the various triple combinations tested, ETH + EMB + SM was purely additive, whereas RMP + SM, followed by RMP + SM + EMB, acted synergistically. No antagonism was observed.

ZIMMER et al. (1982) compared for 49 clinical isolates of the *M. avium* complex the MIC's of INH, RMP, EMB, SM, and KM with those produced by various double combinations in which a quarter of the respective MIC's was applied. Judging from the percentage of strains for which synergy was exhibited at therapeutically relevant MIC's, the activity order of the combinations was as follows: RMP + EMB > SM + EMB > INH + SM = INH + RMP = EMB + KM > RMP + KM > INH + KM. Practically no synergism was observed with INH + EMB. There is no mention of antagonisms.

ISEMAN et al. (1986) studied 90 isolates which were resistant singly to INH, RMP or EMB; 63% were inhibited by these drugs combined. Of 59 isolates with mono-resistance to RMP or EMB 53% were inhibited by the combination of both drugs. In a model simulating the serum kinetics of RMP and EMB in man the combination effect was clearly shown to correlate with the static in vitro inhibition.

Ansamycin (LM 427) is a spiro-piperidyl derivative of rifamycin S which has a special high activity against the *M. avium* complex. The MIC is 2 mg/l for over 90% of the strains (GREENE et al. 1982; WOODLEY and KILBURN 1982; HAWKINS et al. 1984; HEIFETS and ISEMAN 1985). The results obtained by PERUMAL et al.

1985 with the just mentioned pharmacokinetic model are difficult to evaluate because the arbitrarly chosen peak concentration differs widely from that reported for human beings (HEIFETS and ISEMAN 1985).

The sensitivity pattern of *M. avium* has been compared with that of *M. intracellulare* by MEISSNER (1970). Fewer strains of *M. avium* were sensitive to ETH, KM, and EMB, whereas slightly more strains were sensitive to CS. For each of the following drugs the resistance tended to be slightly (but not significantly) higher in *M. avium:* INH, SM, PAS, and TSC.

c) Activity of Other Antimicrobial Agents in Vitro

Resistance to DDS was reported by GANGADHARAM and CANDLER (1977b), whereas DE KANTOR et al. (1985) evaluated the species as sensitive. More than half of the strains are sensitive to clofazimine (EDWARDS 1969; GANGADHARAM and CANDLER 1977b; DAMLE et al. 1978; KUZE et al. 1981; GREENE et al. 1982). Depending on the technique used, the in vitro action was slowly bactericidal or only bacteriostatic (GANGADHARAM et al. 1981). DE KANTOR et al. (1985) considered *M. avium* as resistant to clofazimine. At least half of the strains are sensitive to erythromycin (GUY and CHAPMAN 1961; VIRTANEN 1961; YAMAMOTO et al. 1967; HEJNÝ 1982). Regarding the other macrolides, HEJNÝ (1982) reported that more than half of the strains were sensitive to spiramycin and about half to lincomycin. DE KANTOR et al. (1985) found more strains resistant than sensitive to erythromycin, lincomycin and spiramycin. The majority of strains was sensitive to higher, but therapeutically achievable, concentrations of penicillin G and ampicillin in the experiments of KUZE et al. (1981). This is not very compatible with the reports on resistance to cephalosporins (GARCIA-RODRÍGUEZ and MARTIN-LUENGO 1980; SANDERS et al. 1980; HAAS et al. 1982; DE KANTOR et al. 1985). Some of the third generation cephems have a good activity on extracellular bacilli; however, even the best like cefotaxime or ceftizoxime were practically ineffective against bacilli located in monocytes (NOZAWA et al. 1985). The data of SAKURAI (1983) suggest geographic differences in sensitivity to cephalosporins. There is a general consensus that most, if not all, of the strains are resistant to chloramphenicol (WOLINSKY et al. 1957; LEWIS et al. 1959; GUY and CHAPMAN 1961; VIRTANEN 1961; YAMAMOTO et al. 1967) and to the aminoglycosides (GANGADHARAM and CANDLER 1977a; MARTIN-LUENGO et al. 1978). Half or more of the strains were reported to be resistant to tetracyclines (WOLINSKY et al. 1957; LEWIS et al. 1959; GUY and CHAPMAN 1961; YAMAMOTO et al. 1967; HEJNÝ 1982). TSUKAMURA (1980a, b) tested 10 strains of *M. intracellulare* and 5 strains of *M. avium* against minocycline. All the *M. intracellulare* strains were at least as sensitive as *M. tuberculosis,* whereas 3 of the 5 *M. avium* strains were highly resistant. This corresponds to the higher resistance of *M. avium* to antituberculosis drugs. With regard to sulphonamides, three authors found the majority of the strains to be sensitive (VIRTANEN 1961; HEJNÝ 1982; DE KANTOR et al. 1985), whilst others reported most of the strains to be resistant (LEWIS et al. 1959; LEWIS et al. 1960; YAMAMOTO et al. 1967; DEMOULIN et al. 1982). ENGBAEK et al. (1981) observed sensitivity to co-trimoxazole. For the aminoglycosides the results differ (NAITO et al. 1979; SANDERS et al. 1982; HAAS et al. 1982; NOZAWA et al. 1984; DE KANTOR et al. 1985). This may be due, at least in part, to geographic differences in sensitivity (NAITO et al. 1979). Even the comparative order of these antibiotics is not the same in various investigations (NAITO et al. 1979; NOZAWA et al. 1984). It seems remarkable that dibekacin was bacteriostatic to most strains in monocytes at 12.5 mg/l (NOZAWA et al. 1984). All 3 strains tested by SALFINGER and KAFADER (1986) were sensitive to 0.5 mg/l of the new quinolone Ro 23-6240. 2 mg/l ciprofloxacin and 8 mg/l ofloxacin were found to be the MIC for 90% of 20 clinical isolates of *M. intracellulare* by FENLON and CYNAMON (1986).

d) Activity of Drugs in Animal Experiments

KARLSON (1959) gave 0.1% DDS (a subtoxic dose) in the feed to mice that had been infected intravenously with two different strains of *M. avium*, from the first day after the infection, and observed no influence on the survival time.

HONZA et al. (1966) treated rabbits infected intravenously with Group-III organisms with 200 mg/kg SM for 180 days–210 days. The results were evaluated by the macroscopic findings, the survival time, histopathology, prevention of progress of osteo-articular lesions, and the number of culturable units. The effectiveness was evaluated as good (cited after BURJANOVÁ and URBANCIK 1970).

OLITZKI et al. (1968) treated mice infected intravenously with *M. avium* with subtoxic daily doses (about 250 mg/kg) of streptovaricin C, and found a certain effect on the viable counts from organs.

Extensive investigations were carried out by ROSENFELD (1968) on rabbits infected intravenously. The treatment was started shortly after the infection and was continued for about 3 weeks to 7 weeks. The effect was measured by the survival time. Against a fulminant infection only SM (50 mg/kg) provided some protection, the other drugs – the daily doses are given as mg/kg in brackets – had no effect: INH (20), CS (200 or 500), ETH (50), DATC (200). In a second experiment, with a more protracted course, SM (20) clearly prolonged the survival time and CS (500) extended it for some days. In a third experiment various combinations were tried. The effectiveness was in the following order: SM (20) + CS (20) > SM (20) + INH (5) + PAS (300) > SM (20) + INH (5) + DATC (100) + ETH (20) = SM (20) + INH (5) > SM (20) + EMB (20) = SM. In the fourth experiment the following therapy was nearly or completely ineffective: CS (20), CS (20) + KM (20), CS (20) + ETH (20). Various triple combinations, however, were able to prolong the survival time, the best being CS (20) + KM (20) + DATC (100), followed by ETH (20) + KM (20) + DATC (100) = CS (20) + SM (20) > CS (20) + KM (20) + ETH (20). From all these results it can be concluded that CS, SM, and KM contributed most to the combined effects, but so also did ETH and DATC.

According to BURJANOVÁ and URBANCIK (1970), Burjanová treated mice infected i.v. with *M. avium* for 40 days–50 days. Daily doses of 150 mg/kg EMB and 150 mg/kg VM were ineffective, while CM in doses of 20 mg/kg–40 mg/kg had a good activity as measured by the gross pathology, the survival time and counts of culturable bacilli from lungs.

SHRONTS et al. (1971) treated mice infected i.v. with *M. intracellulare* with daily doses (mg/kg) of INH (25), RMP (25), EMB (125), and INH (25) + RMP

(25) for 50 days, beginning 10 days after the infection. No appreciable effect of the various drugs could be seen on the number of culturable bacilli from heart blood, lungs, and the spleen. In a second experiment, with the translucent and opaque variants of *M. intracellulare*, RMP was tried in a daily dose of 40 mg/kg, but was ineffective. In a third experiment the following daily dosage was used (mg/kg): INH (250 mg/kg), RMP (40 mg/kg and 100 mg/kg), ETH (125 mg/kg), INH (250 mg/kg) + RMP (40 mg/kg), RMP (40 mg/kg) + SM (125 mg/kg), RMP (40 mg/kg) + SM (125 mg/kg) + INH (250 mg/kg), RMP (40 mg/kg) + INH (250 mg/kg) + ETH (125 mg/kg). The therapy was started on day 7 and continued for 45 days. Only RMP + SM showed a reduced number of culturable bacilli in heart blood, but all samples remained positive. The proportion of positive cultures from heart blood plus kidneys was smaller than in the controls only in the groups treated with RMP + SM. Further addition of INH did not improve the results. According to the microbial counts, the number of bacilli in the kidneys was not reduced except by RMP + SM with or without INH. Recultured bacilli did not reveal any significanctly raised resistance to either drug. Altogether, the therapeutic results were clearly inferior to those in the concurrently running infections with *M. kansasii*.

HEJNÝ (1982) mentions briefly two experiments, one on mice and the other on rabbits. The treatment was started some days after the infection, with a combination of CS + erythromycin + sulphamethizole. The doses are not stated. In both species after 30 days of treatment the number of culturable units was reduced to 0.1% and less.

KUZE (1984) carried out an extensive series of experiments on combined treatment of chronic infections in mice. Therapy was evaluated by weight and gross disease of organs, by histology and viable counts from lungs, spleen and kidney. The results demonstrated unequivocally the effectiveness of KM alone, whereas both EMB and RMP alone did not reduce the viable count. The combination of KM + EMB + RMP was slightly advantageous. The triple regimen KM + ETH + CS showed about the same effect as KM + EMB + RMP. A 5-drug combination consisting of KM + EMB + RMP + CS + INH could exert better therapeutic effects than the two triple regimens. There were no clear advantages of adding cephalexin or minocycline to KM + EMB + RMP. Treatment lasted 9 weeks to 12 weeks. The daily dosage was: KM 20 mg/kg, EMB 20 mg/kg, RMP 10 mg/kg, CS 10 mg/kg, INH 10 mg/kg, cephalexin 20 mg/kg, minocycline 4 mg/kg.

ISEMAN et al. (1986) produced an acute infection in immunodeficient mice and compared RMP + EMB with RMP and EMB alone. The combination demonstrated substantially more activity if the mice were infected with a strain inhibited by both drugs.

The animal experiments can be summarized by saying that – as in vitro – the results are worse than the ones obtained in infections due to *M. kansasii*.

e) Treatment of *M. Avium* Complex Infections in Man

The available data have been collected in Table 9, p. 286. Comparison with the therapeutic results in *M. kansasii* infections (see Table 4) shows that on the basis of all parameters used (improvement of the roentgenogram, sputum conversion, cavity closure, proportion of cases still active, proportion of relapses and of patients operated upon), the results for *M. avium* complex infections are worse than those in animal experiments or in vitro. The management of patients with pulmonary diseases due to these organisms thus still presents considerable problems. There is yet no clear evidence that combinations of 5 or 6 drugs are any more effective than combinations of 3 or 4 (DUTT and STEAD 1979; ROSENZWEIG 1979), and even the results with combinations of 5–6 drugs are not very impressive (DAVIDSON et al. 1981). As long as no new drugs with higher activity are available, the main problem is to find patients who are at risk of running an unfavorable course and to reserve rigorous measures with multiple drugs and supplementary resection to this group (ROSENZWEIG 1979). Out of the other antimicrobial agents only clofazimine has been tried, and that without success (HEYWORTH 1967; WATSON and SMYTH 1967; DAVIDSON et al. 1979). In patients with intrinsic (FIEDLER and MÜLLER 1982) or acquired immunodeficiency syndrome (AIDS) chemotherapy usually fails, even as a sixtuple regimen (GREENE et al. 1982; STOVER et al. 1983; WOLLSCHLAGER et al. 1984; FAUCI et al. 1984). Resection has given good long-term results with a relapse rate of only 6% within an average observation period of 94 months (MORAN et al. 1983). The newest guide lines given by an expert committee (ISEMAN et al. 1985) are as follows:

1. For the usual, "moderate severe" case of pulmonary disease, initial therapy should consist of isoniazid, rifampin, and ethambutol for 18 months to 24 months with streptomycin during the initial two to three months.
2. For patients (immunologically intact) with a solitary pulmonary nodule due to *M. avium-intracellulare*, chemotherapy need not be given after resectional surgery.
3. For patients with rapidly progressive, highly symptomatic pulmonary disease, more aggressive initial therapy is indicated employing regimens of five to six drugs, including agents such as ethionamide, cycloserine, or kanamycin (as well as the agents listed previously).
4. For patients with life-threatening disseminated disease due to *M. avium-intracellulare*, initial chemotherapy with five or six drugs is indicated. In this setting, ansamycin (LM 427) and clofazimine should be included in the regimen.
5. For patients with localized pulmonary disease and adequate cardiorespiratory reserve, resectional surgery combined with chemotherapy may offer a better outcome than chemotherapy alone.

2. *M. Haemophilum*

This haemophilic mycobacterium has been responsible for skin and subcutaneous tissue infections in immunologically compromised individuals (SOMPOLINSKY et al. 1978; MOULSDALE et al. 1983). The data on sensitivity to antituberculosis drugs are contradictory. According to Sompolinsky et al. the lesions healed under treatment with INH + SM + EMB, and according to Moulsdale et al. under treatment with cotrimoxazole followed by sulphamethoxazole.

Table 9. Clinical efficacy of antituberculosis drugs in pulmonary infections due to the *M. avium complex*

Authors	No. of patients[a]	Medical treatment	Improved on X-ray	Sputum conversion	Cavity closure	Still active	Relapses	Requiring surgery
			%					
CROW et al. (1957)	64	Various antituberculotic regimens, not specified	51,5	30				20
LEWIS et al. (1960)	116	INH + PAS, later +2 other drugs, depending on susceptibility	47	57	<10	76		33
CARRUTHERS and EDWARDS (1965)	34	INH + SM and/or PAS + additional antituberculotics	44	38				33
JUSTICE and SCHWARTZ (1966)	63	INH + PAS and/or SM; other regimens in some cases	47, + S[b]	57, + S	13; 23, + S	62, + S		38
KREBS (1967)	34	Primary and secondary antituberculotics				100		32
BATES (1967)	60	INH + PAS and/or SM and/or additional drugs (in 43% > 3)	38 (24)[c]		45 (24), + S	59 (12); 52 (24)		38
YAMAMOTO et al. (1967)	45	Combinations of antituberculotics	16 (6)	17 (6)		76 (36)		40
GOLDMAN (1968)	6	INH + PAS and/or SM, in some cases additional antituberculotics		17, + S				
LESTER et al. (1969)	34	5-drug combinations of antituberculotics				26, 5		12

YEAGER and RALEIGH (1973)	45	INH + PAS and/or SM and/or additional drugs (in 47% > 3)			38	19, 6 (60)	42
ADAMS (1974)	21	Antituberculotics, including RMP		41			
CORPE et al. (1975)	413	Antituberculotics in combination	38; 70, + S			17	
KUMAR and VARKEY (1978)	35	21 pat. with 4 or more drugs, 14 ≦ 3 drugs; 34 cases incl. RMP			46 (12)		
DUTT and STEAD (1979)	85	INH + EMB + SM, sometimes + 1 or 2 other antituberculotics		75		23	2, 3
ROSENZWEIG (1979)	82	Combinations of antituberculotics, mostly 3 or more	18	45		11	18
DAVIDSON et al. (1981)	122	Combinations of 5 or 6 antituberculotics		59		16	5
ENGBAEK et al. (1981)	34	Combinations of antituberculotics, mostly 3 or more		44	44, + S	22	20
HUNTER et al. (1981)	26	Most INH + RMP + EMB or SM		58	15	11, 5	11, 5
TSUKAMURA et al. (1981)	12	RMP + enviomycin + minocycline		75 (6)			
	33	Various triple combinations of antituberculotics without minocycline		36 (6)			

[a] Number eligible for evaluation.
[b] + S: operated patients included.
[c] In brackets: months of treatment.

3. *M. Malmoense*

This species has been reported as the causative agent in about 50 cases of pulmonary disease, often with cavities, and 3 cases of cervical adenitis (SCHRÖDER and JUHLIN 1977; JENKINS and TSUKAMURA 1979; BANKS et al. 1983a; 1985; ROBERTS et al. 1985; CONNOLLY et al. 1985). The majority of patients have been observed in Great Britain. Infection predominantly occurs in patients with chronic lung disease or a recognized predisposing factor. Reports on the sensitivity pattern for antituberculotics are not unanimous. It emerges from the published data that all strains are highly resistant to INH and PZA, but sensitive to ETH, CS and CM. The large majority is sensitive to EMB, more than half to RMP and to SM (SCHRÖDER and JUHLIN 1977; SCHRÖDER and MÜLLER 1982; BANKS et al. 1983a; BANKS et al. 1985; CONNOLLY et al. 1985). Efficacy of treatment with antituberculosis drugs in man is difficult to judge. Relapses may occur several years after the end of therapy. It is therefore too early, at the present time, to give any definite figures on healing rates. Regimens including ETH + CS as leading drugs were unsatisfactory, probably due to drug toxicity and poor patient compliance. Best results were obtained in patients receiving triple chemotherapy with RMP + EMB + INH given for between 18 and 24 months. With regard to EMB and RMP all patients who received either one drug with in vitro sensitivity given for at least 16 months or both drugs with in vitro sensitivity given for at least 12 months have done well (BANKS et al. 1985). Resectional surgery was carried out successfully in some patients.

4. *M. Nonchromogenicum* Complex (Including *M. Nonchromogenicum, M. Terrae, M. Novum* and *M. Triviale*)

The four species mentioned in brackets form one cluster in the numerical classification and are therefore called the *M. nonchromogenicum* complex (TSUKAMURA 1980b). The complex has a very low pathogenicity in man, but 3 cases of pulmonary infection and another 3 possible lung infections have been reported recently (TSUKAMURA et al. 1983).

The strains were uniformly resistant to INH, SM, PAS, RMP, CS, KM, CM and TSC. All 6 strains were sensitive to EMB and 2 out of 6 to ETH. Sputum conversion was reported for 3 of the 6 cases after multiple drug treatment with at least 3 agents, most of them found to be ineffective in sensitivity tests. *M. nonchromogenicum* was found to be resistant to minocycline (TSUKAMURA 1980a, b).

A case of localized cavitary lung disease caused by bacteria belonging to the complex has been reported by KUZE et al. (1983). The drug sensitivity pattern was the same as described above for the 6 strains, but with sensitivity to ETH. Treatment with INH + RMP + EMB was unsuccessful. Healing was obtained by resection.

Isolated cases of disseminated infections due to *M. terrae* have been described (CIANCIULLI 1974; EDWARDS et al. 1978). MEISSNER (1970, p 252) tested in vitro 14–30 strains of *M. terrae* per drug. The strains were resistant to INH, PAS, TSC, DATC, and PZA. More than half were resistant to SM, VM, and KM. At least half were sensitive to CS and ETH and nearly all were sensitive to EMB. According to MOLAVI and WEINSTEIN (1971 a, b), most strains are sensitive to RMP and all are to erythromycin. Ansamycin showed the same activity as RMP (HEIFETS and ISEMAN 1985). Resistance to at least 10 mg/l DDS was reported by PATTYN and VAN ERMENGEM (1968).

M. triviale was the only organism cultured from the synovial fluid of an infant with septic arthritis (DECHAIRO et al. 1973). The strain was resistant to INH, PAS, EMB, and erythromycin. It was inhibited by a combination of 10 mg/l SM + 5 mg/l INH. MOLAVI and WEINSTEIN (1971 a, b) reported sensitivity to RMP and erythromycin.

Seven strains of the *M. terrae* complex were found to be uniformly sensitive to 1 mg/l ansamycin by HEIFETS and ISEMAN (1985).

5. *M. Ulcerans (M. Buruli)*

Deeply undermined skin ulcers with extensive necrosis produced by mycobacteria were observed in the 1940's in Australia and in tropical Africa. They were identified as a pathological entity by MACCALLUM et al. (1948). The causative agent with a growth optimum at about 33 °C constitutes a separate species, now known as *M. ulcerans* and included by many authors in Runyon Group III. In its natural course the disease runs for several years and ends in healing with defects that are often severe.

a) Activity of Antituberculosis Drugs in Vitro

The following picture emerges from the available data: The species is uniformly sensitive to RMP. Most strains are sensitive to SM, VM, KM, CM, and CS. One strain tested was sensitive to TC. Most or all of the strains are resistant to INH, PAS, TSC, ETH, EMB, and PZA (CLANCEY 1964; PETTIT et al. 1966; STANFORD and PHILIPPS 1972; SCHRÖDER 1975; ULLMANN et al. 1975; MISGELD et al. 1976).

b) Activity of Other Antimicrobial Agents in Vitro

The species is sensitive to DDS (PATTYN and VAN ERMENGEM 1968), to clofazimine (LUNN and REES 1964), and to co-trimoxazole (DEMOULIN et al. 1982).

c) Activity of Antituberculosis Drugs and Other Antimicrobial Agents in Animals

As for *M. marinum*, the best experimental model is the footpad infection. LEACH and FENNER (1954) treated mice infected by this route with SM, in a dose of about 75 mg/kg/day. The treatment was started at different times. The infection could be controlled, unless the treatment had been started at an advanced stage. FELDMAN and KARLSON (1957) infected mice intravenously and evaluated the effectiveness mainly by microscopic examination of the tails. The treatment started immediately after the infection. SM, 150 mg/kg s.c., and DDS, 150 mg/kg/day in the feed, were markedly effective. INH, 30 mg/kg in the feed, did not alleviate the severity of the lesions but appeared to extend the lifespan of many animals. PETTIT et al. (1966), using the footpad test, were able to show that treatment with clofazimine, the equivalent of 15 mg/kg fed in the feed, completely suppressed the infection when applied from the day of the infection. PATTYN and ROYACKERS (1965) tested INH (0.02% in the feed), CS (0.2% in the feed), DDS (0.1% in the feed), PAS (0.6% in the feed), and SM (about 150 mg/kg s.c.). The treatment was started the day after the infection of the footpads and lasted 48 days. No macroscopic lesions were observed at that time in the mice treated with SM or with DDS. INH was completely ineffective, whereas CS protected some of the mice. 36 days after the end of the treatment all the mice treated with CS or DDS had lesions; only the SM group had remained free. The effect of the various drugs on a severe established footpad infection was studied by STANFORD and PHILIPPS (1972). A course of one month with various regimens of RMP (40 mg/kg 3 or 6 times a week, 160 mg/kg once a week) starting 2 weeks or 5 weeks after the infection led to a clinical improvement, but the disease relapsed 6 weeks–8 weeks after the end of the therapy. Treatment for 10 weeks, however, with 160 mg/kg once a week, produced an apparent cure. Sulphadoxine, 350 mg/kg twice weekly, plus pyrimethamine (14 mg/kg per week) or clofazimine, 15 mg/kg p.o., were ineffective whether the treatment had been instituted 2 weeks or 5 weeks after the infection. Addition of clofazimine or of the combination of sulphadoxine and pyrimethamine to RMP for one month did not improve the results over RMP alone. As HAVEL and PATTYN (1975) have shown, the effectiveness of RMP is much higher if the infection dose is lower than that used by Stanford and Philipps: With an inoculum of 10^3 to 10^4 viable units per footpad – as used in *M. leprae* infections – the minimal effective dose of RMP was between 10 mg/kg and 15 mg/kg, administered 5 days a week, depending on the start of the therapy (10 days or 21 days after the inoculation). The minimal effective dose found is comparable with that obtained by VERBIST and GYSELEN (1968) and by HAVEL and ŠIMONOVÁ (1970) in the treatment of experimental infections of mice with *M. tuberculosis*. SRIVASTAVA et al. (1984) infected rats in the footpad. Treatment started 54 days after infection and was given 6 times weekly for 9 weeks. RMP in a dose of 3 mg/kg was compared with co-trimoxazole (CTM) 10 mg/kg, 20 mg/kg, and 30 mg/kg and with combinations of both drugs in the same dosage. Inflammation was measured by caliper and the therapeutic effect expressed as percentage of decrease in inflammation. 20 mg/kg and 30 mg/kg CTM were nearly as active as RMP alone, but the combination of 20 mg/kg or 30 mg/kg CTM + 3 mg/kg RMP was clearly superior to RMP alone or to the combination of 3 mg/kg RMP + 10 mg/kg CTM. Intravenously infected mice were treated from the day of infection for 10 days. The CTM dose was kept constant at 30 mg/kg, the RMP dose was varied from 2.5 mg/kg to 5 mg/kg, 10 mg/kg, and 15 mg/kg. CTM alone prolonged the mean survival time from 7 days to 12 days, but in combination with RMP survival increased markedly, if the RMP dose was $\geqq 5$ mg/kg; with 15 mg/kg RMP + 30 mg/kg CTM the survival time amounted to 144 days.

d) Treatment of *M. Ulcerans* Infections in Man

Up to now chemotherapy alone has been unsuccessful. Penicillin (JANSSENS 1950; MELENEY and JOHNSON 1950), chlortetracycline, chloramphenicol, and streptomycin (MELENEY and JOHNSON 1950) were all ineffective. Isolated cases are reported in which DDS (AGUILAR et al. 1953) or DDS + SM (REID 1967) did give some relief. The results of a pilot study by LUNN and REES (1964) with clofazimine could not be confirmed by a controlled trial (REVILL et al. 1973). The drug alone did not constitute adequate treatment, even of small and non-ulcerated lesions. In patients treated surgically clofazimine did not shorten the course of the disease nor did it reduce the number of operations required or produce smaller scars. Furthermore, it did not prevent recurrences. No trials with RMP have yet been published except one case treated successfully with RMP systemically and with trypsin and a dextran polymer topically (SONG et al. 1985). At present excision of the nodules in the pre-ulcerative stage (UGANDA BURULI GROUP 1970) or extensive surgery and skin grafting in the ulcerative stage, are the method of choice.

IV. Group IV

1. *M. Fortuitum* Complex (Including *M. Fortuitum* and *M. Chelonei* with Subspecies *Abscessus*)

This complex includes the species *M. fortuitum*, *M. chelonei*, and *M. chelonei* subspecies *abscessus*, which are difficult to differentiate at the present time. The typical disease produced by the complex is soft tissue infection after a penetrating trauma, but other infections, including pulmonary and systemic ones, have also been observed (HAND and SANFORD 1970; DALOVISIO 1981). The spectrum of disease has been described by WALLACE et al. (1983). Microorganisms belonging to the complex are regularly resistant to INH, SM, PAS, EMB, RMP, CS, TSC, and PZA. Many strains are sensitive to ETH, a minority to KM, CM, and VM (WICHELHAUSEN and ROBINSON 1965; HOBBY et al. 1967; HAND and SANFORD 1970; PORTAELS and PATTYN 1970; MOLAVI and WEINSTEIN 1971 a; RYNEARSON et al. 1971; TSUKAMURA et al. 1973; DREISIN et al. 1976; SANDERS Jr et al. 1977; FOZ et al. 1978; JAKSCHIK 1979; SWENSON et al. 1980; YATES and COLLINS 1981; HEJNÝ 1982; HEIFETS and ISEMAN 1985; DE KANTOR et al. 1985).

Many other drugs have been tested. Ansamycin is ineffective (HEIFETS and ISEMAN 1985), also DDS (DE KANTOR et al. 1985) and clofazimine (DAMLE et al. 1978; DE KANTOR et al. 1985). The organisms are resistant to penicillin (BROSBE et al. 1964), oxacillin (DALOVISIO and PANKEY 1978), cefalothin and cefazolin (HAAS et al. 1973; SANDERS Jr et al. 1977; DALOVISIO and PANKEY 1978), and other cephalosporins (SAKURAI 1983), chloramphenicol (WELCH and KELLY 1979), clindamycin, vancomycin (DALOVISIO and PANKEY 1978), and to trimethoprim (LASZLO and EIDUS 1978; WALLACE et al. 1981 a; CASAL and RODRÍGUEZ 1983). MICHEL et al. (1973) reported species differences in the sensitivity to vancomycin: all 11 strains of *M. fortuitum* were sensitive, all 14 strains of *M. abscessus* resistant, *M. borstelense* being in an intermediate position.

Sensitivity to cefoxitin seems doubtful, the test results depending on the technique (SWENSON et al. 1980; CYNAMON and PATAPOW 1981; CASAL and RODRÍGUEZ 1982; STONE et al. 1983; CYNAMON and PALMER 1983; SAKURAI 1983; DE KANTOR et al. 1985; WALLACE et al. 1985 b). By combination of clavulanic acid with amoxicillin most strains came into the usual therapeutic range (CYNAMON and PALMER 1983). N-formimidoyl thienamycin inhibited 10 of 12 strains at 6.25 mg/l, cefmetazole 12 of 13 strains at 12.5 mg/l as compared to cefoxitin, which needed

25 mg/l to inhibit 11 of 13 strains. Moxalactam and cefotetan were even less active than cefoxitin (CYNAMON and PALMER 1982).

Some strains are sensitive to erythromycin (MOLAVI and WEINSTEIN 1971 b; SANDERS Jr et al. 1977; GARCIA-RODRÍGUEZ and MARTIN-LUENGO 1978; DALOVISIO and PANKEY 1978; FOZ et al. 1978; WALLACE et al. 1979; SWENSON et al. 1980; HEJNÝ 1982; STONE et al. 1983; WALLACE et al. 1985 b).

At least half of the strains are sensitive to tetracyclines: tetracycline, doxycycline, and minocycline (BROSBE et al. 1964; GARCIA-RODRÍGUEZ and MARTIN-LUENGO 1978; DALOVISIO and PANKEY 1978; WALLACE et al. 1979; TSUKAMURA 1980 a, b; SWENSON et al. 1980; STONE et al. 1983; WALLACE et al. 1985 b), and about half to gentamicin, sisomicin, and tobramycin (DALOVISIO and PANKEY 1978; WALLACE et al. 1979; WELCH and KELLY 1979). DE KANTOR et al. (1985), however, found their strains resistant to tetracycline and gentamicin. Excepting the report by GANGADHARAM and CANDLER (1977 a), a higher proportion is sensitive to amikacin (DALOVISIO and PANKEY 1978; GARCIA-RODRÍGUEZ and MARTIN-LUENGO 1978; WELCH and KELLY 1979; SWENSON et al. 1980; HEJNÝ 1982; STONE et al. 1983; CASAL and RODRIGUEZ 1983; DE KANTOR et al. 1985; WALLACE et al. 1985 b). Likewise, about three-quarters of the strains are sensitive to sulphonamides (WALLACE et al. 1981 a; HEJNÝ 1982; STONE et al. 1983). DE KANTOR et al. (1985) judged their strains as resistant to various sulphonamides except sulfisoxazole.

The newer quinolones might become of interest, since of the older ones pipemidic acid was shown to be active by CASAL and RODRÍGUEZ (1983) and GAY et al. (1984) found all 20 strains of *M. fortuitum* and about 50% of 20 strains of *M. chelonei* sensitive to ciprofloxacin; norfloxacin was less active. Very few animal experiments have been published. High doses of DDS, 0.1% mixed in with the feed, did prolong the survival time of intravenously infected mice (KARLSON 1959). Tetracycline (100 mg/kg/day i.p.) had a significant protective effect on intravenously infected mice as measured by the survival time and gross renal involvement. Penicillin, in daily doses of 10000 units was ineffective. INH (25 mg/kg/day) slightly prolonged the survival time and alleviated renal disease. Two-drug combinations were no better than the most active single drugs (BROSBE et al. 1964). EMB was reported to be effective (SAKAMOTO and GODA 1966, cited after WOLINSKY 1979). SAITO et al. (1984) tried cefoxitin and cefotetan in intravenously infected mice. A dose dependent effect, increasing from 20 mg/kg/day up to 400 mg/kg/day, was noted. Both drugs suppressed spinning disease and both reduced the severity of renal disease and the numbers of culturable bacilli in the kidneys and liver, but not in the lungs or spleen.

In human medicine, treatment with antituberculosis drugs is ineffective (HAND and SANFORD 1970; NICHOLSON and SEVIER 1971; RADENBACH 1972; TSUKAMURA et al. 1973; AWE et al. 1973; BURKE and ULLIAN 1977; FOZ et al. 1978; SOPKO et al. 1980; IRWIN et al. 1982). The effects of even combinations of 4–6 antituberculotics were not really impressive (DREISIN et al. 1976).

The results obtained with other chemotherapeutic agents are contradictory, as can be seen from Table 10. Combinations of drugs to which the causative organism is susceptible seem to be superior. Surgical intervention is necessary in most cases of soft tissue infections. Especially difficult to treat are disseminated

Table 10. Clinical efficacy of other antimicrobial agents against *M. fortuitum/chelonei* infections

Sulphonamides	
Success:	TICE and SOLOMON (1979)
	WALLACE et al. (1981a)
	HEIRONIMUS et al. (1984)
Failure:	GRAYBILL et al. (1974)
Cotrimoxazole	
Success:	–
Failure:	STANECK et al. (1981)
Erythromycin	
Success:	IRWIN et al. (1982)
	+minocycline: STANECK et al. (1981)
	+streptomycin: ARROYO and MEDOFF (1977)
Failure:	GRAYBILL et al. (1974)
	+kanamycin: GRAYBILL et al. (1974)
	SOPKO et al. (1980)
Cefoxitin	
Success:	BRANNAN et al. (1984)
Failure:	–
Tetracycline	
Success:	RADENBACH (1972)
	DALOVISIO et al. (1981)
Failure:	SOPKO et al. (1980)
Amikacin	
Success:	METCALF et al. (1981)
	DALOVISIO et al. (1981)
	KURITZKY et al. (1983)
	+another bacterial agent: ROLSTON et al. (1985)
Failure:	+another bacterial agent: ROLSTON et al. (1985)

infections due to *M. chelonei* (BEVELAQUA et al. 1981; POTTAGE et al. 1982; CARPENTER et al. 1984). The effect may vary with the immune status of the patient (CARPENTER et al. 1984). Acquired resistance has been observed in both species of the complex which seems to be due to mutational resistance (WALLACE et al. 1985a). On the basis of treatment results in 132 patients with non-pulmonary infections, WALLACE et al. (1985b) give detailed recommendations for therapy specified according to type of disease and causative agent. In serious infections initial empirical treatment with amikacin (15 mg/kg/day) + cefoxitin (200 mg/kg/day up to 12 g/day) with oral probenecid seems the most promising.

2. *M. Smegmatis*

Isolated cases of aspiration pneumonia due to *M. smegmatis* have been described in patients with oesophageal dysfunction, reviewed by SIMON (1970). No case reports from later years came to the knowledge of the present writer. *M. smegmatis* is said to be resistant to INH, PAS, RMP, ETH, CS, TSC, and PZA in vitro and sensitive to SM, EMB, KM, and VM (TACQUET and TISON 1963; RYNEARSON et al. 1971; BARTMANN 1980). Experiments on intravenously infected mice were carried out by ROSENFELD (1968). In monotherapy, the best (but weak) effects were obtained after high doses of DDS, CS, and EMB. Combinations were more active. The survival rate was highest with the four-drug combinations of DDS + sulphonamide + tetracycline + CS or EMB. GUY and CHAPMAN (1961) found one strain to be sensitive to erythromycin and probably also to chloramphenicol, but resistant to tetracyclines.

3. *M. Thermoresistibile*

The first case of pulmonary (cavitary) disease due to this organism was reported by WEITZMAN et al. in 1981. The patient improved rapidly on treatment with RMP + EMB + SM. The culture was found to be sensitive in vitro to SM, EMB, RMP, and CS and resistant to INH, PAS, ETH, CM, and TSC.

References

Adams AR (1974) Mycobacterium "Battey" in western Australia. Bull Int Union Tuberc XLIX:295–296

Aguilar PL, Iturribarria FM, Middlebrook G (1953) Un caso de infeccion humana por *Mycobacterium ulcerans* en el hemisferio occidental nota previa. Int J Lepr 21:469–476

Ahn CH, Lowell JR, Ahn SS, Ahn S, Hurst GA (1981) Chemotherapy for pulmonary disease due to *Mycobacterium kansasii:* efficacies of some individual drugs. Rev Infect Dis 3:1028–1034

Ahn CH, Lowell JR, Ahn SS, Ahn SI, Hurst GA (1983) Short-course chemotherapy for pulmonary disease caused by *Mycobacterium kansasii.* Am Rev Respir Dis 128:1048–1050

Arroyo J, Medoff G (1977) *Mycobacterium chelonei* infection: successful treatment based on a radiometric susceptibility test. Antimicrob Agents Chemother 11:763–764

Awe RJ, Gangadharam PR, Jenkins DE (1973) Clinical significance of *Mycobacterium fortuitum* infections in pulmonary disease. Am Rev Respir Dis 108:1320–1324

Bailey JP Jr, Stevens J, Bell WM, Mealing HG Jr, Loebl DH, Cook EH (1982) *Mycobacterium marinum* infection. A fishy story. JAMA 247:1314

Bailey WC, Albert RK, Davidson PT, Farer LS, Glassroth J, Kendig E Jr, Loudon RG, Inselman LS (1983) Treatment of tuberculosis and other mycobacterial diseases. Am Rev Respir Dis 127:790–796

Banerjee DK, Holmes IB (1976) *In vitro* and *in vivo* studies of the action of rifampicin, clofazimine and B 1912 on *Mycobacterium marinum.* Chemotherapy 22:242–252

Banks J, Smith AP, Jenkins PA (1983a) *Mycobacterium malmoense* – problems with treatment and diagnosis – a case report. Tubercle 64:217–219

Banks J, Hunter AM, Campbell IA, Jenkins PA, Smith AP (1983b) Pulmonary infection with *Mycobacterium kansasii* in Wales, 1970–9: review of treatment and response. Thorax 38:271–274

Banks J, Hunter AM, Campbell IA, Jenkins PA, Smith AP (1984) Pulmonary infection with *Mycobacterium xenopi:* review of treatment and response. Thorax 39:376–382

Banks J, Jenkins PA, Smith AP (1985) Pulmonary infection with *Mycobacterium malmoense* – a review of treatment and response. Tubercle 66:197–203

Barrow GI, Hewitt M (1971) Skin infection with *Mycobacterium marinum* from a tropical fish tank. Br Med J 1:505–506

Bartmann K (1980) Mikrobiologische Grundlagen. In: Jentgens H (Hrsg) Handb Innere Med IV/3 Atmungsorgane 3. Teil. Lungentuberkulose, pp 1–45

Bates JH (1967) A study of pulmonary disease associated with mycobacteria other than *Mycobacterium tuberculosis:* clinical characteristics. Am Rev Respir Dis 96:1151–1157

Bell RC, Higuchi JH, Donovan WN, Krasnow I, Johanson WG Jr (1983) *Mycobacterium simiae.* Clinical features and follow-up of twenty-four patients. Am Rev Respir Dis 127:35–38

Benjamin M, Spagnolo SV (1982) Rifampin in initial therapy of M. kansasii pulmonary disease. Am Rev Respir Dis 125, no 4, part 2:183

Bevelaqua FA, Kamelhar DA, Campion J, Christianson LC (1981) *Mycobacterium fortuitum-chelonei.* Two patients with fatal pulmonary infection. NY State J Med 81:1621–1624

Black MM, Eykyn SJ (1977) The successful treatment of tropical fish tank granuloma (*Mycobacterium marinum*) with co-trimoxazole. Br J Dermatol 97:689–692

Blacklock ZM, Dawson DJ, Kane DW, Mc Evoy D (1983) *Mycobacterium asiaticum* as a potential pulmonary pathogen for humans. Am Rev Respir Dis 127:241–244

Bogaerts Y, Elinck W, van Renterghem D, Pauwels R, van der Straaten M (1982) Pulmonary disease due to *Mycobacterium xenopi.* Eur J Respir Dis 63:298–304

Boisvert H (1974) Contribution a l'étude bactériologique de *Mycobacterium simiae.* Bull Soc Pathol Exot 67:458–465

Brannan DP, Du Bois RE, Ramirez MJ, Ravry MJR, Harrison EO (1984) Cefoxitin therapy for *Mycobacterium fortuitum* bacteremia with associated granulomatous hepatitis. South Med J 77:381–384

Brosbe EA, Sugihara PT, Smith CR, Hyde L (1965) Experimental drug studies on *Mycobacterium fortuitum.* Antimicrob Agents Chemother 1964:733–736

Burjanová B (1970) Not published data. In: Burjanová B, Urbancik R (1970), table II, pp 166–167

Burjanová B, Dornetzhuber V (1967) Isoxyl und T 283 in der Behandlung photochromogener Infektionen bei Mäusen. Z Tuberk 127:123–125

Burjanová B, Urbančík R (1967) Experimentelle Chemotherapie von *Mycobacterium kansasii* – Infektionen im Tierversuch. Beitr Klin Tuberk 135:364–369

Burjanová B, Urbancik R (1970) Experimental chemotherapy of mycobacterioses provoked by atypical macobacteria. Adv Tuberc Res 17:154–188

Burjanová B, Dornetzhuber V (1975) Empfindlichkeit der Stämme des *M. kansasii* auf verschiedene Antibiotika und Chemotherapeutika in vitro and in vivo. Z Erkr Atmungsorgane 142:68–77

Burke DS, Ullian RB (1977) Megaesophagus and pneumonia associated with *Mycobacterium chelonei.* Am Rev Respir Dis 116:1101–1107

Carpenter JL, Troxell M, Wallace RJ Jr (1984) Disseminated disease due to *Mycobacterium chelonei* treated with amikacin and cefoxitin. Arch Intern Med 144:2063–2065

Carruthers KJM, Edwards FGB (1965) Atypical mycobacteria in Western Australia. Am Rev Respir Dis 91:887–895

Casal M, Rodríguez F (1982) *In vitro* susceptibility of *Mycobacterium fortuitum* and *Mycobacterium chelonei* to cefoxitin. Tubercle 63:125–127

Casal MJ, Rodríguez FC (1983) *In vitro* susceptibility of Mycobacterium fortuitum to non-antituberculous antibacterial agents. Ann Microbiol (Paris) 134 A:73–78

Casimir MT, Fainstein V, Papadopolous N (1982) Cavitary lung infection caused by *Mycobacterium flavescens.* South Med J 75:253–254

Chapman JS (1977) The atypical mycobacteria and human mycobacteriosis. Plenum Medical Book Co, New York

Cianciulli FD (1974) The radish bacillus (*Mycobacterium terrae*): saprophyte or pathogen? Am Rev Respir Dis 109:138–141

Citron KM, Smith MJ (1983) Clinical review of pulmonary disease caused by *Mycobacterium xenopi.* Thorax 38:373–377

Clancey JK (1964) Mycobacterial skin ulcers in Uganda: description of a new mycobacterium (*Mycobacterium buruli*). J Path Bact 88:175–187

Clancey JK, Dodge OG, Lunn HF, Oduori ML (1961) Mycobacterial skin ulcers in Uganda. Lancet II:951–954

Connolly MJ, Magee JG, Hendrick DJ, Jenkins PA (1985) *Mycobacterium malmoense* in the North-East of England. Tubercle 66:211–217
Contorer P, Jones RN (1979) Minocycline therapy of aquarium granuloma. Cutis 23:864–868
Corpe RF, Liang JL, Sanchez ES (1975) Early and late results in persons with atypical, group III tuberculosis. Am Rev Repir Dis 111:915 (Abstract)
Cortez LM, Pankey GA (1973) *Mycobacterium marinum* infections of the hand. J Bone Joint Surg 55-A:363–370
Costrini AM, Mahler DA, Gross WM, Hawkins JE, Yesner R, D'Esopo ND (1981) Clinical and roentgenographic features of nosocomial pulmonary disease due to *Mycobacterium xenopi.* Am Rev Respir Dis 123:104–109
Crow HE, King CT, Smith CE, Corpe RT, Stergus I (1957) A limited clinical, pathologic, and epidemiologic study of patients with pulmonary lesions associated with atypical acid-fast bacilli in the sputum. Am Rev Tuberc 75:199–222
Cynamon MH, Patapow A (1981) In vitro susceptibility of *Mycobacterium fortuitum* to cefoxitin. Antimicrob Agents Chemother 19:205–207
Cynamon MH, Palmer GS (1982) In vitro susceptibility of *Mycobacterium fortuitum* to N-formimidoyl thienamycin and several cephamycins. Antimicrob Agents Chemother 22:1079–1081
Cynamon MH, Palmer GS (1983) In vitro susceptibility of *Mycobacterium fortuitum* to amoxicillin or cephalothin in combination with clavulanic acid. Antimicrob Agents Chemother 23:935–937
Dalovisio JR (1981) Treatment of disease caused by organisms of the *Mycobacterium fortuitum* complex. Semin Respir Dis 2:240–242
Dalovisio JR, Pankey GA (1978) In vitro susceptibility of *Mycobacterium fortuitum* and *Mycobacterium chelonei* to amikacin. J Infect Dis 137:318–321
Dalovisio JR, Pankey GA, Wallace RJ, Jones DB (1981) Clinical usefulness of amikacin and doxycycline in the treatment of infection due to *Mycobacterium fortuitum* and *Mycobacterium chelonei.* Rev Infect Dis 3:1068–1074
Damle P, Mc Clatchy JK, Gangadharam PRJ, Davidson PT (1978) Antimycobacterial activity of some potential chemotherapeutic compounds. Tubercle 59:135–138
David HL (1981) Basis for lack of drug susceptibility of atypical mycobacteria. Rev Infect Dis 3:878–884
Davidson PT (1976a) *Mycobacterium szulgai.* A new pathogen causing infection of the lung. Chest 69:799–801
Davidson PT (1976b) Treatment and long-term follow-up of patients with atypical mycobacterial infections. Bull Int Union Tuberc LI, Tome 1:257–261
Davidson PT (1981) The treatment of *Mycobacterium avium-intracellulare* complex disease. Seminars Respir Med 2:233–238
Davidson PT, Goble M, Lester W (1972) The antituberculosis efficacy of rifampin in 136 patients. Chest 61:574–578
Davidson PT, Waggoner R (1976) Acquired resistance to rifampicin by *Mycobacterium kansasii.* Tubercle 57:271–273
Davidson PT, Goble M, Fernandez E, Gangadharam PRJ (1979) Clofazimine (B 663) for the treatment of *M. intracellulare* infections in man. Am Rev Respir Dis 119, Suppl:398
Davidson PT, Khanijo V, Goble M, Moulding TS (1981) Treatment of disease due to *Mycobacterium intracellulare.* Rev Infect Dis 3:1052–1059
Dechairo DC, Kittredge D, Meyers A, Corrales J (1973) Septic arthritis *due to Mycobacterium triviale.* Am Rev Respir Dis 108:1224–1226
De Kantor IN, Barrera L, Di Lonardo M (1985) In vitro susceptibility to antibiotics and sulfonamides of atypical mycobacteria isolated in South America. Zentralbl Bakteriol Mikrobiol Hyg (A) 260:247–253
Demoulin L, Medard M, Kellens J (1982) Étude in vitro de la sensibilité des mycobactéries aux sulfonamides, par les méthodes de disques et des proportions. Pathol Biol 30:201–205

Dreisin RB, Scoggin C, Davidson PT (1976) The pathogenicity of *Mycobacterium fortuitum* and *Mycobacterium chelonei* in man: a report of seven cases. Tubercle 57:49–57

Dutt AK, Stead WW (1979) Long-term results of medical treatment in *Mycobacterium intracellulare* infection. Am J Med 67:449–453

van Dyke JJ, Lake KB (1975) Chemotherapy for aquarium granuloma. JAMA 233:1380–1381

Edwards FGB (1969) Personal communication to Johnston RN. In: Johnston RN (1969) The treatment of infection due to "atypical" mycobacteria. Tubercle 50:88–91

Edwards MS, Huber TW, Baker CJ (1978) *Mycobacterium terrae* synovitis and osteomyelitis. Am Rev Respir Dis 117:161–163

Elston HR, Duffy JP (1973) *Mycobacterium xenopi* and mycobacteriosis. Am Rev Respir Dis 108:944–949

Engbaek HC, Vergmann B, Baess I, Will DW (1967) M. xenopei. A bacteriological study of M. xenopei including case reports of Danish patients. Acta Pathol Microbiol Scand 69:576–594

Engbaek HC, Vergmann B, Bentzon MW (1981) Lung disease caused by *Mycobacterium avium/Mycobacterium intracellulare*. Eur J Respir Dis 62:72–83

Even-Paz Z, Haas H, Sacks T, Rosenmann E (1976) *Mycobacterium marinum* skin infections mimicking cutaneous leishmaniasis. Br J Dermatol 94:435–442

Fauci AS, Macher AM, Longo DL, Lane HC, Rook AH, Masur H, Gelmann EP (1984) Acquired immunodeficiency syndrome: epidemiologic, clinical, immunologic, and therapeutic considerations. Ann Intern Med 100:92–106

Feldman WH, Karlson AG (1957) *Mycobacterium ulcerans* infections. Am Rev Tuberc 75:266–279

Fenlon CH, Cynamon MH (1986) Comparative in vitro activities of ciprofloxacin and other 4-quinolones against *Mycobacterium tuberculosis* and *Mycobacterium intracellulare*. Antimicrob Agents Chemother 29:386–388

Fiedler M, Müller KM (1982) Letale Mykobakterium avium-Sepsis bei Immundefekt, ein Beitrag zur „Mykobakteriellen Histiozytose". Prax Pneumol 36:312–317

Flowers DJ (1970) Human infection due to *Mycobacterium marinum* after a dolphin bite. J Clin Path 23:475–477

Forschbach G (1975) Nichttuberkulöse Infektionen durch Mycobakterien. Internist 16:393–400

Foz A, Roy C, Jurado J, Arteaga E, Ruiz JM, Moragas A (1978) *Mycobacterium chelonei* iatrogenic infections. J Clin Microbiol 7:319–321

Francis PB, Jay SJ, Johanson WG Jr (1975) The course of untreated *Mycobacterium kansasii* disease. Am Rev Respir Dis 111:477–487

Fraser DW, Buxton AE, Naji A, Barker CF, Rudnick M, Weinstein AJ (1975) Disseminated *Mycobacterium kansasii* infection presenting as cellulitis in a recipient of a renal homograft. Am Rev Respir Dis 112:125–129

Gangadharam PRJ, Candler ER (1977a) *In vitro* anti-mycobacterial activity of some new aminoglycoside antibiotics. Tubercle 58:35–38

Gangadharam PRJ, Candler ER (1977b) Activity of some antileprosy compounds against *Mycobacterium intracellulare* in vitro. Am Rev Respir Dis 115:705–707

Gangadharam PR, Pratt PF, Damle PB, Davidson PT (1981) Dynamic aspects of the activity of clofazimine against *Mycobacterium intracellulare*. Tubercle 62:201–206

Garcia-Rodríguez JA, Martin-Luengo F (1978) Activity of amikacin, erythromycin and doxycycline against *Mycobacterium chelonei* and *Mycobacterium fortuitum*. Tubercle 59:277–280

Garcia-Rodríguez JA, Martin-Luengo F (1980) In vitro susceptibility of atypical mycobacteria to cephalosporins. Tubercle 61:39–40

Gay JD, De Young DR, Roberts GD (1984) In vitro activities of norfloxacin and ciprofloxacin against *Mycobacterium tuberculosis, M. avium* complex *M. chelonei, M. fortuitum,* and *M. kansasii*. Antimicrob Agents Chemother 26:94–96

Gernez-Rieux Ch, Tacquet A, Collet A, Martin JC, Devulder B (1967) Activité de différentes substances antibacillaires sur l'infection expérimentale par *Mycobacterium kansasii* du cobaye empoussiére. Proc Vth Intern Congr Chemother Vol V, 511–514

Glasser D (1978) Dimethylsulfoxide (DMSO) "resensibilization" as potential chemotherapy for opportunistic mycobacterial disease. Am Rev Respir Dis 118:969–970
Goldman KP (1968) Treatment of unclassified mycobacterial infection of the lungs. Thorax 23:94–99
Gonzáles Montaner LJ, Abbate EH, Brea A (1983) Initial treatment in M. kansasii pulmonary disease. Am Rev Respir Dis 127, no 4, part 2:202
Good RC (1979) Nontuberculous mycobacteria. Clin Microbiol Newsletter 1:No 20:1–7
Graybill JR, Silva J Jr, Fraser DW, Lordon R, Rogers E (1974) Disseminated mycobacteriosis due to *Mycobacterium abscessus* in two recipients of renal homografts. Am Rev Respir Dis 109:4–10
Greene JF, Gurdip SS, Levine JF, Masur H, Simberkoff MS, Nicholas P, Good RC, Zolla-Pazner B, Pollock AA, Tapper ML, Holzman RS (1982) *Mycobacterium avium-intracellulare:* a cause of disseminated life-threatening infection in homosexuals and drug abusers. Ann Intern Med 97:539–546
Guy LR, Chapman JS (1961) Susceptibility in vitro of unclassified mycobacteria to commonly used antimicrobials. Am Rev Respir Dis 84:746–749
Haas H, Michel J, Sacks TG (1973) In-vitro susceptibility of *Mycobacterium fortuitum* and related strains to cephalosporins. J Med Microbiol 6:141–145
Haas H, Michel J, Sacks TG (1982) In vitro susceptibility of *Mycobacteria* species other than *Mycobacterium tuberculosis* to amikacin, cephalosporins and cefoxitin. Chemotherapy 28:1–5
Hand WL, Sanford JP (1970) *Mycobacterium fortuitum* – a human pathogen. Ann Intern Med 73:971–977
Harris GD, Johanson WG Jr, Nicholson DP (1975) Response to chemotherapy of pulmonary infection due to *Mycobacterium kansasii.* Am Rev Respir Dis 112:31–36
Havel A, Šimonová S (1970) The effect of capreomycin on "atypical" and avian mycobacterial strains *in vitro*. Antibiotica et Chemotherapia 16:17–19
Havel A, Pattyn SR (1975) Activity of rifampicin on *Mycobacterium ulcerans*. Ann Soc Belge Méd Trop 55:105–108
Hawkins JE, Gross WM, Vadney FS (1984) Ansamycin LM 427 activity against mycobacteria *in vitro* (abstract). Am Rev Respir Dis 129 (Suppl:A187)
Hedgecock LW, Blumenthal HT (1965) The effect of isoniazid and para-aminosalicylic acid on infection in mice produced by *Mycobacterium kansasii.* Am Rev Respir Dis 91:21–29
Heifets LB (1982) Synergistic effect of rifampin, streptomycin, ethionamide, and ethambutol on *Mycobacterium intracellulare*. Am Rev Respir Dis 125:43–48
Heifets LB, Iseman MD (1985) Determination of *in vitro* susceptibility of mycobacteria to ansamycin. Am Rev Respir Dis 132:710–711
Heironimus JD, Winn RE, Collins CB (1984) Cutaneous nonpulmonary *Mycobacterium chelonei* infection. Arch Dermatol 120:1061–1063
Hejný J (1982) Mykobakteriologische Grundlagen der Therapie von Mykobakteriosen. Z Erkr Atmungsorgane 158:163–167
Herlitz S, Linell F, Nordén Å (1951) Epidemic of skin lesions produced by a special type of acid-fast bacilli. Intern Congr Clin Path, London 1951. Cited from: Zettergren L (1970) Erkrankungen des Menschen durch *Mycobacterium balnei*. In: Meissner G, Schmiedel A (Hrsg) Mykobakterien und mykobakterielle Krankheiten. Teil VII. Bovine Tuberkulose, aviäre Tuberkulose und andere Mykobakteriosen. Fischer, Jena, pp 281–303
Heyworth F (1967) B 663 in treatment of atypical tuberculous disease. Med J Aust 1:106–107
Hobby GL, Redmond WB, Runyon EH, Schaefer WB, Wayne LG, Wichelhausen RH (1967) A study on pulmonary disease associated with mycobacteria other than *Mycobacterium tuberculosis:* identification and characterization of the mycobacteria. Am Rev Respir Dis 95:954–971
Honza M, Kubin M, Sikorová A, Jankú A (1966) The influence of streptomycin and steroid hormones on the course of experimental osteo-arthritis provoked by non-chromogenous mycobacteria. Rozhl Tuberk 26:240–245; cited from: Burjanová B, Urbancik R (1970) Adv Tuberc Res 17:154–188

Hugh TB, Coleman MJ (1981) "Fish fanciers' finger": tropical fish-tank granuloma. M J Aust 1:614–615
Hui J, Gordon N, Kajioka R (1977) Permeability barrier to rifampicin in mycobacteria. Antimicrob Agents Chemother 11:773–779
Hunter AM, Campbell IA, Jenkins PA, Smith AP (1981) Treatment of pulmonary infections caused by mycobacteria of the Mycobacterium avium-intracellulare complex. Thorax 36:326–329
Irwin RS, Pratter MR, Corwin RW, Farrugia R, Teplitz C (1982) Pulmonary infection with *Mycobacterium chelonei:* successful treatment with one drug based on disk diffusion susceptibility data. J Infect Dis 145:772
Iseman MD, Corpe RF, O'Brien RJ, Rosenzweig DY, Wolinsky E (1985) Disease due to *Mycobacterium avium-intracellulare*. Chest 87, no 2 suppl:139S–149S
Iseman MD, Heifets L, Gangadharam PRJ (1986) Combination of drug effects in the chemotherapy of *M. avium-intracellulare: in vitro* and *in vivo* observations. Am Rev Respir Dis 133, no 4 part 2:A 40
Izumi AK, Hanke W, Higaki M (1977) *Mycobacterium marinum* infections treated with tetracycline. Arch Dermatol 113:1067–1068
Jakschik M (1979) Infektionen durch sogenannte atypische Mykobakterien. Klinische und bakteriologische Gesichtspunkte. Infection 7, Suppl 2:S211–S215
Janssens PG (1950) Discussion remark. Ann Soc Belge Méd Trop XXX:621–627
Jenkins DE, Bahar D, Chofnas I (1960) Pulmonary disease due to atypical mycobacteria: current concepts. Trans 19th Conf Chemother Tuberc, VAAF:224–231
Jenkins PA, Tsukamura M (1979) Infections with *Mycobacterium malmoense* in England and Wales. Tubercle 60:71–76
Johanson WG Jr, Nicholson DP (1969) Pulmonary disease due to *Mycobacterium kansasii*. Am Rev Respir Dis 90:73–85
Justice FK, Schwartz WS (1966) Clinical characteristics of pulmonary infections associated with Battey-bacilli, protocol 6. Trans 25th Res Conf Pulmon Dis, VAAF:83–86
Karasseva V, Weiszfeiler JG, Krasznag E (1965) Occurrence of atypical mycobacteria in *Macacus rhesus*. Acta microbiol Acad Sci Hung 12:275–282
Karlson AG (1959) Diaminodiphenylsulfone (DDS): preliminary observations on its effect in vitro and in mice infected with various species of mycobacterium. Trans 18th Conf Chemother Tuberc, VAAF:247–252
Kass I, Dye WE (1962) The use of viomycin and ethionamide in the chemotherapy of patients with pulmonary disease caused by unclassified mycobacteria (groups I and III), a preliminary report. Trans 21th Res Conf Pulm Dis, VAAF:175–179
Kelly R (1976) *Mycobacterium marinum* infection from a tropical fish tank. Treatment with trimethoprim and sulphamethoxazole. Med J Aust 2:681–682
Kestle DG, Abbott VD, Kubica GP (1967) Differential identification of mycobacteria. II Subgroups of groups II and III (Runyon) with different clinical significance. Am Rev Respir Dis 95:1041–1052
Kettel LJ (1965) Clinical course of 12 patients with pulmonary infection with *M. kansasii*. Trans 24th Res Conf Pulm Dis VAAF:78–82
Kim R (1974) Tetracycline therapy for atypical mycobacterial granuloma. Arch Dermatol 110:299
Kim TC, Arora NS, Aldrich TK, Rochester DF (1981) Atypical mycobacterial infections: a clinical study of 92 patients. South Med J 74:1304–1308
Krebs A (1967) Disposition zur Erkrankung der Lungen durch atypische Mykobakterien, Behandlungsergebnisse und Spätresultate. Z Tuberk 127:133–140
Kubica GP, Gross WM, Hawkins JE, Sommers HM, Vestal AL, Wayne LG (1975) Laboratory services for mycobacterial diseases. Am Rev Respir Dis 112:773–787
Kumar UN, Varkey B (1978) Clinical features, course and treatment of *Mycobacterium intracellulare* pulmonary disease compared to pulmonary tuberculosis. Am Rev Respir Dis 117, no 4, suppl:424
Kuritsky JN, Bullen MG, Broome VC, Silcox VE, Good RC, Wallace RJ Jr (1983) Sternal wound infections and endocarditis due to organisms of the *Mycobacterium fortuitum* complex. Ann Intern Med 98:938–939

Kuze F (1984) Experimental chemotherapy in chronic *Mycobacterium avium-intracellulare* infection of mice. Am Rev Respir Dis 129:453–459
Kuze F, Kurasawa T, Bando K, Lee Y, Maekawa N (1981) In vitro and in vivo susceptibility of atypical mycobacteria to various drugs. Rev Infect Dis 3:885–897
Kuze F, Mitsuoka A, Chiba W, Shimizu Y, Ho M, Teramatsu T, Maekawa N, Suzuki Y (1983) Chronic pulmonary infection caused by *Mycobacterium terrae* complex: a resected case. Am Rev Respir Dis 128:561–565
Laszlo A, Eidus L (1978) Identification of *Mycobacterium phlei* TMC 1523 and *Mycobacterium smegmatis* SN 40 as members of *Mycobacterium smegmatis* and *Mycobacterium fortuitum*, respectively: selective inhibition by trimethoprim. Int J System Bacteriol 28:602–604
Leach RH, Fenner F (1954) Studies of *Mycobacterium ulcerans* and *Mycobacterium balnei*. III. Growth in the semi-synthetic culture media of Dubos and drug sensitivity *in vitro* and *in vivo*. Aust J exp Biol 32:835–852
Lester W Jr, Botkin J, Colton R (1958) An analysis of forty-nine cases of pulmonary disease caused by photochromogenic mycobacteria. Trans 17th Conf Chemother Tuberc, VAAF:289–294
Lester W, Moulding T, Fraser RI, Mc Clatchy K, Fischer DA (1969) Quintuple drug regimens in the treatment of Battey-type infections. Trans 28th Pulmon Dis Res Conf, VAAF:83
Lewis AG Jr, Dunbar FP, Lasché EM, Bond JO, Lerner EN, Wharton DJ, Hardy AV, Davies R (1959) Chronic pulmonary disease due to atypical mycobacterial infections. Am Rev Tuberc 80:188–199
Lewis AG Jr, Lasché EM, Armstrong AL, Dunbar FP (1960) A clinical study of the chronic lung disease due to nonphotochromogenic acid-fast bacilli. Am Rev Tuberc 53:273–285
Lincoln EM, Gilbert LA (1972) Disease in children due to Mycobacteria other than *Mycobacterium tuberculosis*. Am Rev Respir Dis 105:683–714
Lockshin NA (1977) Treatment of *Mycobacterium marinum* infections with minocycline. Arch Dermatol 113:987
Lorber B, Suh B (1983) Bursitis caused by *Mycobacterium gordonae:* is surgery necessary? Am Rev Respir Dis 128:565–566
Loria P (1976) Minocycline hydrochloride treatment for atypical acid-fast infection. Arch Dermatol 112:517–519
Lunn HF, Rees RJW (1964) Treatment of mycobacterial skin ulcers in Uganda with a riminophenazine derivative (B.663). Lancet I:247–249
MacCallum P, Tolhurst JC, Buckle G, Sissons HA (1948) A new mycobacterial infection in man. J Path Bact LX:93–122
MacKellar A (1976) Diagnosis and management of atypical mycobacterial lymphadenitis in children. J Pediatr Surg 11:85–89
Manten A (1959) The occurrence of atypical mycobacterial infections in the Netherlands and the behaviour of the bacteria in vitro. Proc Tuberc Res Council, The Hague, No 46:71–82
Marks J, Schwabacher H (1965) Infection due to *Mycobacterium xenopei.* Br Med J 1:32–33
Marks J, Jenkins PA, Tsukamura M (1972) *Mycobacterium szulgai* – a new pathogen. Tubercle 53:210–214
Martin-Luengo F, Garcia-Rodríguez JA, Saenz-Gonzalez MC, Gomez-Garcia AC (1978) Antimicrobial activity of different aminoglycosides against potentially pathogenic “atypical” mycobacteria. In: Siegenthaler W, Lüthy R (eds) Proc 10th Intern Congr Chemotherapy, Vol 1, 237–238
Mayer RL, Eisman PC, Gisi TA, Konopka EA (1958) The chemotherapeutic activity upon chromogenic mycobacteria of certain derivatives of thiocarbanilide (SU 1906), thiazoline (SU 3068), and thiazolidinone (SU 3912). Am Rev Tuberc 77:694–702
Mc Clatchy JK, Waggoner RF, Lester W (1969) *In vitro* susceptibility of mycobacteria to rifampin. Am Rev Respir Dis 100:234–236
Mc Donald PJ, Tomasovic AA, Evans C (1971) *Mycobacterium xenopei* pulmonary infection in man. Med J Aust 1:873

McGeady SJ, Murphey SA (1981) Disseminated *Mycobacterium kansasii* infection. Clin Immunol Immunopathol 20:87–98
Mc Nutt DR, Fudenberg HH (1971) Disseminated scotochromogen infection and unusual myeloproliferative disorder. Ann Intern Med 75:737–744
Meissner G (1968) Kulturelle Artendifferenzierung. In: Meissner G, Schmiedel A (Hrsg) Mykobakterien und mykobakterielle Krankheiten. Teil IV. Laboratoriumsdiagnose der Mykobakterien. Fischer, Jena, pp 149–237
Meissner G (1970) Erkrankungen des Menschen durch *M. kansasii* und Mykobakterien der aviären Gruppe. In: Meissner G, Schmiedel A (Hrsg) Mykobakterien und mykobakterielle Krankheiten. Teil VII. Fischer, Jena, pp 239–280
Meissner G, Schmiedel A (1970) Mykobakterien und mykobakterielle Krankheiten. Teil VII. Bovine Tuberkulose, aviäre Tuberkulose und andere Mykobakteriosen. Fischer, Jena
Meissner G, Heidelbach H, Schuster H, Wentz D (1970) Lungenerkrankungen mit *Mycobacterium xenopi.* Prax Pneumol 24:564–570
Meissner G, Schröder K-H (1975) Relationship between *Mycobacterium simiae* and *Mycobacterium habana.* Am Rev Respir Dis 111:196–200
Meleney FL, Johnson BA (1951) Supplementary report on the case of chronic ulceration of the foot due to a new pathogenic mycobacterium (MacCallum). Int J Lepr 11:330–333
Metcalf JF, John JF Jr, Wilson GB, Fudenberg HH, Harley RA (1981) *Mycobacterium fortuitum* pulmonary infection associated with an antigen-selective defect in cellular immunity. Am J Med 71:485–492
Michel J, Haas H, Sacks TG (1973) *In vitro* susceptibility of *Mycobacterium fortuitum, M. abscessus* and *M. borstelense* to vancomycin. Chemotherapy 19:299–304
Misgeld V, Albrecht G, Hussels H (1976) Zur Kenntnis der Infektion mit *Mycobacterium ulcerans.* Castellania 4:1–6
Mizuguchi Y, Fukunaga M, Taniguchi H (1981) Plasmid desoxyribonucleic acid and translucent-to-opaque variation in *Mycobacterium intracellulare* 103. J Bact 146:656–659
Mizuguchi Y, Udou T, Yamada T (1983) Mechanism of antibiotic resistance in *Mycobacterium intracellulare.* Microbiol Immunol 27:425–431
Molavi A, Weinstein L (1971 a) In vitro susceptibility of atypical mycobacteria to rifampin. Appl Microbiol 22:23–25
Molavi A, Weinstein L (1971 b) In-vitro activity of erythromycin against atypical mycobacteria. J Inf Dis 123:216–219
Moran JF, Alexander LG, Staub EW, Young WG Jr, Sealy WC (1983) Long-term results of pulmonary resection for atypical mycobacterial disease. Ann Thorac Surg 35:597–604
Moulding T (1978) The relative drug susceptibility of opaque colonial forms of *Mycobacterium intracellulare-avium:* does it affect therapeutic results? Am Rev Respir Dis 117:1142 1143
Moulsdale MT, Harper JM, Thatcher GN (1983) Infection by *Mycobacterium haemophilum,* a metabolically fastidious acid-fast bacillus. Tubercle 64:29–36
Mulder-de Jong MT (1964) Anonymous mycobacteria in Western New Guinea. Selected Papers 8:80–91
Naito Y, Kuze F, Maekawa N (1979) Sensitivities of atypical mycobacteria to various drugs. V. Sensitivities of *Mycobacterium intracellulare* to some aminoglycoside and peptide antibiotics. Kekkaku 54:423–427
Nash DR, Steingrube VA (1982) *In vitro* drug sensitivity of *M. avium-intracellulare* complex in the presence and absence of dimethyl sulphoxide. Microbios 35:71–78
Nicholson DP, Sevier WR (1971) *Mycobacterium fortuitum* as a pathogen. A case report. Am Rev Respir Dis 104:747–750
Nozawa RT, Kato H, Yokota T (1984) Intra- and extracellular susceptibility of *Mycobacterium avium-intracellulare* complex to aminoglycoside antibiotics. Antimicrob Agents Chemother 26:841–844
Nozawa RT, Kato H, Yokota T, Sugi H (1985) Susceptibility of intra- and extracellular *Mycobacterium avium-intracellulare* to cephem antibiotics. Antimicrob Agents Chemother 27:132–134

Olitzki AL, Godinger D, Israeli M, Honigman A (1967) In vitro effects of some chemotherapeutic agents on mycobacteria. Appl Microbiol 15:994–1001

Olitzki AL, Olitzki Z, Davis CL (1968) Chemotherapeutic studies of mycobacterial infections in mice. Appl Microbiol 16:500–505

Pattyn SR, Royackers J (1965) Traitement de l'infection expérimentale de la souris par *Mycobacterium ulcerans* et *Mycobacterium balnei*. Ann Soc Belge Méd Trop 45:31–38

Pattyn SR, Hermans-Boveroulle MT, van Ermengem J (1968) A study on slow growing chromogenic (Runyon's group II) mycobacteria. Zentralbl Bakteriol Mikrobiol Hyg (A) 207:509–516

Pattyn SR, van Ermengem J (1968) DDS sensitivity of mycobacteria. Int J Lepr 36:427–431

Pattyn SR, Dommisse R (1973) Bacteriological study of *Mycobacterium habana*. Ann Soc Belge Méd Trop 53:267–273

Perumal VK, Gangadharam PR, Heifets LB, Iseman MD (1985) Dynamic aspects of the *in vitro* chemotherapeutic activity of ansamycin (rifabutine) on *Mycobacterium intracellulare*. Am Rev Respir Dis 132:1278–1280

Pettit JHS, Marchette NJ, Rees RJW (1966) *Mycobacterium ulcerans* infection. Br J Dermatol 78:187–197

Pezzia W, Raleigh JW, Bailey MC, Toth EA, Silverblatt J (1981) Treatment of pulmonary disease due to *Mycobacterium kansasii:* recent experience with rifampin. Rev Infect Dis 3:1035–1039

Pfuetze KH, Vo LV, Reimann AF, Berg GS, Lester W (1965) Photochromogenic mycobacterial pulmonary disease. Am Rev Respir Dis 92:470–475

Pocza A (1981) Pulmonary infection caused by *Mycobacterium szulgai*. Med J Aust 1:419–420

Portaels F, Pattyn SR (1970) Resistance to ethambutol as an aid to the identification of *Mycobacterium friedmannii (abscessus)* and *M. borstelense*. J Med Microbiol 3:674–676

Pottage JC Jr, Harris AA, Trenholme GM, Levin S, Kaplan RL, Feczko JM (1982) Disseminated *Mycobacterium chelonei* infection: a report of two cases. Am Rev Respir Dis 126:720–722

Radenbach KL (1972) Permanently successful chemotherapy in two cases with severe pulmonary mycobacterial disease due to *Mycobacterium kansasii* and *fortuitum*, respectively. Scand J Respir Dis Suppl 80:23–27

Rastogi N, Frehel C, Ryter A, Ohayon H, Lesourd M, David HL (1981) Multiple drug resistance in *Mycobacterium avium:* is the wall architecture responsible for the exclusion of antimicrobial agents? Antimicrob Agents Chemother 20:666–677

Rauscher CR, Kerby G, Ruth WE (1974) A ten-year clinical experience with *Mycobacterium kansasii*. Chest 66:17–19

Raz J, Katz M, Aram H, Haas H (1984) Sporotrichoid *Mycobacterium marinum* infection. Int J Dermatol 23:554–555

Reid IS (1967) *Mycobacterium ulcerans* infection: a report of 13 cases at the Port Moresby General Hospital, Papua. Med J Aust I:427–431

Revill WDL, Pike MC, Morrow RH, Ateng J (1973) A controlled trial of the treatment of *Mycobacterium ulcerans* infection with clofazimine. Lancet II:873–877

Roberts C, Clague H, Jenkins PA (1985) Pulmonary infection with *Mycobacterium malmoense:* a report of 4 cases. Tubercle 66:205–209

Rogul M, Keller R, Cabelli VJ (1957) The classification and susceptibilities to chemotherapeutic agents of chromogenic acid-fast bacilli. Am Rev Tuberc 76:697–702

Rolston KVI, Jones PG, Fainstein V, Bodey GP (1985) Pulmonary disease caused by rapidly growing mycobacteria in patients with cancer. Chest 87:503–506

Rosenfeld M (1968) Chemotherapie sogenannter atypischer Mycobakteriosen. Beitr Klin Tuberk 137:115–129

Rosenzweig DY (1979) Pulmonary mycobacterial infections due to *Mycobacterium intracellulare-avium* complex. Chest 75:115–119

Runyon EH (1959) Anonymous mycobacteria in pulmonary disease. Med Clin North Am 43:273–290

Rynearson TK, Shronts JS, Wolinsky E (1971 a) Rifampin: *In vitro* effect on atypical mycobacteria. Am Rev Respir Dis 104:272–274
Saito H, Sato K, Jin BW (1984) Activities of cefoxitin and cefotetan against *Mycobacterium fortuitum* infections in mice. Antimicrob Agents Chemother 26:270–271
Sakamoto I, Goda K (1966) Effectiveness of ethambutol against mice infected with atypical mycobacteria. Kekkaku 41:233–238
Sakurai N (1983) *In vitro* susceptibility of atypical mycobacteria to cephem and other antibiotics. Kekkaku 58:355–362
Salfinger M, Kafader F (1986) In vitro activity of a new quinolone (Ro 23-6240) against mycobacteria. Am Rev Respir Dis 133, no 4, part 2:A 71
Sanders WE Jr, Hartwig EC, Schneider NJ, Cacciatore R, Valdez H (1977) Susceptibility of organisms in the *Mycobacterium fortuitum* complex to antituberculous and other antimicrobial agents. Antimicrob Agents Chemother 12:295–297
Sanders WE Jr, Schneider N, Hartwig C, Cacciatore R, Valdez H (1980) Comparative activities of cephalosporins against mycobacteria. In: Nelson JD, Grassi C (eds) Proc 11th Intern Congr Chemother Boston, Vol II:1075–1077
Sanders WE Jr, Hartwig C, Schneider N, Cacciatore R, Valdez H (1982) Activity of amikacin against mycobacteria *in vitro* and in murine tuberculosis. Tubercle 63:201–208
Sanders WJ, Wolinsky E (1980) In vitro susceptibility of *Mycobacterium marinum* to eight antimicrobial agents. Antimicrob Agents Chemother 18:529–531
Schaefer WB, Wolinsky E, Jenkins PA, Marks J (1973) *Mycobacterium szulgai* – a new pathogen. Am Rev Respir Dis 108:1320–1326
Schraufnagel DE, Leech JA, Schraufnagel MN, Pollak B (1984) Short-course chemotherapy for mycobacteriosis kansasii? Can Med Assoc J 130:34–38
Schröder KH (1973) Klassifizierung von Mykobakterien. Ann Soc Belge Méd Trop 53:255–261
Schröder KH (1975) Investigation into the relationship of *M. ulcerans* to *M. buruli* and other mycobacteria. Am Rev Respir Dis 111:559–562
Schröder KH, Hensel J, Scheuch V (1969) Die Sensibilitätsprüfung von *M. tuberculosis* und atypischen Mykobakterien gegen Ethambutol, Capreomycin und Rifampicin. Prax Pneumol 23:683–694
Schröder KH, Juhlin I (1977) *Mycobacterium malmoense* sp. nov. Int J System Bacteriol 27:241–246
Schröder KH, Müller U (1982) *Mycobacterium malmoense* in Deutschland. Zentralbl Bakteriol Mikrobiol Hyg (A) 253:279–283
Selkon JB (1969) "Atypical" mycobacteria: a review. Tubercle 50, Suppl:70–78
Shronts JS, Rynearson TK, Wolinsky E (1971) Rifampin alone and combined with other drugs in *Mycobacterium kansasii* and *Mycobacterium intracellulare* infections of mice. Am Rev Respir Dis 104:728–741
Silcox VA, David HL (1971) Differential identification of *Mycobacterium kansasii* and *Mycobacterium marinum*. Appl Microbiol 21:327–334
Simon C (1970) Seltene mykobakterielle Erkrankungen bei Mensch und Tier. IV. Infektionen durch *Mycobacterium smegmatis*. In: Meissner G, Schmiedel A (Hrsg) Mykobakterien und mykobakterielle Krankheiten. Fischer, Jena, Teil VII, p 312
Smith MJ, Citron KM (1983) Clinical review of pulmonary disease caused by *Mycobacterium xenopi*. Thorax 38:373–377
Sompolinsky D, Lagziel A, Naveh D, Yankilevitz T (1978) *Mycobacterium haemophilum* sp. nov., a new pathogen of humans. Int J System Bacteriol 28:67–75
Song M, Vincke G, Vanachter H, Benekens J, Achten G (1985) Treatment of cutaneous infection due to *Mycobacterium ulcerans*. Dermatologica 171:197–199
Sopko JA, Fieselmann J, Kasik JE (1980) Pulmonary disease due to *Mycobacterium chelonei* subspecies abscessus: a report of four cases. Tubercle 61:165–169
Srivastava A, Singh NB, Gupta SK (1984) Prospective treatment for *Mycobacterium ulcerans* infection (Buruli ulcer) in rat and mice through combined therapy with rifampicin and septran. Current Science (Bangalore) 53:487–488
Staneck JL, Frame PT, Altemeier WA, Miller EH (1981) Infection of bone by *Mycobacterium fortuitum* masquerading as *Nocardia asteroides*. Am J Clin Path 76:216–222

Stanford JL, Phillips I (1972) Rifampicin in experimental *Mycobacterium ulcerans* infection. J Med Microbiol 5:39–45

Steenken W Jr, Smith MM, Montalbine V (1958) In vitro and in vivo effect of antimicrobial agents on atypical mycobacteria. Am Rev Tuberc 78:454–461

Stone MS, Wallace RJ Jr, Swenson JM, Thornsberry C, Christensen LA (1983) Agar disk elution method for susceptibility testing of *Mycobacterium marinum* and *Mycobacterium fortuitum* complex to sulfonamides and antibiotics. Antimicrob Agents Chemother 24:486–493

Stottmeier D (1964) Die Empfindlichkeit von photo- und scotochromogenen Mykobakterien für Pyrazin-2-carboxamid (Pyrazinamid). Beitr Klin Tuberk 129:106–109

Stottmeier D, Woodley C, Kubica GP (1968) The antimicrobial action of combinations of isoniazid, erythromycin, oxacillin and methenamine on the growth of *Mycobacterium intracellulare*. Trans 27th Conf Pulmon Dis, VAAF:18–20

Stover DE, Gellene R, Romano P, White D (1983) Lung diseases associated with the acquired immunodeficiency syndrome (AIDS). Am Rev Respir Dis 127, suppl:81

Swenson JM, Thornsberry C, Silcox V (1980) Susceptibility of rapidly growing mycobacteria to 34 antimicrobial agents. In: Nelson JD, Grassi C (eds) Proc 11th Congr Chemother Boston, 1979, Vol II, pp 1077–1079

Tacquet A, Tison F (1963) Activité *in vitro* et *in vivo* du dextro-2,2'(éthylène diimino)di-1-butanol (éthambutol) utilisé seul ou en association sur les mycobactéries „atypiques". Rev Tuberc Pneumol (Paris) 27:431–444

Tacquet A, Tison F, Devulder B, Roos P (1966) Étude *in vitro* de la sensibilité de *Mycobacterium kansasii* à la 4,4'diisoamyloxythiocarbanilide. Ann Inst Pasteur 110:436–442

Tacquet A, Devulder B, Tison F, Martin JC (1970) Activité de l'isoxyl sur *Mycobacterium kansasii;* études *in vitro* et chez le cobaye pneumoconiotique. Antibiotica et Chemotherapia 16:160–176

Tellis CJ, Beechler CR, Ohashi DK, Fuller SA (1977) Pulmonary disease caused by *Mycobacterium xenopi*. Am Rev Respir Dis 116:779–783

Tice AD, Solomon RJ (1979) Disseminated *Mycobacterium chelonei* infection: response to sulfonamides. Am Rev Respir Dis 120:197–201

Thibier R, Vivien JN, Lepeuple A (1970) Sept cas de pleuro-pneumopathie à „*Mycobacterium xenopei*". Rev Tuberc Pneumol (Paris) 34:623–625

Torres JR, Sands M, Sanders CV (1978) *In vitro* sensitivity of *Mycobacterium marinum* to minocycline and doxycycline. Tubercle 59:193–195

Tsang AY, Bentz RR, Schork MA, Sodeman TM (1978) Combined vs single-drug studies of susceptibilities of *Mycobacterium kansasii* to isoniazid, streptomycin, and ethambutol. Am J Clin Path 70:816–820

Tsukamura M (1980a) *In vitro* antimycobacterial activity of minocycline. Tubercle 61:37–38

Tsukamura M (1980b) A review on the taxonomy of the genus *Mycobacterium*. II. Species within the genus *Mycobacterium* – Trial of new grouping. Kekkaku 55:341–347

Tsukamura M, Nakamura E, Kurita T, Nakamura T (1973) Isolation of *Mycobacterium chelonei* subspecies *chelonei (Mycobacterium borstelense)* from pulmonary lesions of 9 patients. Am Rev Respir Dis 108:683–685

Tsukamura M, Inoue T, Kuwahara T, Yoshimoto K, Nakajima N (1981) Clinical effect of chemotherapy including minocycline on lung infection due to *Mycobacterium avium-intracellulare*. Kekkaku 56:57–61

Tsukamura M, Kita N, Otsuka W, Shimoide H (1983) A study of the taxonomy of the *Mycobacterium nonchromogenicum* complex and report of six cases of lung infection due to *Mycobacterium nonchromogenicum*. Microbiol Immunol 27:219–236

Turner T, Donald GF, Burry JN, Kirk J, Reid JG (1975) *Mycobacterium marinum* infection. Arch Dermatol 111:525

Uganda Buruli Group (1970) Report II Clinical features and treatment of pre-ulcerative Buruli lesions (*Mycobacterium ulcerans* infection). Br Med J II:390–393

Ullmann U, Schubert GE, Kieninger G (1975) Bakteriologische und tierexperimentelle Untersuchungen mit *Mycobacterium ulcerans* (Tübingen 1971). Zentralbl Bakteriol Mikrobiol Hyg (A) 232:318–327

Urbančik R (1959) Chemotherapy of diseases caused by atypical mycobacteria. I. In vitro response to a number of antimicrobial agents in blood agar, 7H9 and Löwenstein media. J Hyg Epidemiol Microbiol (Prague) 3:306–313
Valdivia AJ, Suarez MR (1971) *Mycobacterium habana:* probable nueva especie dentro de las micobacterias no clasificadas. Bol Hig Epid (La Habana) 9:65–73
Verbist L, Gyselen A (1968) Antituberculous activity of rifampin *in vitro* and *in vivo* and the concentrations attained in human blood. Am Rev Respir Dis 98:923–932
Virtanen S (1961) Drug sensitivities of atypical acid-fast organisms. Acta Tuberc Scand 40:182–189
Wallace RA Jr, Dalovisio JR, Pankey GA (1979) Disk diffusion testing of susceptibility of *Mycobacterium fortuitum* and *Mycobacterium chelonei* to antibacterial agents. Antimicrob Agents Chemother 16:611–614
Wallace JR Jr, Jones DB, Wiss K (1981 a) Sulfonamide activity against *Mycobacterium fortuitum* and *Mycobacterium chelonei.* Rev Infect Dis 3:898–904
Wallace RJ Jr, Wiss K, Septimus EJ, Dalovisio JR (1981 b) The in-vitro activity of antibacterial agents against *Mycobacterium marinum.* Am Rev Respir Dis 123, no 4, part 2:260
Wallace RJ Jr, Swenson JM, Silcox VA, Good RC, Tschen JA, Stone MS (1983) Spectrum of disease due to rapidly growing mycobacteria. Rev Infect Dis 5:657–679
Wallace RJ Jr, Hull SI, Bobey DG, Price KE, Swenson JM, Steele LC, Christensen L (1985 a) Mutational resistance as the mechanism of acquired drug resistance to aminoglycosides and antibacterial agents in *Mycobacterium fortuitum* and *Mycobacterium chelonei.* Am Rev Respir Dis 132:409–416
Wallace RJ Jr, Swenson JM, Silcox VA, Bullen MG (1985 b) Treatment of nonpulmonary infections due to *Mycobacterium fortuitum* and *Mycobacterium chelonei* on the basis of in vitro susceptibilities. J Infect Dis 152:500–514
Watson BM, Smyth JT (1967) B 663 and ethambutol in the treatment of Battey disease. Med J Aust 1:261–263
Welch DF, Kelly MT (1979) Antimicrobial susceptibility testing of *Mycobacterium fortuitum* complex. Antimicrob Agents Chemother 15:754–757
Weitzman I, Osadczyi D, Corrado ML, Karp D (1981) *Mycobacterium thermoresistibile:* a new pathogen for humans. J Clin Microbiol 14:593–595
Weiszfeiler JG (1973) (ed) Atypical mycobacteria. Akadémiai Kiadó, Budapest
Weiszfeiler JG, Karczag E (1976) Synonymy of *Mycobacterium simiae* Karasseva et al. 1965 and *Mycobacterium habana* Valdivia et al. 1971. Int J System Bacteriol 26:474–477
Weiszfeiler JG, Karasseva V, Karczag E (1981) *Mycobacterium simiae* and related mycobacteria. Rev Infect Dis 3:1040–1045
Wichelhausen RH, Robinson LB (1965) Classification of and drug-susceptibility determinations on cultures of mycobacteria other than *M. tuberculosis.* Trans 24th Res Conf Pulmon Dis, VAAF:56–64
Williams CS, Riordan DC (1973) *Mycobacterium marinum* (atypical acid-fast bacillus) infections of the hand. J Bone Joint Surg 55-A:1042–1050
Wolinsky E (1959) Chemotherapy and pathology of experimental photochromogenic mycobacterial infections. Am Rev Respir Dis 80:522–534
Wolinsky E (1963) The role of scotochromogenic mycobacteria in human disease. Ann NY Acad Sci 106:67–71
Wolinsky E (1979) Nontuberculous mycobacteria and associated diseases. Am Rev Respir Dis 119:107–159
Wolinsky E, Smith MM, Steenken W Jr (1957) Drug susceptibilities of 20 "atypical" as compared with 19 selected strains of mycobacteria. Am Rev Tuberc 76:497–502
Wolinsky E, Gomez F, Zimpfer F (1972) Sporotrichoid *Mycobacterium marinum* infection treated with rifampin-ethambutol. Am Rev Respir Dis 105:964–967
Wollschlager CM, Khan FA, Chitkava RK, Shivaram U (1984) Pulmonary manifestations of the acquired immunodeficiency syndrome (AIDS). Chest 85:197–202
Wood LE, Buhler VB, Pollak A (1956) Human infection with the "yellow" acid-fast bacillus. Am Rev Tuberc 73:917–929

Woodley CL, Kilburn JO (1982) *In vitro* susceptibility of *Mycobacterium avium* complex and *Mycobacterium tuberculosis* strains to a spiro-piperidyl rifamycin. Am Rev Respir Dis 126:586–587

Yamamoto M, Sudo K, Taga M, Hibino S (1967) A study of diseases caused by atypical mycobacteria in Japan. Am Rev Respir Dis 96:779–787

Yates MD, Collins CH (1981) Sensitivity of opportunist mycobacteria to rifampicin and ethambutol. Tubercle 62:117–121

Yeager H Jr, Raleigh JW (1973) Pulmonary disease due to *Mycobacterium intracellulare*. Am Rev Respir Dis 108:547–552

Yoshida F (1970) Experimental therapy with rifampicin. Antibiotica et Chemotherapia 16:416–423

Zimmer BL, De Young DR, Roberts GD (1982) In vitro synergistic activity of ethambutol, isoniazid, kanamycin, rifampin, and streptomycin against *Mycobacterium avium-intracellulare* complex. Antimicrob Agents Chemother 22:148–150

Zvetina JR (1965) Clinical course of 15 patients with pulmonary infection with *M. kansasii*. Trans 24th Res Conf Pulm Dis, VAAF:74–77

Zvetina JR (1966) Clinical characteristics of pulmonary infections associated with *M. kansasii*, protocol 6. Trans 25th Res Conf Pulm Dis, VAAF:79–82

CHAPTER 5

Experimental Pharmacology and Toxicology of Antituberculosis Drugs

D. TETTENBORN

A. Introduction

The anti-tuberculosis agents are, chemically, a very heterogeneous group exhibiting a wide spectrum of pharmacological and toxicological effects on the various organ systems. These range from the very early recognized ototoxicity and nephrotoxicity of the aminoglycosides, to the question of neurotoxicity, carcinogenicity and mutagenicity of INH, to the oculotoxicity of ethambutol and to effects on neuro-muscular transmission of the aminoglycosides. Whilst for some substances there are enormous numbers of publications, there are other substances where there is a noticeable lack of published pharmacological and toxicological data. With regard to the latter substances it was possible, in some cases, to include in this review previously unpublished results of studies carried out by the manufacturing companies. Since most of the anti-tuberculosis agents were introduced 20 years–30 years ago, it is practically impossible to assess the old publications on the basis of modern standards. It would be misguided, however, to ignore the results of the early studies since they provided important basic data.

The pharmacological and toxicological studies could not always provide precise answers to the problem under consideration. Some of the differences between the results found in man and in laboratory animals are due to species-dependent differences in the type of reaction and to differences in dosage and length of administration period. Thorough clinical and epidemiological studies, exemplified in this case by those concerning the possible carcinogenicity and mutagenicity of INH, were able to indicate safety levels for clinical administration and to settle controversies that had often been raging for years. On the other hand, results can exhibit a good correlation between animal study and man; for example, studies on the nephrotoxicity and ototoxicity of the aminoglycosides. This demonstrates the importance of carefully conducted pharmacological and toxicological investigations for the achievement of the highest possible safety standards for the patient.

B. The Drugs

I. p-Aminosalicylic Acid (PAS)

p-aminosalicylic acid (PAS) is relatively unstable in aqueous solution and decarboxylates with the formation of considerable quantities of toxic m-aminophenol, especially at higher temperatures and under weakly acidic conditions. Independently of the m-aminophenol formation, PAS solutions undergo yellow to brown discoloration in air, and especially on exposure to light (THOMA 1962). Both these phenomena quickly attracted the attention of investigators, and the biological effects of the discolored and aminophenol-containing solutions have been compared with those of PAS in a number of studies. In the solid form, on the other hand, the decomposition of PAS is insignificant.

1. Respiration, Circulation, Heart

Intravenous injection of a freshly prepared solution of PAS sodium to anaesthetized rabbits in a dose of 100 mg/kg produces only a slight and transient increase in the blood pressure. In contrast, the same dose of a 6-months-old solution produced in rabbits and cats a definite increase of the blood pressure that persists for 20 min–30 min. However, the pressure increase cannot be attributed to the m-aminophenol content, as this on its own, or added in the appropriate concentrations to fresh PAS sodium solutions, does not exert any appreciable effect. Since the blood-pressure elevation is not blocked by sympatholytics, it definitely cannot be attributed to sympathetic nervous effects. It may be caused – at least partially – by a direct cardiac effect. In the isolated rabbit heart both freshly prepared and old solutions of PAS sodium gave rise to an increased amplitude of the heart beat without any appreciable increase of the heart rate (BAVIN and JAMES 1952).

PAS has no particular effect on respiration in anaesthetized cats (BAVIN and JAMES 1952).

2. Acute Toxicity

KOELZER and GIESEN (1951) studied the toxicity of free PAS and of its sodium and calcium salts. Table 1 shows that after i.p. administration in mice free PAS exhibits more or less the same toxicity as its salts if the comparison is based on the latter's PAS content. When administered orally, the acid appears to be somewhat more toxic than the salts, but the differences remain within the wide range.

Rats were less sensitive than mice. The development of the toxic reaction is uncharacteristic. No striking alterations were observed in the blood picture, nor did pathological examination of the dying animals reveal any abnormalities. KOELZER and GIESEN (1951) observed a considerable increase in toxicity if PAS sodium solutions had been heated or allowed to stand for a long time. However,

Table 1. Acute toxicity of PAS and its salts. (After KOELZER and GIESEN 1951)

Species	Substance	LD_{50} in mg/kg	
		Per os	Intraperitoneal
Mouse	PAS	5000	4250
	PAS-Na	6900 PAS-Na = 6000 PAS	4600 PAS-Na = 4000 PAS
	PAS-Ca	6500 PAS-Ca = 5750 PAS	5000 PAS-Ca = 4400 PAS
Rat	PAS-Na	8000 PAS-Na = 7000 PAS	4950 PAS-Na = 4300 PAS

the increased toxicity cannot be attributed to the solution – discoloration that occurs in air and especially on exposure to light. During this decomposition only small amounts of aminophenol are formed, and the toxicity increases only slightly. *Heating* of already yellowed solutions does not produce further discoloration, although the toxicity of such solutions increases strongly by the formation of m-aminophenol. Thus, the discoloration and the increased toxicity do not develop in parallel and are due to different decomposition products. SCHONHOLZER (1951) likewise found that the discoloration of the solutions had nothing to do with the increase in toxicity. However, at higher concentrations of m-aminophenol the toxicity of PAS solutions increases as follows:

	LD_{50}, mouse, i.p.
PAS sodium, pure	2800 mg/kg
PAS + 4% m-aminophenol	1740 mg/kg
PAS + 10% m-aminophenol	550 mg/kg
m-Aminophenol	111 mg/kg

BAVIN and JAMES (1952) compared the acute toxicity of freshly prepared solutions of PAS sodium injected i.v. into mice with the toxicity of solutions prepared 1 month and 6 months earlier. Over a 3-day observation period an LD_{50} of 3800 mg/kg was found for the fresh solution. The 1-month-old solution had an LD_{50} of 2600 mg/kg and the 6-month-old solution one of 2300 mg/kg. Thus, there is a clear increase in toxicity within a month, whereas subsequently there is only a slight further increase. However, the authors failed to find any connection of the increase in toxicity with the relatively low increases in m-aminophenol content or with the change in the color of the solutions, which after 6 months were nearly black.

Our own investigations (TETTENBORN 1970) gave an LD_{50} of 4590 (4210–4960) mg/kg after i.v. injection of freshly prepared PAS sodium solutions into male CF_1 mice (20 ml/kg, injection time 30 sec). Higher doses caused transient, tonic convulsions after the injection and later on motility was impaired. After 24 h the symptoms had disappeared. The urine was yellowish-orange for up to 24 h after the administration. Cardiac activity was still present in animals autopsied immediately after the respiratory arrest. An investigation on male Wistar rats revealed that the LD_{50} of orally administered PAS sodium is more than 10000 mg/kg. The orange discoloration of the urine was also observed in rats.

3. Subchronic and Chronic Toxicity

After 15 days–30 days rats treated with 2 × 1000 mg of PAS Na/kg/day administered i.p. or 2 × 1000 mg/kg/day of PAS acid administered orally showed neither macroscopic nor microscopic differences between treated and control animals (KOELZER and GIESEN 1951). However, following longer oral treatment of rats with 1000 mg of PAS Na/kg, BAVIN and JAMES (1952) observed a retardation of growth after 2 months to 3 months. This appeared both in the animals that had received freshly made up solutions and in the animals treated with solutions made up 1 month to 6 months earlier. The retardation was even more pronounced after a further 1 month–2 months. After the treatment had ended the effect on the growth proved to be rapidly reversible. Histological examinations of the thyroid glands revealed pronounced hyperplasia, although the weight of the thyroid had not increased. Long-term administration of m-aminophenol to rats over 20 weeks (7.5 or 150 mg/kg p.o.) showed that the effect on the thyroid was not due to contamination with m-aminophenol but was caused by the PAS.

After administration of PAS in the feed for only 10 days, Kjerulf-Jensen and Wolffbrandt (1951) observed typical cellular hyperplasia of the thyroid in rats, similar to that after thiouracil treatment. The hyperplasia could be prevented by feeding the animals with powdered dried calf thyroid, but not by the administration of sodium iodide. Similar results were obtained in mice and in rabbits but not in guinea pigs. In rats m-aminophenol produced similar effects on the thyroid, but the thyroid-inhibiting effect of PAS and m-aminophenol was only 1% of that of 6-methyl-2-thiouracil. No additive effect was observed on administration of submaximally active doses of PAS and thiouracil.

A study on the antithyroid effect of PAS was carried out by Beattie and Chambers (1953). In rats adapted to an ambient temperature of 29.5 °C treatment with PAS (1000 mg/kg p.o.) for 16 days resulted in a reduction of the ^{131}I uptake and of the oxygen consumption compared with the control animals. Simultaneous administration of thyroxine with the PAS prevented the fall in oxygen consumption and increased the ^{131}I uptake. The structural alterations in the thyroid (absence of colloid in most follicles in the central part of the gland, absence of any cell proliferation, and an increased height of the follicular epithelium at the thyroid centre) point to an increased release of thyreotropic hormone. The primary effect of PAS could therefore be the inhibition of iodine uptake.

In animals kept under normal conditions and treated for 25 weeks with 1000 mg/kg the thyroids exhibited signs of exhaustion (excessive cell proliferation in the follicles and complete degeneration of the follicular epithelium in some animals). Within 2 treatment-free weeks, however, the animals returned completely to normal (Beattie and Chambers 1953).

Mehrotra et al. (1959) reported changes in the liver of rats following chronic treatment with 5% PAS in the feed. Autopsies after 1 month to 12 months revealed that the livers were already enlarged and heavier after 1 month. Although in the first 4 months the appearance and the consistency of the livers were normal, later on small white regions appeared on the surface. Histological and histochemical examinations showed an abnormal increase of the glycogen content of the swollen-looking hepatocytes. In later stages inflammatory cellular infiltrates were observed, together with bile-duct proliferation, periportal fibrosis, and intensive regenerative activity of the liver cells. These alterations proved to be reversible on discontinuation of the treatment.

According to various publications, PAS causes activation of the adrenal cortex by stimulation of the anterior lobe of the hypophysis and an increased release of ACTH (Hetzel and Hine 1951; van Cauwenberge 1951). These results have not been confirmed by the results of other studies (Cronheim et al. 1952; Bavin and James 1952).

References

Bavin EM, James B (1952) Further aspects of the pharmacology of para-aminosalicylic acid. J Pharm Pharmacol 4:856–870
Beattie J, Chambers RD (1953) The anti-thyroid action of para-aminosalicylic acid. J Endocrinol 10:65-72
Cauwenberge H van (1951) The effect of salicylates on the pituitary and suprarenal glands. Lancet 2:686–687
Cronheim G, King JS, Hyder N (1952) Effect of salicylic acid and similar compounds on the adrenal-pituitary system. Proc Soc Exp Biol Med 80:51–55
Hetzel BS, Hine DC (1951) The effect of salicylates on the pituitary and suprarenal glands. Lancet 2:94–97
Kjerulf-Jensen K, Wolffbrandt G (1951) Antithyroid effect of p-aminosalicylic acid and m-aminophenol. Acta Pharmacol Toxicol (Copenh) 7:376–380
Koelzer PP, Giesen J (1951) Untersuchungen zur Toxizität der p-Aminosalicylsäure und ihrer Derivate. Z Naturforsch 6 B:183–190
Mehrotra RML, Chandra S, Singh MP, Gupta NN (1959) Changes in the liver of albino rats after administration of para-aminosalicylic acid. Indian J Med Res 47:500–506
Schonholzer G (1951) Comments on the toxicity of P.A.S. preparations. Aust J Pharm 32:1359–1363
Tettenborn D (1970) Unpublished investigations
Thoma F (1962) Stabilität von PAS-Infusionslösungen und ihre Prüfung durch Papier- und Dünnschichtchromatographie. Tuberk Arzt 16:362–368

II. Streptomycin – Dihydrostreptomycin (SM – DHSM)

1. Respiration, Circulation, Heart

In preliminary toxicological studies on streptomycin (SM) Molitor et al. (1946) observed respiratory disturbances to the point of respiratory arrest after high doses. It was later established by other investigators that these effects are caused by a neuromuscular blockade.

The effects of SM and dihydrostreptomycin (DHSM) on the heart and the circulation in animal experiments have been repeatedly described. As long ago as 1946, Molitor et al. reported the blood pressure lowering effect of high doses of SM, despite the difficulty, always present in the early investigations, of separating the pharmacological effects of the antibiotic from the effects of the large quantities of impurities with histamine-like activity that were often present. Marquardt and Ziegler (1956) observed a pronounced fall in the blood pressure of anaesthetized cats after i.v. injection of SM (38 mg/kg–42 mg/kg). In comparative studies with tetracycline (TC), oleandomycin, DHSM, SM, and chloramphenicol, Leaders et al. (1960) observed a hypotensive effect of these antibiotics (given above in order of decreasing strength) on anaesthetized rabbits following slow infusion. All the antibiotics caused a slowing of the heart rate. The contractility of the isolated rabbit heart was most strongly reduced by SM and DHSM.

According to more recent investigations (Wolf and Wigton 1971), SM produces direct inhibition of the smooth vascular muscle, which can be overcome by calcium chloride. Adams et al. (1973) and Goodman et al. (1974) found that the aminoglycoside antibiotic neomycin restricts the ability of smooth vascular muscle cells to bind and store calcium ions and inhibits the effects of various vasoactive agents (K^+, noradrenaline, histamine, angiotensin II, and serotonin). SM, DHSM, and kanamycin (KM) most probably act in a similar fashion.

Using isolated canine heart-lung preparation, SWAIN et al. (1956) observed that SM and DHSM exerted relatively weak negative inotropic activity in comparison to chloramphenicol, chlortetracycline, oxytetracycline, and TC. High doses caused cardiac failure, which could be antagonized by calcium chloride.

Thus, many findings (see also below) indicate that aminoglycoside antibiotics interfere with the function of calcium ions in various tissues.

COHEN et al. (1970) observed a dose-dependent suppression of the cardiovascular functions in open-thorax dogs after i.v. administration of 2.5 mg/SM/kg, 10 mg/SM/kg, and 40 mg/SM/kg. TC, KM, vancomycin, erythromycin, and colimycin all acted in a similar fashion. In intact dogs intramuscular injection of 2 g SM caused a 26% reduction of the cardiac output and a 22% fall in the mean arterial blood pressure 1 h after the injection. The mean SM concentration at this time was 35 µg/ml and was therefore within the therapeutic range for patients. Using the isolated perfused cat heart (Langendorff) it was shown that SM, TC, KM, vancomycin, and chloramphenicol caused a clear reduction of cardiac contractility.

2. Neuromuscular Blocking Effects of SM, DHSM, and Other Basic Antibiotics

The toxicity picture of lethal doses of SM (see above) in warmblooded animals suggested that an impairment of neuromuscular stimulus conduction may be the cause of the motor effects first discovered experimentally by VITAL BRAZIL and CORRADO (1957). Many subsequent investigations revealed that other basic antibiotics [aminosidine, DHSM, gentamicin, KM, neomycin, paromomycin, and viomycin (VM)] act similarly. Thus, the antibiotics of interest here, SM, DHSM, KM, and VM will be dealt with jointly below, and findings on other antibiotics of this group, e.g., neomycin and gentamicin, can be taken into consideration in the interpretation of their mode of action.

SM, DHSM, KM, and neomycin give rise to a progressive, atonic paralysis of the skeletal muscles to the point of respiratory paralysis. This has been reported in dogs (VITAL BRAZIL and CORRADO 1957; PITTINGER and LONG 1958; CORRADO et al. 1959), rabbits and mice (VITAL BRAZIL and CORRADO 1957; PITTINGER et al. 1958; BEZZI and GESSA 1961) and pigeons (VITAL BRAZIL and CORRADO 1957; PITTINGER et al. 1958). The investigations by VITAL BRAZIL and CORRADO (1957), IWATSUKI et al. (1958), BEZZI and GESSA (1959, 1961), TIMMERMAN et al. (1959), LÜLLMANN and REUTER (1960a, b), and others indicated that SM, DHSM and KM, and the other antibiotics of this group exert curare-like activity and potentiate the effects of d-tubocurarine and diethyl ether while attenuating those of the depolarizing inhibitors suxamethonium and decamethonium (IWATSUKI et al. 1958).

The effects of SM, DHSM, KM, and the other antibiotics in this group are considerably weaker than those of d-tubocurarine, but the quantitative effect is to some extent balanced out by the fact that the doses required for therapeutic purposes are considerably higher than those of d-tubocurarine (LÜLLMANN and REUTER 1960a, b). The simultaneous administration of membrane-stabilizing substances such as d-tubocurarine and diethyl ether during therapy with high doses of basic antibiotics should therefore be avoided (LÜLLMANN and REUTER 1960a, b). Instead, depolarizing drugs such as decamethonium or suxamethonium should be considered for muscle relaxation.

Many individual findings, which will not be dealt with in detail here (see PITTINGER and ADAMSON 1972 for a review) give, however, indications of qualitative differences between the modes of action of curare and the basic antibiotics.

The muscle relaxation effected by the basic antibiotics is slowly and transiently antagonized by neostigmine (VITAL BRAZIL and CORRADO 1957; PITTINGER and LONG 1958; TIMMERMAN et al. 1959; JINDAL and DESPHANDE 1960; KUBIKOWSKI and SZRENIAWSKI 1963; SINGH et al. 1978). The antagonism by calcium ions is particularly noteworthy; its protective effect in cases of SM intoxication had already been observed and further investigated by KELLER et al. (1956). In intact conscious dogs the symptoms induced by 110 mg SM/kg i.v. (muscular weakness, ataxia, atonic paralysis) are immediately eliminated by calcium chloride (50 mg/kg i.v.) (VITAL BRAZIL and CORRADO 1957). The antagonistic effect of Ca^{2+} was subsequently confirmed by other investigators using the phrenic nerve-diaphragm preparation from the rat or the mouse or the sciatic-gastrocnemic-nerve preparation from the dog (PITTINGER and LONG 1958; CORRADO et al. 1959; JINDAL and DESPHANDE 1960; KUBIKOWSKI and SZRENIAWSKI 1963; SINGH et al. 1978).

KELLER et al. (1956) had already noticed the similarity between the intoxication symptoms in rabbits after i.v. injection of SM and the effects induced by magnesium sulphate. Magnesium ions, acting as calcium ion antagonists intensify the acute toxicity of streptomycin.

According to VITAL BRAZIL and PRADO-FRANCESCHI (1969) and others, the aminoglycoside antibiotics compete with Ca^{2+} at the same nerve-ending receptor sites as magnesium ions; as a result there is a reduction in the release of the neurotransmitter substance acetylcholine. The neuromuscular blockade thus takes place presynaptically (PRADO et al. 1978). In addition to the presynaptic effects, however, the aminoglycoside antibiotics evidently also show postsynaptic activity in dependence on the dose or the concentration, as shown by MOLGÓ et al. (1979) on the example of kanamycin.

There are quantitative and qualitative differences between the neuromuscular-blocking effects of the different antibiotics. SM exhibits a stronger neuromuscular paralysing activity than DHSM and its effects set in faster and last longer (JINDAL and DESPHANDE 1960). According to KUBIKOWSKI and SZRENIAWSKI (1963), the neuromuscular blocking activity of the antibiotics decreases in the order SM, DHSM, VM, and KM. The subunits of the SM molecule, streptidine and streptamine, also produce neuromuscular blockade (VITAL BRAZIL et al. 1959).

3. Smooth Muscles

SM inhibits the spontaneous contractions of isolated rabbit ileum and also those induced by methylcholine and histamine (LEADERS et al. 1960). This is also true of the rat and the rabbit uterus (DŽOLJIĆ and BABIĆ 1967). POPOVICI et al. (1965, 1967) found that the effects of SM are concentration-dependent. At concentrations of 5×10^{-5} to 2×10^{-4} SM stimulates the uterus of adult, non-pregnant guinea pigs, while at concentrations higher than 5×10^{-4} the effect is inhibitory.

The effects of DHSM are similar to those of SM (LEADERS et al. 1960). DŽOLJIĆ and BABIĆ (1967) explain the inhibitory action of SM as an effect on the smooth-muscle-cell membrane.

4. Ganglion Blocking Effects

SM exerts a blocking effect on the ganglia of the sympathetic and parasympathetic systems (CORRADO 1958), similar to the inhibition of the ganglionic stimulus conduction caused by magnesium ions. Neostigmine and calcium ions antagonize the ganglioplegic action of SM.

5. Further Pharmacologic Effects

I.p. injections of SM and DHSM induce the release of histamine in guinea pigs (AMANN and RADENBACH 1961).

6. Acute Toxicity

The results of the first toxicologic studies on SM can only be evaluated to a limited extent, since the experiments were initially performed with relatively impure material which caused histamine-like effects (MOLITOR et al. 1946; MOLITOR and KUNA 1949; ROBSON and SULLIVAN 1963). For this reason the older LD_{50} values have not been included in Tables 1 and 2.

Studies on the acute toxicity of SM and DHSM were performed predominantly on mice; i.v. and s.c. administration was most commonly used. MÜCKTER

Table 1. Acute toxicity of streptomycin sulphate

Species	Strain sex	Route of adminis-tration	LD_{50} mg/kg	Confidence interval p=0.05	Literature source
Mouse	A 2 G, ♂	i.v.	85		5
Mouse	GFF, ♀	i.v.	111		5
Mouse	Albino	i.v.	80–92[a]		4
Mouse	A 2 G, ♂	i.p.	610		5
Mouse	GFF, ♀	i.p.	575		5
Mouse	CF_1, ♂	i.p.	495[a]	(433–561)	6
Mouse	Albino	s.c.	640[a]	(555–707,5)	2
Mouse	Albino	s.c.	500[a]		3
Mouse	Albino	s.c.	700[a]		1
Mouse	A 2 G, ♂	s.c.	500		5
Mouse	GFF, ♀	s.c.	550		5
Mouse	A 2 G, ♂	p.o.	15550		5
Mouse	GFF, ♀	p.o.	30000		5
Rat	Wistar	i.p.	997[a]	(893–1113)	6

[1] DUCROT et al. (1956); [2] KELLER et al. (1956); [3] KIMMERLE and GÖSSWALD (1956); [4] HAWKINS et al. (1956–1957); [5] BACHARACH et al. (1959); [6] HOFFMANN (1970)
[a] As the base.

Table 2. Acute toxicity of dihydrostreptomycin sulphate

Species	Strain sex	Route of adminis-tration	LD_{50} mg/kg	Confidence interval $p=0.05$	Literature source
Mouse	Albino	i.v.	172[a]		2
Mouse	Albino	i.v.	147–208[a]		4
Mouse	No data	s.c.	1200[a]		1
Mouse	Albino	s.c.	1200[a]	1100–1310	2
Mouse	Albino	s.c.	890[a]		3

[1] DUCROT et al. (1956); [2] KELLER et al. (1956); [3] KIMMERLE and GÖSSWALD (1956); [4] HAWKINS et al. (1956–1957).
[a] As the base.

(1961) pointed out that i.v. injection gave much more consistent results than s.c. administration and it was preferable for comparative investigations.

Respiratory disturbances and loss of consciousness are observed almost immediately after i.v. injection of lethal doses of SM sulphate. The animals die because of peripheral respiratory paralysis, since the heart carries on beating for a few minutes after the respiratory arrest (MOLITOR et al. 1946). If the animal survives the initial effects, it usually recovers rapidly. If artifical respiration is given, the treatment is usually survived without problems.

If the injection is given by the s.c. route, some 5 times to 10 times the dose is needed to produce the same toxic effects. Irrespective of the route of administration, SM is about twice as toxic as DHSM.

In contrast, orally administered SM and DHSM have virtually no effect, as the antibiotics are only absorbed to a small extent (SM about 3%) (MÜCKTER 1961). However, golden hamsters also respond very sensitively to oral administration of SM (LD_{50} 400 mg/kg), perhaps because of a selective modification of the intestinal flora (DESALVA et al. 1969).

Whereas the acute toxicity picture in the different species is very consistent, the sensitivity varies between different animal species.

Pigeons react very sensitively to streptomycin antibiotics. The i.m. LD_{50} for DHSM is 715 mg/kg (GRAY and PURMALIS 1958) and that for SM is 400–500 mg/kg (MÜCKTER 1961). Frogs, which do not depend exclusively on pulmonary respiration, survive the administration of substantially higher doses than mice if they remain submerged deeply enough in constantly changed water to ensure oxygen exchange through the skin (MOLITOR et al. 1946). There are practically no differences in toxicity between newborn and adult rats given s.c. injections of SM sulphate (MICHAEL and SUTHERLAND 1961).

According to the pharmacological findings, the acute toxic effects of the two antibiotics are definitely due to neuromuscular blockade.

a) Attempts at Reducing the Acute Toxicity

Since the discovery of SM and its toxic side effects many attempts have been made to reduce the toxicity and therefore the side effects of the drug (MÜCKTER 1961).

Initially it was thought that the impurities in SM preparations were the main cause of the side effects and the appropriate measure seemed to be to improve the purity. Thus, the original SM-calcium chloride complex was just changed to SM sulphate and later to DHSM, in which the aldehyde group of SM is hydrogenated to a primary alcohol. As already mentioned, the acute toxicity of DHSM is about half of that of SM. However, one serious disadvantage of DHSM compared with SM is the increased cochlear nerve toxicity; this will be dealt with in detail later on (p. 317).

The acute toxicity of streptomycin and of the other basic streptomyces antibiotics can be very considerably reduced by calcium ions (KELLER et al. 1956). As expected, magnesium ions, being antagonists of calcium ions, intensify the acute toxicity.

Under certain conditions a number of non-ionic substances belonging to various groups of substances can reduce the acute toxicity of SM and DHSM and of the other basic streptomyces antibiotics (review in MÜCKTER 1961; STUPP 1970). These include INH, glycerol, propylene glycol, rutin, etc. and anionic compounds such as certain amino acids (glycine), vitamins (nicotinic acid, p-aminobenzoic acid) and methane sulphonates, or acid compounds related to the mucopolysaccharides (heparin, heparinoids).

Pantothenic acid, whose "detoxifying" effect was first described by KELLER et al. (1956), plays a particular role. These findings were subsequently repeatedly checked and confirmed by DUCROT et al. (1956) and by PRESCOTT et al. (1959), whilst other investigators were unable to observe any effect of pantothenic acid on the acute toxicity of the streptomycins (CHILD et al. 1957; HAWKINS et al. 1957; KIMMERLE and GÖSSWALD 1956). OSTERBERG et al. (1956/1957) reported only a very slight detoxifying effect and BRIGHAM and NIELSEN (1958) established that the toxicity of SM and DHSM was only reduced by Ca pantothenate.

Attempting to explain the discrepancies between the various investigators, MÜCKTER (1961) referred to the different experimental conditions, beginning with the animal strain used and including the purity of the antibiotic (Ca ions!) and the different test conditions (method of administration, concentration, volume, pH of the solution, injection speed), all of which may be responsible for the differing results and the often poor reproducibility.

The effect of pantothenic acid on ototoxicity will be dealt with later.

7. Subchronic Toxicity

It appears that subchronic toxicity studies (in the conventional sense of the term) with SM on various species have only been carried out by MOLITOR et al. (1946). Because of the problems due to the impurities frequently present in the preparation in those days, these investigations will not be discussed further here. At least two important toxic side effects of the streptomyces antibiotics became apparent at that time. There was evidence of nephrotoxicity in dogs and in monkeys, and in dogs neurotoxicity was observed. Later studies by many authors concentrated mainly on the ototoxicity that developed in the course of prolonged administration. This is discussed in detail in the following section.

8. Ototoxicity of the Aminoglycoside Antibiotics

Ever since the first report by HINSHAW and FELDMAN (1945) on the toxic effects of SM on the cochleovestibular apparatus this particular side effect, common to a whole series of antibiotics, has aroused the interest of a large number of clinical and experimental investigators. As early as 1969 Meyer zum Gottesberge and Stupp established that the literature on the ototoxic effects of aminoglycoside antibiotics was almost too extensive to review.

In addition to the substances under consideration here, namely, SM, DHSM, and KM, this class of antibiotics include neomycin, gentamicin, and aminoglycosides, developed later on. VM and CM, being basic polypeptides, do not belong to this group, although they too are ototoxic.

Regarding the morphology of the ototoxic damage they induce, these antibiotics act in a fundamentally similar fashion; the only differences are, for example, that neomycin and gentamicin are more strongly ototoxic than SM and KM, or that a particular antibiotic will damage certain sensory epithelia preferentially (for example, DHSM preferentially damages the cells of the organ of Corti, while SM damages chiefly the vestibular sensory cells). The morphology of the damage of the inner ear by SM, DHSM, and KM can therefore be discussed under one heading.

a) Morphology of Ototoxic Inner Ear Damage

For a long time there was a considerable disagreement regarding the localization of the damage caused by SM and related antibiotics. In the earlier literature in particular there are reports of direct toxic effects on the cerebral centres of the auditory pathway and the vestibular system (WINSTON et al. 1948; FLOHBERG et al. 1949; ESCHER 1949; SECONDI 1954; CHRISTENSEN et al. 1950).

Later on too, various authors considered (HOLZ et al. 1967; STANGE et al. 1967) that, in addition to their toxic effect on the peripheral sensory cells, the aminoglycoside antibiotics also act upon the CNS. Recently ALLEVA and BALAZS (1979) again put forward the suggestion of central effects, having demonstrated in rats that SM-induced dyskinesia can be eliminated by dopaminergic agonists. However, the prevalent opinion is now that the primary damage is confined to the peripheral sensory cells of the cochlea and the labyrinth, as already pointed out by CAUSSE et al. 1949; (GREVEN 1953; BERG 1951; HAWKINS et al. 1957; HAWKINS 1959; CATALANO and MADONIA 1956; NEUMANN and NEUBERT 1958; BECK and KRAHL 1962; SPOENDLIN 1966; KOHONEN 1965; MERKLE et al. 1968, and many others). KOHONEN (1965) suggested that the alterations in the nervous system were caused by secondary, ascending degeneration of neurons following the loss of function of the corresponding sensory cells. According to KELLERHALS et al. (1967), the degeneration reaches the spiral ganglion after about 10 days and then ascends via the axons of the gangliocytes into the cochlear nuclei. This explains why in many cases a progressive loss of hearing occurs despite a discontinuation of the antibiotic therapy. However, the effects on the CNS can also be explained on the basis of the sometimes considerable experimental overdosage of the antibiotics (KELLERHALS 1973).

Morphologically, the ototoxic damage to the inner ear is confined largely to the peripheral sensory cells (KELLERHALS 1973), i.e., to the hair cells of the organ of Corti (mechanoreceptors sensitive to sound vibrations), the hair cells of the two maculae (mechanoreceptors sensitive to linear acceleration), and the hair cells of the three cristae ampullares (mechanoreceptors sensitive to angular acceleration).

KOHONEN (1965) and KOHONEN and TARKKANEN (1966) showed that a characteristic defunctionalization pattern develops in the coils of the organ of Corti. In guinea pigs it was found that after treatment with KM, framycetin, neomycin, and SM the external hair cells at the base of the cochlea are the first to be affected by the damage, which then extends apically along the cochlea, affecting the inner hair cells situated at the base. The inner hair cells, in contrast to the outer ones, are particularly sensitive, especially in the apical segments where the damage and the sensory cell losses begin. This damage spreads in the basal direction until it joins up with the damage proceeding apically from the base of the cochlea. Similar findings have been reported by FARKASHIDY et al. (1963), LUNDQUIST and WERSÄLL (1966), ENGSTRÖM (1967), AKIYOSHI and SATO (1970), and others.

According to KOHONEN (1965), the sensitivity of the hair cells is directly proportional to the number of their nerve endings. However, STUPP (1970) pointed out that it was not only the sensory epithelium that was affected by the toxic effect of streptomyces antibiotics, but that practically all cells of the inner ear (gangliocytes, supporting cells in the organ of Corti, epithelia of the stria vascularis) showed signs of damage. Some investigators (e.g. MÜSEBECK and SCHÄTZLE 1962) believe that this damage is induced even before the damage to the hair cells. HAWKINS (1970, 1973) also refers to the very early appearance of degenerative alterations in the region of the spiral ligament, Reissner's membrane, and the stria vascularis. These could lead to a disturbance of the microhomeostasis and thus, secondarily, to sensory cell damage.

Distinct differences in sensitivity are also found in the sensory epithelium of the vestibular organ. MCGEE and OLSZEWSKI (1962) found that in cats the sensory epithelium of the cristae ampullares is most sensitive after the administration of SM and DHSM.

NAGABA (1968) obtained the same results in squirrel monkeys (Saimiri sciureus) using SM, LINDEMAN (1969) in guinea pigs using KM, and WATANUKI et al. (1972) in guinea pigs using gentamicin. The sensory epithelium of the macula utriculi is the next most sensitive, while the macula sacculi is least affected by sensory cell losses. In all labyrinthine sensory epithelial regions the central parts lose their hair cells first (LINDEMAN 1969; WATANUKI and STUPP 1971). After treatment of guinea pigs with SM it was chiefly the type-I cells which were affected, in contrast to the type-II cells in all the segments, which were considerably more resistant to intoxication (NAGABA 1968; WATANUKI and STUPP 1971; WATANUKI and MEYER ZUM GOTTESBERGE 1971).

The type-II cells are phylogenetically the oldest and least differentiated of the cells, and this may explain their lower sensitivity (WERSÄLL and HAWKINS 1966; SPOENDLIN 1966; WATANUKI et al. 1972).

In guinea pigs treated with SM the ultrastructural alterations to the vestibular sensory cells first take the form of degeneration of the mitochondria and formation of myelin bodies (DUVALL and WERSÄLL 1964). Later on the sensory hairs swell up and the cell surface becomes deformed, until finally the sensory hairs disappear and the ruptured cells and cell detritus are expelled into the endolymph. The nerve fibres and nerve endings remain unaffected. The organ of Corti is less severely damaged. The damage is thus manifested above all by an impairment of the cell membranes and the mitochondrial walls. After treating cats with KM, FARKASHIDY et al. (1963) found that the earliest alterations occurred in the supranuclear, apical region of the sensory cells of the organ of Corti, with mitochondrial and cell-membrane alterations.

In guinea pigs treated with SM JOHNSSON et al. (1980) found limited damage to the crystalline layer of the otolith membrane of the macula utriculi, corresponding in size and position to a sharply defined lesion in the neuroepithelium. According to LODHI et al. (1980), the ototoxicity and possibly also the nephrotoxicity of the aminoglycoside antibiotics are due to their interaction with polyphosphoinositides.

b) Pathophysiology of the Ototoxic Damage

The functional losses can be readily deduced from the morphological findings (KELLERHALS 1973):

The sensory cell losses in the organ of Corti, starting at the base of the cochlea and progressing apically, result in a loss of hearing that at first affects only the high frequencies but thereafter increasingly the middle and low frequencies as well.

In the labyrinth the peripheral sensory cell losses give rise to the clinical picture of a peripheral vestibular disorder in which the slow, progressive functional loss and compensation processes follow largely parallel courses.

From clinical experience it is known that the impairment to both hearing and balance can develop some time after the end of the antibiotic therapy. MCGEE and OLSZEWSKI (1962) also observed a delayed steady loss of hearing a few weeks to several months after treating cats with DHSM.

While the auditory damage is irreversible, the peripheral vestibular sensory cell losses are compensated relatively quickly by accommodation and central substitution (PFALTZ and PIFFKO 1972). For this reason SM with its predominantly vestibular attack has replaced DHSM, which predominantly affects hearing.

c) The Causes of Ototoxicity

α) Pharmacokinetics in the Ear: The ototoxic damage produced by various antibiotics, and especially SM, was initially blamed on impurities in the SM preparations. However, this idea was revised following the investigations by MAHADY et al. (1956), after it had been found that highly purified DHSM preparations were also ototoxic. For a long time the ototoxicity (and nephrotoxicity) was explained by a specific sensitivity of these organs, until it had been shown by several authors that the ototoxic effects of these compounds were due to the special anatomical and physiological characteristics of the inner ear and the particular pharmacokinetic behavior of the antibiotics.

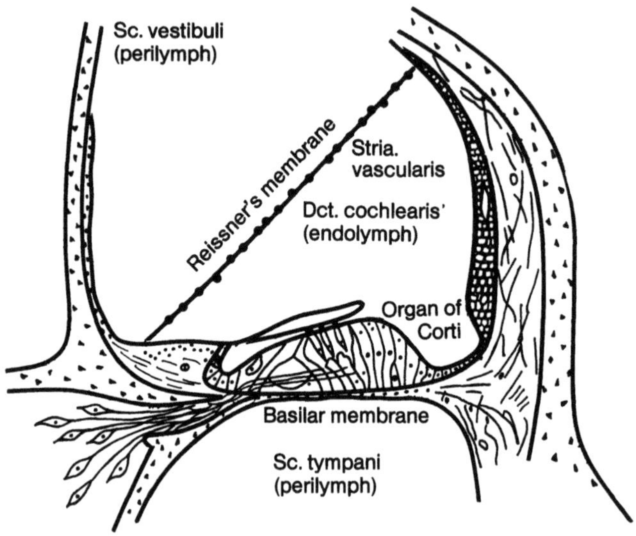

Fig. 1. Anatomy of the inner ear. (After STUPP, 1970)

The complicated anatomical structure of the cochleovestibular apparatus is illustrated in Fig. 1. The two-chamber fluid system (perilymphatic and endolymphatic spaces) separated by Reissner's membrane is particularly characteristic. A further special feature is that the sensory cells protude into the endolymphatic space, so that they are in direct contact with the lymph. The lymph not only fulfils the mechanical function important for the hearing process, namely the conduction of vibrations, but also, according to the current view, supplies the sensory epithelium, which has no intrinsic blood supply, with oxygen and nutrients (STUPP 1970).

After the site of attack and the harmful consequences of the various ototoxically active antibiotics had been determined over a number of years by numerous investigators with the aid of morphological and functional methods of investigation, VRABEC et al. (1965), VOLDŘICH (1965), STUPP et al. (1966, 1967), and STUPP (1970) dealt with the pharmacokinetic behavior of the antibiotics in the blood, organs, endolymph, and perilymph. In particular, STUPP, using KM as an example demonstrated that after parenteral administration of sufficiently high doses measurable concentrations appeared in the inner-ear fluid and that these were only eliminated slowly (Fig. 2). The half-life of kanamycin in the inner-ear fluids, approximately 15 h, is some 10 times as long as that in the blood.

The extremely high KM concentrations reached in the inner-ear fluid can best be seen by comparing them with those in other organs (Table 3).

There was a striking correspondence between the KM concentrations in the endolymph and those in the perilymph, even though these two lymph spaces are separated by Reissner's membrane. Evidently the drug passes the membrane and reaches identical concentrations on both sides.

Whereas in the serum there is a linear relationship between the dose and the concentration reached, the dose/concentration relationship in the perilymph ini-

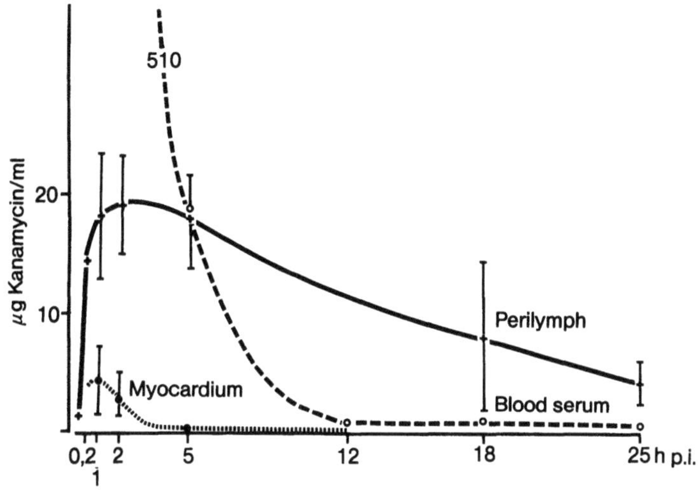

Fig. 2. Kanamycin concentrations in the serum, perilymph, and myocardium of guinea pigs after a single injection of 250 mg/kg. (After STUPP, 1970)

Table 3. Comparison of the KM concentrations in various organs of guinea pigs. (After STUPP 1970)

Time after injection h	Peri-lymph	Endo-lymph	Serum	Heart	Liver	Brain-stem	Cerebrum
5	23,5	18	9,2	0,71	0,65	0,15	0,124
18	13,0	11	0,7	0,44	0,39	0,10	0,055

μg Kanamycin-base/ml or g organs (fresh weight).

tially rises steeply. At doses higher than 50 mg/kg the concentration hardly ever exceeds a certain saturation level (Fig. 3), although dose-proportional blood concentrations are found. It appears that, following an initially short but steep rise, the accumulation of KM in the inner ear comes to a standstill as the dose is increased. The fact that the therapeutic dose range is precisely in this steeply ascending section of the curve explains the relatively narrow therapeutic range of the aminoglycoside antibiotics, since small variations of the serum concentrations can give rise to disproportionately large increases, in the perilymph concentration.

Although the concentration in the perilymph already appears to reach a maximum after a single injection of 250 mg KM/kg, repeated administration at daily intervals can result in a considerable increase of the KM concentration in the inner ear fluid. However, since the serum concentration after the 20th injection behaves exactly as after the first injection, toxic accumulation as a result of kidney damage can be ruled out. The effect cannot be attributed to normal accumulation either, since with higher concentrations in the inner ear the excretion, also speeds up, so that, even though it had been substantially higher, the perilymph level prac-

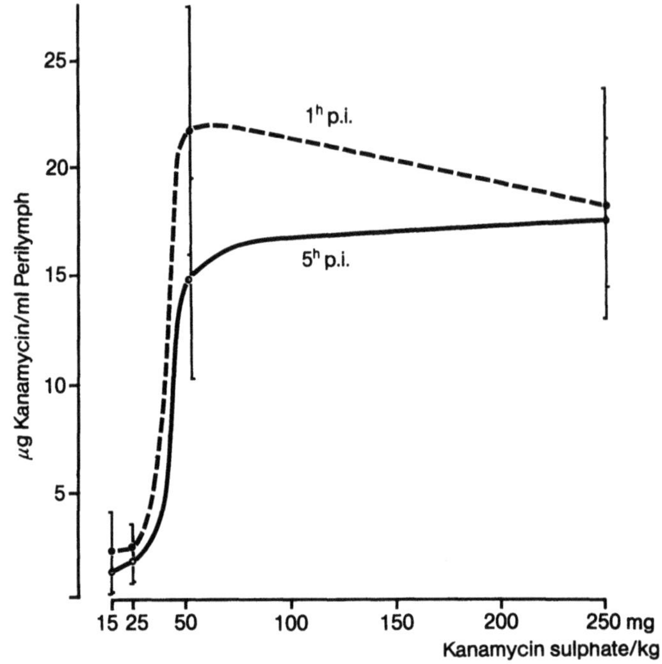

Fig. 3. Correlation between the kanamycin dose and the kanamycin concentration in the perilymph of guinea pigs. (After STUPP, 1970)

tically returns to the same initial value after 18 and after 25 h p.i. The streptomyces antibiotics are therefore probably eliminated by passive diffusion. STUPP (1970) explains the effect of exceeding the saturation concentration after repeated doses as advancing toxic membrane damage, which facilitates the passage of antibiotics into the perilymphatic duct while at the same time preventing them from leaving it.

Thus, the primary cause of the ototoxicity is probably accumulation of the antibiotics in the inner-ear fluid. This precedes the actual inner-ear damage and could be regarded as the initial phase.

The other aminoglycoside antibiotics (SM, DHSM, neomycin) behave in a fundamentally similar fashion to KM (STUPP 1970). They also accumulate in the inner ear and are only slowly excreted, as, for example, VRABEC et al. (1965) demonstrated with SM in cats.

In rabbits, WAGNER et al. (1971) found that SM is eliminated from the perilymph about 3 times as slowly as from the serum.

Figure 4 shows that, when given in the same doses (250 mg/kg), SM reaches perilymph concentrations more or less equal to those of KM, while after DHSM treatment substantially higher levels are reached. The difference in ototoxic activity could therefore be due to these different behavior patterns.

A correlation between the concentrations in the perilymph and the histopathological alterations also appears after local applications of the various antibiotics into the inner ear (STUPP et al. 1973).

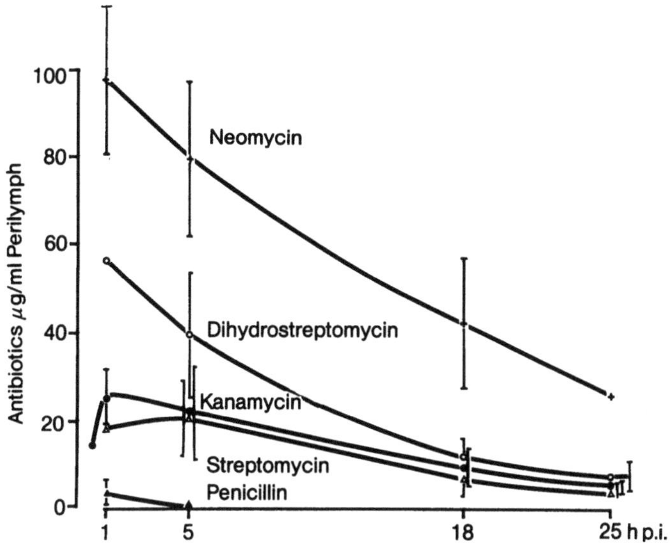

Fig. 4. Antibiotic concentrations in the perilymph of guinea pigs on administration of standard doses of 250 mg/kg each. Neomycin was given in a dose of only 100 mg/kg. (After STUPP, 1970)

β) Biochemical Effects in the Inner Ear: The antibacterial properties of SM are due to effects exerted on the cell membrane and on the protein synthesis. The biochemical effects responsible for the antibacterial activity presumably also play a role in the ototoxicity (THALMANN et al. 1973). Thus, PLESTER (1963) found a reduction of the protein metabolism in the organ of Corti, in Reissner's membrane, and in the stria vascularis after chronic treatment with DHSM. BECK and KRAHL (1962) reported disruption of the protein and RNA metabolism in the sensory cells of the organ of Corti in guinea pigs treated with KM.

According to SPOENDLIN (1966), the primary damage caused by SM treatment occurs in the cell nuclei; this is followed by damage to the ribosomes and the ergastoplasm membranes. These structures play a role in protein synthesis and there appears to be a certain correlation between the level of protein metabolism of the various cells in the inner ear and their sensitivity to SM. KRAUS and DOENNINGS (1969) showed that the sensory cells of the organ of Corti have the highest rate of ribosomal protein synthesis and interpreted this as a possible starting point for the sensitivity of the sensory cells to ototoxic antibiotics. HAWKINS (1970, 1973) postulated that the ototoxic and nephrotoxic effects of these antibiotics might have a common biochemical basis, namely an influence on protein synthesis and membrane functions in tissues responsible for the active transport of ions. The reduction of ATP-ase activity in the stria vascularis and in the spiral ligament in the guinea pig after administration of SM, DHSM, or KM may also be relevant in this context (IINUMA et al. 1976). MENDELSOHN and KATZENBERG (1972) observed a reduction of the sodium level and an increase of the potassium level in the endolymph following the administration of high doses of KM to guinea pigs. Presumably, therefore, KM interferes with the active transport systems in the cochlea. Recently GARCIA-QUIROGA et al. (1978) showed a connection between the ototoxic action of KM and disturbances of the glucose transport mechanisms in the inner ear.

d) Species-Related Sensitivity Differences and Differences in the Activity of the Various Antibiotics

Even though the ototoxicosis follows a similar course in the different species after treatment with the various antibiotics, it is fairly evident from the preceeding discussion that there are clear differences in sensitivity between the various species and in the preferred localization of the damage. Some results of comparative investigations are given below, although the list is by no means complete.

SM has a stronger vestibular toxicity than cochlear toxicity in guinea pigs, rats, and cats (MÜSEBECK 1962; VERNIER and ALLEVA 1968; TETTENBORN 1971). It is less cochleotoxic in the guinea pig than KM or gentamicin (TETTENBORN 1971). In the cat, SM exerts a stronger vestibulotoxic activity than DHSM (EDISON et al. 1948) or KM (TISCH et al. 1958; TETTENBORN 1971), whereas in man DHSM often induces auditory damage (STUPP 1970).

On the other hand, after local intratympanic application SM exerts a stronger cochleotoxic than vestibulotoxic activity in guinea pigs, while conversely, DHSM is more vestibulotoxic than cochleotoxic (RUDNICK 1979). It is therefore concluded that every aminoglycoside antibiotic exerts a cell-specific ototoxic effect, which is modified according to the route of administration. KM is predominantly cochleotoxic. Guinea pigs are about 3 to 4 times more sensitive to the cochleotoxic action of KM than rats (HAWKINS 1959; VERNIER and ALLEVA 1968; TETTENBORN 1971, Fig. 5). Regarding the vestibulotoxicity in the cat, KM is clearly weaker than, for example, SM or DHSM (HAWKINS 1959; TETTENBORN 1971).

e) Attempts to Reduce the Ototoxicity

There have been many attempts to reduce or eliminate the ototoxicity by simultaneous administration of "detoxifying" substances (ascorbic acid, nicotinic acid, vitamin A, lactoflavine, etc.). MÜCKTER (1961) gives a review of the early litera-

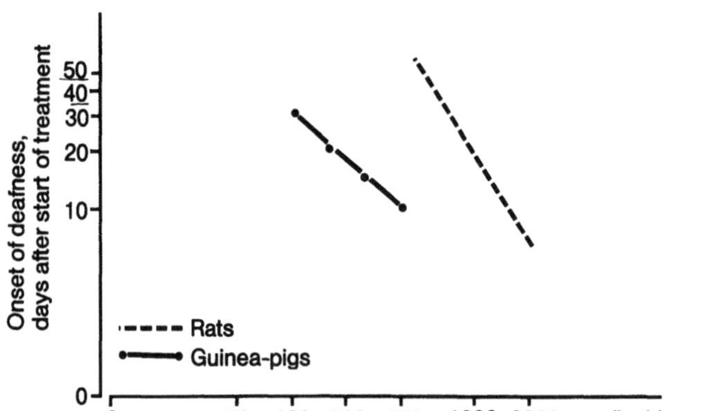

Fig. 5. Time of hearing loss in guinea pigs (after TETTENBORN, 1971) and rats (after VERNIER and ALLEVA, 1968) following treatment with kanamycin

ture. STUPP (1970) also concentrated on this problem. Most of the additives had no practical effect. KELLER et al. (1955, 1956a, b) were the first to report a reduction in the acute toxicity and ototoxicity of SM (and later also KM and VM) in mice and in cats by the addition of pantothenates. These findings have been confirmed in animal experiments by MARQUARDT and ZIEGLER (1956), DUCROT et al. (1956), NEUMANN and NEUBERT (1958), COURVOISIER and LEAU (1956), TYBERGHEIN and OSTJIN (1961), and others.

The importance of pantothenic acid as a detoxifier of streptomyces antibiotics has been disputed. OSTERBERG et al. (1957) found only a weak effect on cochleotoxicity and no effect at all on the vestibular damage. KIMMERLE and GÖSSWALD (1956), HAWKINS et al. (1957), CHILD et al. (1957), BRIGHAM and NIELSEN (1958), KUSCHINSKY et al. (1959), and WERSÄLL and HAWKINS (1962) obtained completely negative results.

With the aid of the latest experimental methods and improved, standardized, experimental conditions, a limited (though significant) improvement in tolerance was demonstrated for pantothenic acid (TYBERGHEIN 1967; PLATTIG et al. 1967; MERKLE et al. 1968). However, according to Müsebeck's estimates (cited in STUPP 1970), this protective effect only represents at best a 30% improvement. This relatively small difference may perhaps explain why the protective effect of pantothenic acid has been detected by only some of the investigators. On the basis of his pharmacokinetic studies, STUPP (1970) came to the conclusion that the toxicity differences of the various pantothenate and sulphate compounds of the aminoglycoside antibiotics can be attributed to their different concentrations in the inner-ear fluid.

The same evidently applies also to ozothin, a combination of oleum terebinthinae and terpentinum hydratum, which according to STANGE et al. (1967) and STANGE (1969) inhibits the cochleotoxic effect of SM and of the other aminoglycoside antibiotics but is unable to protect the vestibular sensory cells (LANGE 1968). STUPP et al. (1970) found that simultaneous administration of ozothin to guinea pigs lowered the SM cocentration in the blood by 20%–25%. Thus, we are evidently not dealing with true detoxification but merely with a reduction in concentration (and therefore in effect) of the toxic antibiotics.

9. Nephrotoxicity

Astonishingly enough, relatively few experimental studies have been done specifically on the nephrotoxicity of SM and DHSM, although this problem was frequently referred to, particularly in the earlier studies.

In the preliminary toxicological studies on dogs with prolonged administration (50 mg–100 mg of SM/kg s.c. or i.m.) MOLITOR et al. (1946) observed proteinuria as well as casts, epithelial cells, and leucocytes in the urinary sediment.

Several days of treatment with 100 mg/kg–200 mg/kg also gave rise to proteinuria and a slight increase of the plasma urea level in monkeys. MUSHETT and MARTLAND (1946) found morphological alterations in the tubules and glomeruli in monkeys, dogs, and cats. These were not observed in guinea pigs, mice, and rats treated with 100 mg/kg for 2½ months. Acidophilic colloid-like droplets were observed in the cytoplasm of the tubule epithelial cells in dogs and in rats after a week of SM and DHSM treatment (400 mg/kg) (MUSHETT and STEBBINS 1949).

Investigations by GROSS et al. (1969) on partially nephrectomized rats revealed an increased incidence of functional-morphological renal damage of various kinds in these insufficient animals after SM and DHSM (40 mg/kg i.m. for 90 days). Whereas SM caused both glomerular and tubular damage and reduced the glomerular filtration and tubular absorption of water, DHSM had no effect on the water absorption. DHSM also caused less tubule damage.

RAAB (1970) clearly demonstrated the effects exerted on rat kidneys by a single dose of 100 mg SM/kg i.p. These took the form of an increased renal excretion of leucine aminopeptidase, alkaline phosphatase, and lactate dehydrogenase. KM exerted similar effects after a dose of 500 mg/kg.

Like other aminoglycoside antibiotics, SM and DHSM are stored in the renal tubules (ANDRÉ 1956). However, LAGLER et al. (1960) showed that much less DHSM and SM is stored compared, for example, to KM.

10. Reproductive Toxicity

SUZUKI and TAKEUCHI (1961) treated rats and mice with respectively 200 DHSM/kg–600 DHSM/kg and 800 mg DHSM/kg, administered intraperitoneally throughout gestation. As expected, the high doses gave rise to a high degree of maternal and neonatal toxicity. No malformations were found in the offspring, and the Preyer reflex test did not reveal any hearing loss.

ERICSON-STRANDVIK and GYLLENSTEIN (1963) treated mice from the 9th to the 13th day of gestation with 250 mg SM/kg i.m. and failed to observe any increase in embryonic mortality or any external or internal malformations of the CNS, although passage of SM into the foetuses via the placenta was detected. BOUCHER and DELOST (1964), on the other hand, observed an impairment of growth after birth in the young of mice treated with 25 mg/kg or 250 mg/kg on the 14th day of gestation.

11. Biochemical Effect of SM

According to MASCITELLI-CORIANDOLI (1962), SM and DHSM influence to different extents the coenzyme A contents of the liver, kidneys, heart, and the adrenals, while the coenzyme A level in the brain remains unaffected. After parenteral administration the coenzyme A content decreases, particularly in the liver and the adrenals, the reduction being more noticeable after 14 days of treatment than after a single injection. As the site of coenzyme A synthesis, the mitochondria exhibit the strongest reduction.

In the adrenal glands the decrease in the coenzyme A level results in a reduced corticosteroid synthesis. MOSONYI et al. (1956) also found evidence of an influence on steroid synthesis. After treating rabbits with SM, these authors observed a reduced 11-hydroxy steroid excretion, both after ACTH and in the absence of stimulation of the adrenal cortex. The significance of these findings for the toxicology of the aminoglycoside antibiotics does not appear to have been followed up.

Later, POPOVICI et al. (1970) reported elevated concentrations of NAD and NADP in the liver and kidneys of rats after 6 days of treatment with SM (60 mg/kg i.p.).

References

Adams HR, Goodman FR, Lupean VA, Weiss GB (1973) Effects of neomycin on tension and ^{45}Ca movements in rabbit aortic smooth muscle. Life Sci Part I Physiol Pharmacol 12:279–287

Akiyoshi M, Sato K (1970) Reevaluation of the pinna reflex test as screening for ototoxicity of antibiotics. In: Progress in Antimicrobiol and Anticancer Chemotherapy; Proc 6th Intern Congr Chemotherapy, Vol I:621–627

Alleva FR, Balazs T, Morris SO, Crowley WR, O'Donohue TL, Jacobowitz DM (1979) Reversal of streptomycin-induced dyskinesia in rats by dopaminergic agonists. Toxicol Appl Pharmacol 48:A 36

Amann R, Radenbach KL (1961) Akute Kanamycin-Nebenwirkungen und Histaminfreisetzung. Beitr Klin Tuberk 123:208–210

André T (1956) Studies on the distribution of tritium-labelled dihydrostreptomycin and tetracyclin in the body. Acta Radiol Suppl 142:1–89

Bacharach AL, Clark BJ, McCulloch M, Tomich EG (1959) Comparative toxicity studies on ten antibiotics in current use. J Pharm Pharmacol 11:737–741

Beck Ch, Krahl P (1962) Experimentelle und feingewebliche Untersuchungen über die Ototoxizität von Kanamycin. Arch Otorhinolaryngol 179:594–610

Berg K (1951) The toxic effect of streptomycin on the vestibular and cochlear apparatus. Acta Otolaryng Suppl 97:5–77

Bezzi G, Gessa GL (1959) Neuromuscular blocking action of some antibiotics. Nature 184:905–906

Bezzi G, Gessa GL (1961) Influence of antibiotics on the neuromuscular transmission in mammals. Antibiot Chemotherap 11:710–714

Boucher D, Delost P (1964) Développement post-natal des descendants issus de mères traitées par la streptomycine au cours de la gestation chez la souris. CR Soc Biol (Paris) 158:2065–2069

Brigham RS, Nielsen JK (1958) The effect of calcium pantothenate on the acute and chronic toxicity of streptomycin and dihydrostreptomycin in mice. Anbiot Chemother 8:122–129

Catalano GB, Madonia T (1956) Ulteriore contributo sperimentale sulle lesioni istologiche labyrinthiche da streptomicina. Clin Otorinolaryng 8:51

Caussé R, Gondet I, Vallancien B (1949) Action de la streptomycine sur les cellules ciliées des organes vestibulaires de la souris. CR Soc Biol 144:619–620

Child KJ, Davis B, Sharpe HM, Tomich EG (1957) Toxicologic studies on the sulfates and pantothenates of streptomycin and dihydrostreptomycin. Antibiot Annu 1956–1957: 574–580

Christensen E, Hertz H, Riskaer N, Vraa-Jensen G (1950) Experiments on the neurotoxic effect of streptomycin. Acta Otolaryng Suppl 95:165–176

Cohen LS, Wechsler AS, Mitchell JH, Glick G (1970) Depression of cardiac function by streptomycin and other antimicrobial agents. Am J Cardiol 26:505–511

Corrado AP (1958) Ganglioplegic action of streptomycin. Arch Int Pharmacodyn 114:166–178

Corrado AP (1963) Respiratory depression due to antibiotics: calcium in treatment. Anesth Analg 42:1–5

Corrado AP, Ramos AO, De Escobar CT (1959) Neuro-muscular blockade by neomycin potentiation by ether anesthesia and d-tubocurarine and antagonism by calcium and prostigmine. Arch Int Pharmacodyn Ther 121:380–394

Courvoisier S, Leau O (1956) Study of the onset of deafness in rats treated with streptomycin, dihydrostreptomycin and neomycin. Antibiot Chemother 6:411–419

DeSalva SJ, Evans RA, Marcussen HW (1969) Lethal effects of antibiotics in hamsters. Toxicol Appl Pharmacol 14:510–514

Dretchen KL, Sokoll MD, Gergis SD, Long JP (1973) Relative effects of streptomycin on motor nerve terminal and endplate. Eur J Pharmacol 22:10–16

Ducrot R, Leau O, Cosar C (1956) Protective action of pantothenic acid against toxic effects of streptomycin and dihydrostreptomycin. Antibiot Chemother 6:404–410

Duvall AJ, Wersäll J (1964) Site of action of streptomycin upon inner ear sensory cells. Acta Otolaryng 57:581–598

Dzoljić M, Babić M (1967) Action of streptomycin on the uterus. Eur J Pharmacol 2:123–126
Edison AO, Frost BM, Graessle OE, Hawkins JE Jr, Kuna S, Mushett CW, Silber RH, Solotorovsky M (1948) An experimental evaluation of dihydrostreptomycin. Am Rev Tuberc 58:487–493
Engström H (1967) The pathological sensory cell in the cochlea. Acta Otolaryng Appendix to Vol 63:20–26
Ericson-Strandvik B, Gyllenstein L (1963) The central nervous system of foetal mice after administration of streptomycin. Acta Pathol Microbiol Scand 59:292–300
Escher F (1949) Das Streptomycin in der Otolaryngologie unter besonderer Berücksichtigung der Vestibularisstörungen. Praxis:141–146
Farkashidy J, Black RG, Briant TDR (1963) The effect of kanamycin on the internal ear: an electrophysiological and electron microscopic study. Laryngoscope 73:713–727
Flohberg C, Hamberger CA, Hyden H (1949) Inhibition of nucleic acid production in vestibular nerve cells by streptomycin. Acta Otolaryng Suppl 75:36
Garcia-Quiroga J, Norris CH, Glade L, Bryant GM, Tachibana M, Guth PS (1978) The relationship between kanamycin ototoxicity and glucose transport. Res Commun Chem Pathol Pharmacol 22:535–547
Goodman FR, Weiss GB, Adams HR (1974) Alterations by neomycin of ^{45}Ca movements and contractile responses in vascular smooth muscle. J Pharmacol Exp Ther 188:472–480
Gray JE, Purmalis A (1958) The acute toxicity of procaine penicilline G and of dihydrostreptomycin sulfate in the pigeon and the chicken. Avian Dis 2:187–196
Greven H (1953) Die toxische Wirkung von Streptomycin auf den Cochlear- und Vestibularapparat. Z Laryng Rhinol 32:109–117
Gross A, Legait E, Delabroise AM (1969) Etude de la néphrotoxicité de la streptomycine et de la dihydrostreptomycine chez le rat blanc porteur d'une insufficance rénale expérimentale. Thérapie 24:327–341
Hawkins JE Jr (1959) The ototoxicity of kanamycin. Ann Otol 68:698–715
Hawkins JE Jr (1970) Biochemical aspects of ototoxicity. In: Paparella MM (ed) Biochemical mechanisms in hearing and deafness. Thomas Publ, pp 323–339
Hawkins JE Jr (1973) Ototoxic mechanisms. A working hypothesis. Audiology 12:383–393
Hawkins JE Jr, Wolcott H, O'Shanny WJ (1957) Ototoxic effects of streptomycin and dihydrostreptomycin pantothenates in the cat. Antibiot Annu 1956–1957:554–563
Hinshaw HC, Feldman WH (1945) Streptomycin in treatment of clinical tuberculosis: A preliminary report. Mayo Clin Proc 20:313
Hoffmann K (1970) unpublished investigations
Holz E, Hoffmann M, Beck Ch (1967) Morphologische und bakteriologische Befunde zur Minderung der Ototoxicität basischer Streptomycesantibiotika. Arch Otorhinolaryngol 188:236–242
Iinuma T, Mizukoshi O, Daly JF (1976) Possible effects of various ototoxic drugs upon the ATP-hydrolyzing system in the stria vascularis and spiral ligament of the guinea pig. Laryngoscope 77:159–169
Iwatsuki K, Ueda T, Yamada A, Nishimura S, Kanemura K (1958) Effects of certain antibiotics on the action of muscle relaxants. Far East J Anesth 2:106–115; cited from Ber Ges Physiol 213 (1960):121
Jindal MN, Desphande VR (1960) Neuromuscular blockade by streptomycin and dihydrostreptomycin. Brit J Pharmacol 15:506–509
Johnsson L-G, Wright CG, Preston RE, Henry PJ (1980) Streptomycin-induced efects of the otoconial membrane. Acta Otolaryngol (Stockh) 89:401–406
Keller H, Krüpe W, Sous H, Mückter H (1955) Versuche zur Toxizitätsminderung basischer Streptomyces-Antibiotika. 1. Mitt. Arzneimittelforsch 5:170–176
Keller H, Krüpe W, Sous H, Mückter H (1956a) Versuche zur Toxizitätsminderung basischer Streptomyces-Antibiotika. 2. Mitt. Arzneimittelforsch 6:61–66
Keller H, Krüpe W, Sous H, Mückter H (1956b) Versuche zur Toxizitätsminderung basischer Streptomyces-Antibiotika. 3. Mitt. Arzneimittelforsch 6:585–591

Kellerhals B, Engström H, Ades HW (1967) Die Morphologie des Ganglion spirale cochleae. Acta Otolaryng (Stockh) Suppl 226:1–78
Kellerhals B (1973) Zur Ototoxizität der Aminoglykosid-Antibiotika. MMW 115:1667–1672
Kimmerle G, Gösswald R (1956) Versuche zur Entgiftung von Streptomycin und Dihydrostreptomycin. Arzneimittelforsch 6:379–383
Kohonen A (1965) Effect of some ototoxic drugs upon the pattern and innervation of cochlear sensory cells in the guinea pig. Acta Otolaryngol (Stockh) Suppl 208:1–70
Kohonen A, Tarkkanen JV (1966) Dihydrostreptomycin and kanamycin ototoxicity. An experimental study by surface preparation technique. Laryngoscope 76:1671–1680
Kraus H, Doenning G (1969) Cytophotometrische RNA- und Eiweißbestimmungen am häutigen Innenohr des Meerschweinchens als Grundlage zur Beurteilung des Eiweißstoffwechsels und der Streptomycinototoxizität. Arch Otorhinolaryngol 194:1551
Kubikowski P, Srzeniawski Z (1963) The mechanism of the neuromuscular blockade by antibiotics. Arch Int Pharmacodyn Ther 146:549–560
Kuschinsky G, Lüllmann H, Pracht W (1959) Über den Einfluß von Pantothensäure auf die vestibularisschädigende Wirkung von Streptomycin. Dtsch Med Wochenschr 84:363–366
Kuschinsky G, Lüllmann H (1963) Tierexperimentelle Untersuchungen zur Abhängigkeit der Ototoxicität von der Dosierung des Kanamycin und zur Schutzwirkung durch Vitamine. Klin Wochenschr 41:230–233
Lagler F, Osterloh G, Mückter H (1960) Studies on the pharmacology of kanamycin. Antibiot Annu 1959–1960: 862–867
Lange G (1968) Die quantitative Auswertung von Streptomycinschäden des vestibulären Sinnesepithels beim Meerschweinchen mit Hilfe des Cytovestibulogramms und der calorischen Erregbarkeitsprüfung. Arch Otorhinolaryngol 192:249–257
Leaders F, Pittinger CB, Long JP (1960) Some pharmacological properties of selected antibiotics. Antibiot Chemotherap 10:503–507
Lindeman HH (1969) Regional differences in sensitivity of the vestibular sensory epithelia to ototoxic antibiotics. Acta Otolaryngol (Stockh) 67:177–189
Lodhi S, Weiner ND, Mechigian J, Schacht J (1980) Ototoxicity of aminoglycosides correlated with their action on monomolecular films of polyphosphoinositides. Biochem Pharmacol 29:597–601
Lüllmann H, Reuter H (1960a) Über die Hemmung der neuromuskulären Übertragung durch einige Antibiotika. Chemotherapia 1:375–383
Lüllmann H, Reuter H (1960b) Die curare-artigen Nebenwirkungen einiger Antibiotika. Klin Wochenschr 38:771–772
Lundquist P-G, Wersäll J (1966) Kanamycin-induced changes in cochlear hair cells of the guinea pig. Z Zellforsch 72:543–561
Mascitelli-Coriandoli E (1962) Der Einfluß basischer Antibiotica auf das Coenzym A-System. Arzneimittelforsch 12:597–601
Mahady SCF, Armstrong FL, Monroe J (1956) Purified dihydrostreptomycin. Am Rev Tuberc 73:776–778
Marquardt P, Ziegler E (1956) Zur Pharmakologie von Streptomycinsulfat und -pantothenat. Arzneimittelforsch 6:213–214
McGee TM, Olszewski J (1962) Streptomycin sulfate and dihydrostreptomycin toxicity. Arch Otolaryngol 75:295–311
Mendelsohn M, Katzenberg I (1972) The effect of kanamycin on the cation content of the endolymph. Laryngoscope 82:397–403
Merkle U, Plattig KH, Keidel UO (1968) Histologische Untersuchungen zur ototoxischen Wirkung des Kanamycins am Cortischen Organ der Katze. Zschr Mikrosk Anat Forsch 78:441–460
Meyer zum Gottesberge A, Stupp HF (1969) Streptomycinspiegel in der Perilymphe des Menschen. Acta Otolaryngol 67:171–176
Michael AF, Sutherland JM (1961) Antibiotic testing in newborn and adult rats. Am J Dis Child 101:442–446

Molgó J, Lemeignan M, Uchiyama T, Lechat P (1979) Inhibitory effect of kanamycin on evoked transmitter release. Reversal by 3,4-diaminopyridine. Eur J Pharmacol 57:93–97
Molitor H, Graessle OE, Kuna S, Mushett ChW, Silber RH (1946) Some toxicological and pharmacological properties of streptomycin. J Pharmacol Exp Ther 86:151–173
Molitor H, Kuna S (1949) Pharmacologic studies of the neurotoxic properties of streptomycin. Arch Int Pharmacodyn Ther 76:197–202
Mosonyi L, Pollák L, Zulik R, Károlyházi G (1956) Streptomycin and endocrine system. Experientia 12:311–313
Mückter H (1961) Zur Pharmakologie der basischen Streptomyces-Antibiotika. Antibiotica et Chemotherapia Separatum Vol 9:83–144
Müsebeck K, Schätzle W (1962) Experimentelle Studien zur Ototoxicität des Dihydrostreptomycins. Arch Otorhinolaryngol 181:41–48
Mushett ChW, Martland HS (1946) Pathologic changes resulting from the administration of streptomycin. Arch Pathol 42:619–629
Mushett ChW, Stebbins RB (1949) Renal cytoplasmic inclusions following the administration of large doses of streptomycin. Fed Proc 8:363
Nagaba M (1968) Electron microscopic study of semicircular canal organs and otolith organs of squirrel monkeys after administration of streptomycin sulfate. Acta Otolaryngol (Stockh) 66:541–552
Neumann G, Neubert K (1958) Die Sensularien des Innenohres unter der Einwirkung von Streptomycin – Experimentelle Untersuchungen am Corti'schen Organ und an der Macula utricula des Meerschweinchens. Arzneimittelforsch 8:63–72
Osterberg AC, Oleson JJ, Yuda NN, Rauh CE, Parr HG, Will LW (1957) Cochlear, vestibular and acute toxicity studies of streptomycin and dihydrostreptomycin pantothenate salts. Antibiot Annu 1956–1957: 564–573
Pfaltz CR, Piffko P (1972) Central compensation of retrolabyrinthine vestibular lesions. Acta Otolaryngol (Stockh) 73:183–189
Pittinger CB (1970) pH and streptomycin influences upon ionic calcium in serum. Anesth Analg 49:540–545
Pittinger CB, Long JP (1958) Neuromuscular blocking action of neomycin sulfate. Antibiot Chemother 8:198–203
Pittinger CB, Long JP, Miller JR (1958) The neuromuscular blocking action of neomycin. Anesth Analg 37:276–282
Pittinger C, Adamson R (1972) Antibiotic blockade of neuromuscular function. Annu Rev Pharmacol 12:169–184
Plattig KH, Keidel UO, David E (1967) Minderung der Ototoxizität des Kanamycins durch Pantothensäure. Dtsch Med Wochenschr 92:1391–1397
Plester D (1963) Discussion remark. Arch otorhinolaryngol 182:587
Popovici GG, Moisă L, Negoită M, Manoilă V, Botez E, Hafner R, Gumeni N (1965) The influence of certain antibiotics on intestinal motor activity. Arch Int Pharmacodyn Ther 154:374–381
Popovici GG, Negoită M, Moisă L, Manoilă V, Hafner R, Botez E (1967) The influence of some antibiotics on uterine motor activity in the guinea pig. Arch Int Pharmacodyn Ther 166:20–25
Popovici GG, Mungiu C, Filip M, Botez E, Ababei L (1970) Influence of some antibiotics on stationary NAD and NADP concentrations in rat liver and kidney. Arch Int Pharmacodyn Ther 188:73–78
Prado WA, Corrado AP, Marseillan RF (1978) Competitive antagonism between calcium and antibiotics at the neuromuscular junction. Arch Int Pharmacodyn Ther 231:297–307
Prescott B, Kauffmann G, James WD, Stone HJ (1959) Means of increasing the tolerated dose of streptomycin in mice. Antibiot Chemother 9:369–375
Raab WP (1970) Renal effects of streptomycin in rats. Clin Chim Acta 29:451–454
Ritter R, Chou J, v Ilberg C, Wagner WH (1971) Eine neue Möglichkeit zur Verhinderung der Ototoxizität des Streptomycins. Arch Otorhinolaryngol 199:573–577
Robson JM, Sullivan FM (1963) Antituberculous drugs. Pharmacol Rev 15:169–223

Rudnick MD (1979) A quantitative and qualitative study of aminoglycoside antibiotic ototoxicity in the vestibulo-cochlear apparatus following intratympanic administration in guinea pig (Cavia cobaya). Dissertation Abstr Intern B 39:4145–4146
Saito H, Daly JF (1971) Quantitative analysis of acid mucopolysaccharides in the normal and kanamycin intoxicated cochlea. Acta Otolaryngol (Stockh) 71:22–26
Secondi U (1954) Ancora sull'effetto neurotossico della streptomicina. L'importanza del fattore dose-tempo. Arch Ital Otol 65:165
Singh YN, Harvey AL, Marshall IG (1978) Antibiotic-induced paralysis of the mouse phrenic nerve-hemidiaphragm preparation, and reversibility by calcium and by neostigmine. Anesthesiology 48:418–424
Sokoll MD, Diecke FPJ (1969) Some effects of streptomycin on frog nerve in vitro. Arch Int Pharmacodyn Ther 177:332–339
Spoendlin H (1966) Zur Ototoxizität des Streptomycins. Pract Oto-Rhino-Laryng (Basel) 28:305–322; 374–375
Spoendlin H (1967) Acute streptomycin intoxication of the labyrinth. Acta Otolaryngol (Stockh) 63:26–38
Stange G (1969) Minderung bzw. Verhütung der Ototoxizität basischer Streptomyzes-Antibiotika. Therapiewoche 19:106–117
Stange G, Soda T, Beck Ch (1967) Elektrophysiologische Ergebnisse bei Ototoxizitätsminderung basischer Streptomyces-Antibiotika. Arch Otorhinolaryngol 188:242–249
Stupp HF (1970) Untersuchung der Antibiotikaspiegel in den Innenohrflüssigkeiten und ihre Bedeutung für die spezifische Ototoxizität der Aminoglykosidantibiotika. Acta Otolaryngol (Stockh) Suppl 262
Stupp H, Rauch S, Sous H, Lagler F (1966) Untersuchungen über die Ursache der spezifisch ototoxischen Wirkung der basischen Streptomycesantibiotika unter besonderer Berücksichtigung des Kanamycins. Acta Otolaryngol (Stockh) 61:435–444
Stupp H, Rauch S, Sous H, Brun JP, Lagler F (1967) Kanamycin dosage and levels in ear and other organs. Arch Otolaryngol 86:515–521
Stupp H, Küpper K, Lagler F, Sous H, Quante M (1973) Inner ear concentrations and ototoxicity of different antibiotics in local and systemic application. Audiology 12:350–363
Suzuki Y, Takeuchi S (1961) Etude expérimentale sur l'influence de la streptomycine sur l'appareil auditif du foetus après administration de doses variées a la mère enceinte. Keio. J Med 10:31–41
Swain HH, Kiplinger GF, Brody TM (1956) Action of certain antibiotics on the isolated dog heart. J Pharmacol Exp Ther 117:151–159
Tettenborn D (1971) Unpublished investigations
Thalmann R, Miyoshi T, Kusakari J, Thalmann J (1973) Quantitative approaches to the ototoxicity problem. Audiology 12:364–382
Timmerman JC, Long JP, Pittinger CB (1959) Neuromuscular blocking properties of various antibiotic agents. Toxicol Appl Pharmacol 1:299–304
Tisch DE, Huftalen JB, Dickison HL (1958) Pharmacological studies with kanamycin. Ann NY Acad Sci 76:44–65
Tyberghein J (1962) Influence of some streptomyces antibiotics on the cochlear microphonics in the guinea pig. Acta Otolaryngol (Stockh) Suppl 171
Tyberghein J (1967) Einfluß der Pantothensäure auf die Ototoxizität des Kanamycins beim Meerschweinchen. Med Welt:2017–2020
Tyberghein J, Ostjin F (1961) L'ototoxicité de la streptomycine. Acta Tuberc Pneumol Belg 52:139–146
Vernier VG, Alleva FR (1968) The bioassay of kanamycin auditory toxicity. Arch Int Pharmacodyn Ther 176:59–73
Vital Brazil O (1961) Streptomycin effect on the skeletal muscle stimulation produced by acetylcholine. Arch Int Pharmacodyn Ther 130:136–140
Vital Brazil O, Corrado AP (1957) The curariform action of streptomycin. J Pharmacol Exp Ther 120:452–459
Vital Brazil O, Corrado AP, Berti FA (1959) Neuromuscular block produced by streptomycin and some of its degradation products. In: Bovet D, Bovet-Nitti F, Marini-Bettolo (eds) Curare and curare-like agents. Elsevier, Amsterdam

Vital Brazil O, Prado-Franceschi J (1969) The nature of neuromuscular block produced by neomycin and gentamicin. Arch Int Pharmacodyn Ther 179:78–85
Voldřich L (1965) The kinetics of streptomycin, kanamycin and neomycin in the inner ear. Acta Otolaryngol (Stockh) 60:243–248
Vrabec DP, Cody DT, Ulrich JA (1965) A study of the relative concentrations of antibiotics in the blood, spinal fluid, and perilymph in animals. Ann Otol Rhinol Laryngol 74:688–703
Wagner WH, Chou JTY, Ilberg v. C, Ritter R, Vosteen KH (1971) Untersuchungen zur Pharmakokinetik von Streptomycin. Arzneimittelforsch 21:2006–2016
Watanuki K, Meyer zum Gottesberge A (1971) Toxic effect of streptomycin and kanamycin upon the sensory epithelium of the crista ampullaris. Acta Otolaryngol (Stockh) 72:59–67
Watanuki K, Stupp H (1971) Haarzellenschädigungsmuster an Crista und Maculae bei Ototoxikose durch Antibiotika. Arch Otorhinolaryngol 199:569–573
Watanuki K, Stupp H-F, Meyer zum Gottesberge A (1972) Toxic effects of gentamycin upon the peripheral vestibular sensory organs. Laryngoscope 82:363–371
Wersäll J, Hawkins JE Jr (1962) The vestibular sensory epithelia in the labyrinth and their reactions in chronic streptomycin intoxication. Acta Otolaryngol (Stockh) 54:1–23
Winston J, Lewey FH, Parentease A, Marden PA, Cramer FB (1948) An experimental study of the toxic effects of streptomycin on the vestibular apparatus of the cat. Ann Otol Rhinol Laryngol 57:738–753
Wolf GL, Wigton RS (1971) Vasodilatation induced by streptomycin in the perfused canine kidney. Arch Int Pharmacodyn Ther 194:285–289

III. Thiosemicarbazone – Thioacetazone, Thiacetazone (TSC)

1. Acute Toxicity

Investigations on the acute toxicity of TSC revealed considerable differences between the sensitivities of different animal species and between different modes of administration. In many cases there were also no clear dose-effect relationships (HECHT 1950). According to HECHT (1950), the oral LD_{50} for rats is above 6 g/kg and for mice it is around 6 g/kg. GINOULHIAC (1950) gives the oral LD_{50} for mice as 3.53 g/kg and for rats as 2.73 g/kg. In contrast, SAVINI (1950) found a substantially higher toxicity in mice after oral administration (LD_{50} about 0.95 g/kg). Guinea pigs usually survive doses of 0.5 g/kg p.o. and frequently also ones of 1.0 g/kg, though individual deaths may occur after as little as 0.2 g/kg (HECHT 1950). In experiments carried out by RÁVNAY et al. (1954) guinea pigs survived single oral doses of 1.0 g/kg without exhibiting any symptoms. The most sensitive species was the rabbit, with an oral LD_{50} of around 0.2 g/kg (HECHT 1950).

In rabbits, autopsies revealed pulmonary oedema or severe pleural exudation. In the dog 0.5 g/kg p.o. proved fatal; the intoxication picture was similar to that in the rabbit (HECHT 1950).

After i.p. administration TSC is absorbed only slowly (GÜLZOW 1950; HECHT 1950). Despite this, the i.p. toxicity is higher than the toxicity after oral administration. Studies of the intoxication picture after i.p. injection of an oil-based solution to dogs revealed that doses of 20 to 50 mg/kg administered in this way can be fatal (GÜLZOW 1950). Vomiting, loss of appetite, diarrhoea, lack of motility, dyspnoea, tracheal wheezing, unconsciousness, tonoclonic twitching of the limbs and tachycardia are among the intoxication symptoms that regularly occur. Haemoconcentration, oedema in the lung, the mediastinal connective tissue, and the pericardium, and pleural effusions follow severe intoxication. Death occurs as a result of circulatory failure. Thus, the principal effect is a permeability disturbance due to capillary damage. An oil-based TSC suspension evidently exerts stronger action on oral or intraperitoneal administration than the active substance suspended in distilled water.

2. Subchronic and Chronic Toxicity

Repeated administration (both i.p. and oral) of TSC to dogs leads to the development of tolerance, as a result of which higher doses can be tolerated if the dose is increased gradually (GÜLZOW 1950). Whereas a 30 mg/kg i.p. dose will kill animals that have not received previous treatment with the substance, dogs started on low doses can tolerate up to 140 mg/kg i.p. Laboratory tests on animals intoxicated by repeated administration showed symptoms of haemoconcentration, hyperglycaemia, and anaemia, a shift of the granulocytes to the left, leucocytosis, and eosinopenia. The pulmonary oedema fluid is very rich in protein, and the blood thickens considerably as a result of loss of plasma (GÜLZOW and SCHLICHT 1950).

Following repeated oral administration of higher doses to dogs, MOYER and PERKINS (1951) observed a considerable cumulative toxicity. 5 out of 7 dogs treated with 100 mg/kg/day died within 48 h. The autopsies usually revealed pleural effusions, mediastinal oedemas, and foamy exudation in the bronchi. In contrast, the animals survived a 50 mg/kg dose administered for 5 days.

In a chronic toxicity study MOYER and PERKINS (1950) treated 10 dogs daily with 10 mg TSC/kg p.o. One dog died within 24 h and another (presumably intercurrently) after 7 weeks. After 3 months the dose was increased to 20 mg/kg for 2 months. 2 of the animals died as a result and 3 had to be sacrificed. The remaining dogs were given 50 mg/kg for one month. In some of the dogs increased bromthalein retention was observed and fatty infiltrations were found in the liver; these normalized, however, even though treatment was continued. The erythrocyte sedimentation rate was slowed down, especially in the first month, and the haematocrit decreased. In most of the dogs the haematocrit stabilized at a subnormal level, although in a few others it fell steadily during the 6-month treatment period. However, the bone marrow was not aplastic and there was no evidence of intravascular haemolysis. There were no signs of toxic kidney damage. Thus, GÜLZOW's (1950) findings on the development of tolerance to the drug through the administration of increasing doses were confirmed.

3. Liver Toxicity

RÁVNAY et al. (1954) investigated the question of liver damage induced by TSC. Treatment of guinea pigs for 19 days to 27 days with oral doses of 100 mg/kg/day led to the death of all the animals; liver and kidney damage was established. Repetition of the experiment during the summer months revealed a substantially better tolerability.

Fatty degeneration of the liver after TSC has also been observed in various animal experiments by DOMAGK (1948), SAVINI (1950) and EMMRICH and PETZOLD (1952).

References

Domagk G (1948) Die experimentellen Grundlagen einer Chemotherapie der Tuberkulose. Beitr Klin Tuberk 101:372–394
Emmrich R, Petzold H (1952) Experimentelle Untersuchungen zur Frage der Leberschädigung durch TB I. Z Ges Inn Med 7:625–628
Ginoulhiac E (1950) Toxicity of certain chemotherapeutics. Boll Soc Ital Biol Sper 26:574–577
Gülzow M (1950) Experimentelles zur TB I-Wirkung. I. Mitteilung: Intoxikationserscheinungen. Z Ges Exp Med 116:26–39
Gülzow M, Schlicht A (1950) Experimentelles zur TB I-Wirkung. II. Mitteilung: Aminosäure-Untersuchungen des Serum- und Organeiweiß im Verlauf von TB I (Conteben)-Intoxikationen. Z Ges Exp Med 116:40–55
Hecht G (1950) Unpublished Investigations
Moyer JH, Perkins RB (1951) Experimental studies on the toxicity of amithiozone in dogs. Am Rev Tuberc 64:659–668
Rávnay TH, Forró L, Szegö L (1954) Untersuchungen über den Wirkungsmechanismus der Thiosemikarbazone. Z Tuberk 104:249–255
Savini E (1950) Recherches expérimentales sur la toxicité du thiosemicarbazone. CR Soc Biol 144:1310–1313

IV. Pyrazinamide (PZA) and Morphazinamide (MZA)

1. Pyrazinamide (PZA)

a) Respiration and Blood Pressure

In doses of 200 mg/kg i.p. or 400 mg/kg p.o. pyrazinamide had no effect on the blood pressure or on the respiration in cats (ROBINSON et al. 1954).

b) Acute Toxicity

Pyrazinamide has a low acute toxicity. According to the data of ROBINSON et al. (1954), an LD_{50} of 3.4 (3.18–3.64) g/kg was determined for male mice following oral administration. In male rats the LD_{50} was above 4.0 g/kg. BONATI and BERTONI (1962) report an oral LD_{50} of about 2.75 g/kg and an i.p. LD_{50} of 1.68 (1.30–2.18) g/kg for mice. Doses up to 1.5 g/kg were tolerated by mice and by rats without any symptoms. Higher doses resulted in excitation, rapidly followed by depression. Deaths, which usually occurred within the first 2 days after the treatment, are attributed to respiratory paralysis (ROBINSON et al. 1954).

c) Subchronic Toxicity

Rats given oral treatment for 90 days tolerated doses up to 0.62 g/kg/day without any symptoms. After higher doses (1.25 and 2.5 g/kg) the weight gain was impaired (ROBINSON et al. 1954). ZITKOVÁ et al. (1970) also reported reduced weight gain in rats as a toxic effect after 7 days of oral treatment with 3.0 g/kg. Dogs tolerated up to 0.5 g/kg/day without any symptoms in a study lasting for 90 days (ROBINSON et al. 1954). Doses of 1.0 g/kg, however, caused anorexia, vomiting, and a rapid deterioration of the general condition. After 21 and 58 days the dogs were in a moribund state and had to be sacrificed. The liver of one of these animals showed pronounced zonal necrosis of the liver cord cells, especially in the pericentral lobular and periportal areas. The periportal and subcapsular lymphatic pathways of the liver were dilated and macroscopically visible on the surface. An elevation of alkaline phosphatase and icterus were observed before death. In the dogs treated with 0.25 g/kg the livers were normal.

Histopathologically detectable kidney lesions were found in the dogs treated with 1.0 g/kg and 0.5 g/kg. These were in the form of irregular, bluish-red, largely amorphous masses in endothelial-lined channels, probably lymphatic vessels. There were no pathological findings in any of the other organs and tissues examined. In rats corresponding kidney alterations were found in only one animal, treated with 2.5 g/kg. The other rats had numerous small vacuoles in the epithelium of the proximal convoluted tubules. The cells of the loops of Henle and of the distal convoluted tubules had small compact nuclei and a vacuolated cytoplasm.

d) Liver Toxicity

Following repeated reports of the hepatotoxic action of pyrazinamide, GRUSS and NICKLING (1967) studied the tolerability of PZA in rabbits and found good tolerability on repeated administration of relatively low doses (up to 0.25 g/kg). Biochemical and histopathological examinations failed to reveal any toxic liver damage.

On the other hand, ŠŤASTNÁ et al. (1970) showed that in rats an elevation of the serum GPT occurs after 3 days of oral treatment with 3.0 g/kg, while histologically detectable liver alterations first appear on the 7th day. These take the form of an infiltration of the periportal space and isolated, diffuse regions of fatty degeneration. After treatment with 1.5 g/kg no liver damage was found either biochemically or histologically.

Further investigations by ČELIKOVSKÁ et al. (1970) revealed that 7 days of administration of 3.0 g PZA/kg to rats caused an increase of the total serum cholesterol in addition to a significant rise of the GPT. The phospholipid and cholesterol contents of the liver were elevated. Focal fatty degeneration occurred, predominantly in the vicinity of the central veins.

Thus, the liver damage observed in dogs and in rats obviously represents the experimental equivalent of the hepatotoxic symptoms that occur in man.

e) Carcinogenicity

After 7 months of administration of 3% PZA with the feed, MORI et al. (1960) observed an increased incidence of pulmonary tumours in mice.

References

Bonati F, Bertoni L (1962) Derivati basici dell'acido pirazin-2-carbonico ad azione antimicobatterica. Minerva Med 53:1704–1708

Čelikovská G, Šťastná J, Zitková L, Březinová H, Kürti V (1970) Leberschädigung nach Verabreichung von Pyrazinamid im Tierversuch. III. Biochemische Veränderungen im Lebergewebe und im Blutserum. Arzneimittelforsch 20:155–157

Gruss JD, Nickling HG (1967) Vergleichende funktionelle und bioptische Untersuchungen der normalen Kaninchenleber während der Applikation von Pyrazincarbonsäureamid. Arzneimittelforsch 17:1565–1568

Mori K, Yasuno A, Matsumoto K (1960) Induction of pulmonary tumors in mice with isonicotinic acid hydrazid. Gann 51:83–89
Robinson HJ, Siegel H, Pietrowski JJ (1954) Toxicity of pyrazinamide. Am Rev Tuberc 70:423–429
Šťastná J, Čelikovská G, Zitková L, Viklický J (1970) Leberschädigung nach Verabreichung von Pyrazinamid im Tierversuch. II. Untersuchungen über die zeitlichen Veränderungen der Konzentrationen von Pyrazinamid im Blut und der Aktivität der Serum-Transaminasen. Arzneimittelforsch 20:153–155
Zitková L, Šťastná J, Čelikovská G, Kürti V (1970) Leberschädigung nach Verabreichung von Pyrazinamid im Tierversuch I. Änderungen des Körpergewichtes von Ratten unter Einwirkung von Pyrazinamid. Arzneimittelforsch 20:151–153

2. Morphazinamide (MZA)

a) Acute Toxicity

After oral administration to mice the LD_{50} is 3.55 (3.0–4.0) g/kg. After intraperitonael injection the LD_{50} is 2.75 (2.47–3.05) g/kg (BONATI and BERTONI 1962).

b) Subchronic Toxicity

No effect on weight gain or on the blood picture was detectable after oral administration of 1 g/kg (BONATI and BERTONI 1962).

When morphazinamide was administered to rabbits at doses corresponding to the therapeutic dose in man there were no liver alterations; the double dose caused only slight degenerative alterations which were clearly milder than the damage caused by pyrazinamide under the same conditions (MARCHIONI et al. 1963).

References

Bonati F, Bertoni L (1962) Derivati basici dell'acido pirazin-2-carbonico ad azione antimicobatteria. Minerva Med 53:1704–1708
Marchioni CF, Monzali G, Velluti G, Corato P (1963) Indagine comparative sul comportamento del parenchima epatico dopo somministrazione di morfazinamide e pirazinamide nel coniglio. Boll Soc Med Chir Modena 63:769–778

V. Isoniazid (INH)

1. Respiration, Circulation, Heart

Isoniazid (INH) exhibits only weak pharmacodynamic effects in the usual pharmacological tests. The respiration and blood pressure of anaesthetized dogs were unaffected by an intravenous dose of 100 mg INH/kg (REINHARDT et al. 1952). Similarly, the dogs' normal circulatory response to vagus stimulation, carotid occlusion, or injections of acetylcholine and adrenaline were unaffected by i.v. doses of up to 8 mg INH/kg (BENSON et al. 1952). However, in the cat a dose of 8 mg/kg causes a slight and transient reduction of the blood pressure (BENSON et al. 1952). No significant effects were observed in conscious dogs either (RUBIN and BURKE 1953), as the cumulative administration of 1 mg/kg to 32 mg/kg i.v. was tolerated without any changes in the blood pressure, the heart rate, or the ECG.

In isolated guinea pig, rat, and rabbit Langendorff heart preparations the frequency and the amplitude of the ventricular contractions were not affected by the injection of doses up to 100 μg into the perfusion system (REINHARDT et al. 1952). After higher doses (10 mg–250 mg), however, ALLMARK et al. (1953) observed a positive inotropic effect and an increased coronary flow in isolated rabbit heart.

2. Smooth Muscles

The spontaneous movements of the ileum and bladder in anaesthetized dogs are not affected by i.v. injection of 1 mg–32 mg INH/kg (RUBIN and BURKE 1953). Concentrations of 100 μg INH/ml bath fluid have no effect on the normal function of isolated guinea pig ileum and uterus (REINHARDT et al. 1952); only at a concentration of 1000 μg/ml is the amplitude of the spontaneous contractions of isolated rabbit ileum reduced (RUBIN and BURKE 1953). The effect of INH on the acetylcholine induced contractions of isolated rabbit intestine proved to be 100 times weaker than that of atropine (BENSON et al. 1952). RUBIN and BURKE (1953) reported a still weaker activity. According to BENSON et al. (1952), the antihistaminic effect on isolated guinea pig intestine is only $^{1}/_{1000}$ of that of β-dimethylaminoethyl benzhydryl ether hydrochloride (Benadryl). RUBIN and BURKE (1953) also observed only a slight inhibitory effect on the histamine- and barium-induced spasm in isolated guinea pig ileum. INH is about $^{1}/_{20}$ as effective as atropine on methacholine-induced bronchospasm in the guinea pig (BENSON et al. 1952). The broncholytic activity, however, does not affect histamine-induced bronchospasm.

3. Other Pharmacological Effects

A very weak ganglion-blocking effect was established in the cat. Neuromuscular conduction is not affected. The salivation induced in the rabbit by pilocarpine and the metacholine-stimulated tear secretion in the rat are not inhibited by INH. The local application of a 1% solution into the rabbit eye induces neither mydriasis nor local anaesthesia (BENSON et al. 1952). The ciliated epithelium in the trachea is unaffected by 10% concentrations of INH (REINHARDT et al. 1952). Doses up to 16 mg/kg, administered orally, do not act antipyretically in rabbits (BENSON et al. 1952) and doses up to 500 mg/kg do not act analgesically (RUBIN and BURKE 1953). No irritation of the gastric mucosa was observed in the rat after doses up to 200 mg/kg (REINHARDT et al. 1952).

The pharmacological investigations therefore failed to provide any evidence of parasympatholytic or sympathomimetic effects, or indeed of any other notable pharmacodynamic activity of INH.

4. Central Stimulation Effects

Although, unlike nicotine, INH is pharmacodynamically very inactive, like nicotine it has a stimulating effect on the central nervous system (ALLMARK et al. 1953). In acute toxicity studies it emerged for the first time that INH, like other hydrazides (semicarbazide, thiosemicarbazide, carbohydrazide, etc.) and hy-

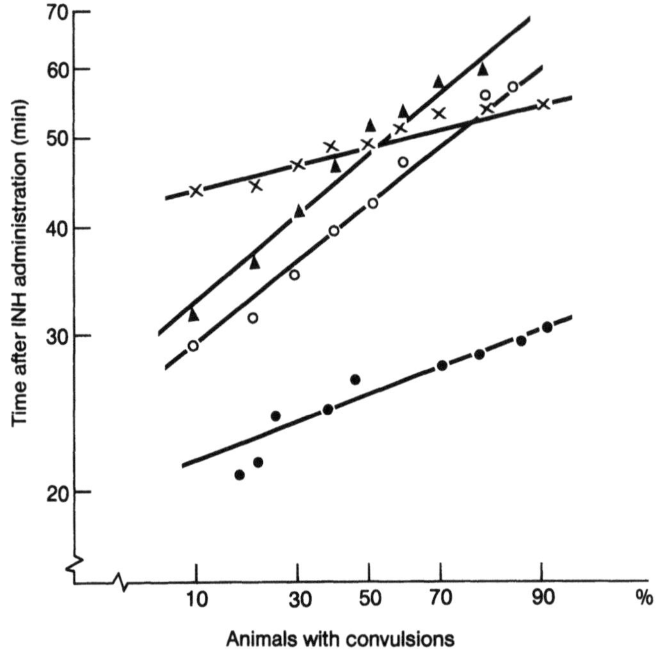

Fig. 1. Time of occurrence of convulsions in mice ●, chicks; ○, rats ▲; and guinea pigs; ×, following treatment with 2.2 mmol INH/kg. (After CASEY and WOOD, 1973)

drazine itself, leads to convulsions. In addition, it lowers the convulsion threshold of other substances such as amidopyrine, nikethamide, pentetrazole, and procaine (DIENEMANN and SIMON 1953).

Compared with chicks, rats, and guinea pigs, mice react most sensitively to the convulsant effect of INH, as can be seen in Fig. 1 (CASEY and WOOD 1973). Interaction between INH and vitamin B_6 is thought to play an important part in the development of the convulsions.

5. INH and Vitamin B_6 Metabolism

The action of INH on vitamin B_6 metabolism is complex. As a "carbonyl reagent", INH, like other hydrazides, reacts with the carbonyl oxygen to form a hydrazone. As a result of this reaction among other things the functionally important aldehyde group of pyridoxal 5′-phosphate is blocked. This group represents the active form of vitamin B_6 and plays an important role as a coenzyme in decarboxylation and transamination processes (review in HOLTZ and PALM 1964). In addition, both INH and INH hydrazone act – the latter considerably more strongly – as inhibitors of pyridoxal kinase, which phosphorylates the vitamin to the cofactor pyridoxal 5′-phosphate (MCCORMICK and SNELL 1961). On the other hand, DIXON and WILLIAMS (1962) found that on intracerebral injection of an INH-pyridoxal phosphate complex, which does not inhibit pyridoxal kinase, the convulsant effect in mice is unchanged or even increased in comparison to the effect of unphosphorylated complexes or of pure INH. This makes it clear that neither the effect on the pyridoxal-phosphate bond nor the inhibition of pyridoxal kinase is entirely responsible for the convulsions. All the same, the various effects on vitamin B_6 metabolism suggest that under the influence of INH a pyridoxal-phosphate depletion occurs in the organism, and this is also indicated by clinical observations.

It seemed sensible, as in the attempts at reducing the convulsant action of hydrazides with pyridoxine (review in WILLIAMS and BAIN 1961), to also try and attenuate the convulsant effect and the toxicity of INH by means of vitamin B_6. According to BALZER et al. (1960), however, INH occupies a special position among the hydrazides, since even in a molar ratio of 1:2 pyridoxine failed to eliminate INH-induced convulsions in the mouse; QUADBECK and SARTORI (1957) arrived at the same conclusion, again using mice. According to LECHAT et al. (1963), pyridoxine does not suppress the INH-induced tendency towards audiogenic convulsions in rats, but it does reduce the mortality rate. DUBNICK et al. (1960) actually observed an increase in the toxicity of INH after administration of pyridoxal, and BALZER et al. (1960) reported an earlier onset of the convulsions after treating mice with pyridoxal 5'-phosphate and INH. On the other hand, PRESCOTT et al. (1957d) observed that pyridoxal in one- or two-molar equivalent concentrations exerted a protective effect in mice. MANTHEI (1960) found that increasing doses (25 mg/kg–150 mg/kg) of pyridoxine had an increasingly protective effect against the lethal action of INH in adult mice, whereas in doses greater than 25 mg/kg pyridoxal increased the toxicity of sublethal doses of INH. In younger mice pyridoxal in low doses proved to be more active than pyridoxine. LECHAT et al. (1963) reported a reduction in the number of convulsions and a reduction of the mortality in mice after pyridoxine treatment. The effect of a subconvulsant dose of INH, which in the conditioned reflex test in rats enables a reduced CNS function to be detected, can be eliminated by pyridoxine (FÖLDI et al. 1970). The antagonistic activity of pyridoxine on the lethal and convulsant effects of INH was also established in guinea pigs (TIRUNARAYANAN and VISCHER 1956) and in dogs (WILLIAMS and WIEGAND 1960).

CHIN et al. (1978) reported dose-dependent anticonvulsant and mortality-reducing effects of pyridoxine in dogs, but found it to be ineffective in rats. Combination with diazepam, on the other hand, gave a protective effect in both species, which is of significance for the treatment of INH intoxications in man.

6. INH and the γ-Aminobutyric Acid Metabolism

Attempts to correlate the convulsant and anticonvulsant effects of the hydrazines and hydrazides with interaction with individual stages of γ-aminobutyric acid (GABA) metabolism [GABA plays an inhibitory role in the CNS; reviews by KRNJEVIC (1971) and ROBERTS (1974)], have not as yet yielded any consistent results (BALZER et al. 1960; FREY 1976). Problems in the interpretation of the experimental results are due not least to the GABA metabolism differences observed in the various species (CASEY and WOOD 1973).

7. Protective Action of Various Substances

In addition to vitamin B_6, many other substances were investigated to see if they exerted a protective effect against INH.

BARRETO and MANO (1961) observed in rabbits a reduction of the pyruvate concentration in the blood as a result of the formation of a non-toxic isonicotinyl hydrazone with pyruvic acid after administration of INH. The convulsant and lethal effects of INH could be eliminated by injection of pyruvate. However, DAUPHINEE et al. (1975) were unable to confirm this antidote action of pyruvate. According to WIEZOREK et al. (1977), diazepam, chlordiazepoxide, and methaqualone reduce the acute toxicity of INH in mice by a factor of 2–3 when administered simultaneously. It is thought that the benzodiazepines protect against convulsions by re-establishing the γ-aminobutyric acid levels in the brain, which are reduced by INH in subtoxic and toxic doses. Diazepam, especially in combination with pyridoxine, clearly causes a reduction of the toxicity in rats and in dogs, which is particularly important with respect to acute INH intoxication (CHIN et al. 1978).

The following substances are also reported to act protectively: vitamin B_{12} (ATA and TANAKA 1952), glutamic acid (CEDRANGOLO et al. 1953), cycloserine (PRESCOTT et al. 1957a), glycine and sodium glucuronate (PRESCOTT et al. 1954), L-cysteine (PRESCOTT et al. 1957c), calcium pantothenate (MANTHEI 1957), p-aminobenzoic acid and nicotinic acid (PRESCOTT et al. 1957c), glycerol (PRESCOTT et al. 1957b), glycerol-formol (PRESCOTT and STONE 1969), and coumarin (FÖLDI et al. 1970). RUBIN and BURKE (1952) were unable to confirm the protective effect of vitamin B_{12}. Furthermore, they tested 50 other substances, including amino acids and vitamins (no further details available), and found that none of them showed a protective effect. Barbiturates and other central suppressants were the only substances with any antagonistic activity.

a) Barbiturates

According to P'AN et al. (1952), phenobarbital and pentobarbital in small doses eliminate the central nervous excitation induced by INH in mice and in dogs and reduce its toxicity. REINHARDT et al. (1952) also found phenobarbital and chloral hydrate to be effective. GOLDIN et al. (1955) confirmed the effect of pentobarbital. ALLMARK et al. (1953) found that the toxicity of INH was reduced by hexobarbital in rats and in rabbits; WOLF et al. (1965) observed the same thing in mice. However, the hypnotic effect of the barbiturates is prolonged in rats (ALLMARK et al. 1953).

b) Alcohol

In mice the action of INH corresponding to the LD_{50} is quite considerably attenuated, and the mortality is actually eliminated, when the substance is administered simultaneously with ethanol in a dose equal to one-quarter of the LD_{50}.

However, following the administration of toxic doses equivalent to the LD_{50} of both substances, the effects are potentiated; the alcohol is obviously the more toxic (GLASS et al. 1964). Prolonged administration of INH and alcohol in the drinking water also showed that low doses of alcohol had a protective effect against the long-lasting INH intoxication (GLASS and MALLACH 1965).

8. Acute Toxicity

Many studies have been carried out on the acute toxicity of INH. The results are summarized in Table 1.

The summary shows a particularly good agreement between the toxicity data reported by the various investigators. Mice are most sensitive to INH and, surprisingly, the method of administration has scarcely any effect on toxicity in this species. The small variations generally found in the LD_{50} occur as a result of the very extensive absorption and distribution of the INH. Guinea pigs react in a similar fashion, although they tolerate INH better. Up to 30 min after the treatment mice appear normal. Symptoms of central nervous stimulation then develop. The animals become excited, convulsive tremor appears, then convulsions and terminal tonic spasms. Respiratory arrest precedes cardiac arrest. Most of the deaths occur within 2 h of the treatment (BENSON et al. 1952; FUST et al. 1952; P'AN et al. 1952; REINHARDT et al. 1952; RUBIN et al. 1952).

The rat proved to be the least sensitive species. Parenterally administered INH is about twice as toxic as orally administered INH. Convulsions also occur in rats and in rabbits. Death comes as a result of respiratory paralysis (BENSON et al. 1952). HARPER and WORDEN (1966) found that the nature of the solvent or suspension medium has an essential influence on the oral toxicity in rats. Administration in acacia gum yielded an LD_{50} of 3300 (2900–3750) mg/kg, administration in gelatin an LD_{50} of around 2650 mg/kg, and administration in water one of 2000 (1675–2390) mg/kg.

Dogs react to 25 mg/kg i.v. only with salivation (REINHARDT et al. 1952). A dose of 50 mg/kg causes salivation, vomiting, and defaecation after about 30 min. 100 mg/kg is lethal, death being preceded by central intoxication symptoms (fear, tonoclonic spasms) (RUBIN et al. 1952).

In monkeys (Macaca mulatta) clonic spasms developed within 90 min–120 min of oral administration of 80 mg/kg–160 mg/kg in 4 out of 10 animals. After 240 mg/kg–320 mg/kg they occurred within the same time in 7 out of 8 animals. 10 min–20 min previously the animals had been anxious and overexcited. The initial fit of convulsions was usually the most severe one, and was followed by two or more attacks of shorter duration and lower intensity. Complete recovery occurred within 3 h (SCHMIDT et al. 1953).

Intracisternal injection of 6 mg INH/kg to rabbits caused violent tonoclonic convulsions after about 20 min, preceded by transient excitation and strong salivation and interspersed with short spasm-free intervals (LEOPOLD et al. 1966). According to FUST et al. (1952), the intracisternal LD_{50} in rabbits is >12 mg/kg.

The INH-glucuronic acid derivatives isonicotinoyldrazone-d-glucuronic acid lactone and isonicotinoylhydrazine sodium glucuronide are considerably less toxic than INH itself (ORLOWSKI et al. 1976).

9. Subchronic and Chronic Toxicity

a) Rats

BENSON et al. (1952) administered INH to young male rats in concentrations up to of 0.05% in the feed for 14 weeks. The growth and the red blood picture were not affected. No macroscopic pathological alterations were found.

Table 1. Acute toxicity of isoniazid

Species	Strain, sex	Route of adminis-tration	LD_{50} mg/kg	Confidence interval	Literature source
Mouse	CF1, ♂	i.v.	150		4
	–	i.v.	153	± 16,8	1
	–	i.v.	165	± 4	5
	–	i.v.	152		2
	–	i.v.	165	(155–170)	3
	CF1, ♂	i.p.	159		4
	–	i.p.	186		2
	–	i.m.	137	± 15,1	1
	–	i.m.	162		2
	–	s.c.	177	± 19,5	1
	–	s.c.	170	± 5	5
	–	s.c.	138		2
	– ♀	s.c.	282	(260–306)	7
	–	s.c.	150	(120–160)	3
	CF1, ♂	p.o.	205		4
	–	p.o.	133	± 14,0	1
	–	p.o.	190	± 6	5
	–	p.o.	141		2
	–	p.o.	170	(165–175)	3
Rat	CF, ♂	i.v.	425		2
	–	i.p.	380		4
	–	i.p.	335		2
	–	i.m.	425		2
	–	s.c.	412		2
	Sprague-Dawley, ♂+♀	p.o.	2000–3300		7
	–	p.o.	1849		2
	–	p.o.	1435		1
	CF, ♂	p.o.	650		4
Guinea-pig	– ♂	i.v.	220	(210–231)	8
	CF, ♂	i.p.	200		4
	–	i.p.	295		2
	–	i.m.	255		2
	–	s.c.	195		2
	CF, ♂	p.o.	280		4
	–	p.o.	255		2
Rabbit	–	i.v.	94		1
	–	i.v.	155		2
	–	i.p.	147		2
	–	i.m.	155		2
	–	s.c.	135		2
	–	p.o.	200		1
	–	p.o.	295		2
Dog	–	i.v.	~ 50		5
	Mongrel	p.o.	~ 100		9
Monkey	Macaca mulatta	p.o.	> 320		6

[1] BENSON et al. (1952); [2] FUST et al. (1952); [3] P'AN et al. (1952); [4] REINHARDT et al. (1952); [5] RUBIN et al. (1952); [6] SCHMIDT et al. (1953); [7] Harper and WORDEN (1966); [8] LEOPOLD et al. (1966); [9] NOEL et al. (1967).

RUBIN et al. (1952) treated groups of 5 rats with 40 mg/kg, 160 mg/kg, 320 mg/kg, and 640 mg/kg p.o. for a period of 21 days. The doses were divided into 2–4 portions per day. Only the rats treated with 40 mg/kg put on weight to the same extent as the control animals. The rats treated with the higher doses lost weight and several rats on 320 and 640 mg/kg died. Histopathological examinations revealed necrotic alterations, slight granular or fatty degeneration in the liver, and slight granular degeneration of the proximal tubules.

After treating rats for 10 days and 25 days with 10 mg/kg–90 mg/kg s.c., WEISS et al. (1954) observed adrenal hypertrophy and a reduction of the sudanophilic lipids. After 14 weeks of treatment with 0.001%–0.05% in the feed no toxic symptoms or any haematological changes were observed in rats (BENSON et al. 1952).

HARPER and WORDEN (1966) treated groups of 30 Sprague-Dawley rats with INH concentrations of 0.025%–0.5% in the feed for up to 52 weeks. The highest concentration proved to be lethal. All the rats in this group lost weight and most of them died within the first month. The symptoms consisted of piloerection, weakness, anorexia, and diarrhoea. Autopsies and histological examinations revealed hypotrophy of the gonads and liver necroses. After treatment with 0.25% reduced growth and gonadal hypotrophy were established. The latter was also found, independently of the dose, in the lower-dose groups.

b) Dogs [1]

13 weeks of intravenous administration of 1 mg, 5 mg, and 20 mg INH/kg caused anorexia, reduced weight gain, and liver alterations in the highest-dose group (BENSON et al. 1952).

Oral administration of daily doses of 25 and 17.5 mg/kg was lethal within about 30 days. The symptoms observed were anorexia, weight loss, ataxia, tremor, convulsions, and icterus (RUBIN et al. 1952).

In general, a dose of 4 mg/kg was tolerated without any symptoms. Histopathological and biochemical investigations revealed that the icterus caused by the higher doses was due to fatty degeneration of the liver. There were various signs suggesting that the damage was reversible. Plasma concentration measurements showed that concentrations of 9 µg/ml–35 µg/ml lead to anorexia, central nervous stimulation, liver damage, and death within one month. Concentrations of 6 µg/ml–8 µg/ml only resulted in anorexia and transient central nervous excitation.

In a comparative study using isoniazid methanosulphonate (NOEL et al. 1967) dogs reacted so badly to the higher dose of INH (50 mg/kg p.o.) that after 3 days it had to be reduced to 40 mg/kg. Vomiting, gait disturbances, and convulsions still occurred, and consequently after a break of one week the treatment was continued with 5 mg/kg and 25 mg/kg. Within a week 2 of the animals on 25 mg/kg had died, with the result that the dose was further reduced to 15 mg/kg. In the end it was found that 5 mg/kg was tolerated over a total experimental period of 195 days. On the other hand, 5 out of the 6 dogs treated with 15 mg/kg died. The clinical symptoms were loss of appetite, vomiting, central nervous excitation,

[1] It should be noted at this point that the dog, unlike most other species, including man, is unable to acetylate and therefore to detoxify INH.

muscular twitching, and epileptiform fits. Slight and transient anaemia was detected after 3 months of treatment. The histopathological alterations to the CNS are presented on p. 346.

c) Monkeys

Oral administration of INH in divided daily doses of 2.5 mg/kg for 14 days, 10 mg/kg for 52 days, 40 mg/kg for 38 days, and 80 mg/kg for 20 days failed to induce any toxic symptoms (SCHMIDT et al. 1953). Similarly, 2 months of treatment with 5 mg/kg followed by 7 months at 20 mg/kg failed to produce any toxic symptoms in a large group of monkeys (Macacus rhesus, 169 animals). On the contrary, the general condition, weight gain, and the activity of the tuberculin-positive animals, many of which had been in a poor condition at the start of the study, were improved. No toxic changes affecting the haematopoietic system, the liver, the kidneys, or the endocrine system could be found. Monkeys are therefore substantially less sensitive than dogs to INH.

d) Rabbits and Guinea Pigs

Subcutaneous administration of INH (30 mg/kg) 5 days a week had no effect on the body weight in rabbits and in guinea pigs in a study lasting 4 weeks. The haemoglobin concentration fell slightly (FUST et al. 1952). CERIOTTI and FRANCESCHINI (1953) treated rabbits for 7 days with 35 mg/kg and observed a reduced bromthalein excretion as a sign of damage to the liver. HARPER and WORDEN (1966) confirmed this result in a similar series of experiments.

e) Ducks

Ducks proved to be very sensitive to parenteral and oral administration of INH (BOTTA and CARLTON 1967a). After 7 days on INH administered in the feed Peking ducks showed an LD_{50} (7 days) of 0.13% (0.118%–0.142%). The toxic symptoms were excitation, ataxia, convulsions, lassitude, and a comatose state before death. After 7 days of i.p. administration an LD_{50} of 57 mg/kg (53.0 mg/kg–61.3 mg/kg) was determined. Chronic administration of INH with the feed produced no clinical symptoms and no differences in the mortality rate after 12 weeks with concentrations of up to 0.005%. After 0.01% INH 20% of the animals died within 3 months. The characteristic neuropathological alterations observed in the duck are dealt with on p. 346.

10. Liver Toxicity

The liver damage induced by INH in man, which appears after treatment for a prolonged period, can be reproduced in rats and in guinea pigs. In rats fatty degeneration and midzonal liver-cell necrosis were observed, associated with elevated GOT levels although there were no signs of hepatitis. Ultrastructural alterations consisted of a reduction in the smooth endoplasmic reticulum and increased membrane fragments and liposomes (RAISFELD 1975). The fatty degeneration of the liver develops in two stages after i.p. administration of 150 mg INH/kg: the initial rise in the liver triglycerides is apparently the result of inhibited hepatic secretion of the pre-β-lipoproteins into the serum. This is followed by a blockade of the triglyceride breakdown with further accumulation of fat (BLACK 1977). The hepatotoxicity is due to covalent binding of acetylhydrazine, formed by hydrolysis of acetylisoniazid, the principal metabolite of INH, to the liver proteins (TIMBRELL et al. 1980). Pretreatment of the animals, which leads to the induction of microsomal drug-metabolizing enzyme systems, results in an intensification of the hepatic toxicity. Inhibition of the microsomal enzyme systems, on the other hand, reduces hepatic toxicity. Pretreatment with ethanol increases the liver toxicity in rabbits (WHITEHOUSE et al. 1978).

11. Neurotoxic Effects

KLINGHARDT (1954) was the first to induce in rats a disease picture analogous to the previously established INH neuritis in man. This was produced by prolonged overloading with INH and manifested itself by sensitivity disturbances and pareses. Histopathological examinations revealed focal primary degeneration of the peripheral nerve fibres, which chiefly affected the myelin sheaths though the axons were also involved. After oral treatment of rats with 200 mg–250 mg INH/kg ZBINDEN and STUDER (1955a) observed paresis of the extremities only after 7 months–8 months of treatment, whereas severe focal degeneration of the myelin sheaths, and often disintegration of the axis cylinders and proliferation of the Schwann cells, were already detectable after 15 days. The gangliocytes of the dorsal spinal ganglia showed sporadic, low-grade degeneration phenomena only after months-long treatment. The nerve fibres of the dorsal roots were affected in form of small, isolated foci only in the most severe cases. The spinal cord and the brain degenerative changes were completely absent.

According to CAVANAGH (1967), the motor and sensory fibres are equally affected, fibres of medium diameter being particularly subject to damage. Distal fibres are evidently more severely changed than proximal ones. In the electron microscope the nerve alterations first become evident by swelling of the axonal mitochondria and coarse-granular separation of the axoplasmic ground substance (SCHLAEPFER and HAGER 1964a). During the first phase of axonal alteration the myelin sheaths and the Schwann cells appear to be intact. The early disintegration of the axoplasm is followed by changes in the myelin sheaths (SCHLAEPFER and HAGER 1964b). These lose their continuity and irregularly-shaped myelin spheres form within the cytoplasm of the Schwann cells. This is followed by reactive alterations and the appearance of phagosome-like vacuoles in the Schwann cells. Finally, the myelin degradation products are engulfed by macrophages.

The degenerative changes are associated with reparative and regenerative processes of the parenchymal and mesenchymal elements (SCHLAEPFER and HAGER 1964c). They are characterized by fibrosis of the endoneurium, proliferation of Schwann cells, regeneration of the axons, and new myelin sheath formation. The considerable capacity to regenerate new nerve fibres from undamaged cells is also emphasized by ZBINDEN and STUDER (1955a) and by CAVANAGH (1967).

In all, according to SCHLAEPFER and HAGER (1964a) and to CAVANAGH (1967), the neural alterations correspond to those encountered in Wallerian degeneration.

SCHRÖDER (1970a, b) also points out many aspects in common with Wallerian degeneration, though he also emphasizes certain differences. Thus, in INH neuropathy he observed, in addition to marked permeability changes affecting the endoneural blood vessels, erythrodiapedesis that had not previously been found either in Wallerian degeneration or in the other forms of distally accentuated neuropathies. In contrast to CAVANAGH (1967), SCHRÖDER (1970b) also observed changes affecting the lumbosacral spinal ganglia, the anterior horn cells of the spinal cord, and the sensory nerve endings in the muscle spindles.

INH neuropathy differs in many respects from the neurotoxic damage caused by organic phosphoric esters (CAVANAGH 1967, 1973; SCHRÖDER 1970a).

KLINGHARDT (1954) did not succed in preventing or reducing the nerve damage by simultaneously treating rats with nicotinic acid amide (50 mg/animal), pyridoxine (25 mg/animal), or total vitamin B complex; ZBINDEN and STUDER (1955a, b), on the other hand were able to prevent peripheral nerve degeneration almost completely for the first 15 days and largely in the next 15 days by treating rats daily with 50 mg pyridoxine or pyridoxamine/kg body weight i.m. However, when the treatment lasted for more than 4 weeks the difference between the animals which were and those which were not treated with vitamin B_6 gradually disappeared. Thus, during chronic intoxication the neurotoxic effect of INH can only be delayed by vitamin B_6 but not permanently prevented. ZBINDEN and STUDER (1955c) subsequently showed that pyridoxal 5′-phosphate also exerts a protective effect. Glutamic acid, on the other hand, proved completely ineffective against the neurotoxic action of INH on the peripheral nerves (ZBINDEN and STUDER 1956). ROSEN (1955) was able to eliminate the symptoms induced by INH in rats on a vitamin-B_6-deficient diet (inhibition of growth and convulsions) by simultaneously giving pyridoxine.

In contrast to rats, dogs treated with INH develop cerebral lesions that are very similar to those caused by some monoamine oxidase inhibitors (phenelzine, indanylcarbethoxyhydrazine) (PALMER and NOEL 1965; WORDEN et al. 1967), even though INH is not a potent MAO inhibitor (ZELLER et al. 1952). Histopathological examination reveals separation of the fibres in certain regions of the subcortical myelin. Fissures and spaces appear and there is an activation of the microglia and hypertrophy of the astrocytes. The myelin becomes pale and the myelin sheaths are swollen. However, there are no myelin disintegration products. The neurites remain intact and the majority of the cortical neurons appear healthy, although microcavity formation does occur. The same alterations are produced by INH methanesulphonate.

Under the electron microscope these alterations appear in dogs as a vacuolation of the myelin, hypertrophy of the astrocytes, and degeneration of the oligodendrocytes (BLAKEMORE et al. 1972).

In ducklings the administration of INH leads to a neurological syndrome characterized by tremor, convulsions, ataxia, and pareses (CARLTON et al. 1965; CARLTON and KREUTZBERG 1966; BOTTA and CARLTON 1967a). Demyelination and vacuolation are observed particularly in the white matter of the cerebellum but also in the optic lobe and the spinal cord. All these alterations are representative of spongy degeneration. The axis cylinders also degenerate in the affected regions, and this is accompanied by the appearance of lipid macrophages. One finds proliferation of the microglia and macroglia and swelling of the astrocytes, and there is degeneration of the nuclei of cerebellar Purkinje cells, the motor neurons, the dental horn of the spinal cord, and the neurons of the medulla oblongata (CARLTON et al. 1965). The administration of pyridoxine, niacin, glutamic acid, or arginine together with the INH to ducklings had no protective effect against either the clinical symptoms or the neurological damage (BOTTA and CARLTON 1967b). INH gives rise to similar effects in chicks (CARLTON 1967).

Despite our knowledge of the biochemistry of INH, the way in which the specific peripheral neuropathy is induced is unknown (CAVANAGH 1973).

It is also unclear why in the dog, the duck, and the chick alterations develop in the oligodendroglia of the white matter in the brain, whereas a characteristic peripheral neuropathy develops in the rat and in man.

12. Ototoxicity

No signs of vestibulotoxicity were found after 19 days of treating guinea pigs with doses up to 100 mg/kg s.c. (CREMA and FABRIS 1954).

13. Reproductive Toxicity

HELLRIEGEL and KRAUS (1955) treated male mice for 20 days–50 days with about 125 mg INH/kg administered subcutaneously. Examination revealed increased amounts of connective tissue in the interstitium of the testicles and a microscopically visible reduction of spermatogenesis. However, the procreative capacity and the libido were maintained. In addition, many giant cells were found, together with disruption of mitosis and atrophy of the germinal epithelium. The alterations were thought to represent a weak temporary cytostatic effect. Permanent damage was not observed. STEINBRÜCK (1959), on the other hand, reported that the treatment caused reduced male fertility as a result of suppressed spermatogenesis in a study performed over 5 generations of mice.

Female rats treated for 50 days with 30 mg INH/kg p.o. did not exhibit any disturbance of the ovarian function or of the vaginal cycle (HESS 1954). Treatment of rats before mating and during gestation with 30 mg/kg had no effect either on fecundity or on the course of gestation. The intrauterine development of the foetuses was not impaired. Neither was extrauterine development during the suckling period adversely affected by treatment of the dams. No delayed damage was discernible.

In a study performed over 5 reproductive cycles in which male and female rats were continually given high (no further data available) doses of INH, HARPER and WORDEN (1966) did not observe any damage to the offspring.

After injection of INH into embryonated hen eggs, beak malformations (crossed beak or shortened upper and deformed lower beak) developed in 21.6% of the chicks (SEIFERT 1966). Because of the special circumstances of embryonic development in chicks it is virtually impossible to extrapolate these findings to mammals and in particular to man. According to JANSEN et al. (1980), teratogenic effects can largely be ruled out for INH.

14. Carcinogenic Effects

a) In Mice

The possibility of INH carcinogenicity has been the subject of many, and in some cases controversial, publications. Stimulated by a report by BERENCSI et al. (1952) of unusually rapid tumour development and the striking metastatic spread of a bronchial carcinoma under INH therapy, TIBOLDI et al. (1955) carried out animal studies on this problem. They investigated the effect of INH on the growth of Brown-Pearce carcinomas in rabbits and found that 10 mg/kg had a stimulating effect on the formation, number, and size of the metastases. However, there was no significant difference in the number of mitoses between the treated animals and the controls. The carcinogenic effect was therefore attributed to a modification of the protective mechanism by INH. In the same year BERENCSI et al. studied the action of INH on squamous-epithelial carcinomas on rabbit ears induced by painting with tar. There were no differences between the treated and the untreated animals. In 1957 JUHÁSZ et al. found that 3-month treatment of mice with a total dose of 82 mg caused tumours to develop. In 7 out of 45 animals solitary and multiple pulmonary adenomas developed within 61–225 days, and 7 other animals showed lymphoid and myeloid leukaemias, histiocytic leukaemia, and reticulosarcoma of the liver. JUHÁSZ's study inspired many further investigations on mice (MORI and YASUNO 1959; MORI et al. 1960; BIANCIFIORI and RIBACCHI 1962; WEINSTEIN and KINOSITA 1963; BIANCIFIORI and SEVERI 1966; ENGBAEK et al. 1965; JUHÁSZ et al. 1963; TOTH and SHUBIK 1966 a–c; TOTH and RUSTJA 1967; PEACOCK and PEACOCK 1966; SEVERI and BIANCIFIORI 1968; KELLY et al. 1969; TOTH and TOTH 1970; YAMAMOTO and WEISBURGER 1970; JONES et al. 1971; TOTH and SHIMIZU 1973; BHIDE et al. 1978). In these studies predominantly pulmonary adenomas were found, but also lymphosarcomas, reticulosarcomas, myeloid leukaemias, and other tumour forms.

It was not possible to demonstrate the carcinogenicity of INH in all the experiments on mice. For example, using the same experimental methods as JUHÁSZ, HACKMANN (1957) was unable to detect any carcinogenic action in 125 mice treated with INH after a total dose of 1.44 g/mouse and an observation period of either 6 or more than 12 months. In an extensive series of experiments VIALLIER and CASANOVA (1960) were also unable to induce any increased incidence of tumours in Swiss mice by i.p. and s.c. injection, inhalation, or administration of the substance in the drinking water.

b) In Other Animal Species

Tests for carcinogenicity of INH in other animal species gave mainly negative results. In experiments on 50 rabbits PANSA and BIKFALVI (1960) observed papillomatous changes of the bronchial mucosa after intratracheal administration of total doses of 2250 or 4500 mg INH over a period of 15 weeks. The hyperplastic effect of the INH depended on the duration of treatment and on the concentration given.

HECHT (1953) failed to observe any carcinogenic effect after oral treatment of rats over about 8 months with a total dose of 1.3 g INH/rat. In rats treated with INH by inhalation or by i.p. administration for one year PANSA et al. (1962) observed hyperplasia of the epithelium, particularly in the small bronchi, in the respiratory bronchioles, in the terminal segment bronchioles, and in the alveoli. Apart from the hyperplasia, which should not be regarded as a carcinogenically-induced effect, no morphological alterations were observed in other organs. On administration of 0.25% INH with the drinking water (about 90 mg/kg) 1 out of 8 rats was found to have alveolar hyperplasia and a papillary adenoma in a study by PEACOCK and PEACOCK (1966). Another group of 14 male and 14 female rats was treated with INH in drinking water or the feed for a total of 55 weeks. The surviving rats were sacrificed after 2 years. Only one hyperplastic and neoplastic subpleural alteration was observed. 1 out of 49 male Cb/Se rats treated with 0.35% of INH in the drinking water for 48 weeks had a liver carcinoma and 2 out of the 49 had lung tumours. 11 out of 40 females had fibroadenomas in the mammary glands (SEVERI and BIANCIFIORI 1968).

LOSCALZO (1964) treated 60 rats daily with about 30 mg INH/kg administered in the drinking water for 290 days or 355 days. No tumours developed. The development of transplanted myelomas of the Oberling-Guérin and Guérin types was not affected in comparison to control animals. In addition, TOTH and TOTH (1970) failed to find any carcinogenic effect in MRC rats treated throughout their lives with 0.1% INH administered in the drinking water ($\approx$ 20 mg/day–30 mg/day).

No evidence of carcinogenicity was found in voles (Clethrionomys g. Glariolus Schreb), gerbils (Meriones lybicus) or golden hamsters (ENGBAEK et al. 1965; PEACOCK and PEACOCK 1966; TOTH and BOREISMA 1969; TOTH and SHUBIK 1969).

On the basis of comparative studies with INH, isoniazid-methanesulphonate pyrazinamide, and semicarbazide, MORI et al. (1960) came to the conclusion that in view of the structural similarity to urethane, a known carcinogen, the carbamyl group NH_2-CO-R present in the aforementioned compounds was responsible for the carcinogenic activity.

BIANCIFIORI and RIBACCHI (1962), on the other hand, believed that the carcinogenic hydrazine H_2N-NH_2 split off from the INH was responsible for the tumorigenic effect. This opinion is supported by the findings of BRAUN et al. (1976), which show that in mice the carcinogen hydrazine is the metabolite with the longest elimination half-life ($t_{1/2}$ = 517 min), whereas in golden hamsters hydrazine has a half-life of only 11 min. This would also explain why the substance is not carcinogenic or mutagenic in the latter species.

Summarizing, many authors working independently and using different experimental methods (oral, subcutaneous, intramuscular, or intraperitoneal administration) on various mouse strains have detected INH carcinogenicity, often after very high doses of the substance. In general pulmonary adenomas were induced, and in a few cases also pulmonary adenocarcinomas and carcinomas, leukaemias, and other adenocarcinomas. However, in some other strains there were no carcinogenic effects. In other animal species too, e.g. rats and golden hamsters, the detection of INH carcinogenicity was sometimes quite uncertain or gave definitely negative results.

Since for various biological reasons the suitability of the mouse as a species for carcinogenicity tests is increasingly called into question (see, for example,

GRASSO and CRAMPTON 1972), and because of the species-specific metabolization, the relevance of carcinogenicity demonstrated predominantly in this species to man should not be overestimated. Many careful epidemiological studies on patients who had been treated for a long time with INH have, at any rate, failed to reveal any increased risk of cancer (IARC Monographs, Lyon 1974; HAMMOND et al. 1967; JANSEN et al. 1980).

15. Cytostatic Effects

In addition to the aforementioned reports on the cytostatic effects of INH on germinal epithelium there are reports on investigations into the inhibitory effects on the growth of normal or neoplastic tissue. SIMON (1952) established a cytostatic effect on Ehrlich's ascites carcinoma in the mouse. SIEGEL and IWAINSKY (1960), investigating the same tumour type, observed only a "prophylactic" effect if the INH treatment had been commenced 8 days before the implantation of the tumour. No cytostatic effect occurred if the treatment was initiated after the implantation. The number and the course of the mitoses also revealed a cytostatic effect of INH on this tumour (SIEGEL 1960). The DNA content of the tumour cells is significantly reduced (SIEGEL 1961). Similarly, INH causes a considerable inhibition of de novo production of DNA in rat livers regenerating after partial resection (SIEGEL and BERSCHNEIDER 1960).

BUCHER (1953) observed only a very weak toxic effect in chicken and mouse fibrocyte and osteoblast cultures in vitro. GROSS (1956) established an inhibition of tumour growth in Walker's rat carcinomas and BRAMBILLA and BALDINI (1959) in Galliera's rat sarcomas. According to MATSUMOTO et al. (1960), the development of p-dimethylaminoazobenzene (DAB)-induced liver carcinomas is also inhibited by INH. The growth of Jensen's sarcomas, Joshida's sarcomas, and Walker's carcinomas in vitro is stimulated by low concentrations of INH. Higher concentrations inhibit the tumour growth in vivo and in vitro (WAGNER and MORITZ 1962).

All in all, the cytostatic effects of INH are so weak that it has not been possible to utilize them therapeutically. It is also unlikely that they are of any significance in the therapeutic doses used in man (BUCHER 1953).

16. Mutagenic Effects

a) Reactions with DNA

Using E. coli, ROSENKRANZ and CARR (1971) showed that INH reacts with the DNA of living cells, so that there is a possibility of mutagenicity. However, in rabbit spermatocytes and spermatides BÜRGIN et al. (1979) failed to find any unscheduled DNA synthesis after i.v. injection of even high doses of INH, and in spermatogonia there was no effect on DNA synthesis. This suggests that the substance is not mutagenic. WADE et al. (1980) also failed to observe in human fibroblasts any inhibition of DNA synthesis as a result of DNA damage. On the other hand, they did find inhibition due to a metabolic block.

b) Gene Mutations in Bacteria

Various results were obtained in the Salmonella test using different test strains. In some cases only weak mutagenic effects were found (RÖHRBORN et al. 1972; HERBOLD and BUSELMAIER 1976; WADE et al. 1980; TOSK et al. 1979). Other investigators reported that INH is non-mutagenic in the absence of activation by liver microsomes (MILLER and STOLTZ 1978; NODA et al. 1978; RÖHRBORN et al. 1972; BRAUN et al. 1976). NELSON et al. (1976) and ASHBY and PURCHASE (1977) consider the Salmonella test to be unsuitable for testing hydrazines. Some investigators have attributed the mutagenicity to contamination of the INH with hydrazine. In all, INH is at worst an extremely weak mutagen in the Salmonella plate test (JANSEN et al. 1980). A detailed review has been given by WADE et al. (1980).

Host-Mediated Assay: An increased incidence of mutations was found in Salmonella typhimurium G 46 incubated in the abdominal cavity of INH-treated mice (RÖHRBORN et al. 1972). Hydrazine, which is regarded as a mutagenic metabolite, provoked a substantially higher mutation rate in the same test. On the basis of comparative studies BRAUN et al. (1976) also came to the conclusion that hydrazine, as a metabolite of INH, is the mutagenic agent in mice.

c) Gene Mutations in Mammalian Cells

BEYER et al. (1979) induced mutagenic effects in the somatic cells by treating pregnant mice with embryos heterozygotic for various locations that determine fur color.

It is extremely difficult to evaluate the mutagenic potential of INH on the basis of the published literature (BÜRGIN et al. 1979). JANSEN et al. (1980) largely rule out the possibility of significant clastogenic effects on peripheral lymphocytes in patients and laboratory animals. The situation is more complicated with regard to the induction of gene mutations. In the Salmonella test INH is evidently weakly mutagenic, though a substantial proportion of the mutagenicity can probably be attributed to metabolites. Gene mutations have, however, been observed not only in bacteria but also in mice, so that the possibility of inducing gene mutations in mammals cannot be entirely ruled out (JANSEN et al. 1980).

d) Cytogenetic Investigations

The early and in some cases contradictory findings on the influence of INH on cytogenesis have been reviewed by BRAUN et al. (1976) and by KIMBALL (1977). To clarify these contradictory results RÖHRBORN et al. (1978) carried out extensive studies in 13 laboratories, the results of which can be summarized as follows: although the majority of the short- and long-term studies using the micronucleus test on golden hamsters and on rats were negative, the possibility of a weak mutagenic effect on bone-marrow cells could not be ruled out entirely. No chromosomal aberrations were found in the bonemarrow cells of golden hamsters or rats or in the spermatogonia or primary spermatocytes of the golden hamster and the mouse. Similarly, no chromosomal damage was found in the lymphocytes of patients who had been treated prophylactically or therapeutically with INH.

e) Dominant Lethal Test

Various investigations based on the dominant lethal test in mice failed to reveal mutagenicity (RÖHRBORN et al. 1972, 1978).

17. Lathyrogenic Activity

In chick embryos INH exerts a lathyrogenic activity after being applied to the chorioallantoic membrane (LEVENE 1961; SAID and AHMED 1967). Pyridoxal was largely able to eliminate this effect, but vitamin K did not.

References

Allmark MG, Lu FC, Carmichael E, Lavallee A (1953) Some pharmacological observations on isoniazid and iproniazid. Am Rev Tuberc 68:199–206
Ashby J, Purchase IFH (1977) The selection of appropriate chemical class controls for use with short term tests for potential carcinogenicity. Ann Occup Hyg 20:297–301
Ata S, Tanaka K (1952) Vitamin B_{12} and isoniazid. Lancet II:589
Balzer H, Holtz P, Palm D (1960) Untersuchungen über die biochemischen Grundlagen der konvulsiven Wirkung von Hydraziden. Naunyn Schmiedebergs Arch Pharmacol 239:520–552
Barreto RCR, Mano DB (1961) Prevention of the convulsant and lethal effects of isonicotinic acid hydrazide by pyruvic acid. Biochem Pharmacol 8:409–412
Benson WM, Stefko PL, Roe MD (1952) Pharmacologic and toxicologic observations on hydrazine derivatives of isonicotinic acid (Rimifon, Marsilid). Am Rev Tuberc 65:376–391
Berencsi G, Entz A, Vajkóczy A (1957) Kongreß der Ungarischen Phthisiolog Gesellsch, Szeged 1952, cited from Juhász J, Baló J, Kendrey G. Z Krebsforsch 62:188–196
Beyer E, Braun R, Schöneich J (1979) Genetic activity of isoniazid in the mammalian spot test. Mutat Res 64:152
Bhide SV, Maru GB, Sawai MM, Ranadive KJ (1978) Isoniazid tumorigenicity in mice under different experimental conditions. Int J Cancer 21:381–386
Biancifiori C, Ribacchi R (1962) Pulmonary tumors in mice induced by oral isoniazid and its metabolites. Nature 194:488–489
Biancifiori C, Severi L (1966) The relation of isoniazid (INH) and allied compounds to carcinogenesis in some species of small laboratory animals. A review. Br J Cancer 20:528–538
Black SLD (1977) Hepatic triglyceride metabolism and aminoacid pools in isonicotinic acid hydrazide treated rats. Dissertation Abstr Intern B 38:1668–1669
Blakemore WF, Palmer AC, Noel PRB (1972) Ultrastructural changes in isoniazid-induced brain oedema in the dog. J Neurocytol 1:263–278
Botta JA Jr, Carlton WW (1967a) Studies of the toxicity of isonicotinic acid hydrazide (Isoniazid) to ducklings. Toxicol Appl Pharmacol 11:35–48
Botta JA Jr, Carlton WW (1967b) Isoniazid toxicosis in ducklings-studies on pyridoxine, niacin, glutamic acid, and arginine supplementation. Avian Dis 11:621–633
Brambilla G, Baldini L (1959) Azione inibitrice dell'acido isonicotinico sullo sviluppo del sarcoma Galliera del ratto. Boll Soc Ital Biol Sper 35:1169–1171
Braun R, Schubert J, Schöneich J (1976) On the mutagenicity of isoniazid. Biol Zbl 95:423–436
Bucher O (1953) Zur Frage der cytotoxischen Wirkung von Rimifon. Schweiz Med Wochenschr 83:1206–1208
Bürgin H, Schmid B, Zbinden G (1979) Assessment of DNA damage in germ cells of male rabbits treated with isoniazid and procarbazine. Toxicology 12:251–257
Carlton WW (1967) Neural toxicity of isonicotinic acid hydrazide (isoniazid) for chickens. Avian Dis 11:241–254

Carlton WW, Hunt CE, Newberne PM (1965) Neural lesions induced by isonicotinic acid hydrazide and semicarbazide hydrochloride. Exp Mol Pathol 4:438–448
Carlton WW, Kreutzberg G (1966) Isonicotinic acid hydrazide-induced spongy degeneration of the white matter in the brains of peking ducks. Am J Pathol 48:91–105
Casey RE, Wood JD (1973) Isonicotinic acid hydrazide-induced changes in the metabolism of γ-aminobutyric acid in the brain of four species. Comp Biochem Physiol B 45:741–748
Cavanagh JB (1967) On the pattern of change in peripheral nerves produced by isoniazid intoxication in rats. J Neurol Neurosurg Psychiat 30:26–33
Cavanagh JB (1973) Peripheral neuropathy caused by chemical agents. CRC Crit Rev Toxicol 2:365–417
Cedrangolo F, Gioia A, Bagnulo R (1953) Un meccanismo enzimatico, per il quale si puo'abbassare in vivo la tossicità dell' idrazide dell'ac. isonicotinico. Enzymologia 16:41–50
Ceriotti G, Franceschini J (1953) Dati biologici e microbiologici su un nuvo derivato della idrazide dell'acido isonicotinico a bassa tossicatà e ad alta attività (metansulfonato dell' idrazide isonicotinica). Arch Int Pharmacodyn Ther 93:105–117
Chin L, Sievers ML, Laird HE, Herrier RN, Picchioni AL (1978) Evaluation of diazepam and pyridoxine as antidotes to isoniazid intoxication in rats and dogs. Toxicol Appl Pharmacol 45:713–722
Chin L, Sievers M, Herrier RN, Picchioni AL (1979) Convulsions as the etiology of lactic acidosis in acute isoniazide toxicity in dogs. Toxicol Appl Pharmacol 49:377–384
Cirnu-Georgian L, Lenghel V (1971) Isoniazid-induced chromosome aberrations. Lancet 2:93
Crema A, Fabris L (1954) Sulla tossicatà per il vestibolo dell'idrazide dell' acido isonicotinico. Boll Soc Ital Biol Sper 30:120–121
Dauphinee KR, Paynters S, Russell DW (1975) Failure of pyruvate to counteract isonazid toxicity in rabbits. J Pharm Pharmacol 27:884–886
Dienemann G, Simon K (1953) Mitteilung eines Todesfalles nach kombinierter Verabreichung von Irgapyrin und Neoteben (INH). MMW 95:221–222
Dixon RH, Williams HL (1962) The toxicity of pyridoxal and pyridoxal phosphate hydrazones in mice. Fed Proc 21:338
Dubnick B, Leeson GA, Scott CC (1960) Effect of forms of vitamin B_6 on acute toxicity of hydrazines. Toxicol Appl Pharmacol 2:403–409
Emmrich R, Petzold H (1952) Tierexperimentelle Untersuchungen zur Frage einer Leberschädigung durch Rimifon (Isonicotinylhydrazin). Klin Wochenschr 30:1081–1083
Engbaek HC, Bentzon H, Heegård H, Christensen O (1965) Har isoniazid en tumorfremkaldende virkning? Nord Med 74:1326
Földi M, Zoltán ÖT, Maurer M (1970) Die Wirkung von Isonicotinsäurehydrazid (INH) auf das Zentralnervensystem und der Antagonismus zwischen dieser Substanz und Pyridoxin, Pantothensäure sowie Cumarin aus Melilotus officinalis bei Ratten. Arzneimittelforsch 20:1620–1623
Frei H-H (1976) Elevation of central γ-aminobutyric acid levels by isoniazid in mice and convulsant thresholds. Biochem Pharmacol 25:1216–1219
Fust B, Studer A, Böhni E (1952) Experimentelle Erfahrungen mit dem Antituberculotikum „Rimifon". Schweiz Z Tuberk 9:226–242
Glass F, Gossow H, Mallach HJ (1964) Beobachtungen und Untersuchungen über die gemeinsame Wirkung von Alkohol und Isonicotinsäurehydrazid. Arzneimittelforsch 14:1203–1208
Glass F, Mallach HJ (1965) Tierexperimentelle Untersuchungen über die Alkoholwirkung nach längerer Belastung mit Isonicotinsäurehydrazid. Arzneimittelforsch 15:1069–1070
Goldin A, Dennis D, Venditti JM, Humphreys SR (1955) Potentiation of pentobarbital anesthesia by isonicotinic acid hydrazide and related compounds. Science 121:364–365
Grasso P, Crampton RF (1972) The value of the mouse in carcinogenicity testing. Fd Cosmet Toxicol 10:418–426
Gross W (1956) Ein Beitrag zur cytostatischen Wirkung des Isonicotinsäurehydrazids (INH). Klin Wochenschr 34:495

Hackmann CH (1957) Unpublished data
Hammond EC, Selikoff IJ, Robitzek EK (1967) Isoniazid therapy in relation to later occurence of cancer in adults and infants. Br Med J 2:792–795
Harper KH, Worden AN (1966) Comparative toxicity of isonicotinic acid hydrazide and its methanosulfonate derivative. Toxicol Appl Pharmacol 8:325–333
Hecht G (1953) Unpublished data
Hellriegel W, Kraus R (1955) Über die zytostatische Wirkung des Isonikotinsäurehydrazins. Tuberk Arzt 9:653–660
Herbold B, Buselmaier W (1976) Induction of point mutations by different chemical mechanisms in the liver microsomal assay. Mutat Res 40:73–84
Hess M (1954) Über den Einfluß von Isonicotinsäurehydrazid (Neoteben) auf die Genitalfunktion und die Gestation. Arch Gynäkol 185:315–324
Holtz P, Palm D (1964) Pharmacological aspects of Vitamin B_6. Pharmacol Rev 16:113–178
IARC (1974) Monographs on the evaluation of carcinogenic risk of chemicals to man, vol 4. International Agency for Research on Cancer, Lyon
Jansen JD, Clemmesen J, Sundaram K (1980) Isoniazid – an attempt at retrospective prediction. Mutat Res 76:85–112
Jones LD, Fairchild DG, Morse WC (1971) The induction of pulmonary neoplasms in mice by isonicotinic acid hydrazide. Am Rev Respir Dis 103:612–617
Juhász J, Baló J, Kendrey G (1957) Über die geschwulsterzeugende Wirkung des Isonicotinsäurehydrazid (INH). Z Krebsforsch 62:188–196
Juhász J, Baló J, Szende B (1963) Neue experimentelle Angaben zur geschwulsterzeugenden Wirkung des Isonicotinsäurehydrazid (INH). Z Krebsforsch 65:434–438
Kelly MG, O'Gara RW, Yancey ST, Gadekar K, Botkin C, Oliviero VT (1969) Comparative carcinogenicity of N-isopropyl-α-(2-methylhydrazino)-p-toluamide HCl (procarbazine hydrochloride), its degradation products, other hydrazines, and isonicotinic acid hydrazide. J Natl Cancer Inst 42:337–344
Kimball RF (1977) The mutagenicity of hydrazine and some of its derivatives. Mutation Res 39:111–126
Klinghardt GW (1954) Experimentelle Nervenfaserschädigung durch Isonicotinsäurehydrazid und ihre Bedeutung für die Klinik. Verh Dtsch Ges Inn Med 60:764–768 (Kongress München)
Krnjevic K (1971) Synaptic transmission in the brain. Klin Wochenschr 49:519–523
Lechat P, Deleau D, Devillechabrolle A (1963) Etude expérimentale du pouvoir protecteur de la pyridoxine vis-à-vis des effets toxique de l'isoniazide. Thérapie 18:63–67
Leopold D, Röthig W, Wehran H-J, Wolf P (1966) Verteilung und Wirkung des Isoniazid nach Applikation therapeutischer und toxischer Dosen im Tierversuch. Arch Toxicol 22:80–91
Levene CJ (1961) The lathyrogenic effect of isonicotinic acid hydrazide (INAH) on the chick embryo and its reversal by pyridoxal. J Exp Med 113:795–811
Loscalzo B (1964) Hydrazide de l'acide isonicotinique et neoplasies. Arch Int Pharmacodyn Ther 152:249–251
Lüers H, Obe G (1971) Action of isoniazid on human chromosomes in vitro. EMS Newsletter:36
Manthei RW (1957) Effect of calcium pantothenate on isoniazid toxicity in the guinea pig. Proc Soc Exp Biol Med 95:402–404
Manthei RW (1960) Vitamin B_6 and isoniazid toxicity. Fed Proc 19:414
Matsumoto K, Mori K, Yasuno A (1960) Effect of isonicotinic acid hydrazide on hepatocarcinogenesis. Gann 51:91–95
McCormick DB, Snell EE (1961) Pyridoxal phosphokinases. J Biol Chem 236:2085–2088
Miller CT, Stoltz DR (1978) Mutagenicity induced by lyophilization or storage of urine from isoniazid-treated rats. Mutat Res 56:289–293
Mori K, Yasuno A (1959) Preliminary note on the induction of pulmonary tumors in mice by isonicotinic acid hydrazide feeding. Gann 50:107–110
Mori K, Yasuno A, Matsumoto K (1960) Induction of pulmonary tumors in mice with isonicotinic acid hydrazide. Gann 51:83–89

Nelson SD, Snodgrass WR, Mitchell JR (1976) Chemical reaction mechanisms responsible for the tissue injury caused by monosubstituted hydrazines and their hydrazide drug precursors. In: De Serres, Fouts, Bend and Philpot (eds) In vitro metabolic activation in mutagenesis testing. Elsevier, Amsterdam, pp 257–276
Noda A, Goromaru T, Matsuyama K, Sogabe K, Hsu KY, Iguchi S (1978) Quantitative determination of hydrazines derived from isoniazid in patients. J Pharmacol Dyn 1:132–141
Noel PRB, Worden AN, Palmer AC (1967) Neuropathologic effects and comparative toxicity for dogs of isonicotinic acid hydrazide and its methanosulfonate derivative. Toxicol Appl Pharmacol 10:183–198
Orlowski EH, Rosenfeld M, Wolter H, Schunk R (1976) Experimentelle vergleichende Untersuchung der tuberkulostatischen Wirksamkeit und Toxizität von INH, INHG und INHG-Na. Arzneimittelforsch 26:409–416
Palmer AC, Noel PRB (1965) Neuropathological effects of dosing dogs with isonicotinic hydrazide and with its methanosulphonate derivative. Nature 205:506–507
P'an SY, Markaroglu L, Reilly J (1952) The effects of barbiturates on the toxicity of isoniazid (isonicotinic acid hydrazide). Am Rev Tuberc 66:100–103
Pansa E, Bikfalvi A (1960) Über die Wirkung hoher Dosen Isonikotinsäure-Hydrazid (INH) auf die Bronchusschleimhaut der Kaninchen. Thoraxchirurgie 8:451–457
Pansa E, Picco A, Gnavi M (1962) Sul problema del supposto effecto carcinogenetico dell'idrazide dell'acido isonicotinico (IAI). Richerchi sperimentali sul ratto. Minerva Med 53:3162–3168
Peacock A, Peacock PR (1966) The results of prolonged administration of isoniazid to mice, rats and hamsters. Br J Canc 20:307–325
Prescott B, Kauffmann G, James WD (1954) A means of increasing the tolerated dose of isoniazid in mice. Proc Soc Exp Biol Med 86:682–685
Prescott B, Kauffmann G, James WD (1957a) Increase in tolerated dose of isoniazid in mice by use of cycloserine. Proc Soc Exp Biol Med 94:94–96
Prescott B, Kauffmann G, James WD (1957b) Effect of glycerine on toxicity of isoniazid in mice. Proc Soc Exp Biol Med 94:272–276
Prescott B, Kauffmann G, James WD (1957c) Means of increasing the tolerated dose of isoniazid in mice. II. Certain amino acids. Proc Soc Exp Biol Med 95:687–690
Prescott B, Kauffmann G, James WD (1957d) Means of increasing the tolerated dose of isoniazid in mice. III. Certain vitamins. Proc Soc Exp Biol Med 95:705–708
Prescott B, Stone HJ (1969) Glycerol formol as a solvent for detoxification of isoniazid. Chemotherapy 14:227–231
Quadbeck G, Sartori GD (1957) Über den Einfluß von Pyridoxin und Pyridoxal-5-Phosphat auf den Thiosemicarbazid-Krampf der Ratte. Naunyn Schmiedebergs Arch Pharmacol 230:457–461
Raisfeld IH (1975) Drug-induced liver disease: guinea pig model for isoniazid (INH) hepatitis – the predictive value of urinary d-glucaric acid excretion. Gastroenterology 69:A54/854
Reilly RH, Killam KF, Jenney EH, Marshall WH, Tausig T, Apter NS, Pfeiffer CC (1953) Convulsant effect of isoniazid. JAMA 152:1317–1321
Reinhardt JF, Kimura ET, Schachter RJ (1952) Some pharmacologic characteristics of isonicotinyl hydrazide (Pyricidin®), a new antituberculosis drug. Science 116:166–167
Roberts E (1974) γ-Aminobutyric acid and nervous system function – a perspective. Biochem Pharmacol 23:2637–2649
Röhrborn G, Propping P, Buselmaier W (1972) Mutagenic activity of isoniazid and hydrazine in mammalian test systems. Mutat Res 16:189–194
Röhrborn G et al. (1978) A correlated study of the cytogenetic effect of isoniazid (INH) on cell systems of mammals and man conducted by thirteen laboratories. Hum Genet 42:1–60
Rosen F (1955) Effect of isonicotinic acid hydrazide on niacin and pyridoxine metabolism in rats. Proc Soc Exp Biol Med 88:243–246
Rosenkranz HS, Carr HS (1971) Hydrazine antidepressants and isoniazid: potential carcinogens. Lancet I:1354–1355

Rubin B, Hassert GLJr, Thomas BGH, Burke JC (1952) Pharmacology of isonicotinic acid hydrazide (Nydrazid). Am Rev Tuberc 65:392–401
Rubin B, Burke JC (1952) Vitamin B_{12} and isoniazid. Lancet II:937
Rubin B, Burke JC (1953) Further observations on the pharmacology of isoniazid. Am Rev Tuberc 67:644–651
Said AH, Ahmed AAS (1967) Connective tissue changes induced in the chick embryo by isonicotinic acid hydrazide and vitamin K. Zbl Veterinarmed (A) 14:78–84
Schlaepfer WW, Hager H (1964a) Ultrastructural studies of INH-induced neuropathy in rats. I. Early axonal changes. Am J Pathol 45:209–219
Schlaepfer WW, Hager H (1964b) Ultrastructural studies of INH-induced neuropathy in rats. II. Alteration and decomposition of the myelin sheath. Am J Pathol 45:423–433
Schlaepfer WW, Hager H (1964c) Ultrastructural studies of INH-induced neuropathy in rats. III. Repair and Regeneration. Am J Pathol 45:679–689
Schmidt LH, Hoffmann R, Hughes HB (1953) The toxicity of isoniazid for the rhesus monkey. Am Rev Tuberc 67:798–807
Schöneich J (1976) Safety evaluation based on microbial assay procedures. Mutat Res 41:89–94
Schröder JM (1970a) Zur Pathogenese der Isoniazid-Neuropathie. I. Eine feinstrukturelle Differenzierung gegenüber der Wallerschen Degeneration. Acta Neuropath 16:301–323
Schröder JM (1970b) Zur Pathogenese der Isoniazid-Neuropathie. II. Phasenkontrast- und elektronenmikroskopische Untersuchungen am Rückenmark, an Spinalganglien und Muskelspindeln. Acta Neuropathol 16:324–341
Seifert S (1966) Die teratogene Wirkung von Isonikotinsäurehydrazid (INH) auf den Hühnerembryo. Diss Freiburg i Br
Severi L, Biancifiori C (1968) Hepatic carcinogenesis in CBA/Cb/Se mice and Cb/Se rats by isonicotinic acid hydrazide and hydrazine sulfate. J Natn Cancer Inst 41:331–340
Siegel D, Iwainsky H (1960) Über den Einfluß von Iso-Nicotinsäure-Hydrazid (INH) auf die Metastasierungsquote des Ehrlichschen Ascitescarcinom der Maus. Klin Wochenschr 38:769
Siegel D (1960) Beitrag zur Frage der cytostatischen Wirkung des Iso-Nicotinsäure-Hydrazids (INH). Naturwissenschaften 47:307–308
Siegel D (1961) Veränderungen des Nucleinsäuregehaltes tumorösen Gewebes durch Iso-Nikotinsäure-Hydrazid (INH). Naturwissenschaften 48:55–56
Siegel D, Berschneider F (1960) Untersuchungen zum Nucleinsäurestoffwechsel der regenerierenden Leber nach Isonicotinsäurehydrazid (INH). Z Gesamte Exp Med 134:59–64
Simon K (1952) Untersuchungen von Derivaten des Hydrazins auf ihre cytostatische Wirkung am Ascitestumor der Maus. Z Naturforsch 7b:531–536
Steinbrück P (1959) Der Einfluß über lange Zeit fortgeführter INH-Gaben auf die Fruchtbarkeit der weißen Maus. Z Tuberk 113:281–284
Tiboldi T, Dávid M, Kovács K, Molnár P (1955) Die Wirkung des Isonikotinsäurehydrazid auf das Brown-Pearce-Karzinom des Kaninchens. Z Tuberk 106:257–260
Timbrell JA, Mitchell JR, Snodgrass WR, Nelson SD (1980) Isoniazid hepatotoxicity: the relationship between covalent binding and metabolism in vivo. J Pharmacol Exp Ther 213:364–369
Tirunarayanan MO, Vischer WA (1956) Effect of vitamines on the acute toxicity of hydrazine derivatives. Experientia 12:291–292
Tosk J, Schmeltz I, Hoffmann D (1979) Hydrazines as mutagenes in a histidine – requiring auxotroph of Salmonella typhimurium. Mutat Res 66:247–252
Toth B, Shubik P (1966a) Inhibition of tumor development and carcinogenesis by isonicotinic acid hydrazide (INH) in C3H und AKR mice. Abstract, p 124. Presented at the IX International Cancer Congress, Tokyo
Toth B, Shubik P (1966b) Mammary tumor inhibition and lung adenoma induction by isonicotinic acid hydrazide. Science 152:1376–1377
Toth B, Shubik P (1966c) Carcinogenesis in swiss mice by isonicotinic acid hydrazide. Cancer Res 26:1473–1475

Toth B, Rustja A (1967) The effect of isonicotinic acid hydrazide on the development of tumors. Int J Cancer 2:413–420
Toth B, Shubik P (1969) Lack of carcinogenic effects of isonicotinic acid hydrazide in the syrian golden hamster. Tumori 55:127–135
Toth B, Boreisha J (1969) Tumorigenesis with isonicotinic acid hydrazide and urethan in the syrian golden hamsters. Eur J Cancer 5:165–171
Toth B, Toth T (1970) Investigation on the tumor producing effect of isonicotinic acid hydrazide in ASW/Sn mice and MCR rats. Tumori 56:315–324
Toth B, Shimizu H (1973) Lung carcinogenesis with 1-Acetyl-2-Isonicotinoylhydrazine, the major metabolite of isoniazid. Eur J Cancer 9:285–289
Viallier J, Casanova F (1960) L'isoniazide a-t-il des propriétés cancérigènes? Essai sur l'animal. CR Soc Biol 154:985–987
Wade DR, Lohman PHM, Mattern IE, Berends F (1980) The mutagenicity of isoniazid in Salmonella and its effects on DNA repair and synthesis in human fibroblasts. Mutat Res 89:9–20
Wagner H, Moritz R (1962) Beeinflussung des Tumorwachstums durch INH in Tierversuch und Gewebekultur. Arch Geschwulstforsch 19:123–129
Weinstein HJ, Kinosita R (1963) Isoniazid induction of pulmonary tumors in mice. Am Rev Respir Dis 88:124–125
Weiss P, Gáti T, Forrai G (1954) Die Wirkung von Isonikotinsäurehydrazid auf das Hypophysen-Nebennierenrindensystem bei weißen Ratten. Z Inn Med 9:808–809
Whitehouse LW, Tryphonas L, Thomas BH, Paul CP, Zeitz W (1978) Isoniazid toxicity alone and in combination with ethanol in the rabbit. I. Pathologic and biochemical factors. Toxicol Appl Pharmacol 45:351
Wiezorek WD, Kermes U, Wolf P (1977) Experimentelle Untersuchungen über die Wirkung von Barbituraten, Methaqualon und Benzodiazepinen bei der akuten Isoniazidintoxikation. Pharmazie 32:37–39
Williams HL, Wiegand RG (1960) Xanthurenic acid excretion and possible pyridoxine deficiency produced by isonicotinic acid hydrazide and other convulsant hydrazides. J Pharmacol Exp Ther 128:344–348
Williams HL, Bain JA (1961) Convulsive effects of hydrazides: relationship to pyridoxine. Int Rev Neurobiol 3:319–348
Wolf P, Ellert T, Gröger H (1965) Zur Frage der Beeinflußbarkeit der Isoniazid-Intoxikation durch einige Barbiturate, Chloralhydrat und Methylpentinol im Tierexperiment. Acta Biol Med German 15:184–186
Worden AN, Palmer AC, Noel PRB, Mawdesley-Thomas LE (1967) Lesions in the brain of the dog induced by prolonged administration of mono-amine oxidase inhibitors and isoniazid. Proc Eur Soc Study Drug Tox 8:149–161
Yamamoto RS, Weisburger JH (1970) Failure of arginine glutamate to inhibit lung tumour formation by isoniazid and hydrazine in mice. Life Sci 9(II):285–289
Zbinden G, Studer A (1955a) Zur Wirkung von Vitaminen der B-Gruppe auf die experimentelle Isoniazid-„Neuritis". Schweiz Z Path Bakt 18:1198–1211
Zbinden G, Studer A (1955b) Experimenteller Beitrag zur Frage der Isoniazid-Neuritis und ihrer Beeinflussung durch Pyridoxin. Z Tuberk 107:97–107
Zbinden G, Studer A (1955c) Vergleichende Untersuchungen über die Wirkung von Pyridoxin, Pyridoxal-5'-phosphat und Pyridoxal-isonicotinylhydrazon auf die experimentelle Isoniazid-„Neuritis" der Ratte. Int Z Vitaminforsch 26:130–137
Zbinden G, Studer A (1956) Wirkung der Glutaminsäure auf die experimentelle Isoniazid-Schädigung peripherer Nerven bei Ratten. Experientia 12:442–443
Zeller EA, Barsky J, Fouts JR, Kirchheimer WF, Van Orden LS (1952) Influence of isonicotinic acid hydrazide (INH) and 1-isonicotinyl-2-isopropyl hydrazide (IIH) on bacterial and mammalian enzymes. Experientia 8:349–350

VI. Tetracyclines: Tetracycline, Oxytetracycline (TC, OTC)

1. Respiration, Circulation, Heart

The i.v. injection of TC or OTC in doses of up to 100 mg/kg had no effect on respiration, blood pressure, heart rate, or the circulatory responses to adrenaline, histamine, acetylcholine, or vagal stimulation in anaesthetized dogs (CUNNINGHAM et al. 1953; P'AN et al. 1950).

In contrast, TUBARO et al. (1964) observed a considerable blood-pressure reduction in experiments on anaesthetized cats and dogs treated with 25 mg/kg.

SWAIN et al. (1956) observed negative inotropic effects of chlortetracycline, oxytetracycline, and tetracycline on isolated canine hearts (given in order of descending intensity). This is attributed to complex formation with calcium, since the inotropy can be eliminated by substitution with Ca^{2+} ions. LEADERS et al. (1960) carried out comparative studies with tetracycline, oleandomycin, dihydrostreptomycin, and chloramphenicol on anaesthetized rabbits and found a hypotensive effect and a reduction of the heart rate (substances given in order of descending effectiveness). In the isolated rabbit heart doses of 250 µg TC caused a reduction in contractility, while doses of up to 125 µg had a positive inotropic effect.

COHEN et al. (1970) obtained similar findings in the open-chest dog and in isolated cat hearts; here again high doses of TC caused a reduction of the contractile force of the heart.

2. Neuromuscular Blocking Effect of Tetracyclines

In higher doses tetracyclines inhibit neuromuscular transmission (BEZZI and GESSA 1961; KUBIKOWSKI and SZRENIAWSKI 1963). The effects are curare-like and the effect of d-tubocurarine is intensified by these antibiotics. Overall, neuromuscular blocking by the tetracyclines is stronger than that by streptomycin or by kanamycin.

Calcium ions, though not cholinesterase inhibitors like e.g., prostigmin, act antagonistically, indicating that the mode of action differs from the neuromuscular blockade caused by aminoglycoside antibiotics (see p. 312) (BEZZI and GESSA 1961; PITTINGER and ADAMSON 1972). It is likely that the ability of tetracyclines to form calcium chelates (KELLY and BUYSKE 1960) plays an important part in the inhibition of neuromuscular transmission (PITTINGER and ADAMSON 1972).

3. Smooth Muscles

Acccording to CUNNINGHAM et al. (1953) and P'AN et al. (1950), TC and OTC do not act spasmolytically on isolated rabbit intestine. However, LEADERS et al. (1960) found that in concentrations of 1×10^{-3} to 9.6×10^{-6} TC is able to prevent the acetylcholine- and histamine-induced contractions of isolated rabbit ileum to about the same extent as streptomycin, dihydrostreptomycin, and chloramphenicol.

A number of the pharmacological effects of the tetracyclines can thus be attributed to their calcium-binding abilities.

4. Acute Toxicity

Studies on the acute toxicity of tetracyclines were carried out on mice and on rats. Following intravenous injection the LD_{50} in mice is between 145 mg/kg and 200 mg/kg and that in rats between 129 mg/kg and 220 mg/kg. After oral administration the LD_{50} in mice is between 2130 mg/kg and >5900 mg/kg, while in rats it is >3000 mg/kg. The i.p. LD_{50} is similar to the i.v. LD_{50} (CUNNINGHAM et al. 1953; ENGLISH et al. 1953; BACHARACH et al. 1959; KUCK and REDIN 1960; TUBARO et al. 1964). Evidently there are no essential differences in sensitivity between mice and rats.

GIOVANNINI (1962) gives a comparative list of LD_{50} values for the various tetracyclines.

Acute toxicity of tetracyclines in mg/kg (after GIOVANNINI, 1962)

	LD_{50} in albino mice				LD_{50} in rats		
	i.v.	s.c.	i.p	Oral	i.v.	i.p.	Oral
Chlortetracycline	134	3500			118		
Oxytetracycline	178	650–892		6696–7200	260		
Tetracycline	162–170		190–330	2130–3000	129–220	320	3000

In earlier toxicological investigations of TC the cause of death following high doses had not been clarified. GREENBERGER et al. (1967) discovered severe metabolic acidosis in rats within 4 h–8 h of i.p. injection of 400 mg/kg. In addition, severe hyperkalaemia and azotaemia developed. The metabolic acidosis or cardiac arrhythmias due to the hyperkalaemia were considered as possible causes of death. MAFFII et al. (1957) pointed out that the toxicity of tetracyclines in mice, rats, and guinea pigs is strongly influenced by the type of the solvent used. Tetracycline solutions in physiological saline are substantially less toxic than solutions in distilled water. Similar findings were made by SURGEN and NIELSEN (1960) using TC, OTC, and chlortetracycline. The influence of the pH of the solution and the vehicle used on toxicity was also investigated by WIVAGG et al. (1976).

Following intramuscular or subcutaneous injection TC acts as a local irritant and causes considerable tissue irritation, to the point of extensive necroses (HANSON 1961).

5. Subacute Toxicity

Male mice tolerated daily treatment with 100 mg/kg p.o. for 6 weeks without any signs of toxic damage. However, they did put on more weight than the control animals (CUNNINGHAM et al. 1953).

Rats treated with 100 mg/kg, 200 mg/kg, and 400 mg/kg p.o. also failed to exhibit any particular symptoms after 4 weeks of treatment, apart from an increased weight gain (ENGLISH et al. 1953).

8 dogs tolerated quite well 17 and 32 i.v. injections of 10 mg/kg–30 mg/kg. Liver and kidney function tests and measurements of the blood sugar, urea, blood

coagulation, and haematological parameters did not reveal any toxic effects. Autopsies and histopathological investigations also failed to bring to light any unusual features (CUNNINGHAM et al. 1953). Dogs tolerated 13 weeks of twice daily oral treatment with 10 or 100 mg TC/kg without displaying any toxic symptoms (CUNNINGHAM et al. 1953).

According to MIKAELYAN and ULYANOV (1971), oral treatment of rabbits with 10 mg/kg, 40 mg/kg, or 100 mg TC/kg for 20 days caused a reduction of platelets in the blood and a reduction of megakaryocytes in the bone marrow. In addition, haemorrhages and oedemas developed as a result of increased capillary permeability (MIKAELYAN et al. 1973). However, blood coagulation was uninfluenced in rabbits after 7 days of treatment with 100 mg TC/kg (ZOLOTUKHIN 1958).

Oxytetracycline was tolerated by rats in doses of up to 200 mg/kg s.c. given for 2 weeks (SCHOENBACH et al. 1950). Dogs tolerated a dose of 250 mg/OTC/kg administered for 99 days without any pathological symptoms (NELSON and RADOMSKI 1954).

6. Liver Toxicity

Although no liver toxicity was found in the earlier subacute toxicity studies on TC, cases of fatty degeneration of the liver in man after high-dose tetracycline therapy attracted attention to this side effect. Indications that the risk of intensified fatty infiltration of the liver might be particularly high in pregnant women were investigated by LEWIS and SCHENKER (1966) and by LEWIS et al. (1967). Pregnant and non-pregnant rats were given i.v. infusions of 100 mg of TC/kg on 3 successive days. There was an increase in the total-lipid and triglyceride levels in the livers of the treated rats compared with the controls. However, there was no significant difference between the pregnant and the non-pregnant rats. The ATP content of the livers was the same in all groups. Thus, at least in rats, pregnancy does not constitute a predisposing factor for the lipogenetic effect of TC (LEWIS et al. 1967). MILLER et al. (1967) and GRAY et al. (1974) also found no difference in the extent of the fatty degeneration after tetracycline therapy in pregnant and non-pregnant rats.

The increased triglyceride levels in the livers of rats treated with tetracyclines is probably due to impairment of the hepatic triglyceride secretion due to reduced synthesis of the acceptor proteins (apoprotein, very low density lipoprotein) which remove the triglycerides from the liver. As a result, fat accumulates in the hepatocytes (HANSEN et al. 1968; SCHENKER et al. 1968; BREEN et al. 1972a, b). However, the reduced secretion of triglycerides from the hepatocytes is only responsible for 30%–50% of the lipid accumulation, so that other mechanisms must also be involved (BREEN et al. 1975).

MUKHERJEE and MUKHERJEE (1969) used rats to show that in addition to the impaired release of triglycerides from the liver, there is a stimulation of triglyceride synthesis in the liver after just one injection of TC in a therapeutic dose (35 mg/kg i.m.). The phospholipids are only slightly reduced by the treatment, while the free and esterified cholesterol content of the liver remains unchanged (MUKHERJEE et al. 1969). In addition, there is a significant increase of the free fatty acids in rat plasma, which is due to increased mobilization from adipose tissue and to a simultaneous decrease in the utilization by the body (MUKHERJEE et al. 1969).

In adrenalectomized rats treatment with TC does not produce either increased triglyceride synthesis in liver homogenates (MUKHERJEE and MUKHERJEE 1969) or an increase of the free fatty acids in the plasma (MUKHERJEE et al. 1969). MUKHERJEE et al. (1971) also showed that the synthesis of fatty acids and cholesterol is dose-dependently variably affected in rats. Low doses of TC stimulate and high doses inhibit the hepatic fatty acid synthesis. Injection of sublethal doses (250 mg/kg i.p.) revealed that the endoplasmic reticulum and the mitochondria were the principal target organelles (DAMJANOV and SOLTER 1971).

Comparatively speaking, the ultrastructural alterations correspond to those induced by other protein-synthesis inhibitors, such as orotic acid and ethionine (DAMJANOV and SOLTER 1971). Thus, STEINER et al. (1965) and MILLER et al. (1967) came to the conclusion that the striking vacuolation of the liver cells during the various stages is not a sign of fatty degeneration. STEINER et al. (1965) assumed instead that as a result of protein-synthesis inhibition osmotically active substances (amino acids, peptides) accumulate in the liver cells, and it is this that causes the vacuolation. In comparative studies with various tetracyclines OTC and DMTC were found to produce the least fatty degeneration of the liver (EGER and ILBAGIAN 1962).

7. Nephrotoxicity

At high serum and tissue concentrations tetracyclines exert antianabolic activity in man and in animals. Among other things, this leads to a prerenal elevation of the urea concentration in the blood plasma. In addition, high doses of these antibiotics are directly nephrotoxic. FARHAT et al. (1958) found that in rabbits given repeated i.p. injections of high doses of TC (250 mg/kg–300 mg/kg) the antibiotic accumulates in the serum. This accumulation correlates with the increased level of non-protein nitrogen. 20 μg/ml proved to be the minimum toxic serum concentration, while 80 μg/ml–320 μg/ml was lethal. The kidneys of the rabbits exhibited pronounced tubular degeneration and contained casts and cystine-like crystals. In rats and dogs doses of 25 mg TC/kg–50 mg TC/kg i.v. also caused an increase in the blood urea level (POLEC et al. 1971). Furthermore, higher doses caused increased creatinine levels, increased diuresis, and tubular necroses. Previous or simultaneous i.v. injection of ascorbic acid prevented the kidney damage in both species. In the dog mannitol also afforded protection. The protective effect of these substances is attributed to the osmotic diuresis and thus to the accelerated elimination of TC. According to CLAUSEN et al. (1975), in dogs TC causes an obstruction of the renal tubules distal to the Na-reabsorbing segments. The foetal kidney is evidently more sensitive to TC than the adult kidney. BARKALAYA (1964) observed fatty degeneration of the tubuli contorti in rat foetuses after administering 4 doses of 100 mg TC/kg p.o. to the dams; the mother's kidneys did not exhibit any corresponding alterations.

A reversible Fanconi-type syndrome was observed in man following oral administration of tetracycline capsules that had not been stored correctly. This resulted in BENITZ et al. (1964) investigating various degradation products of TC in rats and in dogs. It was found that anhydro-4-epitetracycline (AET) induced renal dysfunctions in the form of proteinuria, glucosuria, enzymuria, increased excretion of cells with the urine, and necroses of the convoluted tubuli. Intravenous injection of one-tenth of the oral, nephrotoxically-active dose of AET is sufficient to induce tubular necroses of comparable severity (LOWE and TAPP 1966). LINDQUIST and FELLERS (1966) observed corresponding alterations to the renal function in rats not only after AET but, to a smaller extent, also after TC.

8. Effects on the Intestinal Epithelium

Since gastrointestinal irritation is common in patients who have been treated with tetracyclines, HAHN et al. (1970) used the electron microscope to examine the intestinal epithelium of rats treated orally with 5 mg–500 mg of tetracycline/kg. After just 10 min–30 min the inner chondrioplasma appeared lighter and signs of cristolysis were observed in the affected mitochondria. However, the most noticeable change consisted of vacuole-like, membrane bound dilatations of the external chondrioplasma containing electron-dense material in the form of myelin bodies. After 4 h to 6 h the number of intact mitochondria was clearly reduced. The majority had degenerated to vacuoles containing myelin-like or fat-like substances. This stage is also apparent under a light microscope as vacuolation of the cytoplasm. The selective localization of TC in the mitochondria of various organs was detected by fluorescence measurements (DU BUY and SHOWACRE 1961).

9. Tetracyclines and Bone Metabolism

HELANDER and BÖTTIGER reported the storage of oxytetracycline in bones as early as 1953 by the detection of typical tetracycline fluorescence; initially, however, this phenomenon was ignored. TC accumulation in the bone and teeth of mice was rediscovered by ANDRÉ (1956), who was working with tritiated TC, and by RALL et al. (1957). The latter showed that tetracyclines can be detected in tumours and bone as a fluorescing complex. The problem of tetracycline accumulation in the bones has been studied from various standpoints, not least because tetracyclines were widely used in obstetrics and pediatrics. Thus, the question of a possible influence on foetal development and the possibility of teratogenicity was investigated.

MILCH et al. (1957, 1958) found that TC is detectable in soft tissues for about 24 h–48 h, but that it persists in regions of new bone proliferation for weeks or months, where it is recognizable by its golden-yellow fluorescence.

According to KÄMMERER and EGER (1965), like certain heavy metals, alizarin, and the radioisotopes of some elements, tetracyclines are stored in bone. Stable tetracycline accumulation essentially only occurs in the bone tissue fraction which, as so-called metabolic bone, is directly involved in the overall metabolism of the organism. For this reason the apposition zones of osteons, where the calcium complex is bound to acidic mucopolysaccharides, are the principal sites of tetracycline deposition (KÄMMERER and EGER 1965). The tetracyclines themselves form complexes known as chelates with metal ions (KELLY and BUYSKE 1960). However, in addition to the chelation with metal ions there must be another factor decisive for permanent deposition of tetracyclines in the tissues, since calcium complex formation on its own is evidently insufficient to anchor the TC firmly in the bone tissue. MILCH et al. (1961) believed that the D-ring of the tetracycline nucleus was bound by calcium to the phosphate oxygen of apatite, this last being a solid component of the collagen fibrils. The firm binding of the tetracycline molecules in bone is thus understandable. A similar idea was developed by IBSEN and URIST (1962).

However, TC is bound not only to apatite but also to other calcium complexes, e.g., calcium carbonate in fish scales (BEVELANDER and GOSS 1962), egg shells (HARCOURT et al. 1962), and the skeleton of Pinna, a species of marine mollusc (BEVELANDER 1963), and to calcifying cartilage and calluses (URIST and IBSEN 1963) and calcifying metastases of experimentally induced tumours (HAKKINEN 1958).

Accumulation of TC disrupts bone formation and mineralization. The effects are most clearly discernible in the teeth, and appear in children as discoloration and enamel hypoplasia; this can also be shown in animal experiments (BEVELANDER et al. 1961; OWEN 1961).

MCINTOSH and STOREY (1970) showed in comparative studies that the different tetracyclines cause varying degrees of dental alteration. TC is one of the drugs that causes the most serious damage to teeth.

The disruption of foetal bone growth and mineralization is dealt with in the section on teratogenicity.

10. Reproductive Toxicity

Preliminary investigations on the teratogenicity of TC were carried out by FILIPPI and MELA (1957). After oral treatment of pregnant rats with a dose of about 25 mg/kg cleft palate, hypoplasia of the mandibula, syndactyly, and shortening of the extremities were observed in the foetuses. Later studies by FILIPPI (1967) confirmed this result. About one-third of the foetuses of rats treated with about 25 mg/kg p.o. from the 5th to the 20th day of gestation showed these malformations. When B complex vitamins were added to the tetracyclines, no malformations were observed, so that these could be attributed to hypovitaminosis.

There is some criticism of Filippi's findings. HURLEY and TUCHMANN-DUPLESSIS (1963) refer to insufficient controls and to a lack of data on experimental details such as diet. In experiments on rats treated from the 1st to the 18th day of gestation and on rats treated with doses of 150 mg–200 mg/animal administered with the feed during the whole of gestation and for 28 days after birth, Hurley and Tuchmann-Duplessis did not observe any teratogenic effects. However it was shown that TC does cross the placental barrier, since tetracycline fluorescence was detected in the foetuses. In 5 young rats treated up to the 28th day, however, there was a significant shortening of the lower part of the hind legs in comparison with untreated controls. TUBARO et al. (1964) also failed to observe any malformations after treatment of pregnant rats and rabbits with 10 mg/kg i.v. According to MENNIE (1962), 5000 mg TC/kg administered with the feed did not cause any limb malformations in one generation of rats. MCCOLL et al. (1965) also did not observe any leg malformations in rats treated with 500 mg TC/kg. However, the incidence of hydroureters was increased.

STEINER et al. (1965) treated rats from the 14th day of gestation onwards with 85 mg TC/kg i.p. and found an increased incidence of abortions. The degree and the extent of the necrobiotic and degenerative alterations in the trophoblasts depended on the duration of the treatment. DETYUK et al. (1971) treated rats from the 7th to the 15th day of gestation with daily doses of 50 mg or 85 mg TC/kg i.m. The incidence of resorptions was dose-dependently increased in the treated animals, growth and development of the foetuses were inhibited. In some foetuses there were teratogenic effects (defects of the spinal column, the CNS, the eyes, and the respiratory and digestive apparatus) and cranial anomalies. OTC is said to be teratogenic in the dog (SAVINI et al. 1968). BEVELANDER and COHLAN (1962) and COHLAN et al. (1963) observed growth retardation in rat foetuses but no malformations after treatment of the dams with TC.

In chick embryos BEVELANDER et al. (1960) observed growth retardation, bending of the bones, and disruption of mineralization of the cartilage ground substance after injection of TC into the yolk sac on the 8th day of incubation. SMITH and CHAPMAN (1963) found that embryonic growth was retarded from 4 mg or 5 mg onwards after injecting increasing doses of tetracycline into 11-day-old incubated eggs. Up to this dose the bone formation appeared to be normal. However, higher doses gave rise to deformed embryos and to liver damage. Under UV light extensive skeletal deposits of the antibiotic were observed. Similar findings were made with OTC by VERRET and MUTCHLER (1964) and with OTC, chlortetracycline, and demethylchlortetracycline by HUGHES et al. (1965).

In-vitro studies by SAXÉN (1966) on embryonic mouse bone revealed inhibition of bone growth and of ^{45}Ca incorporation.

KOHONEN et al. (1968) also observed inhibition of calcification and retarded growth at the calcification zones in mouse foetuses after treatment of the dams with TC. The incorporation of ^{45}Ca in the tibia on the 16th, 17th, and 18th days of gestation was about 50% less than in the controls. In addition to the reduced deposition of ^{45}Ca, the incorporation of ^{14}C-hydroxyproline in foetal bone and skin was also reduced. Thus, the primary effect of TC may be an inhibition of collagen synthesis (HALME and AER 1968; HALME et al. 1969).

The foetal bone deformities and growth retardation reported by various authors after treatment of the dams with TC, although variable, can thus be interpreted as being due to a disruption of foetal bone growth and mineralization.

BROWN et al. (1968) believed that another mode of action was the cause of the embryotoxicity. They attributed the abortive and embryotoxic effects of some antibiotics, including TC, in the rabbit to changes in the intestinal flora which, by having a harmful effect on the mother, could give rise to secondary foetal damage. To support this theory young New Zealand albino rabbits were treated with increasing doses of the antibiotics up to a daily dose of 100 mg/kg; this treatment was maintained throughout pregnancy. Although some of the dams died before the dose of 100 mg/kg had been reached, no abortions or teratogenic effects were observed in the surviving animals.

11. Inhibition of Protein Synthesis

Tetracycline antibiotics inhibit protein synthesis in bacteria (HASH 1963) and in homogenates of bacteria and mammalian cells (RENDI and OCHOA 1961; FRANKLIN 1963); this inhibition occurs at the translation stage (RENDI and OCHOA 1961;

FRANKLIN 1964). SUAREZ and NATHANS (1965) showed that, in E. coli, TC prevents the specific binding of aminoacyl-tRNA to the mRNA-ribosome complex and thus inhibits protein synthesis.

In experiments on whole animals YEH and SHILS (1966) found that TC also impairs ^{14}C-leucine incorporation in various tissues in the rat. The incorporation of the substance into the proteins was more strongly inhibited in the gastrointestinal tract, the pancreas, and the skeletal muscles than in the liver and kidney. This inhibition occurred after both oral and parenteral administration and was unaffected by food intake, local trauma, or stress factors.

GREENBERGER (1967) also reported a reduced incorporation of ^{14}C-leucine into the protein of sections of the jejunum in rats previously treated with TC (400 mg/kg i.p.).

12. Ototoxicity

Local application of tetracycline into the bullae of guinea pigs proved to be strongly ototoxic. Parenteral administration, on the other hand, produced no harmful effects on the hearing, as tetracycline evidently does not pass through the blood-perilymph barrier (KÜPPER et al. 1970).

Chlortetracycline and oxytetracycline were less ototoxic than tetracycline itself when applied locally (PARKER et al. 1978).

13. Phototoxicity

Like other tetracycline derivatives, TC is phototoxic in man (SCHORR and MONASH 1963; CULLEN et al. 1966).

This effect was demonstrated on hairless mice previously treated with TC, using long-wave (300 nm–400 nm) UV light, natural sunlight, and sunlight filtered through glass (ISON and BLANK 1967). Natural sunlight was found to be most effective in this respect.

References

André T (1956) Studies on the distribution of tritium-labeled dihydrostreptomycin and tetracycline in the body. Acta Radiol Suppl 142:52–73

Bacharach AL, Clark BJ, McCulloch M, Tomich EG (1959) Comparative toxicity studies on ten antibiotics in current use. J Pharm Pharmacol 11:737–741

Barkalaya AJ (1964), Transplacental effect of antibiotics of tetracycline group on kidneys of fetuses of pregnant rats. Fed Proc 23:T 753–754

Benitz K-F, Diermeier HF (1964) Renal toxicity of tetracycline degradation products. Proc Soc Exp Biol 115:930–935

Bevelander G (1963) Effect of tetracycline on crystal growth. Nature 198:1103

Bevelander G, Nakahara H, Rolle GK (1960) The effect of tetracycline on the development of the skeletal system of the chick embryo. Dev Biol 2:298–312

Bevelander G, Rolle GK, Cohlan SQ (1961) The effect of the administration of tetracycline on the development of teeth. J Dent Res 40:1020–1024

Bevelander G, Cohlan SQ (1962) The effect on the rat fetus of transplacentally acquired tetracycline. Biol Neonat 4:365–370

Bevelander G, Goss RJ (1962) Influence of tetracycline on calcification in normal and regenerating teleost scales. Nature 193:1098–1099

Bezzi G, Gessa GL (1961) Influence of antibiotics on the neuromuscular transmission in mammals. Antibiot Chemotherap 11:710–714
Breen KJ, Schenker S, Heimberg M (1972a) Pathogenesis of tetracycline fatty liver. Clin Res 20:74
Breen K, Schenker S, Heimberg M (1972b) The effect of tetracycline on the hepatic secretion of triglyceride. Biochem Biophys Acta 270:74–80
Breen KJ, Schenker S, Heimberg M (1975) Fatty liver induced by tetracycline in the rat. Dose-response relationship and effect of sex. Gastroenterology 69:717–723
Brown DM, Harper KH, Palmer AK, Tesh SA (1968) Effects of antibiotics upon pregnancy in the rabbit. Toxicol Appl Pharmacol 12:295
Du Buy HG, Showacre JL (1961) Selective localization of tetracycline in mitochondria of living cells. Science 133:196–197
Clausen G, Nagy Z, Szalay L, Aukland K (1975) Mechanism in acute oliguric renal failure induced by tetracycline infusion. Scand J Clin Lab Invest 35:625–633
Cohen LS, Wechsler AS, Mitchell JH, Glick G (1970) Depression of cardiac function by streptomycin and other antimicrobial agents. Am J Cardiol 26:505–511
Cohlan SQ, Bevelander G, Tiamsic T (1963) Growth inhibition of prematures receiving tetracycline. Am J Dis Child 105:453–461
Cullen SJ, Catalano PM, Helfman RJ (1966) Tetracycline sun sensitivity. Arch Derm 93:77
Cunningham RW, Hines LR, Stokey EH, Vessey RE, Yuda NN (1953) Pharmacology of tetracycline. Antibiot Annu 1953–1954:63–69
Damjanov J, Solter D (1971) Ultrastructure of acute tetracycline induced liver change. Experientia 27:1204–1205
Detyuk ES, Vdovichenko IA, Kartysh GA (1971) Tetracycline effect on embryogenesis of albino rats. Antibiotiki (Moskau) 16:923–926
Eger W, Ilbagian K (1962) Untersuchungen über die Wirkung von Tetracyclinen auf die Leber. Arzneimittelforsch 12:285–289
English AR, P'an SY, McBride TJ, Gardocki JF, Van Halsema G, Wright WA (1953) Tetracycline-microbiologic, pharmacologic and clinical evaluation. Antibiot Annu 1953–1954:70–80
Farhat SM, Schelhart DL, Musselman MM (1958) Clinical toxicity of antibiotics correlated with animal studies. AMA Arch Surg 76:762–765
Fillippi B, Mela V (1957) Malformazioni congenite facciali e degli arti da tetraciclina. Minerva Chir 12:1–15
Fillippi B (1967) Antibiotics and congenital malformations: Evaluation of the teratogenicity of antibiotics. Adv Teratol 2:239–256
Franklin TJ (1963) The inhibition of incorporation of leucine into protein of cell-free systems from rat liver and Escherichia coli by chlortetracycline. Biochem J 87:449–453
Franklin TJ (1964) The effect of chlortetracycline on the transfer of leucine and "transfer" ribonucleic acid to rat-liver ribosomes in vitro. Biochem J 90:624–628
Giovannini M (1962) Toxizität (der Tetracycline). In: Brunner R, Machek G (eds) Die Antibiotika, Band I, Teil 2. Carl, Nürnberg, pp 506–510
Gray JE, Weaver RN, Skinner P, Mathews J, Day CE, Stern K (1974) Effects of tetracycline on ultrastructure and lipoprotein secretion in the rat hepatocyte. Toxicol Appl Pharmacol 30:317–322
Greenberger NJ, Perkins RL, Cuppage FE, Ruppert RD (1967) Severe metabolic acidosis in the rat induced by toxic doses of tetracycline. Proc Soc Exp Biol Med 125:1194–1197
Greenberger NJ (1967) Inhibition of protein synthesis in rat intestinal slices by tetracycline. Nature 214:702–703
Hahn KJ, Morgenstern E, von Puttkamer K, Weber E (1970) Schädigungen der Mitochondrien von Darmepithelzellen bei oraler Therapie mit Tetrazyklinen. Naunyn Schmiedebergs Arch Pharmacol 266:347
Hakkinen JPT (1958) The fluorescence of tetracycline in rats treated with dihydrotachysterol, AT 10. Acta Physiol Scand 42:282–287
Halme J, Aer J (1968) Inhibition of collagen synthesis and bone calcification in the foetal rat by tetracycline. Scand J Clin Lab Invest 21, Suppl 101:4

Halme J, Kivirikko KJ, Kaitila J, Saxen L (1969) Effect of tetracycline on collagen biosynthesis in cultured embryonic bones. Biochem Pharmacol 18:827–836
Hansen CH, Pearson LH, Schenker S, Combes B (1968) Impaired secretion of triglycerides by the liver; a cause of tetracycline-induced fatty liver. Proc Soc Exp Biol Med 128:143–146
Hanson DJ (1961) Local toxic effects of broad-spectrum antibiotics following injection. Antibiot Chemotherap 11:390–404
Harcourt JK, Johnson NW, Storey E (1962) Incorporation of tetracycline antibiotics in bone, teeth, and egg shells. J Dent Res 41:511
Hash JH (1963) Effects of tetracyclines on the incorporation of C^{14}-alanine into staphylococcus aureus. Fed Proc 22:301
Helander S, Böttiger L (1953) On the distribution of terramycin in different tissues. Acta Med Scand 147:71–75
Hughes WH, Lee WR, Flood DJ (1965) A comparative study of the actions of six tetracyclines on the development of the chick embryo. Br J Pharmacol 25:317–323
Hurley LS, Tuchmann-Duplessis H (1963) Influence de la tétracycline sur le développement pré-et post-natal du rat. CR Acad Sci 257:302–304
Ibsen KH, Urist MR (1963) Complexes of calcium and magnesium with oxytetracycline. Proc Soc Exp Biol Med 109:797–801
Ison A, Blank H (1967) Testing drug phototoxicity in mice. J Invest Dermatol 49:508–511
Kämmerer H, Eger W (1956) Tetracycline und Knochenstoffwechsel. Med Welt 1:986–991
Kelly RG, Buyske D (1960) Metabolism of tetracycline in the rat and the dog. J Pharmacol Exp Ther 130:144–149
Kohonen J, Guile EE, Plosila A (1968) Effects of tetracycline on osteogenesis in embryos of mice. Scand J Clin Lab Invest 21, Suppl 101:4
Kubikowski P, Szreniawski Z (1963) The mechanism of the neuromuscular blockade by antibiotics. Arch Int Pharmacodyn Ther 146:549–560
Kuck NA, Redin GS (1960) Comparison of demethylchlortetracycline with tetracycline in the control of experimental infections in mice. J Pharmacol Exp Ther 129:350–355
Küpper K, Stupp H, Orsulakova A, Quante M (1970) Vergleichende Untersuchungen der Ototoxizität verschiedener antibiotischer Substanzen bei lokaler Applikation am Innenohr des Meerschweinchens. Arch Otorhinolaryngol 196:169–172
Leaders F, Pittinger CB, Long JP (1960) Some pharmacological properties of selected antibiotics. Antibiot Chemotherap 10:503–507
Lewis M, Schenker S (1966) Studies on the pathogenesis of tetracycline-induced fatty liver. Clin Res 14:48
Lewis M, Schenker S, Combee B (1967) Studies on the pathogenesis of tetracycline-induced fatty liver. Am J Digest Dis 12:429–438
Lindquist RR, Fellers FX (1966) Degraded tetracycline nephropathy. Lab Invest 15:864–876
Lowe MB, Tapp E (1966) Renal damage caused by anhydro-4-epitetracycline. Arch Pathol 81:362–364
Maffii G, Semenza F, Soncin E (1957) Saline solutions as a factor affecting the toxicity of intravenously injected tetracyclines in mice. J Pharm Pharmacol 9:105–112
McColl JD, Globus M, Robinson S (1965) Effect of some therapeutic agents on the developing rat fetus. Toxicol Appl Pharmacol 7:409–417
McIntosh HA, Storey E (1970) Tetracycline-induced tooth changes, Part 4. Discoloration and hypoplasia induced by tetracycline analogues. Med J Aust 1:114–119
Mennie AT (1962) Tetracycline and congenital limb abnormalities. Br Med J II:480
Mikaelyan NP, Ulyanov MI (1971) On some shifts in thrombocytopoiesis systems in rabbits treated with tetracyclin. Antibiotiki 16:624–626
Mikaelyan NP, Eingorn AG, Ulyanov MI (1973) Morphological changes induced by tetracycline in rabbits. Antibiotiki 18:906–910
Milch RA, Rall DP, Tobie JE (1957) Bone localization of the tetracyclines. J Natl Cancer Inst 19:87–93

Milch RA, Rall DP, Tobie JE (1958) Fluorescence of tetracycline antibiotics in bone. J Bone Joint Surg 40 A:897–910
Milch RA, Tobie JE, Robinson J (1961) A microscopic study of tetracycline localization in skeletal neoplasms. J Histochem Cytochem 9:261–270
Miller SEP, MacSween RNM, Glen ACA, Tribedi K, Moore FML (1967) Experimental studies on the hepatic effects of tetracycline. Br J Exp Pathol 48:51–57
Mukherjee D, Mukherjee S (1969) Studies on the effect of tetracycline on triglyceride synthesis in experimental rats. J Antibiotics 22:45–48
Mukherjee D, Ghosh H, Mukherjee S (1969) Studies on the effect of administration of tetracycline on free fatty acid metabolism in adrenalectomised and control rats. J Antibiotics 22:480–483
Mukherjee D, Ghosh HN, Mukherjee S (1971) The effect of tetracycline on synthesis of fatty acid and cholesterol in the liver of control and experimental rats. J Antibiotics 24:263–265
Nelson AA, Radomski JL (1954) Comparative pathological study in dogs of feeding of six broadspectrum antibiotics. Antibiotics Chemother 4:1174
Owen LN (1961) Fluorescence of tetracyclines in bone tumors, normal bone teeth. Nature 190:500–502
P'an SY, Scaduto L, Cullen M (1950) Pharmacology of terramycin in experimental animals. Ann New York Acad Sci 53:238–244
Parker FL, James GWL (1978) The effect of various topical antibiotics and antibacterial agents on the middle and inner ear of the guinea-pig. J Pharm Pharmacol 30:236–239
Pittinger Ch, Adamson R (1972) Antibiotic blockade of neuromuscular function. Annu Rev Pharmacol 12:169–184
Polec RB, Yeh SDJ, Shils ME (1971) Protective effect of ascorbic acid, isoascorbic acid and mannitol against tetracycline-induced nephrotoxicity. J Pharmacol Exp Ther 178:152–158
Rall DP, Loo TL, Lane M, Kelly MG (1957) Appearance and persistence of fluorescent material in tumor tissue after tetracycline administration. J Natl Cancer Inst 19:79–85
Rendi R, Ochoa S (1961) Enzyme specificity in activation and transfer of amino acids to ribonucleoprotein particles. Science 133:1367
Savini EC, Moulin MA, Herrou MFJ (1968) Effets tératogènes de l'oxytetracycline. Thérapie 23:1247–1260
Saxén L (1966) Effect of tetracycline on osteogenesis in vitro. J Exp Zool 162:269–294
Schenker S, Hansen C, Combes B (1968) Impaired secretion of hepatic triglycerides – a cause of tetracycline-induced fatty liver. Gastroenterology 54:1268
Schoenbach EM, Bryer MS, Long PH (1950–1951) The pharmacology of terramycin in animals and man with reference to its clinical trial. Ann NY Acad Sci 53:245–252
Shauer BA, Lukacs L, Zimmerman HJ (1974) Biochemical indices of tetracycline hepatic injury in rats. Proc Soc Exp Biol Med 147:868–872
Schorr WF, Monash S (1963) Photo-irradiation studies of two tetracyclines. Arch Dermatol 88:440–444
Smith H, Chapman IV (1963) Use of the living chick embryo as a biological indicator of the effectiveness of chelating agents. Nature 198:32–33
Steiner G, Bradford W, Craig JM (1965) Tetracycline-induced abortion in the rat. Lab Invest 14:1456–1463
Suarez G, Nathans D (1965) Inhibition of aminoacyl-sRNA binding to ribosomes by tetracycline. Biochem Biophys Res Comm 18:743–750
Surgen RC, Nielsen JK (1960) Some factors influencing the toxicity (safety) test for antibiotics. Antibiot Chemotherap 10:169–173
Swain HH, Kiplinger GF, Brody TM (1956) Actions of certain antibiotics on the isolated dog heart. J Pharmacol Exp Ther 117:151–159
Tubaro E (1964) Possible relationship between tetracycline stability and effect on foetal skeleton. Br J Pharmacol 23:445–448
Tubaro E, Barletta M, Banci F (1964) Some pharmacological aspects of a new water-soluble tetracycline. J Pharm Pharmacol 16:33–37

Urist MR, Ibsen KH (1963) Chemical reactivity of mineralized tissue with oxytetracycline. Arch Pathol 76:484–496
Verret MJ, Mutchler MK (1964) Teratogenic effects of antibiotics in the chick embryo. Fed Proc 23:104
Wivagg RT, Jaffe JM, Colaizzi JL (1976) Influence of pH and route of injection on acute toxicity of tetracycline in mice. J Pharm Sci 65:916–918
Yeh SDJ, Shils ME (1966) Tetracycline and incorporation of amino acids into proteins of rat tissues. Proc Soc Exp Biol Med 121:729–734
Zolotukhin SI (1958) The effect of the tetracycline group of antibiotics on the coagulation of the blood. Antibiotics 4:324–327

VII. Viomycin (VM)

1. Respiration, Blood Pressure

Slow intravenous injection (10 mg/kg/min) of 100 mg VM sulphate/kg did not cause any noteworthy reduction in the blood pressure or any modification of the respiration in anaesthetized cats and dogs (P'AN et al. 1951).

2. Neuromuscular Blocking Effect

Like streptomycin, neomycin, kanamycin, and other basic antibiotics, VM causes a neuromuscular blockade (ADAMSON et al. 1960; VITAL BRAZIL et al. 1961; KUBIKOWSKI and SZRENIAWSKI 1963) which can be antagonized by calcium ions.

3. Ganglion Blocking Effect

VM induces a ganglionic blockade (VITAL BRAZIL et al. 1961).

4. Smooth Muscles

VM exerts a relaxing effect on isolated rat duodenum and guinea pig ileum (VITAL BRAZIL et al. 1961).

5. Acute Toxicity

The acute toxicity of VM is low. The i.v. and s.c. LD_{50} in mice are 241 mg/kg (207 mg/kg–276 mg/kg) and 1381 mg/kg (1278 mg/kg–1491 mg/kg) respectively. Mice tolerated oral doses of 7500 mg/kg (P'AN et al. 1951). The symptoms that followed i.v. injection were central excitation phenomena such as increased irritability, limb tremors, the Straub tail reaction, clonic convulsions, and finally atonic paralysis.

Death, which usually occurs within 5 to 10 min of administration, is caused by respiratory paralysis ultimately due to the neuromuscular blockade.

KELLER et al. (1956) studied the toxicity of VM pantothenate in parallel with attempts to reduce the toxicity of streptomycin by the administration of its pantothenate. Whereas the LD_{50} of VM sulphate following s.c. injection is 1375 mg/kg (1250 mg/kg–1510 mg/kg) in mice, the corresponding value for VM pantothenate was found to be 1750 mg/kg (1532 mg/kg–1995 mg/kg). Thus, there does not appear to be any major detoxifying effect.

6. Subacute Toxicity

Rats treated with 200 mg VM sulphate/kg administered subcutaneously 6 days a week for 6 weeks gained a little less weight than the control animals. Doses of 50 mg/kg and 100 mg/kg were well tolerated (P'AN et al. 1951).

KELLER et al. (1956) observed toxic symptoms in rats in the course of 7 days of treatment with 300 mg VM sulphate/kg i.p. These symptoms grew stronger from one injection to the next and resulted in states of collapse and polydipsia. There were serious alterations of the kidneys, in the form of tubule necroses, severe cast formation in the tubules, and some fatty degeneration and hydropic alterations of the tubuli recti and contorti. There was no discernible difference in the severity of the alterations in comparison with a group of animals treated simultaneously with VM pantothenate.

Dogs treated intramuscularly with 50 mg or 100 mg VM sulphate/kg for 150 days did not exhibit any haematological alterations or any disturbances of the liver and kidney function. No protein or sugar were found in the urine (P'AN et al. 1951).

Rabbits tolerated 40 days of treatment with 200 mg VM sulphate or pantothenate/kg without showing any symptoms. No liver or kidney damage could be established (KELLER et al. 1956).

7. Nephrotoxicity

Following early reports of nephrotoxic effects in patients after the administration of the high doses of VM that were usual at that time, MOYER and HANDLEY (1953) investigated the tolerability of VM in a special study on dogs using i.m. doses of 15 mg/kg–60 mg/kg. Viomycin did not appear to produce any evidence of renal toxicity as estimated by renal function tests.

Nevertheless, like KELLER et al. (1956), STAEMMLER and KARHOFF (1956) found evidence of nephrotoxicity of VM in rats after several days of intraperitoneal treatment with 300 mg/kg. The kidneys were enlarged, mostly pale glassy-yellow in color, and oedematous. Microscopic examination revealed extensive necroses in the medullary region, which bore some resemblance to the damage caused by mercuric chloride. However, they were distinguishable from the latter by a strong tendency towards hyaline-droplet accumulations in the epithelia of the tubules and glomeruli, by the strong fall of the alkaline phosphatase levels, and by certain differences between the clinical and the anatomical findings, since despite the severe kidney damage the general condition of the animals was usually not too poor. At the height of the VM intoxication, i.e., after 6 days of treatment with 300 mg/kg, renal function disturbances were discernible in the form of an elevation of non-protein nitrogen (STAEMMLER and KARHOFF 1956). There was no increase in the quantities of protein and sugar in the urine.

The necroses were very rapidly followed by an extensive two-phase regeneration of the tubular epithelium (STAEMMLER 1957). The first phase consisted of relining of the basal tubes that had remained intact with a single layer of smooth undifferentiated epithelium. In the second phase, which was complete by the 15th day–20th day, the newly produced epithelium matured into functional cells.

Electronmicroscopic studies reported by CAESAR (1965) indicate that the cell necrosis in VM nephrosis is preceded by rupture of lysosomal membranes, leading to an intracellular release of hydrolytic enzymes. GÖSSNER (1962) also regards the effects on the lysosomes as the decisive damage which ultimately triggers cell death.

8. Ototoxicity

Strangely enough, although VM is an ototoxic antibiotic, there are virtually no publications dealing with its vestibulotoxic and cochleotoxic effects in animals. After 25 days–32 days of daily treatment of cats with 100 mg VM sulphate/kg P'AN et al. (1951) found, as signs of vestibular toxicity, initially weakness in the hind legs, followed by a weaving gait, loss of righting reflex, and a reduction of post-rotatory nystagmus. With 50 mg/kg similar symptoms appeared only after 40 days–53 days of treatment.

In squirrel monkeys (Saimiri sciureus) and cats ataxia developed after about 3 weeks of intramuscular treatment with VM sulphate (150 mg/kg or 200 mg/kg–300 mg/kg) (KANDA and IGARASHI 1969). The cells of the crista ampullaris were more severely damaged than those of the macula utricula; vacuolation, vesicle formation, mitochondrial degeneration, and nuclear chromatin accumulation were observed more often in the type-I than in the type-II hair cells. The free surface was usually unaffected.

For data on the ototoxicity of basic antibiotics see the section on streptomycin.

Overall, the ototoxic action of VM seems to be considerably weaker than that of the other basic streptomyces antibiotics (MÜCKTER 1961).

References

Adamson RH, Marshall FN, Long JP (1960) Neuromuscular blocking properties of various polypeptide antibiotics. Proc Soc Exp Biol Med 105:494–497

Caesar R (1965) Die Bedeutung der Lysosomen für die formale Genese der Viomycin-Nephrose. Verh Dtsch Ges Pathol 49:157–161

Gössner W (1963) Nebenwirkungen der modernen Chemotherapeutika vom Standpunkt des Pathologen. Antibiot Chemother 11:285–300

Kanda T, Igarashi M (1969) Ultra-structural changes in vestibular sensory and organs after viomycin sulfate intoxication. Acta Otolaryngol 68:474–488

Keller H, Krüpe W, Sous H, Mückter H (1956) Versuche zur Toxizitätsminderung basischer Streptomyces-Antibiotica. 2. Mitteilung. Arzneimittelforsch 6:61–66

Klein HJ, Steinbach E, Schümmelfeder N (1966) Ultrastrukturelle und histochemische Untersuchungen zur Entstehung der Viomycin-Nephrose. Frankfurter Z Pathol 75:432–445

Kubikowski P, Szreniawski Z (1963) The mechanism of the neuromuscular blockade by antibiotics. Arch Int Pharmacodyn Ther 146:549–560

Moyer JH, Handley CA (1953) Renal function during viomycin administration to dogs. Proc Soc Exp Biol Med 82:761–763

Mückter H (1961) Zur Pharmakologie der basischen Streptomyces-Antibiotika. Antibiot Chemother 9 Sep:83–144

P'an SY, Halley TV, Reilly JC, Pekich AM (1951) Viomycin. Acute and chronic toxicity in experimental animals. Am Rev Tuberc 63:44–48

Staemmler M, Karhoff B (1956) Die akuten Nephrosen. II. Mitteilung. Nierenschäden durch Antibiotica. Virchows Arch 328:481–502
Staemmler M (1957) Die akuten Nephrosen. IV. Mitteilung. Tubuläre Schädigung und Wiederherstellung. Virchows Arch 330:139–155
Vital Brazil O, Ramos AO, Sperandio LG, Martinez AL (1961) Viomycin. Pharmacological actions on myoneural junction, ganglionic synapse and smooth muscle. Chemotherapia 3:521–531

VIII. Cycloserine (CS) and Terizidone (TZ)

1. D-Cycloserine (CS)

a) Respiration, Circulation, Heart

Intravenous doses of 75 mg–100 mg D-cycloserine/kg have little or no effect on the blood pressure of anaesthetized cats (FUST et al. 1958; ROBINSON et al. 1956; BYKOVA et al. 1965). Doses of 200 mg/kg–600 mg/kg, administered intravenously, cause a rapid but transient fall in the blood pressure by 30 mm Hg to 60 mm Hg (ROBINSON et al. 1956). The ECG remains unaffected during this time. Doses of 40 mg/kg or more cause the respiration to deepen without affecting the respiratory rate. After 400 mg/kg i.v. the respiratory minute volume is roughly doubled (ROBINSON et al. 1956). The bronchi of the artificially ventilated cat are not affected by cycloserine. But a dose of 400 mg/kg administered i. v. eliminates pilocarpine-induced bronchospasm. Oral administration of 1000 mg/kg to anaesthetized cats has no effect on the blood pressure (ROBINSON et al. 1956). In anaesthetized dogs doses of 50 mg/kg–100 mg/kg i.v. cause a fall in blood pressure and an acceleration of the heart and respiratory rate (ANDERSON et al. 1956).

In the cat in situ i.v. doses of 100 mg/kg temporarily reduce the blood flow in the carotid artery; doses of 1000 mg/kg lead to the same effect, but for a longer time. Under the low dose the blood flow in the femoral artery decreases, while under the higher dose it increases (FUST et al. 1958). In the isolated cat heart a 1‰ solution induced increased coronary flow. At the same time the heart contractions decreased strongly, with only a slight change in the heart rate (FUST et al. 1958).

b) Smooth Muscles

D-Cycloserine reduces the tone of the isolated guinea pig and rabbit ileum (ROBINSON et al. 1956; FUST et al. 1958), but does not antagonize either the neural spasms induced by acetylcholine or the muscular spasms induced by $BaCl_2$ (FUST et al. 1958). According to ANDERSON et al. (1956), the tone of the isolated rabbit uterus is not affected by concentrations of 4×10^{-3} in the bath medium, whereas FUST et al. (1958) observed clear excitation at a concentration of 5×10^{-3}.

c) Central Nervous Effects

A number of central nervous effects were recorded in the very first toxicity studies on cycloserine, following its introduction as an antituberculotic drug. These findings caused more comprehensive pharmacological tests to be performed, in which the various optical isomers were subjected to comparative analysis, after it had been found that the L-form and the racemic form exerted stronger neurotoxic effects in man compared to the D-form.

The motility of mice excited by the administration of pervitin or caffeine decreases under the influence of D-cycloserine (FUST et al. 1958). D-cycloserine also reduces the motility and the reaction time measured in the hot-plate test, although to a much smaller degree than e.g. L-cycloserine (LANGE and OEHME 1964). Only after the administration of 800 mg/kg of CS is the exploratory behaviour of mice clearly reduced (MAYER et al. 1971). The conditioned avoidance reaction of rats is not inhibited by 180 mg/kg p.o. (BONAVITA et al. 1964). DL-Cycloserine also exerts a stronger antagonistic effect than D-cycloserine against isoniazid convulsions (LANGE and OEHME 1964). In rats and dogs no significant change is observed in the EEG (FUST et al. 1958; LANGE and OEHME 1964). D-cycloserine has a moderate anticonvulsant effect in fatal penetrazole shock in mice (FUST et al. 1958; MAYER et al. 1971). The anaesthetic effect of ethanol is potentiated by D-cycloserine in mice (FUST et al. 1958), and the toxicity of higher ethanol doses is increased by low doses of D-cycloserine (GLASS et al. 1965). Conversely, small doses of ethanol suppress the lethal effect of high doses of D-cycloserine.

In vitro, DENGLER (1962) observed an inhibition of the pyridoxal-5-phosphate-dependent L-glutamic acid decarboxylase and L-dopa decarboxylase by D-cycloserine. It may well be that the inhibition of L-glutamic acid decarboxylase and the associated disturbance of the glutamic acid-γ-aminobutyric acid metabolism are partly responsible for the convulsions observed after cycloserine.

d) Other Pharmacological Effects

In mice and in rats high i.v. doses of D-cycloserine lower the body temperature. In yeast fever in rats and pyrifer fever in rabbits the compound has a weak antipyretic effect (FUST et al. 1958). Even high doses do not act analgesically or diuretically in experimental animals (ANDERSON et al. 1956). 1% solutions cause neither irritation nor local anaesthesia in the rabbit eye (ROBINSON et al. 1956).

D-cycloserine is not a histamine antagonist (ANDERSON et al. 1956) and has only a slight anti-inflammatory effect (FUST et al. 1958).

Overall, D-cycloserine has relatively few pharmacological properties. According to FUST et al. (1958), it can be regarded as a chlorpromazine-type tranquillizer in view of the inhibition of the postural reflexes observed in mice, the reduction of induced excitability, and the anticonvulsant and anaesthesia-potentiating effects. Similar results were obtained by MAYER et al. (1971).

e) Acute Toxicity

Single oral, subcutaneous, intraperitoneal, or intravenous doses of cycloserine are well tolerated by experimental animals. The range between lethal doses and doses that do not induce any symptoms is very wide (FUST et al. 1958). The LD_{50} values determined by various authors are in good agreement with one another (Table 1).

The intoxication symptoms are determined by the dose and the route of administration (FUST et al. 1958; ANDERSON et al. 1956). In mice, ataxia, trembling, and convulsions appear almost immediately after i.v. injection, followed by apa-

Table 1. Acute toxicity of D-cycloserine

Species	Route of administration	LD_{50} (mg/kg)	Confidence interval	Literature source
Mouse	i.v.	1810	1730–1890	1
		2500		3
		2400	–	4
		2150–2850	–	5
	i.p.	2870	2690–3050	1
		4300	3947–4653	3
		3900	3480–4360	6
	s.c.	2800	2650–2950	1
		>5000		3
		4700		4
	p.o.	5290	5090–5490	1
		>5000	–	2
		>5000	–	3
		8400	–	4
Rat	s.c.	>3000	–	1
		>5000	–	3
	p.o.	>5000	–	1
		~4000	–	2
		>5000		3
Guinea pig	s.c.	>1000	–	1
	p.o.	>2000	–	1
Dog	s.c.	<2000		3
	p.o.	>2000	–	1
Monkey	s.c.	>2000		3

[1] ANDERSON et al. (1956); [2] ROBINSON et al. (1956); [3] SPENCER and PAYNE (1956); [4] FUST et al. (1958); [5] BYKOVA et al. (1965); [6] MAYER et al. (1971).

thy, increasing relaxation, and muscular weakness. Death occurs within a few minutes. After s.c. and oral administration similar symptoms are observed with a latency of 20–30 min. The intoxication symptoms in rats and in guinea pigs are similar to those in mice. Rabbits often react to oral or i.v. administration of cycloserine with convulsions (ROBINSON et al. 1956). The maximum i.v. dose that rabbits can tolerate without any symptoms is 200 mg/kg. Twice this dose causes a slight respiratory depression and "tranquillization" (FUST et al. 1958). 10 mg administered intracisternally is lethal in rabbits (ROBINSON et al. 1956).

In dogs 2 g/kg, administered orally, act as an emetic (ANDERSON et al. 1956). Also in dogs, an s.c. injection of 1 g/kg causes salivation, vomiting, defaecation, pallor, lethargy, and weakness. A 2 g/kg dose is lethal (SPENCER and PAYNE 1956).

Rhesus monkeys tolerate D-cycloserine better than dogs. 1 g/kg s.c. produces no symptoms, while a 2 g/kg dose merely causes pallor, slight nausea, and apathy. The substance is only lethal at a dose of 4 g/kg (SPENCER and PAYNE 1956).

Higher, non-lethal doses of cycloserine reduce the toxic effect of simultaneously administered isoniazid (PRESCOTT et al. 1957). Prolonged administration of cycloserine in the feed, however, failed to inhibit the damage to the peripheral nerves provoked by isoniazid (FUST et al. 1958).

Studies on rats have shown that the toxicity of cycloserine in this species is apparently unconnected with a vitamin B_6 deficiency (EPSTEIN et al. 1958/59). The antagonistic role of pyridoxine was attributed more to a pharmacological effect than to a purely vitamin activity.

f) Subchronic Toxicity

Juvenile mice treated for 30 days with 100 mg/kg of orally or subcutaneously administered cycloserine did not show any symptoms of intoxication and put on more weight than control animals of the same age (FUST et al. 1958). Even after i.v. injection of 50 mg/kg and 30 mg/kg for one month no effect on growth could be observed in mice (BYKOVA et al. 1965).

Rats tolerated oral doses up to 300 mg/kg over periods as long as 17 weeks without any essential toxic symptoms (FUST et al. 1958; ROBINSON et al. 1956). Doses of 600 and 1200 mg/kg caused a slight to moderate reduction in the weight gain in rats, but no other toxic symptoms (ROBINSON et al. 1956).

Rabbits treated for 4 weeks with 100 mg/kg p.o. did not display any externally visible symptoms. However, at the start of the treatment in particular, there were signs of anaemia and in some cases leucocytopenia and bilirubinaemia, polychromasia, punctate basophilia, anisocytosis, Howell-Jolly bodies, normoblasts, bone-marrow hyperplasia, hyperaemia, and haemosiderosis of the spleen (FUST et al. 1958). Conversely, BYKOVA et al. (1956) failed to observe any alterations in the peripheral blood or the bone marrow in rabbits after intramuscular administration of 5, 10, and 50 mg/kg. According to ROBINSON et al. (1956), dogs tolerated twice-daily administration of 200 mg/kg p.o. over a 4 month period without any symptoms developing.

Dogs given 250 mg/kg or 125 mg/kg s.c. showed greatly increased salivation from the 7th to 10th day onwards, setting in 20–30 min after the injection. 250 mg/kg caused a significant reduction of the haemoglobin and the erythrocytes. One dog died after 50 injections of 250 mg/kg. The local tolerability at the site of injection was good. In the bone marrow the erythroid elements were increased and there was a simultaneous reduction of the myeloid cell lines (SPENCER and PAYNE 1956).

Oral doses of 500 mg/kg produced tremor, ataxia, and nausea in 2 monkeys within 2 h of the second administration. By the 4th day the animals were anorectic, pale, and weak and were suffering from diarrhoea. Both animals died on the 10th and on the 14th day. Treatment with 100 mg/kg p.o., on the other hand, did not cause any notable toxic symptoms. On the 60th day of the treatment there was an increased reticulocyte count and autopsy after 3 months of treatment revealed bone marrow hyperplasia (SPENCER and PAYNE 1956).

g) Chronic Toxicity

Female rats were treated for one year with cycloserine administered in the feed in concentrations of 0.5%, 1.0%, 3.0%, and 5.0% (ANDERSON et al. 1956). Concentrations up to 3% were well tolerated, whereas from 5% the food was refused owing to the unpleasant taste.

The same authors treated dogs for one year with 50 mg/kg–100 mg/kg i.v. Although the animals usually vomited an hour after the injection and showed a slight fall in the haemoglobin, together with reticulocytosis in the first phase of the study, all the dogs gained weight and survived the one-year treatment period (ANDERSON et al. 1956).

After one year of treatment with 100 mg/kg or 300 mg/kg monkeys (Macaca mulatta) temporarily exhibited changes in the blood similar to those in the dogs and the bone marrow was hyperplastic. Otherwise, however, the one year of treatment was well tolerated (ANDERSON et al. 1956).

h) Nephrotoxicity

In rabbits, FUST et al. (1958) observed slight degenerative renal symptoms in the form of granular degeneration of the renal epithelium after 4 weeks of treatment with 100 mg/kg p.o.

BYKOVA et al. (1965) also found evidence of a nephrotoxic effect in rats (proteinuria, granular casts, and erythrocytes) after 14 days of treatment with 285 mg/kg. In cats and in dogs they found proteinuria, fatty degeneration, and necrosis of the renal epithelium after doses of 50 and 100 mg/kg. These findings contradict those of other authors, who failed to observe pathological changes in the kidneys even after chronic administration. These differences may be due to differences in the quality of the cycloserine used, although BYKOVA et al. (1965) obtained similar results with material from another origin.

i) Ototoxicity

Cycloserine did not exhibit vestibulotoxicity in cats when given in doses of 20–50 mg/kg i.m. over a period of 30–83 days (ANDERSON et al. 1956; BYKOVA et al. 1965). The hearing of guinea pigs was not noticeably impaired by one month of treatment with 140 mg/kg (BYKOVA et al. 1965).

j) Local Tolerability

Only slight local reactions are observed after parenteral administration (BYKOVA et al. 1965; FUST et al. 1958).

2. Terizidone (TZ)

a) Acute Toxicity

The acute oral toxicity of terizidone was studied in mice, rats and rabbits (BONATI et al. 1965). The toxicity was found to be very low (Table 1).

Table 1. Acute toxicity of terizidone

Species	LD_{50} g/kg	Confidence interval
Mouse	8.1	(7.4–8.9)
Rat	7.0	(6.1–8.0)
Rabbit	2.4	(2.0–2.7)

b) Subacute Toxicity

After treatment with 1 g/kg p.o. for one month rats showed an inhibition of weight gain; 0.4 g/kg was tolerated without symptoms (BONATI et al. 1965).

c) Chronic Toxicity

After administration of 0.35 g/kg or 0.7 g/kg to rats for 4 months, a dose-dependent increase in relative liver weight was detected. In the animals treated with the higher dose, histological examination revealed slight fatty degeneration of the liver. 0.35 g/kg was tolerated without any objectively detectable damage (BONATI et al. 1965).

References

Anderson RC, Worth HM, Welles JS, Harris PN, Chen KK (1956) Pharmacology and toxicology of cycloserine. Antibiot Chemother 6:360–368
Bonati F, Bertoni L, Rosati G, Zanichelli V (1963) Caratteristiche biologiche ed attività antibatterica del teridizone. Il Farmaco Prat 20:381–395
Bonavita V, Lettieri M, Monaco P (1964) Behavioural studies on rats injected with L-cycloserine and other compounds. Psychopharmacologia 5:234–238
Bykova MA, Storozhev IA, Berezin EA (1965) Zur Pharmakologie des D-Cycloserin. Antibiotiki 10:626–629
Dengler HJ (1962) Zur Hemmung der L-Glutaminsäure- und L-Dopadecarboxylase durch D-Cycloserin und andere Isoxazolidone. Naunyn Schmiedebergs Arch Pharmacol 243:366–381
Epstein IG, Nair KGS, Mulinos MG, Haber A (1959) Pyridoxine and its relation to cycloserin neurotoxicity. Antibiot Annu 1958–1959:472–481
Fust B, Böhni E, Pellmont B, Zbinden G, Studer A (1958) Experimentelle Untersuchungen mit D-Cycloserin. Schweiz Z Tuberk 15:129–157
Glass F, Mallach HJ, Simsch A (1965) Beobachtungen und Untersuchungen über die gemeinsame Wirkung von Alkohol und D-Cycloserin. Arzneimittelforsch 15:684–688
Lange P, Oehme P (1964) Zentralnervöse Wirkungen von D- und D,L-Cycloserin. Arch Int Pharmacodyn Ther 152:466–473
Mayer O, Janků I, Kršiak M (1971) Die zentralen Wirkungen des Cycloserins im Tierexperiment. Arzneimittelforsch 21:298–303
Prescott B, Kauffmann G, James WD (1957) Increase in tolerated dose of isoniazid in mice by use of cycloserine. Proc Soc Exp Biol Med 94:94–96
Robinson HJ, Mason RC, Siegel H (1956) Toxicity and pharmacology of cycloserine. Am Rev Tuberc 74:972–976
Spencer JN, Payne HG (1956) Cycloserine. Experimental Studies. Antibiot Chemother 6:708–716

IX. Thioamides (Ethionamide, Protionamide)

1. Ethionamide (ETH)

a) Circulation, Heart

In intact cats intravenous injection of ethionamide induces a fall in blood pressure. In spinal cats the same dose produces a temporary rise in blood pressure. Higher doses inhibit the changes in blood pressure caused by noradrenaline. Ethionamide has a negative inotropic effect on the heart which in its time course and intensity corresponds to the blood-pressure reduction. The reduction in the blood pressure is evidently the consequence of a cardiac and a direct vascular effect (BAEDER et al. 1962).

b) Acute Toxicity

After oral administration of ethionamide to mice in the form of an aqueous suspension in gum arabic, DUBOST et al. (1964) determined an LD_{50} of 760 mg/kg. Death occurred as a result of respiratory arrest. Similarly, in mice BARGETON (1964) found an LD_{50} of 776 mg/kg (746 mg/kg–807 mg/kg) on administration of a suspension in carboxymethylcellulose. BAEDER et al. (1962) report an oral LD_{50} of 1000 mg/kg in the mouse. Dogs vomit after doses of 1600 mg/kg, so that it is impossible to establish the lethal oral dose (WOODARD 1960).

c) Subchronic Toxicity

Rats were treated for 12 weeks with concentrations of 1280, 2560, and 5120 ppm in the feed, corresponding to daily doses of around 100 mg/kg, 235 mg/kg, and 560 mg/kg body weight. In the animals treated with the highest and the middle dose the weight gain was reduced during the study. After the end of treatment the animals were observed for a further 6-week treatment-free period; the retardation of weight development was completely made up during this time. At the end of the study leucocytosis and neutrophilia were observed in the rats treated with 560 mg/kg. No histopathological alterations were observed.

Two dogs were given ethionamide in a dose of 30 mg/kg and two in a dose of 90 mg/kg the substance being given as a suspension by a stomach tube (DUBOST et al. 1964). Whereas the lower dose was maintained for 3 months, the higher dose was increased to 120 mg/kg in the third month. Neither the clinical tests nor the extensive laboratory tests or the autopsies and histopathological examinations of the animals yielded any evidence of toxic damage.

d) Chronic Toxicity

In the course of 53 weeks of administration of 2000 ppm, 1000 ppm, or 500 ppm of ethionamide in the feed, corresponding to about 120 mg/kg, 60 mg/kg, and 30 mg/kg body weight, the male rats in the highest-dose group put on less weight (WOODARD 1960). Dogs exhibited gastro-intestinal symptoms (anorexia, diarrhoea) during 28 weeks of treatment with 100 mg/kg p.o. Dogs treated with 30 mg/kg tolerated the treatment without any symptoms.

e) Reproductive Toxicity

Rats were treated orally with doses of 10 mg/kg, 50 mg/kg, or 200 mg/kg from the 6th to the 16th day of gestation (LORKE 1963/64). The high dose had a clearly adverse effect on the dams. The autopsies showed that all the foetuses of the dams in the highest-dose group had died. After treatment with 10 mg/kg and 50 mg/kg, on the other hand, there were no differences in embryological parameters in comparison to the control animals. Studies by ROUX (1962, 1963, 1965) revealed that no teratogenic effects appeared in rats treated with 60 mg/kg, a dose already poorly tolerated by the dams. Doses of 120 mg/kg or more induced abortions and inconsistent teratogenic effects. Doses of up to 240 mg/kg, on the other hand, were not teratogenic in mice.

In experiments on rabbits, treated from the 8th to the 15th day of gestation with doses of about 15 mg/kg, 100 mg/kg, and 250 mg/kg p.o., INGHAM (1963) observed skeletal anomalies (limb malformations and cleft palate) after the dose of 100 mg/kg. After 250 mg/kg practically all the foetuses were resorbed. In rabbits treated orally with 50 mg/kg from the 8th to the 16th day of gestation KHAN and AZAM (1969) observed an increase of the gestation period from 31.2 ± 0.4 (controls) to 33.4 ± 0.4 days. After 100 mg/kg and 200 mg/kg the weight of the offspring was significantly reduced and the numbers of dead and premature foetuses increased. In mice treated with the same doses from the 6th to the 14th day of gestation the number of resorptions was also dose-dependently increased and the number of foetuses accordingly reduced.

f) Carcinogenicity

BIANCIFIORI et al. (1964) treated BALB/c/Cb/Se mice a total of 300 times in the course of some 50 weeks, the total orally administered dose being 600 mg. The treatment failed to induce any lung tumours.

2. Protionamide (PTH)

a) Acute Toxicity

DUBOST et al. (1964) determined an LD_{50} of 780 mg/kg in mice on oral administration of protionamide in the form of an aqueous suspension in gum arabic. According to BARGETON (1964), the oral LD_{50} for mice is 1056 mg/kg (1010 mg/kg–1104 mg/kg). ILIIN (1975) gives an oral LD_{50} of 1000 mg/kg (760 mg/kg–1310 mg/kg) for mice, one of 1320 mg/kg (1150 mg/kg–1530 mg/kg) for rats, and one of >1000 mg/kg for cats.

b) Subchronic Toxicity

Rats were treated for 12 weeks with concentrations of 1400 ppm, 2800 ppm, and 5600 ppm administered in the feed, corresponding to daily doses of 165 mg/kg, 300 mg/kg, and 530 mg/kg (BARGETON 1964). The rats treated with 5600 ppm put on less weight but made up the weight retardation fully during a subsequent treatment-free observation period lasting 6 weeks. No haematological or histopathological alterations were observed.

DUBOST et al. (1964) treated two dogs orally with 30 mg/kg and two with 90 mg/kg of protionamide in the form of a suspension. Whereas the lower dose was maintained for 3 months, the higher dose was increased to 120 mg/kg in the third month. The treatment was well tolerated and there were no toxic symptoms or any alterations in the blood picture, the various biochemical parameters, or the organs.

c) Reproductive Toxicity

Rats were treated with 90 mg/kg, 180 mg/kg, and 270 mg/kg p.o. from the 1st to the 15th day of gestation (ROUX 1965). The highest dose was toxic to the dams and induced abortions. However, no malformations were found. The two lower doses were well tolerated by both dams and foetuses. In mice treated orally with the same doses from the 1st to the 14th day of gestation an abortive effect was again observed after the 270 mg/kg dose, while the other doses were well tolerated (Roux 1965). Rabbits tolerated oral treatment with 50 mg (equivalent to about 16 mg/kg) from the 8th to the 15th day of gestation without developing any symptoms (Ingham 1963). Some signs of embryotoxicity and teratogenicity appeared after 300 mg (about 100 mg/kg). A dose of 750 mg (about 250 mg/kg) was toxic to the dams (anorexia, weight losses, mortality). There was an increased incidence of resorptions in this group.

d) Carcinogenicity

Maral and Ganter (1967) used XVII Rho mice to study the carcinogenicity of protionamide. This strain has a spontaneously elevated incidence of pulmonary adenomas, whereas mammary tumours and leukaemias do not occur. The mice were treated with 30 mg of protionamide/kg body weight, administered with the feed, over a period of 17 months. No carcinogenic effects were observed.

References

Baeder DH, Ledaux G, Marier G (1962) The pharmacology and toxicology of ethionamide. Fed Proc 21:452

Bargeton D (1964) Etude toxicologique du 1321 TH. Unpublished investigations

Biancifiori C, Milia U, Di Leo FP (1964) Lav Ist Anat Istol patol Univ Perugia 24:145, cited from:

Biancifiori C, Severi C (1966) The relationship of isoniazid (INH) and allied compounds to carcinogenesis in some species of small laboratory animals: A review. Br J Cancer 20:528–538

Dubost P, Fournel J, Ganter P, Julou L, Laville J, Myon J, Pascal S (1964) Produits 1314 TH (8.545 R.P.) ou ethionamide (Trecator, N.D. Theraplix) et 1321 TH (9.778 R.P.). Toxicité aigue et toxicité à terme (3 mois). Unpublished investigations

Iliin AM (1975) Pharmaco-toxicogical study of the antituberculous preparation prothionamide Farmakol Toksikol 38:471–472

Ingham B (1963) Personal communication

Khan J, Azam A (1969) Study of teratogenic activity of trifluorperazine, amitriptyline, ethionamide and thalidomide in pregnant rabbits and mice. Proc Eur Soc Study Drug Tox 10:235–241

Lorke D (1963/64) Bericht über die Prüfung der embryotoxischen Wirkung von Iridocin (1314 TH). Unpublished investigations

Maral R, Ganter P (1967) Etude de l'activité cancerogène de: l'isoniazide (5.015 R.P.), du prothionamide (9.778 R.P. = 1321 TH), de l'urethane (10.506 R.P.) et de l'hydrazine (14.377 R.P.). Unpublished investigations

Roux CH (1962) Rapport sur l'étude du pouvoir teratogène du 1314 TH et du 2162 TH. Unpublished investigations

Roux CH (1963) Rapport sur l'étude du pouvoir teratogène du 1314 TH et du 2162 TH. Unpublished investigations

Roux CH (1965) Rapport sur l'étude du pouvoir teratogène du 1314 TH et du 2162 TH. Unpublished investigations

Roux CH (1965) Rapport sur l'étude de l'effect teratogène du 1321 TH. Unpublished investigations

Woodard G (1960) Toxicity of TH-1314 following single and repeated daily doses in rats and dogs. Unpublished investigations

X. Kanamycin (KM)

1. Respiration, Circulation, Heart

Kanamycin (KM) causes peripheral respiratory paralysis, since after lethal doses (about 250 mg/kg i.v.) respiratory arrest is followed by cardiac arrest, whereas these doses are survived with artificial respiration (TISCH et al. 1958; GOLDBERG 1964). Calcium chloride eliminates the respiratory depression (GOLDBERG 1964). Doses up to 100 mg/kg i.v., on the other hand, increase the rate and depth of respiration in anaesthetized dogs (TISCH et al. 1958).

In anaesthetized dogs and cats doses of 100 mg KM/kg–200 mg KM/kg, administered intravenously, brought about a temporary blood-pressure reduction. The amplitude and the frequency of the cardiac contractions remained essentially unaffected (TISCH et al. 1958; GOLDBERG 1964). Deaths were recorded only at intravenous doses of around 250 mg/kg. Neither antihistamines nor atropine were able to eliminate the blood-pressure-lowering effect in cats whereas calcium ions brought the reduced blood pressure back to its initial level (GOLDBERG 1964).

Like streptomycin (SM), KM exerts a constrictive effect on the coronary vessels (GOLDBERG 1964).

In comparative studies on the isolated cat heart with SM, tetracycline (TC), KM, vancomycin, and chloramphenicol, COHEN et al. (1970) observed a pronounced reduction of the contraction force of the heart after treatment with all these antibiotics. KM also exerted negative inotropy on the isolated frog heart. At a concentration of 1×10^{-2} the substance caused cardiac arrest during the diastole (GOLDBERG 1964).

TISCH et al. (1958) did not observe any significant ECG alterations in conscious or anaesthetized dogs after intravenous administration of 100 mg/kg. After higher doses depression of the T wave and prolongation of the ST segment were observed. Since sublethal doses had been given, the alterations were thought to be due to reduced coronary perfusion.

According to more recent investigations the effects of KM on respiration, heart, and circulation, as with the other aminoglycoside antibiotics (see the section on streptomycin), can be explained on the basis of calcium antagonism.

2. Neuromuscular Blocking Effects

Like other related antibiotics (SM, DHSM, neomycin), kanamycin causes a neuromuscular blockade, although to a smaller extent than the other drugs (SINGH et al. 1978). Because of the fundamental similarity that exists between KM and the other basic Streptomyces antibiotics, the reader is referred to the corresponding section on streptomycin (p. 312).

3. Smooth Muscles

A KM concentration of 4×10^{-4} causes a reduction in the contractions of isolated rabbit intestine and a concentration of 1×10^{-3} leads to complete blocking of the intestinal contractions and loss of tone. The tone of isolated guinea pig uterus is unaffected by concentrations up to 5×10^{-3}. KM exerts a weak antihistaminic effect on isolated, atropinized guinea pig intestine (GOLDBERG 1964).

4. Other Pharmacologic Effects

In rats and guinea pigs KM causes release of histamine, this effect being much weaker than that of SM or DHSM but stronger than that of viomycin or neomycin. The effects of the released histamine can be partially eliminated by antihistamines (AMANN and RADENBACH 1961).

5. Acute Toxicity

The acute toxicity of KM has been studied by various authors, predominantly in mice. Table 1 illustrates the good agreement between the findings obtained by the different authors.

LAGLER et al. (1960) and GOLDBERG (1964) pointed out that the pH of the KM solution has a considerable bearing on the toxicity of the substance. The acute toxicity increases with decreasing pH.

As expected, the toxicity is directly proportional to the speed of injection in the case of intravenous administration (GOLDBERG 1964; PINDELL and LEIN 1964). With injections lasting 5 sec or less the LD_{50} was 257 mg/kg (228 mg/kg–290 mg/kg), while with injections lasting 30 sec it was 356 mg/kg (309 mg/kg–409 mg/kg). When the injection was given over 60 sec the LD_{50} was 433 mg/kg (396 mg/kg–476 mg/kg) (GOLDBERG 1964).

Immediately after intravenous injection convulsions occur, followed by exophthalmos, dyspnoea, paresis or paralysis of the hind legs, opisthotonos, and erection of the tail. Death usually occurs within 3 min–5 min.

Table 1. Acute toxicity of kanamycin sulphate in mice

Strain sex	Route of adminis-tration	pH	LD_{50} mg/kg	Confidence interval $p>0.05$	Literature source
Swiss-Webster, ♂	i.v.	7.2	316.3 ± 24.4		1
	i.p.	7.2	1679 ± 186.4		
	s.c.	7.5	1648 ± 54.4		
	p.o.	7.2	>10000		
Albino, ♂	i.v.	8.2	225[a]	(217– 233)	2
	s.c.	8.2	1850[a]	(1740–1965)	
	p.o.	8.2	>10000[a]		
dd	i.v.	7.0	214		3
	i.p.	7.0	1583		
	s.c.	7.0	1883		
Albino	i.v.	7.0	205	(183– 229)	4
	i.v.	8.0	257	(228– 290)	
	i.p.	8.0	2200	(1788–2770)	
	s.c.	8.0	2030	(1610–2557)	
Swiss-Webster	i.v.	–	243[a] ± 13		5

[1] TISCH et al. (1958); [2] LAGLER et al. (1960); [3] OWADA (1962); [4] GOLDBERG (1964); [5] PINDELL and LEIN (1964)

[a] As the base.

In the case of s.c. and i.p. injections substantially higher doses are necessary to produce the same intoxication picture. However, the symptoms set in somewhat faster after intraperitoneal than after s.c. administration. After high doses (1500 mg/kg–3000 mg/kg) weakness, paresis and paralysis of the hind legs, and respiratory symptoms were observed within 5 min–10 min. The animals died within an hour or recovered quickly after 1 h to 2 h (GOLDBERG 1964). When administered orally KM is virtually non-toxic, as it is only absorbed to a very slight extent.

LAGLER et al. (1960) showed that, as in the cases of SM and VM, the acute toxicity of KM is reduced by calcium ions.

However, the toxicity-reducing effect of calcium relates only to the acute toxic effects due to the neuromuscular blockade. Calcium ions have no effect on the damage induced by longer administration.

As a continuation of their experiments on the detoxification of SM by pantothenates, LAGLER et al. (1960) studied the acute toxicity of the mono-, di- and tripantothenates of KM as compared to that of the sulphate. On i.v. injection the pantothenates proved slightly less toxic than the sulphate, although the toxicity-reducing effect is not very considerable.

The methane sulfonates of KM also caused only an apparent reduction of the acute toxicity. This is a result of the lower blood levels, and is associated with a lower antibacterial effect (PINDELL and LEIN 1964).

6. Subchronic and Chronic Toxicity

TISCH et al. (1958) were the first to publish a detailed report on long-term studies with prolonged administration of KM sulphate.

No toxic symptoms were found in rats treated for 5½ months with 100 mg or 200 mg KM sulphate/kg s.c.

Rabbits tolerated doses of 100 mg and 200 mg KM sulphate/kg administered intravenously for 8 months. On the other hand, 2 out of 3 rabbits treated with 100 mg of SM sulphate/kg for comparative purposes died.

Doses of 200 mg to 400 mg KM sulphate/kg proved to be toxic in cats. Some of the animals did survive treatment with the high dose for 30 days, but their general condition deteriorated and they were atactic and lost the righting reflex. Tubular alterations were found in the kidneys, in the form of cloudy swelling to necrosis. A direct comparison with SM (200 mg/kg) revealed that KM has a weaker cochleotoxic effect.

In dogs intramuscular treatment with 200 mg KM sulphate/kg exerted a nephrotoxic effect within 2 weeks–3 weeks. Albuminuria, haematuria, uraemia and later anuria were observed. There were no signs of cochleotoxicity. The kidneys of animals dying during the experiments or sacrificed when evidence of renal damage had been obtained showed histologically cloudy swelling of the proximal tubules up to acute necrosis of the proximal and distal tubules in the animals with anuria. None of the dogs that had received 50 mg or 100 mg KM sulphate/kg for up to 9 months showed any toxic symptoms. GOLDBERG (1964) also reports good tolerability of KM sulphate in doses below 100 mg/kg.

Further subchronic toxicity studies were performed by OWADA (1962). Mice were found to tolerate 20 days of s.c. treatment with doses up to 1250 mg KM sulphate/kg without toxic symptoms. By contrast, LAGLER et al. (1960) observed a reduced weight gain in mice after 400 mg KM sulphate/kg and, after about 45 days, a mortality of 30%. In mice treated with KM monopantothenate the mortality was 20% and in a group treated with tripantothenate 5%. In the dipantothenate group there were no deaths. The mortality differences were evaluated by the authors as an expression of the protective action of pantothenic acid.

7. Ototoxicity

KM is one of the ototoxic aminoglycoside antibiotics, damage to the hearing being in the foreground. In animal experiments HAWKINS (1959), TYBERGHEIN (1962), OWADA (1962), PLATTIG et al. (1967), and STEBBINS et al. (1969) used electrophysiological methods to detect hearing damage.

Extensive histological examinations by HAWKINS (1959), BECK and KRAHL (1962), FARKASHIDY et al. (1963), KOHONEN (1965), AKIYOSHI and SATO (1970), and others revealed damage to the outer hair cells particularly in guinea pigs and cats, and to a smaller extent in rats. This damage occurred especially in the basal coils of the cochlea, and there was loss of the inner hair cells in all the coils. TOYODA et al. (1978) described pronounced vestibular damage which continued to advance after the end of the treatment. Progression and, in some cases, subsequent improvement were reported by ORR (1980). The simultaneous administration of kanamycin and ethacrynic acid or furosemide to guinea pigs potentiates the ototoxic effect of the two substances (WEST et al. 1973; BRUMMETT et al. 1976; RUSSELL et al. 1979). Strong acoustic stimulation with simultaneous administration of KM can also result in a potentiation of the ototoxic effect (BROWN et al. 1979). During prenatal and postnatal development guinea pigs and rats proved to be substantially more sensitive to the ototoxic noxa than during later stages of life (RAPHAEL and FEIN 1980; OSAKA et al. 1979).

Because of the basic similarity between the pathogenesis of kanamycin- and streptomycin-induced ototoxicosis, the reader is referred to the more detailed discussion of this symptom in the section on streptomycin (p. 317).

8. Nephrotoxicity

Subchronic investigations have shown that KM is generally tolerated in doses up to 100 mg/kg. On the other hand prolonged administration of higher doses is nephrotoxic and leads to albuminuria, haematuria, uraemia, anuria, and tubular necroses in dogs, cats, and rats. The pars convoluta of the proximal tubule is the site primarily affected (LUFT et al. 1978).

LAGLER et al. (1960) and STAEMMLER and DUDKOWIAK (1961) were the first to show that the kidneys are able to store KM for prolonged periods. Pronounced tubular damage occurs after high doses (600 mg/kg–1000 mg/kg) administered for 3 days, which can extend beyond vacuolar-droplet degeneration to complete necrosis. The alterations are associated with severe functional disturbances and can give rise to uraemia with a strong elevation of the non-protein nitrogen. The glomeruli remain completely intact during this process. The tubular damage can be rapidly eliminated by regeneration of the necrotic epithelium.

The tubular damage evidently arises as a result of the fact that KM is excreted by the glomeruli and at least partly reabsorbed and stored in the tubule epithelium.

In comparative studies with other aminoglycosides KM proved to be one of the less nephrotoxic substances (LUFT et al. 1978). However, according to SACK and ZÜLLICH (1978) in the rat the tubulotoxic threshold dose on repeated administration is 5 mg/kg.

The simultaneous administration of a plasma expander during KM treatment leads to a clearly increased nephrotoxicity (KINOSHITA et al. 1970; NAKAZONO et al. 1970). In contrast, the nephrotoxicity of SM, which is not as strong anyway is not increased by a plasma expander. Stress (induced through immobilization) gave rise to increased mortality and nephrotoxicity in rats treated with KM, these effects being largely preventable by the administration of NaCl (RENAUD 1960).

9. Reproductive Toxicity

Only relatively small amounts of KM pass through the rat placenta. Following subcutaneous administration of 150 mg/kg to pregnant rats the maximum concentrations in the maternal serum were measured after 30 min and in the foetal tissue and serum after 2 h–3 h. The maximum serum concentrations in 20-day old foetuses and in the tissue fluid of 16-day and 20-day foetuses were respectively 3, 7, and 15 times as low as those in the serum of the dams. Later, however, i.e. 6 h after administration, the concentrations in the foetuses were between 1.4 and 3.4 times as high as those in the maternal serum. Increasing doses led to increasing permeability of the placenta. After the administration of the (therapeutic) dose of 15 mg/kg, however, no antibiotic could be detected in the foetuses. Thus, it may be that, with equal sensitivity, the risk to the foetus is lower than that to the dam (GOLDBERG and ILYUSHINA 1968).

BEVELANDER and COHLAN (1962) did not find any malformations in rats whose dams had been treated with 100 mg KM/kg from the 8th to the 16th day of gestation.

References

Akiyoshi M, Sato K (1970) Reevaluation of the pinna reflex test as screening for otoxicity of antibiotics. In: Progress in antimicrobial and anticancer chemotherapy. Proc 6th Intern Congr Chemotherapy, Vol I:621–627

Amann R, Radenbach KL (1961) Akute Kanamycin-Nebenwirkungen und Histaminfreisetzung. Beitr Klin Tuberk 123:208–210

Beck CHL, Krahl P (1962) Experimentelle und feingewebliche Untersuchungen über die Otoxicität von Kanamycin. Arch Otorhinolaryngol 179:594–610

Bevelander G, Cohlan SQ (1962) The effect on the rat of transplacentally aquired tetracycline. Biol Neonate 4:365–370

Brown JJ, Brummett RE, Fox KE (1979) Combined effects of noise and kanamycin: Cochlear pathology and pharmacokinetics in the guinea pig. Pharmacologist 21:144

Brummett RE, Traynor J, Brown R, Himes D (1975) Cochlear damage resulting from kanamycin and furosemide. Acta Oto-Laryngol (Stockh) 80:86–92

Cohen LS, Wechsler AS, Mitchell JH, Glick G (1970) Depression of cardiac function by streptomycin and other antimicrobial agents. Am J Cardiol 26:505–511
Farkashidy J, Black RG, Briant TDR (1963) The effect of kanamycin on the internal ear: an electrophysiological and electron microscope study. Laryngoscope 73:713–727
Goldberg LE (1964) Pharmakologische Prüfung des Antibiotikums Kanamycin (russ.). Antibiotiki (Moskau) 9:414–420
Goldberg LE, Ilyushina NG (1968) Experimental investigation of kanamycin circulation between mother and fetus. Byul Eksp Biol Med 66:994–996
Hawkins JE Jr (1959) The otoxicity of kanamycin. Ann Otol 68:698–715
Kinoshita Y, Yamasaku F, Takeda H, Usuda Y, Kitahara K (1970) Nephrotoxicity of kanamycin with a combination of plasma expander. In: Progress in antimicrobiol and anticancer chemotherapy. Proc 6th Intern Congr Chemotherapy, Vol I:586–590
Kohonen A (1965) Effect of some ototoxic drugs upon the pattern and innervation of cochlear sensory cells in the guinea pig. Acta Otolaryng (Stockh) Suppl 208:9–70
Lagler F, Osterloh G, Mückter H (1960) Studies on the pharmacology of kanamycin. Antibiot Annu 1959–1960: 862–867
Luft F, Bloch R, Sloan RS, Yum MN, Costello R, Maxwell DR (1978) Comparative nephrotoxicity of aminoglycoside antibiotics in rats. J Infect Dis 138:541–545
Mückter H (1961) Zur Pharmakologie der basischen Streptomyces-Antibiotika. Antibiot Chemotherap 9 Sep:83–114
Nakazono M, Naide Y, Ohkoshi M (1970) Biochemical studies on nephrotoxicity of kanamycin. In: Progress in antimicrobial Chemotherapy. Vol I:591–595
Orr JL (1980) Behavioral toxicology of kanamycin. Dissertation Abstr Intern B 40:5068
Osaka S, Tokimoto T, Matsuura S (1979) Effects of kanamycin on the auditory evoked responses during postnatal development of the hearing of the rat. Acta Oto-Laryngol (Stockh) 88:359–368
Owada K (1962) Experimental studies on the toxicity of kanamycin, its hydrolyzed products and neomycin. Chemotherapia 5:277–293
Pindell MH, Lein J (1964) Comparison of biological and toxicological properties of methane sulfonate and sulfonate derivatives of antibiotics. Chemotherapia 8:163–174
Plattig KH, Keidel UO, David E (1967) Minderung der Otoxizität des Kanamycin durch Panthothensäure. Elektrophysiologische Untersuchungen an der Katze. Dtsch Med Wochenschr 92:1391–1397
Raphael Y, Fein A (1980) Kanamycin otoxicity in utero. Isr J Med Sci 16:554–555
Renaud S (1960) The toxicity of kanamycin and bacitracin as influenced by stress and sodium chloride. Toxicol Appl Pharmacol 2:708–714
Sack K, Züllich B (1978) Differenzierung der nephrotoxischen Potenzen von Aminoglykosiden und Cephalosporinen im Tierexperiment. Therapiewoche 28:2107–2114
Singh YN, Harvey AL, Marshall IG (1978) Antibiotic-induced paralysis of the mouse phrenic nerve-hemidiaphragm preparation, and reversibility by calcium and by neostigmine. Anesthesiology 48:418–424
Staemmler M, Dudkowiak V (1961) Über Wirkungen des Kanamycin auf die Nieren. Med Welt:1296–1299
Stebbins WC, Miller JM, Johnsson L-G, Hawkins JE Jr (1969) Ototoxic hearing loss and cochlear pathology in the monkey. Ann Otol 78:1007–1025
Tisch DE, Huftalen JB, Dickison HL (1958) Pharmacological studies with kanamycin. Ann NY Acad Sci 76:44–65
Toyada Y, Saito H, Matsuoka H, Takenaka H, Oshima W, Mizukoshi O (1978) Quantitative analysis of kanamycin ototoxicosis. Acta Oto-Laryngol (Stockh) 84:202–212
Russel NJ, Fox KE, Brummett RE (1979) Ototoxic effects of the interaction between kanamycin and ethacrynic acid. Cochlear ultrastructure correlated with cochlear potentials and kanamycin levels. Acta Oto-Laryngol (Stockh) 88:369–381
Tyberghein J (1962) Influence of some streptomyces antibiotics on the cochlear microphonics in the guinea pig. Acta Otolaryng (Stockh) Suppl 171
West BA, Brummett RE, Himes DL (1973) Interaction of kanamycin and ethacrynic acid. Arch Otolaryngol 98:32–37

XI. Thiocarlide (DATC)

1. Acute Toxicity

On i.m. or i.p. injection, thiocarlide is hardly absorbed by rats, guinea pigs, or rabbits. The absence of toxic symptoms is therefore not surprising. Even oral administration of doses up to 10 g/kg is tolerated by mice and by rats without any symptoms (LAMBELIN and PARMENTIER 1963).

2. Subacute Toxicity

In rats no signs of toxicity were observed after 15 days of treatment with 2 g/kg in the form of an aqueous suspension administered by a stomach tube. After 2 months of treatment with 2.5% and 3.5% of thiocarlide in the feed, corresponding to daily doses of 1.8 g/kg–2.2 g/kg or 2.5 g/kg–3 g/kg body weight, the weights of the thyroid glands and the liver of the treated rats were increased. Histological examination revealed hyperplasia of the thyroid without degenerative alterations, thus resembling the condition observed after administration of thyroid inhibitors such as propylthiouracil (LAMBELIN and PARMENTIER 1966).

3. Chronic Toxicity

The same authors carried out chronic toxicity studies on rats with 6 and 18 months of treatment with 0.6%, 1.25%, or 2.5% thiocarlide in the feed (LAMBELIN and PARMENTIER 1963, 1966). These doses correspond to a daily intake of around 300 mg/kg–1400 mg/kg body weight.

The growth, the mortality rate, and the blood picture were not affected by 6 months of treatment. However, in this experiment enlargement of the liver and increased thyroid weight as a result of hyperplasia were also observed after the high doses. Mating experiments in the 3rd month of the treatment yielded no evidence of fertility impairment and no decrease in the weight at birth or in the number of stillbirths. After one month, however, the weight of the treated young was lower than that of the controls. No malformations were observed.

In the course of 18 months of treatment a slight liver enlargement and thyroid hyperplasia (the latter not always dose-dependent) was found in the treated animals in addition to an elevation of alkaline phosphatase in the blood plasma; the cause of this last effect is unknown. Morphological and biochemical investigations failed to provide any explanation for the liver enlargement. There was no cholestasis and no evident skeletal alterations.

Monkeys even tolerated doses up to 3 g/kg body weight over a one-year treatment period without toxic effects (LAMBELIN 1970).

4. Reproductive Toxicity

There was no evidence of impaired fertility or impaired maternal behaviour on the part of the mothers. No malformations at all were recorded. The foetal thyroids were unaffected and no evidence of carcinogenicity was found.

References

Lambelin G (1970) Pharmacology and toxicology of Isoxyl. Antibiotica et Chemotherapia 16:84–95
Lambelin G, Parmentier R (1963) Etude toxicologique de l'Isoxyl sur l'animal. Acta Tuberc Pneumol Belg 54:476–493
Lambelin G, Parmentier R (1966) Study of the toxicity of isoxyl. Arzneimittelforsch 16:881–886

XII. Capreomycin (CM)

1. Respiration, Circulation, Heart

In two anaesthetized dogs doses of 4 mg and 8 mg of CM/kg, administered intravenously, caused an increase in the heart rate and the respiration rate. The effect on the arterial blood pressure varied and was not dose-dependent (WELLES et al. 1966).

2. Acute Toxicity

Acute toxicity studies on mice, rats (newborn, just weaned and adult), guinea pigs, and mongrel dogs were reported by WELLES et al. (1966). The results of the toxicity studies are shown in Table 1.

The acute toxicity of capreomycin is of the same order as those of streptomycin and kanamycin.

The majority of the deaths occurred immediately or within a few hours of administration. Death may be due to circulatory failure, while some late deaths may presumably be attributed to kidney damage. There are no differences in sensitivity between newborn, just weaned, and adult rats.

In guinea pigs CM does not exert antigenic effects. A 1% solution did not irritate the rabbit eye.

Table 1. Acute toxicity of capreomycin

Species	Strain sex, age	Route of administration	LD_{50} mg/kg
Mouse	Cox ICR, ♀	i.v.	250.2 ± 9.2
		s.c.	513.9 ± 27.4
		p.o.	>6000
Rat	Harlan, ♀, adult	i.v.	325.3 ± 14.9
		i.p.	157.4 ± 24.1
		s.c.	1191 ± 160
		p.o.	>6000
	just weaned (30–35 g)	s.c.	984 ± 112
		i.p.	194.1 ± 7.9
	newborn	i.p.	165.3 ± 11.3
Guinea pig	–	s.c.	> 550
	–	p.o.	>6000
Dog	Mongrels	i.v.	> 62

3. Chronic Toxicity

WELLES et al. (1966) also reported on long-term studies in rats and in dogs.

Daily s.c. injections of 50 mg/kg did not have a negative effect on the weight gain of female rats over a 2-year treatment period, whereas 100 mg/kg and 250 mg/kg resulted in slightly reduced weight gain. Male rats only put on less weight after 250 mg/kg. The dose of 250 mg/kg, given 3 times a week, caused a reduced weight gain in male rats. There were no haematological or clinico-chemical alterations. However, the kidneys of all the treated rats were significantly heavier and the majority of the animals had nephroses and chronic pyelonephritis. During chronic (2–3 years) administration several dogs from the various dose groups died after doses of 25 mg/kg and 62 mg/kg. Whereas some dogs died after only about 7–8 weeks, others tolerated the same dose for 2 years. Death was preceded by anorexia, loss of weight, dehydration and haemoconcentration as well as by considerable increases in the urea level. All the treated animals exhibited various degrees of pathological alterations of the tubuli contorti in some cases with extensive regeneration of the tubules. After higher doses impaired hearing was observed, sometimes to the point of deafness.

Two other groups of dogs survived doses of 50 mg/kg or 100 mg/kg 3 times a week for over 2 years without developing any clinical symptoms.

4. Reproductive Toxicity

Reproduction studies on rats revealed that doses of 50 mg/kg and 100 mg/kg s.c. had no effect on fertility or the size of the litters or on the viability and growth of the young during lactation. No teratogenic effects were observed (WELLES et al. 1966).

5. Ototoxicity

In studies on the ototoxic effect of CM cats tolerated doses of up to 33 mg/kg s.c. given for 91 days without exhibiting any systemic toxic symptoms (WELLES et al. 1966). After doses of 65 mg/kg and 130 mg/kg weight loss, reduction of post-rotatory nystagmus, and ataxia were observed shortly before death, and the hearing was impaired in individual animals. The renal tubules showed necroses and there was extensive regeneration. AKIYOSHI et al. (1971) observed toxic damage to the hair cells of the organ of Corti after 28 days of treatment with 400 mg CM/kg i.m.

6. Nephrotoxicity

WELLES et al. (1966) had already drawn attention to the nephrotoxicity of capreomycin in rats, dogs, and cats. MURAOKA et al. (1968) showed that in rats capreomycin has mast cell degranulating properties. The 5-hydroxytryptamine which is released in the blood, from the mast cells causes vasoconstriction, ischaemia, and necrosis in the kidneys. However, the possibility of direct action on the kidney cannot be ruled out.

References

Akiyoshi M, Sato Y, Shoji T, Sugahiro K, Tamura H (1971) Histological changes in the stria vascularis of the inner ear in the case of auricular toxicosis by antibiotics (in Japanese). J Otolaryngol (Jap) 74:476–477

Muraoka Y, Hayashi Y, Minesita T (1968) Studies of capreomycin nephrotoxicity. Toxicol Appl Pharmacol 12:350–359

Welles JS, Harris PN, Small RM, Worth HM, Anderson RC (1966) The toxicity of capreomycin in laboratory animals. Ann NY Acad Sci 135:960–973

XIII. Ethambutol (EMB)

1. Acute Toxicity

DIERMEIER et al. (1966) described acute toxicity studies in mice and in rats with various routes of administration. As can be seen from Table 1, a single administration of ethambutol has only a low toxicity.

To investigate any possible interactions between ethambutol and simultaneously administered antituberculotic drugs DIERMEIER et al. (1966) carried out a number of acute toxicity studies on mice and on rats, using combinations of ethambutol and streptomycin or isoniazid. The ratios of the substances used in the various combinations corresponded to those used in clinical practice. Some of the combinations gave rise to a statistically significant reduction or increase in mortality, but in view of the relatively small improvement in tolerability and the high doses administered the effects were of no more than marginal practical significance. Combination studies with capreomycin in rats did not reveal any reciprocal effects on toxicity.

THOMAS et al. (1961) also found no contraindication for the combined use of ethambutol with isoniazid, PAS, capreomycin or streptomycin.

2. Chronic Toxicity

KAISER (1964) carried out a chronic toxicity study on beagles. The histopathological examinations of this study were reported by CAPPIELLO and LAYTON (1965), and later DIERMEIER et al. (1966) summarized all the experimental results.

37 beagles were treated for up to one year with oral doses of 25 mg/kg, 50 mg/kg, 100 mg/kg, 200 mg/kg, 400 mg/kg, 800 mg/kg, or 1600 mg/kg. With the ex-

Table 1. Acute toxicity of ethambutol

Species	Strain sex	Route of adminis- tration	LD_{50} (mg/kg)	Confidence interval
Mouse	Carworth CF_1, ♀	i.v.	230	(200– 250)
		s.c.	1800	(1700–2000)
		p.o.	8900	(8200–9600)
Rat	Sherman, ♂	i.v.	300	(280– 320)
		i.p.	1200	(1100–1300)
		p.o.	6800	(6200–7400)

ception of one dog, which died after treatment with 100 mg/kg, the animals all survived doses up to and including 400 mg/kg. 2 of the 3 animals treated with 800 mg/kg died after the 14th and 69th dose respectively and the dog treated with 1600 mg/kg died after the 19th dose.

After treatment with 400 mg/kg and 800 mg/kg increased bromthalein retention and an increased GPT level in the serum were seen as signs of a liver impairment. However, the histopathological examination failed to establish any morphological correlate in the liver (CAPPIELLO and LAYTON 1965).

High doses caused cardiac damage, this being manifested in the ECG as a depression or elevation of the ST segment and an inversion of the P waves and the QRS complex. Morphological cardiac alterations were found in all the dogs treated with doses of 200 mg/kg or more and in one dog treated with 100 mg/kg. These consisted of eosinophilic hyalinization, vacuolization, and necrosis of the myocardial fibres, and focal interstitial and perivascular inflammatory infiltration. The cardiac alterations were more strongly pronounced in the dogs that had died.

Neurological changes took the form of ataxia and stiffness of the hind legs after doses of 400 mg/kg and 800 mg/kg (KAISER 1964). However, the brain, spinal cord, and the peripheral nerves were histopathologically normal (CAPPIELLO and LAYTON 1965). Studies on ethambutol levels in the serum showed that serious toxic damage occurs at concentrations of around 50 μg/ml, i.e. ones 10 times the maximum therapeutic serum concentration (about 5 μg/ml).

Notable ophthalmoscopic alterations were found in the tapetum lucidum in dogs (KAISER 1964; DIERMEIER et al. 1966). Daily doses of 50 and 100 mg ethambutol/kg caused partial depigmentation of the tapetum and after higher doses there was a complete depigmentation of the canine eye ground, which is normally of a luminous greenish color. There were no alterations to the cornea, lens, the vitreous body or fundus, and vision was seemingly unimpaired. Individual doses of 100 mg/kg–1600 mg/kg caused transient depigmentation of the tapetum lucidum, the color intensity and the distribution being restored within a few hours (VOGEL and KAISER 1963). In long-term studies too the color changes proved to be largely reversible a few days to weeks after discontinuation of the treatment. Electron-microscopic examinations revealed that the bundles of parallel rods densely packed in the canine tapetum cells swell up after administration of ethambutol and lose their original arrangement. VOGEL and KAISER (1963) suggested that EMB acts as a chelating agent on the high concentrations of zinc present in the tapetum lucidum of the canine eye, leading to a modification of the intracellular structure of the tapetum cells and interference with light refraction in the eye.

BUYSKE et al. (1966) then actually discovered in dogs a dose-dependent reduction of the zinc content of the eye, and to a smaller extent also of the heart and the liver, after one year of treatment. The excretion of zinc with the urine in these dogs could be increased by 60% after a single dose of 400 mg EMB/kg. By giving a single oral dose of 1600 mg EMB/kg to dogs, FIGUERA et al. (1971) produced depigmentation of the tapetum lucidum and a clear decrease in its zinc content. A decrease in the zinc content of the eye was also found in rhesus monkeys treated regularly for 6 months with 400 mg/kg or 800 mg/kg and in rats given about

100 mg/kg with the feed for 10 months. Additional analyses of the copper concentrations revealed a decrease in the canine myocardium and in the eye, liver, and skin in the rat (BUYSKE et al. 1966). The reduction of the copper content of the dog heart occurred in parallel with a fall of the cytochrome C oxidase level in the heart (BUYSKE et al. 1966). The toxic alterations occurring in the canine heart may possibly be due to a reduced activity of this enzyme.

In rhesus monkeys clinical symptoms (ataxia, loss of the grip reflex, muscular weakness, blindness) were observed after several months of treatment with doses of 800 mg/kg–1600 mg/kg, and these effects could be correlated with changes in the brain and the spinal cord (SCHMIDT and SCHMIDT 1964; SCHMIDT 1966). These morphological correlations consisted of myelin swelling and demyelination of the pyramidal fibres in the lower medulla, central necrosis, and extensive glial cell proliferation, increasing in severity from the upper cervical marrow to the caudal part of the olive, and in necroses and massive glial proliferation in the chiasma opticum and the tractus opticus. Since monkeys do not have a tapetum lucidum, no changes could be found which corresponded to the eye alterations in the dog.

After 6 months of treatment with 200 mg EMB/kg, however, neither clinical nor histopathological toxic alterations were observed (SCHMIDT 1966).

As in the toxicity studies on dogs, there was also a clear connection between the dose given, the EMB concentration in the serum, and the toxic symptoms in monkeys. Doses up to 400 mg/kg, which gave rise to mean serum peak-levels of 30 μg/ml, were tolerated by monkeys. At serum peak-levels of 80 μg/ml, following doses of 800 mg/kg, loss of the sense of touch and ataxia developed in the course of 4 months of treatment. At serum concentrations higher than 100 μg/ml the aforementioned neuroanatomical symptoms were followed by death. The doses necessary for this are, however, 12 to 48 times the therapeutically effective dose (SCHMIDT 1966). According to HARA and BABA (1970), a metabolite (monobutyric acid) may be responsible for neurological and ocular side effects.

3. Reproductive Toxicity

Studies on the teratogenicity of ethambutol were carried out using mice, rats, and rabbits (YADA 1965; YAMAMURA and TANAKA 1965; CHIESA 1966; SCARINCI 1966: unpublished work cited in BRUCKSCHEN 1970). According to these studies, mouse foetuses whose dams had been treated with 250 mg or 2500 mg EMB/kg p.o. from the 7th to the 12th day of gestation did not exhibit any malformations; delayed ossification of the middle phalanges and of the caudal vertebrae were the only effects observed.

Rats were treated during pregnancy with 0.2%–0.8% ethambutol administered with the feed and with doses of 10 mg/kg–70 mg/kg s.c. Again no teratogenic effects were observed.

In rabbits treated from the 8th to the 16th day of gestation with 100 mg or 500 mg EMB/kg some malformations occurred in the higher-dose group (monophthalmia, shortening of the right forepaw by joint contraction, cleft palate), although according to the authors these effects corresponded to the normal malformation rate in the rabbit strain used.

Testicular lesions and sterility were observed by BOTTICELLI et al. (1971) in rats treated for a prolonged period with high doses of ethambutol. After doses of 300 mg/kg–600 mg/kg the males became sterile as a result of atrophy of the seminiferous tubules and progressive damage and necrosis of the seminal epithelium. After discontinuation of the ethambutol treatment the damage regressed to some extent. The functional and morphological alterations are attributed to a blockade of nucleoprotein synthesis. Similar observations have been reported by ASOLE et al. (1976).

Treated female rats mated with untreated male rats did become pregnant, but the fertilization was delayed by up to 20 days. No histopathologically detectable changes were found in the ovaries. The pregnancy itself and the offspring were unaffected.

4. Ototoxicity

Oral administration of doses of 200 mg ethambutol/kg had no vestibulotoxic effect in cats, nor did it potentiate the vestibulotoxic action of simultaneously administered streptomycin (DIERMEIER et al. 1966).

5. Pharmacology

High doses of EMB inhibit neuromuscular transmission (GRIFA et al. 1967). According to BORCHARD (1974) EMB stabilizes the nerve membrane, reducing the Na^+ permeability. FANTOLI et al. (1968) detected inhibition of serum cholinesterase activity.

References

Asole A, Panu R, Palmieri G (1976) Effetti dell'etambutolo sull'epitelio seminale di ratto e pollo. Boll Soc Ital Biol Sper 52:846–848

Borchard U (1974) Untersuchungen über den Einfluß von Ethambutol auf peripheres und zentralnervöses Gewebe. Thesis, University of Cologne

Botticelli A, Trentini GP, Barbolini G (1971) Lesioni testicolari nel ratto trattato con etambutolo. Boll Soc Ital Biol Sper 47:72–75

Bruckschen EG (1970) Myambutol. Experimentelle und klinische Ergebnisse. Arzneimittelforsch, 20. Beiheft 2. Aufl.

Buyske DA, Sterling W, Peets E (1966) Pharmacological and biochemical studies on ethambutol in laboratory animals. Ann NY Acad Sci 135:711–725

Cappiello VP, Layton WM Jr (1965) A one-year study of the toxicity of ethambutol in dogs: results of gross and histopathologic examinations. Toxicol Appl Pharmacol 7:844–849

Diermeier HF, Kaiser JA, Yuda N (1966) Safety evaluation of ethambutol. Ann NY Acad Sci 135:732–746

Fantoli U, Sebastiani M, Cattaneo C, Sbampato M (1968) Comportamento dell' attività colinesterasica sierica in soggeti trattati con Etambutolo. Ann Inst C Forlanini 28:164

Figueroa R, Weiss H, Smith JC Jr, Hackley BM, McBean LD, Swassing ChR, Halsted JA (1971) Effect of ethambutol on the ocular zinc concentrations in dogs. Am Rev Resp Dis 104:592–594

Grifa P, Jotti D, Benatti G (1967) Ricereche sperimentali sulla tossicità dell' Etambutolo sul sistema nervoso centrale di alcuni animali. Giorn It Chemiother 14:65

Hara T, Baba H (1970) Incorporation and metabolism of ethambutol in rat organs. Kekkaku 45:129
Kaiser JA (1964) A one-year study of the toxicity of ethambutol in dogs: results during life. Toxicol Appl Pharmacol 6:557–567
Schmidt J, Schmidt LH (1964) Neurotoxicity of ethambutol, an anti-tuberculosis drug. Anat Rec 148:333
Schmidt JG (1966) Central nervous system effects of ethambutol in monkeys. Ann NY Acad Sci 135:759–774
Thomas JP, Baughn CO, Wilkinson RG, Sheperd RG (1961) A new synthetic compound with antituberculous activity in mice: ethambutol (dextro-2,2′-(ethylenediimino)-di-1-butanol). Am Rev Respir Dis 83:891–893
Vogel AW, Kaiser JA (1963) Ethambutol-induced transient change and reconstitution (in vivo) of the tapetum lucidum color in the dog. Exp Mol Pathol Suppl 2:136–149

XIV. Rifampicin (RMP)

1. Acute Toxicity

The acute toxicity of rifampicin was investigated in four species using various routes of administration. It was found that the substance has a relatively low toxicity when administered only once. No intoxication symptoms were reported by the authors. The results are shown in Table 1.

2. Subchronic Toxicity

FURESZ (1970) reports on a subchronic toxicity study performed on rabbits. The animals were treated with oral doses of 100 mg or 400 mg RMP/kg 7 days a week

Table 1. Acute toxicity of rifampicin

Species	Route of administration	LD_{50} mg/kg	Confidence interval	Literature source
Mouse	i.v.	260		1
	i.p.	640		1
	i.p.	620.8	595.1– 674.4)	2
	p.o.	885		1
	p.o.	858.4	(829.3– 888.4)	2
Rat	i.v.	330		1
	i.v.	329.5	280 – 390)	3
	i.p.	550		1
	i.p.	533.5	(515.4– 552.1)	2
	i.p.	416.3	(397.9– 435.4)	3
	p.o.	1720		1
	p.o.	1668.4	(1303.3–2135.5)	2
	p.o.	~ 900		3
Guinea pig	i.p.	639		1
Rabbit	p.o.	2120		1
	p.o.	~1500		2

[1] FURESZ (1970); [2] SENSI et al. (1967); [3] SCHIATTI et al. (1967).

for 4 weeks. The dose of 100 mg/kg was tolerated without any symptoms. After 400 mg/kg 3 of the 5 animals died. Considerable weight loss, pronounced icterus, fatty and hydropic degeneration of the liver and kidneys, and haemorrhagic enteritis were observed in one of the dead animals.

3. Chronic Toxicity

Chronic toxicity studies involving 6 months of treatment were carried out on rats, rabbits, and dogs (Furesz 1970).

Rats were treated 6 times a week with 50 mg/kg, 100 mg/kg, and 200 mg/kg, administered orally. Doses up to and including 100 mg/kg were tolerated without any symptoms. The 200 mg/kg dose caused a slight increase in the liver weight as well as slight cloudy swelling and/or hydropic degeneration of the liver epithelium.

Dogs tolerated repeated administration of rifampicin less well. One dog died on the 44th day with necrotic haemorrhagic enteritis after receiving 25 mg/kg p.o. After 50 mg/kg p.o. one dog died of severe liver and kidney damage on the 33rd day. The dogs in this dose group displayed a slight weight reduction and a fall in the haemoglobin concentration and the erythrocyte count. In two dogs there were alterations of the megakaryocytes in the bone marrow. Other symptoms included loss of appetite, vomiting, transient sedation and polydipsia, glucosuria, bilirubinuria, and casts in the urinary sediment in some of the animals.

The general, though not always dose-dependent, effects consisted of an increase of bilirubin, the transaminases and alkaline phosphatase, degenerative renal and hepatic alterations, fatty degeneration of the liver, and slight hyperplastic lymphadenitis.

Monkeys (Macaca irus) tolerated doses up to 75 mg/kg without any effects. After 105 mg/kg some of the animals vomited and their general condition deteriorated. Another animal exhibited loss of appetite, loss of weight, and an increased alkaline phosphatase level in the serum.

4. Microsomal Enzyme Induction

Proliferation of the smooth endoplasmic reticulum was observed in the hepatocytes in guinea pigs and in man.

This was regarded as a morphological manifestation of the induction of microsomal, drug-degrading enzymes caused by rifampicin (Jezequel et al. 1971).

5. Reproductive Toxicity

Rats were treated orally with doses of 50 mg/kg, 100 mg/kg, 200 mg/kg, and 300 mg/kg from the 2nd to the 21st day of gestation (Furesz 1970). The 300 mg/kg dose exerted toxic effects on the dams. All the foetuses died in utero and were resorbed. The number of resorptions was also increased after 200 mg/kg. In the foetuses of this group there were 3 malformations and minor skeletal anomalies. The foetal weights were reduced. Doses of 50 mg/kg and 100 mg/kg were not embryotoxic.

In rabbits doses of 200 mg/kg were toxic to the dams when administered orally from the 6th to the 18th day of gestation. The incidence of resorptions was increased, and the number of foetuses correspondingly reduced. Two foetuses had severe malformations. In the lower dose groups (50 mg/kg and 100 mg/kg) the number of malformations was only slightly above the malformation rate normally encountered in the rabbit strain used.

In teratogenicity studies carried out by TUCHMANN-DUPLESSIS and MERCIER-PAROT (1969) doses of up to 100 mg/kg administered orally, were not harmful to mouse, rat, or rabbit embryos, whereas after 150 mg/kg and 200 mg/kg the number of resorptions was increased in mice and in rats. Malformations (cleft palate and spina bifida) were found in 5%–22% of the rat foetuses and in 5%–10% of the mouse foetuses. JAEGER et al. (1974) also observed cleft palate, rib and vertebral deformities, an increased number of resorptions, and retardation and increased weights at birth on treating pregnant mice with 2×250 mg/kg on the 9th and 10th days of gestation. The cytochrome oxidase activity was reduced and the embryonic mitochondria appeared swollen. In rabbits too, the higher doses of 150 and 200 mg/kg were embryotoxic. However, in contrast to the mice and the rats, teratogenic effects were not found.

After administration by inhalation, rifampicin was found to pass through the placenta in rats, without at the same time causing teratogenic damage (ANUFRIEVA et al. 1980a, b).

6. Ototoxicity

Subacute studies on mice and on rabbits lasting 8 days and chronic studies on mice with treatment lasting 3 months revealed that rifampicin does not damage the organs of hearing and balance (KLUYSKENS 1969). FELGENHAUER and LAGLER (1970) did not observe any significant effect on post-rotatory nystagmus follow-

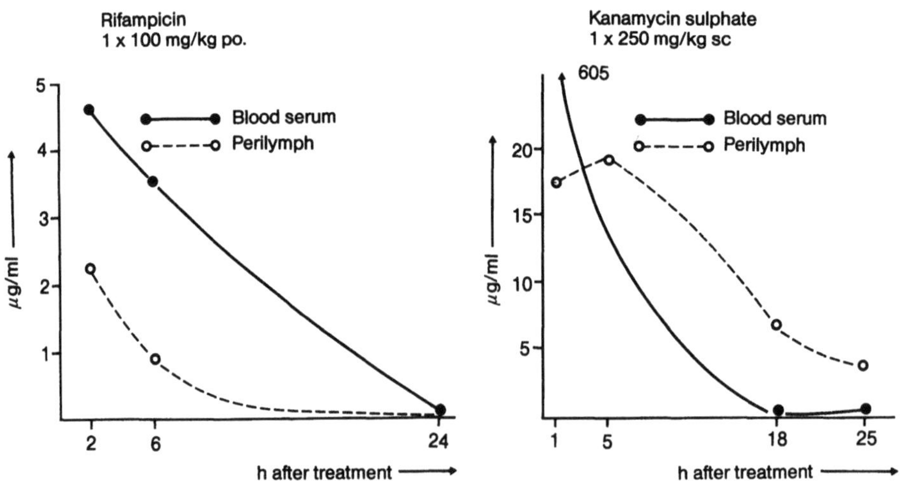

Fig. 1. Concentrations of rifampicin and kanamycin in guinea pig serum and perilymph (after FELGENHAUER and LAGLER, 1970). This shows the substantially higher and longer-lasting concentration of kanamycin in the perilymph as compared to rifampicin

ing oral administration of 50 mg/kg and 150 mg/kg for 31 days. Thus, these investigations showed rifampicin to be non-vestibulotoxic. In contrast to Kluyskens, however, Felgenhauer and Lagler observed penetration of rifampicin into the perilymph in guinea pigs, although only to a small extent (Fig. 1). However, the substance is eliminated from the perilymph much faster than from the blood serum, so that it does not accumulate and reach toxic concentrations. This is an essential difference between rifampicin and the ototoxic antibiotics streptomycin, kanamycin, viomycin, and neomycin.

7. Carcinogenicity

During a follow-up observation period of 10 months BICHL (1973) did not observe any increase in the incidence of malignant tumours in BALB/c mice after 20 subcutaneous injections of 0.3 mg RMP. However, DELLA PORTA et al. (1978) observed an increased incidence of hepatomas in female C3Hf mice after the administration of increasing doses of RMP in the drinking water. In males of the same strain, in BALB/c mice, and in Wistar rats, however, the spontaneous tumour incidence remained the same. An influence on hormonal mechanisms by RMP is suggested as a possible explanation for the difference between the sexes in C3Hf mice.

8. Mutagenicity

Mutagenicity studies with RMP in Drosophila melanogaster (lethal recessive X-chromosome mutations) and in human leucocyte chromosomes in vitro revealed no evidence of genetic effects caused by this substance (VOGEL and OBE 1973). SRB et al. (1974) also failed to find any chromosomal aberrations in HeLa and HEp-2 cells, although RNA synthesis was inhibited.

9. Interactions with Other Drugs

After 14 days of combined treatment of rats with 15 mg/kg or 30 mg/kg RMP plus 5 mg/kg INH HUGUES et al. (1969) observed, besides steatosis, cellular damage of the liver in 7 out of 31 animals. However, treatment with RMP alone was devoid of toxicity. INH (5 mg/kg) alone or in combination with PTH (10 mg/kg) as well as RMP (15 mg/kg) in combination with PTH (10 mg/kg) produced similar degrees of steatosis but no hepatocellular injuries as seen after combined treatment with INH + RMP (HUGUES et al. 1970). In contrast, in healthy and tuberculous mice no drug releated fatty degeneration of the liver was observed after the administration of rifampicin alone or in combination with isoniazid (BALEA et al. 1970).

References

Anufrieva RG, Zeltser IZ, Svinogeeva TP (1980a) Placenta permeability by rifampicin (Russ.). Antibiotiki 25:199–201

Anufrieva RG, Zeltser IZ, Balabanova EL, Lapchinskaya AV, Baru RV, Svinogeeva TP (1980b) Experimental study of rifampicin effect on albino rat embryo genesis (Russ.). Antibiotiki 25:280–284

Balea T, Marche C, Marche J (1970) Effets hépato-biliaires de l'association rifampicine-isoniazide. II. Etude histologique chez la souris tuberculisée. Thérapie 25:125–130
Bichl J (1973) Rifampicin in a carcinogenic experiment. Lancet 2:1209
Della Porta G, Cabral JR, Rossi L (1978) Carcinogenicity study of rifampicin in mice and rats. Toxicol Appl Pharmacol 43:293–302
Epstein SS, Arnold E, Andrea J, Bass W, Bishop Y (1972) Detection of chemical mutagens by the dominant lethal assay in the mouse. Toxicol Appl Pharmacol 23:288–325
Felgenhauer F, Lagler F (1970) Experimental animal investigations with rifampicin on the question of its influence on the vestibular system and its period of retention in the perilymph of the inner ear. Antibiot Chemother 16:361–368
Furesz S (1970) Chemical and biological properties of rifampicin. Antibiot Chemother 16:316–351
Hugues F-C, Marche C, Marche J (1969) Effets hépato-biliaires de l'association rifampicine-isoniazide. I. Etude histologique chez le rat. Thérapie 24:899–906
Hugues F-C, Marche C, Marche J (1970) Effets hépato-biliaires de l'association rifampicine-prothionamide. I. Etude histologique chez le rat. Thérapie 25:131–136
Jaeger E, Merker HJ, Bass R (1974) Investigations on the mode of teratogenic action of high doses of rifampicin. Teratology 10:312
Jezequel AM, Orlandi F, Tenconi LT (1971) Changes of the smooth endoplasmic reticulum induced by rifampicin in human and guinea-pig hepatocytes. Gut 12:984–987
Kluyskens P (1969) Recherches expérimentales de toxicité otovestibulaire des rifamycines. Acta Tuberc Pneumol Belg 60:323–326
Piriou A, Warnet JM, Jacqueson A, Claude JR, Truhaut R (1979) Fatty liver induced by high doses of rifampicin in the rat: possible relation with an inhibition of RNA polymerase in eukaryotic cells. Arch Toxicol Suppl 2:333–337
Schiatti P, Maggi N, Sensi P, Maffii G (1967) Biliary excretion rate of semisynthetic rifamycins in the rat. Chemotherapia 12:155–171
Sensi P, Maggi N, Füresz S, Maffii G (1967) Chemical modifications and biological properties of rifamycins. Antimicrob Agents Chemother 1966:699–714
Srb V, Puza V, Spurna V, Kerptova J (1974) The action of rifampicin on stabilized cell lines HEp-2 and HeLa. Experientia 30:484–486
Tuchmann-Duplessis H, Mercier-Parot L (1969) Influence d'un antibiotique, la rifampicine, sur le développement prénatal des rongeurs. CR Acad Sc (Paris) Série D 269:2147–2149
Vogel E, Obe G (1973) Testing of rifampicin on possible genetic effects on Drosophila melanogaster and human leukocyte chromosomes in vitro. Experientia 29:124–125

CHAPTER 6

Mode of Action, Biotransformation and Pharmacokinetics of Antituberculosis Drugs in Animals and Man

H. IWAINSKY

Abbreviations

SM	= streptomycin	CM	= capreomycin
TSC	= thiacetazone, thiosemicarbazone	RMP	= rifampicin
PAS	= p-aminosalicylic acid	ATP	= adenosine triphosphate
INH	= isoniazid	-(P)	= -phosphate
PZA	= pyrazinamide	Glu-6-(P)	= glucose-6-phosphate
CS	= D-cycloserine	Glu-1-(P)	= glucose-1-phosphate
TC	= tetracyclines	Fru-6-(P)	= fructose-6-phosphate
KM	= kanamycin	NAD	= nicotinamide-adenine dinucleotide
DATC	= dithiocarbanilide, thiocarlide	m-RNA	= messenger-RNA
VM	= viomycin	t-RNA	= transfer-RNA
ETH/PTH	= ethionamide, protionamide	MIC	= minimal inhibitory concentration
EMB	= ethambutol	$t_{50\%}$	= half-life

A. General Part

The biological activity of a drug determined in vitro (e.g., the minimal inhibitory concentration) is a parameter decisive in determining the effect of antituberculotics on mycobacteria in a disease focus. Knowledge of the mode of action yields further therapeutically important information, such as whether intervention of the agent in the bacterial metabolism has any serious consequences or whether the damage is reversible within limits, depending on concentration or time. In addition, the risk of the development of resistance and the incidence of certain side effects in the host organism can be assessed, though it is currently possible only to a moderate extent to derive a proposal for a useful combination therapy on the basis of the mode of action of the drugs in question (Table 1).

The dose to be used in man or in animals will be influenced very strongly by biotransformation processes and by the pharmacokinetics of the original substance and their products of biotransformation. Because of the loss of biological activity often associated with these biotransformation processes, in the case of antituberculotics that undergo strong biotransformation such as INH, PAS, or ETH, the concentration of the active compound falls off very rapidly and to a considerable extent. When conventional combination therapy is used, the biotransformation processes of the combination partners are influenced by interaction only in a few cases. However, when RMP, with its inducing action, is repeat-

Table 1. Type of activity of antituberculosis drugs, determined in vitro. (After EULE et al. 1973; DÜRCKHEIMER 1975; KÄPPLER 1986)

Bacteriostatic	Bactericidal
TSC	SM, INH, PZA
PAS, CS	KM, VM
TC, EMB[a]	ETH/PTH, RMP
DATC, CM	

[a] The classification of EMB is disputable; see pp 199, 200

edly administered over a prolonged period, its own biotransformation is initially intensified and the inducing effect extended also to other drugs (NOCKE-FINK et al. 1973; POWELL-JACKSON et al. 1982; TEUNISSEN and BAKKER 1984). Conversely, a number of inducing drugs exert an influence on the biotransformation of RMP.

As a rule, biotransformation processes also alter the pharmacokinetics of the newly formed products, depending on their structure. It is by these processes that the course of the concentration of the biologically active fraction in the individual organs and compartments is determined. The concentration and its variation at the site of action, which are further influenced by the mode of administration, the administration interval, and the dose, are thus established.

Sufficient efficacy of the concentration attainable at the desired site of action is undoubtedly provided by the doses normally used today, the administration interval, and the duration of therapy. There are evidently close correlations between the concentration of antituberculosis drugs and the induction of adverse reactions (EULE et al. 1974a, b; MITCHELL et al. 1975; GOLDSHTEIN et al. 1977; SOLOVIEV et al. 1977; NAKAGAWA et al. 1981). Specific effects, such as the ototoxicity of SM and other antibiotics, can be attributed to an accumulation of these drugs in the respective compartments.

Serious alterations must ultimately be expected in patients with kidney and liver function disorders or a reduced excretion, when the organs responsible for these processes are damaged (KAMINSKAYA and KARACHUNSKY 1975; TYTOR 1976; ACOCELLA 1978).

I. Mode of Action of Antituberculosis Drugs

1. Type of Effect and Primary Site of Attack

a) Type of Effect

The effect of antituberculosis drugs determined in vitro depends on a large number of factors, among which the metabolic activity of the microorganism depending on the cell cycle is particularly important – continously respectively slowly or intermittent metabolising, semidormant bacilli – (MCCARTHY 1981;

ACOCELLA 1984; GIRLING 1984). While inhibition of the logarithmic phase of growth can be determined without any special experimental problems, an effect on nonproliferating microorganisms (socalled persisters) can only be detected under special conditions. The effect of INH even on non-proliferating mycobacteria was reliably confirmed at a relatively early stage (BARTMANN 1960). In model studies on short-term therapy with intermittent medication the sterilizing effect of RMP was attributed to its special effect on "resting" mycobacteria (GROSSET 1978; DICKINSON and MITCHISON 1981).

Even with bactericidal agents a phase of reversible inhibition of the metabolic processes precedes the irreversible damage. The relevance of the concentration-time product, or of an "effect factor" derived from it, for the extent of damage is thus again confirmed. In the case of INH there is a good correlation with in-vivo results (JENNE and BEGGS 1973). However, testing the MIC under different conditions – e.g., with a constant concentration, with rapidly falling off concentration or with pulsed exposure (PERUMAL et al. 1985) – even though the concentration-time product remains the same, the intensity of the effect is modified, especially with regard to the lag phase before the recommencement of growth of sensitive microorganisms or with regard to the effect on resistant pathogens (BEGGS and JENNE 1969; AWANESS and MITCHISON 1973; BONDAREV and BOLGAYA 1980).

Despite this detailed knowledge, in classification of the type of effect it is still considered expedient to carry out a subdivision into antituberculotics with bacteriostatic or bactericidal activity (Table 1).

b) Experimentally Determined Problems in the Search for the Primary Site of Attack

At the end of the 1950's comprehensive studies were commenced with great engagement into the action mechanism of antituberculosis drugs. It was hoped to replace rapidly the hitherto semi-empirical approach to the development of new chemotherapeutics by planned syntheses based on concepts derived from molecular-biology. The aim of producing tailor-made drugs was evidently evaluated more optimistically at that time than today (ZÄHNER 1977; KÖNIG 1980; GROS et al. 1981; VON DER HAAR et al. 1981; HAMACHER 1981).

Particular problems arose during studies on antituberculotic agents that don't interfere with protein synthesis.

In conventional whole-cell cultures three processes influenced in different ways by the structure of the drug used were regarded as a single magnitude (inhibitory concentration), namely the binding of the drug to the bacterial surface, its permeation through cell wall and membrane and the chemical reaction within the bacterial cells (NODZU and WATANABE 1961). The dependence of the activity of PZA on the pH of the nutrient medium, has long been known (GROSSET 1978). Furthermore, with some antituberculotics it was suspected that the active compound proper was only formed once the drug had penetrated the cell. Recently, by using highly sensitive methods, it has been possible to determine the fraction absorbed by the microorganism and thus to resolve the overall process into individual sub-processes.

Compared with the effort invested the results of this work were unsatisfactory, and this for the following reasons:

1. Inappropriate experimental procedure: to obtain demonstrable effects excessively long incubation periods were used with high antituberculotic concentrations, as a result of which differentiation between the effect at the primary point of attack, secondary metabolic dysfunction, and the breakdown of the metabolism is no longer possible.
2. One-sided or erroneous interpretations: a change in the parameter under determination need not indicate the primary site of attack. Only by measuring several parameters within a metabolic process with time-related differentiation can erroneous interpretation be largely excluded.
3. Inadequate reproducibility: experience has shown that the growth of mycobacteria in a liquid nutrient medium depends on many factors, not all of which are yet known. In addition to this, for difficulties in timing, microorganisms of various subcultures from the solid nutrient medium often have to be used as inoculum. This makes an evaluation of experiments carried out at different times for technical reasons extremely difficult, since the reference values rarely remain constant.
4. Incomplete knowledge of the metabolism of mycobacteria: in the course of investigations essential gaps in our knowledge of the metabolic processes in this type of bacteria have emerged, and our insights into their regulation cannot be said to be more than sporadic (ROBSON and SULLIVAN 1963; GOLDBERG 1965; YOUATT 1969; IWAINSKY 1970; IWAINSKY and KÄPPLER 1974; KRÜGER-THIEMER et al. 1975; REUTGEN 1975; WHITE 1975; RATLEDGE 1977; WINDER 1984).
5. Inappropriate statement of the problem: a number of working hypotheses were based on inapplicable notions to molecular-biological processes. In many cases it was not until the rapid development of biochemistry in the 'sixties and 'seventies that the prerequisites for target-oriented studies were created. On the other hand, some of the gaps in our knowledge of the metabolism of mycobacteria have been filled by studies on the mode of action.

c) Consequences of Studies on the Primary Site of Attack

At the end of 1950's many structurally analogous compounds and in some cases INH and PAS derivatives that had already been introduced into therapy were included in these studies. Essential information was thus obtained concerning the influence exerted by the changes made in the molecular structure on the absorption process and the structure-effect relationships, resulting, inter alia, in the abondonment of the use of INH and PAS derivatives for clinical purposes. With regard to the side effects of antituberculotics it very quickly became evident that a primary site of attack on microorganisms and on the macroorganism, quantitatively different but fundamentally the same, is not the sole reason for the occurrence of side effects. It is more likely that the apparently minor modifications of the pharmacokinetics are responsible. The development of a combination therapy based on the mode of action (MIŠON AND TRNKA 1973) did not get beyond the first few steps.

Reliably effective standard therapeutic programmes with treatment periods of 12 months to 18 months were developed and outstanding successes were thus achieved in the highly industrialized countries. After the introduction of RMP in the early 1970's the experimental basis for intermittent therapy was worked out (MITCHISON 1979) before optimization of the chemotherapy could be tackled. At present questions relating to short-term therapy are at the focus of interest (EULE et al. 1974b, 1985; GROSSET 1978, 1981; ZIERSKI 1981; ACOCELLA 1984; GIRLING 1984; BARTMANN et al. 1985; O'BRIEN and SNIDER 1985).

In the last years several new drugs respectively derivatives of RMP with improved pharmacokinetics have been developed. Beside amikacin, a semisynthetic rifamicin – FCE 22250 –, cyclopentyl-rifamicin – DL 473 –, ansamycin, a spiropiperidyl derivative of rifamicin S – LM 427 – and the group ciprofloxacin, ofloxacin, norfloxacin (TRUFFOT-PERNOT et al. 1985; O'BRIEN and SNIDER 1985; TSUKAMURA 1985a, b; TSUKAMURA et al. 1985, 1986; MADSEN et al. 1986; UNGHERI et al. 1986) have been tested against a variety of mycobacteria. Now they all are under investigation in animal models, only a few in clinical trials. If possible they will be used for treatment of drug resistant tuberculosis, of other mycobacterial diseases including lepra, for intermittent chemotherapy of tuberculosis once weekly and for treatment of other life threatening infectious diseases (LLORENS-TEROL et al. 1981; OBERTI et al. 1981; WATTEL et al. 1981; EULE et al. 1985; ISEMAN et al. 1986). The concentration of work on finding an effective and reliable, intermittent short-term therapy, preferably to be given to out-patients, yielded excellent results and improved acceptability to the patient. The resulting financial savings, despite the relatively high price of RMP, also opened up new ways for young nations to initiate effective treatment of tuberculosis.

2. Transport of Antituberculotics to the Site of Action

a) Permeation Through the Cell Membrane

As is well known, the structure, the lipid-solubility, and the pKa value are important for permeation of substances through the cell membrane. Besides the uptake due to diffusion, active transport processes counter concentration gradients have been detected, which are accelerated to a greater or lesser extent by the addition of energy-supplying nutrients. In mycobacteria the alteration of the cell membrane occurring as a secondary effect after exposure to INH, CS, or ETH/PTH (loss of stability to acids) certainly also results in a modification of the permeation processes, whose extent and consequences have so far scarcely been investigated.

b) Uptake of Antituberculosis Drugs by the Microorganisms

Apart from these factors (2. a), the following are important for the uptake of antituberculotics: the drug concentration in the nutrient medium and the age of the pathogens and their metabolic activity, which is influenced by the supply of oxygen and nutrients (ARIMA and IZAKI 1963; EDA 1963a; IZAKI and ARIMA 1965; VIDEAU 1968; BEGGS and JENNE 1969; YOUATT 1969; YOUATT and THAM 1969a; MCCARTHY 1981). Antituberculotics are incorporated very rapidly. For example, the SM-depending induction of a permease necessary for the incorporation of SM is completed within minutes. Addition of chloramphenicol inhibits the synthesis of this permease, but only when this takes place simultaneously with the incorporation of SM does it protect the microorganism from the bactericidal effect of SM. Addition of the chloramphenicol 10 min later is no more effective (HURWITZ and ROSANO 1962). 3 min after its addition the effect of RMP is manifested in phages incorporated in mycobacteria (JONES and DAVID 1971). A few minutes after making contact with RMP the incorporation of nucleotides in the microbial nucleic acids is also inhibited (WHITE et al. 1971).

c) Biotransformation of Antituberculosis Drugs by Mycobacteria

The biotransformation products of antituberculosis drugs are difficult to isolate from mycobacteria and to identify. However, investigations of this kind allow useful conclusions to be drawn about the permeation of the original substance and the subsequently formed biotransformation products, about the enzymes intervening in these processes, and about the mode of action.

d) Distribution of Antituberculosis Drugs in Mycobacteria

The distribution of antituberculotics can be exactly determined only by using radiolabelled compounds, and even then it is very difficult to separate and to identify any biotransformation products formed. As can be seen from studies reported by a number of working groups, the bulk of PAS, INH, or of the corresponding biotransformation products is localized in the acid-soluble fraction of mycobacteria (EDA 1963b; TSUKAMURA et al. 1963) or can be extracted from the cell contents with water (ZEYER et al. 1960; YOUATT and THAM 1969b). In addition to a variable EMB fraction a second relatively small but firmly bound pool has been detected (BEGGS and AURAN 1972; BEGGS and ANDREWS 1973a, b).

e) Uptake and Biotransformation of Antituberculosis Drugs in the Development of Resistance against Antituberculotics

Studies performed in parallel on drug-sensitive, resistant, and dependent strains have proved very informative about the mechanisms underlying the development of resistance, about the secondary metabolic alterations, and in some cases also about the mode of action (UDOU et al. 1986).

3. Mode of Action of Antituberculosis Drugs

In correspondence with their primary site of attack the antituberculotics can be divided into three groups:

- drugs that primarily attack the nucleic-acid or protein synthesis (RMP, SM, KM, VM, CM, TC);
- drugs that primarily attack the biosynthesis of the microbial cell wall (CS);
- drugs with sites of attack localized predominantly in the soluble fraction of microorganisms (TSC, DATC, ETH/PTH, PAS, INH, PZA, EMB).

a) Nucleic Acid and Protein Synthesis as the Primary Site of Attack

Whereas it is possible to have a disturbance of protein synthesis without a simultaneous disturbance of the nucleic-acid synthesis, interference with the formation or the metabolism of nucleic acids inevitably leads to disturbances in protein synthesis in view of the matrix function of the nucleic acids.

The nucleic acids, divisible into DNA, (m)-RNA and (t)-RNA, all have the same structural principle. A certain number of nucleotides are bonded to one another by phosphate residues in diester bonding (KÜCHLER 1976; KARLSON 1984; RAPOPORT 1985). In the double helix of the DNA, the carrier of genetic information, specific purine or pyrimidine bases connected by hydrogen bridges are always situated opposite one another (guanine-cytosine and adenine-thiamine or adenine-uracil). The base sequence that results from this structural principle on the double helix constitutes the genetic code for the amino acid sequence of the protein to be synthesized. Each three neighbouring bases (codons) determine one amino acid, further codons functioning as start and stop signals.

With the aid of a polymerase a second strand of complementary structure is synthesized in the course of identical replication on a single strand of DNA. The use of radiolabelled nucleotides allows an elegant demonstration that each of the two molecules newly formed from a DNA double helix contains one daughter and one mother strand.

Transcription, the transfer of information to the ribosomes, the site of protein synthesis, takes place with the aid of the m-RNA. Its synthesis proceeds in the same way as the identical replication, with uncoiling of part of the DNA double helix (Fig. 1 – HARTMANN et al. 1968; RÜGER 1972; RICHARDSON 1975). A DNA-dependent RNA polymerase (RNA-nucleotidyl-transferase, transcriptase) is necessary for this purpose.

Protein synthesis takes place in the ribosomes by the collaboration of ribosomal RNA, m-RNA synthesized at the location of the DNA, and several t-RNA, each of them specific to one amino acid. The m-RNA carrying the start codon (AUG or GUG) is attached to a 30-S ribosome subunit. A t-RNA carrying

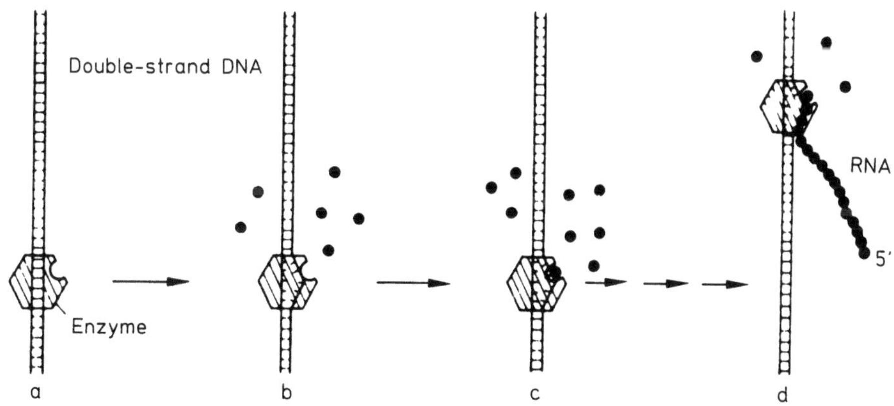

Fig. 1. Synthesis of m-RNA from ribonucleotides with the aid of DNA-dependent RNA polymerase (HARTMANN et al. 1968). • ˙. ˙. Ribonucleotides

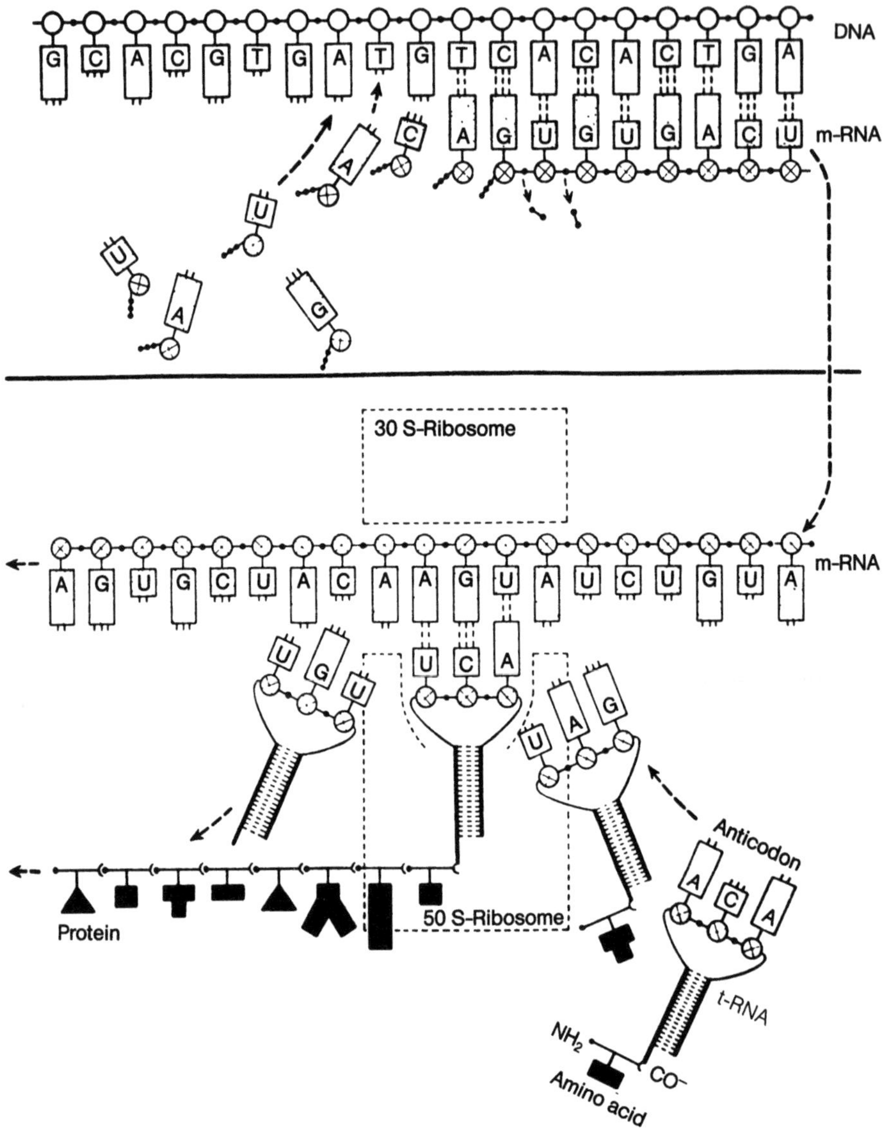

Fig. 2. Schematic representation of protein synthesis (DUBININ 1965). *Top,* Synthesis of m-RNA on a DNA strand (cf. Fig. 1); – – →, Transport of m-RNA to the ribosomes; A C, Purine and pyrimidine bases of DNA, m-RNA, and t-RNA; Y ■, Amino acids bound to t-RNA or to the polypeptide chain

the appropriate anticodon and laden with formylmethionine is added on. The energy supplying positioning of a 50-S ribosome subunit with the release of initiation factors leads to a functional initial complex. As a result of this arrangement of the two ribosomal subunits, an A-attachment site for aminoacyl-t-RNA is simultaneously produced. The next t-RNA bearing a corresponding amino acid is bound to this A-attachment site and with the aid of a peptidyl-transferase the peptide bond between the amino acid and the N-formylmethionine is formed, setting free the t-RNA bound to this compound. The resulting dipeptidyl-t-RNA is displaced to a P-attachment site in a translocation reaction and protein synthesis continues with the addition of the next aminoacyl-t-RNA to the A-attachment site. Besides the peptidyl-transferase and a transport factor, 3 initiation factors are necessary. Once the synthesis is over, the ribosomes, which are built up from 53 proteins and 3 nucleic acids, break down again into their subunits (Fig. 2 – DUBININ 1965; KÜCHLER 1976; GASSEN 1982; KARLSON 1984; RAPOPORT 1985).

RMP inhibits the DNA-dependent polymerases of bacterial origin (HONIKEL et al. 1968), while the remaining antibiotics, interfere with the bacterial protein synthesis. The protein synthesis taking place on 80-S ribosomes in eukaryotic cells remains undisturbed. TC has been shown to act both on 70-S and on 80-S ribosomes, the synthesis inhibition at the 80-S ribosomes being, however, far smaller than that at the 70-S ribosomes.

b) Biosynthesis of the Microbial Cell Wall as the Primary Site of Attack

A number of antibiotics, such as penicillins and CS, inhibit the synthesis of murein, which stabilizes the cell membrane (Fig. 3 – WEIDEL 1964). The requisite precursors consist of a lactic acid N-acetylglucosamine ether linked to a pentapeptide. The first three amino acids in most microorganisms are L-alanine, D-glutamic acid, and L-lysine, and in mycobacteria L-alanine, D-glutamic acid, and meso-diaminopimelic acid. This tripeptide is extended by the dipeptide D-alanyl-D-alanine. For this to happen 2 molecules of L-alanine are transformed by a racemase and the dipeptide is formed with the aid of a synthetase (Fig. 4 – STROMINGER and TIPPER 1965; DICKINSON and MITCHISON 1985). As a result of inhibition of these enzymes, as after exposure to CS, precursors begin to accumulate. Other antibiotics, such as penicillin, interfere with the cross-linking. The peptidoglycan skeleton then has only a low degree of cross-linking and weakened stabilizing function.

c) Antituberculosis Drugs Attacking in the Acid-Soluble Fraction of Microorganisms are Dealt with in the Special Part

II. Biotransformation

The biotransformation processes taking place as the drug passes through the organism influence pharmacokinetic parameters and thus the intensity and duration of the drug's action. As a result of such processes relatively lipophilic drugs are converted into hydrophilic, faster and easier eliminated biotransformation products. These newly formed compounds are distributed predominantly in the extracellular space, renal absorption being extensively inhibited.

1. Site of the Biotransformation

Biotransformation processes can take place in the liver, the gastro-intestinal tract, lungs, kidneys, and adrenals. However, normally some two-thirds of the biotrans-

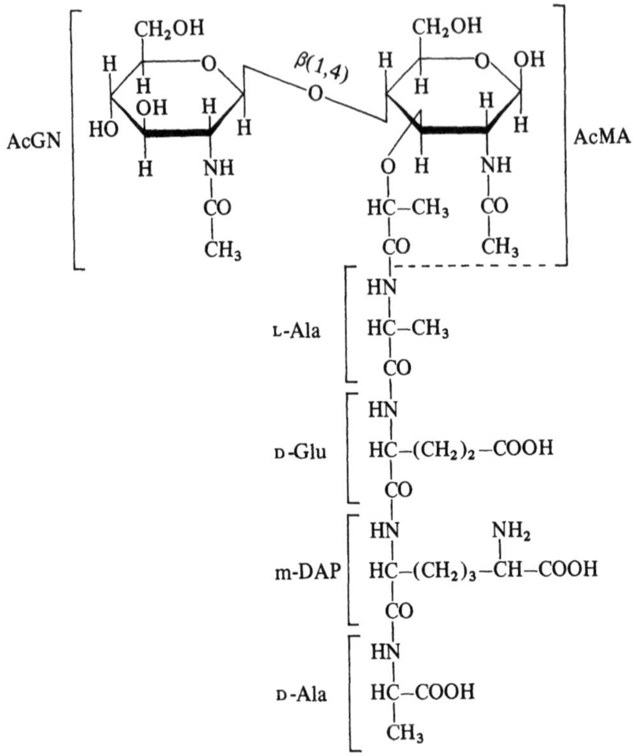

Fig. 3. Structure of a mucopeptide (using E. coli as an example – WEIDEL 1964)
AcGN, acetylglucosamine; *AcMA*, acetylmuraminic acid; *L-Ala, D-Ala*, L-, D-Alanine; *D-Glu*, D-glutamic acid; *mDAP*, m-2,6-diaminopimelic acid

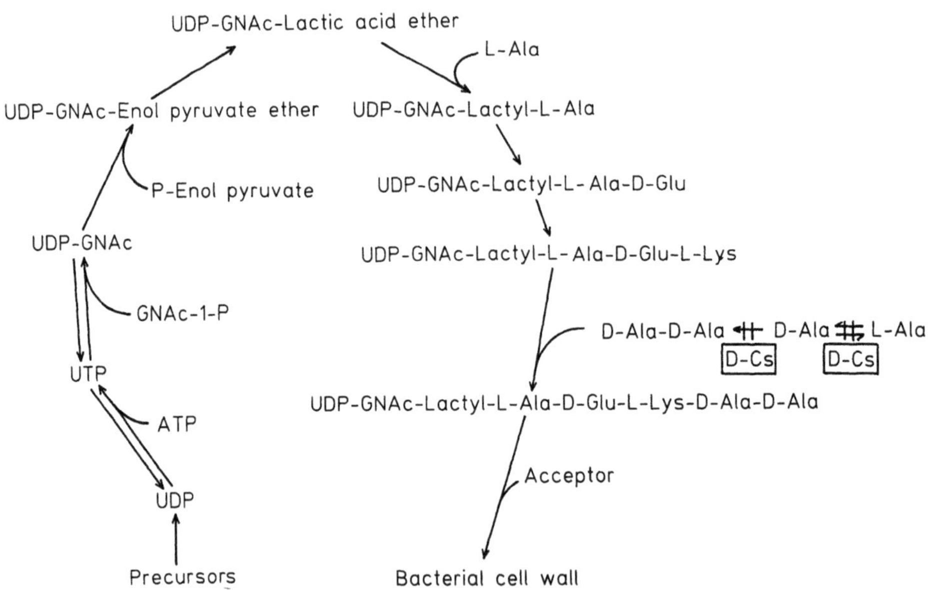

Fig. 4. Intervention of CS in mucopeptide synthesis necessary for formation of the bacterial cell wall (after STROMINGER and TIPPER 1965)
GNAc, Acetylglucosamine; *L-LYS*, L-lysine; *UDP*, Uridine diphosphate; *UTP*, Uridine triphosphate; otherwise as in Fig. 3

formation capacity resides in the hepatic endoplasmic reticulum (DARNIS 1976). Only in exceptional cases are comparable P-450 concentrations measured in certain cell groups of other organs (such as the Clara cells of the bronchial epithelium – SERABJIT-SINGH et al. 1980; DEVEREUX et al. 1981), the enzyme occurring here in several forms.

2. Possible Reactions

Biotransformation takes place as a result of enzymatically regulated catabolic and synthetic processes (PFEIFER and BORCHERT 1978; REICHERT 1981). A wide variety of chemical reaction types have been detected.

In the first stage they include ring-, side-chain-, and N-hydroxylations, hydrolysis reactions, reductions, N-demethylations, N-methylations, and dealkylations. These are followed in the second stage by conjugations with glucuronate, sulphate, acetate, or various amino acids, especially glycine. As a result of a reduced lipid solubility, by the loss or structural changes of the group responsible for the biological activity the biotransformation is in many cases a process of inactivation (HOLDINESS 1984). Especially conjugations lead to a loss of the biological effect. In the case of antituberculotics too the therapeutic effect, i.e., the concentration of biologically active compounds prevailing at the site of action, is often determined far more by biotransformation than by the distribution and elimination processes. With some antituberculosis drugs most of the administered dose is inactivated by biotransformation.

3. Factors Influencing Biotransformation

The biotransformation patterns and rates are usually constant in a given individual and are hereditary. Genetic control appears to be more active than environmental factors (VESELL 1972; ROOTS 1982). In studies on large groups of patients a genetically differently determined enzyme equipment, usually within the range of "health", is regarded as the range of biological variation, and adaptation of the dose to the concentration of biologically active compounds actually present in the macroorganism is rarely believed to be necessary. Only in the case of a few antituberculosis agents, such as RMP, has an additional influence of age or sex on the pharmacokinetics so far been found and the possibility of a modified biotransformation discussed (PORVEN and CANETTI 1968; IWAINSKY et al. 1974; VESELL 1981; WINSEL et al. 1985).

Induction of drug-degrading enzymes such as cytochrome Pm 450 can, however, influence the biotransformation of an inducing drug and/or of other drugs (NOCKE-FINK et al. 1973; EDWARDS et al. 1974; PETERS et al. 1974; SYVÄLÄHTI et al. 1974; SELF and MANN 1975). The excretion of RMP and of its biotransformation products with the urine falls off after only a few days of daily or intermittent administration (Fig. 5 – GRASSI 1971; IOFFE 1973; HOLDINESS 1984; LOOS et al. 1985; WINSEL et al. 1985). When certain fast-growing test strains no more inhibited by deacetyl-RMP are used for the determination, the serum $t_{50\%}$ also becomes shorter (CANETTI et al. 1970; GRASSI 1971). This so-called induction phase lasts between 4 weeks and 8 weeks, depending on the rhythm of administration.

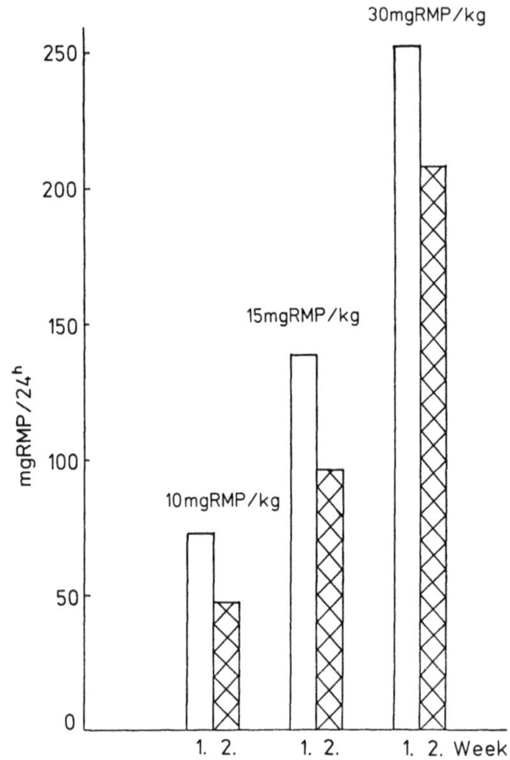

Fig. 5. Reduction of RMP excretion in the urine during the inducing phase. □, Excretion on the 1st day of treatment; ⊠, Excretion on the 8th day of treatment

After a 7-day drug-free interval values like those found at the start of the treatment can once again be measured. If, on the other hand, mycobacteria also sensitive to deacetyl-RMP are used in tests, the antituberculotic activity falls off only slightly during the induction phase in clinical therapy (IWAINSKY et al. 1974; KÖHLER and WINSEL 1982).

Induction of microsomal liver enzymes is thought to be the cause, as is indicated – though this has been contested – by the accelerated biotransformation after induction with phenobarbital, by the increase in NADPH-cytochrome C-reductase and in cytochrome Pm 450 concentration observed after treatment with RMP, and by the absence of an induction phase in patients with liver damage (SCHOENE et al. 1972; OTANI and REMMER 1975; HERKEN and GROSS 1982).

4. Influence of the Inductive Effect of RMP on the Biotransformation of Other Drugs

More than 200 drugs are known to have an inductor effect, but only in a few cases is it necessary to consider the effects of induction on the clinical results (LAMPE et al. 1981). In animal experiments RMP and its quinone exert an inductor activity dependent on the test strain used, manifested by an enlargement of the smooth endoplasmic reticulum of the hepatocytes (JEZEQUEL et al. 1971), and changes in the wavelenght of the P 450-CO complex.

The transient change is identical with that caused by phenobarbital or 3-methylcholanthrene, whereas a wavelength shift specific to RMP remains permanently (STOLTZ 1981).

This induction has only a very little effect on the biotransformation and pharmacokinetics of other antituberculotics administered side by side (PERRY et al. 1981). On the other hand, interference of RMP with endogenous compounds such as the bile acids and with drugs is repeatedly described (KROKER and HEGNER 1980; OKOLICSANYI et al. 1980; TEUNISSEN and BAKKER 1984), namely with cardiac glycosides, oral contraceptives (BOLT et al. 1974, 1975, 1976), oral antidiabetic drugs, dapsone, anticoagulants, narcotics and analgesics, corticosteroids, and others. It is usually sufficient to adjust the dose also in the case of steroid-dependent asthma (POWELL-JACKSON et al. 1982); only oral contraceptives have to be withdrawn (ACOCELLA and CONTI 1980). Specifically, there have been reports of interference between RMP and quinidine (AHMAD et al. 1979), between RMP and tolbutamide (ZILLY et al. 1977), between RMP and chlorpropamide (SELF 1980), between RMP and phenprocoumon (HELD 1979), and between RMP and methadone (BENDING and SKACEL 1977), between RMP and corticosteroids (BUFFINGTON et al. 1976; HENDRICKSE et al. 1979; SARMA et al. 1980; MCALLISTER et al. 1983).

5. Antituberculosis Treatment and Biotransformation

With the majority of antituberculosis drugs biotransformation processes reduce the biologically active fraction, even at therapeutic doses. In recovery studies with the antibiotics SM, CS, TC, KM, VM, and CM a 10 to 50% reduction of the original dose has been found, though it has not yet always been possible to detect the corresponding biotransformation products. The reactions responsible for the inactivation are also only incompletely known so far, the same is true for TSC.

In the case of EMB only about 10% of the administered quantity is converted. With RMP, despite the quantitatively modified biotransformation as a result of induction, the antimycobacterial activity in the serum remains largely intact (GRASSI 1971; IWAINSKY et al. 1976; KÖHLER and WINSEL 1982). With PAS, INH, PZA, and ETH the activity is distinctly reduced by biotransformation, the transformation processes being the same in each case (acetylation, coupling with glycine, and hydrolysis – Fig. 6). Moreover, in the case of ETH clear correlations with the biotransformation of nicotinamide or nicotinic acid can be deduced from the biotransformation pattern (GRUNERT 1969). However, in the event of equimolar administration of these 4 antituberculotics the individual biotransformation processes take place to different extents. In clinical use, in addition to the dose actually administered further factors such as the given combination partner, and in the case of INH polymorphism, are of importance for the biotransformed and thus inactivated fraction (RMP constituting an exception).

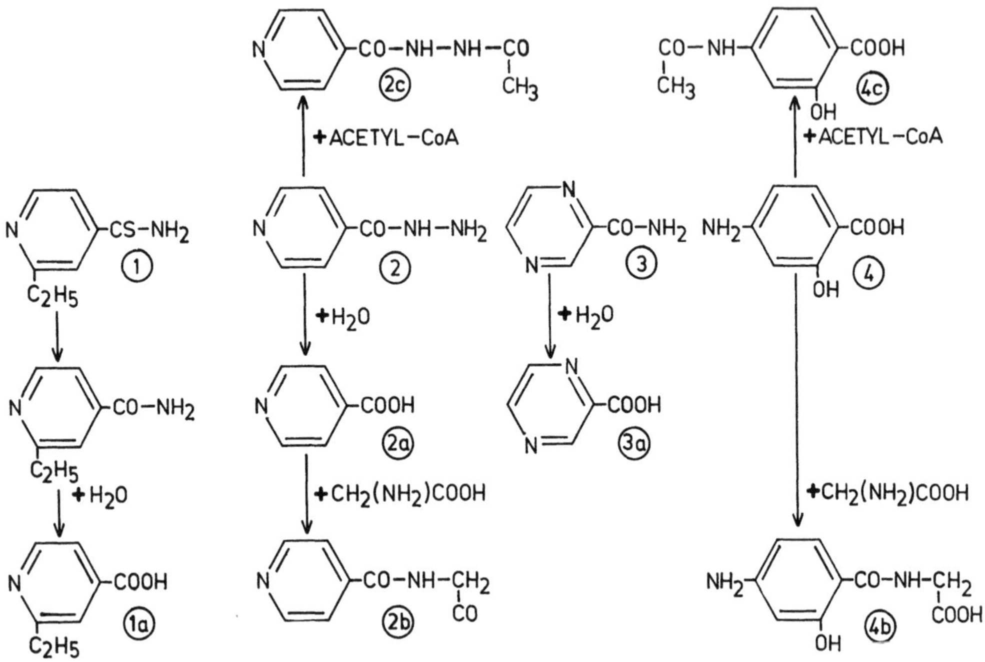

Fig. 6. Similar biotransformation processes (hydrolysis, acetylation, conjugation with glycine) of various antituberculosis drugs. 1:ETH; 2:INH; 3:PZA; 4:PAS; 1a, 2a: hydrolysis; 2b, 4b: conjugation; 2c, 4c: acetylation

III. Pharmacokinetics

1. Absorption of Antituberculosis Drugs

After parenteral administration the quantity of a substance introduced into the macroorganism is known and the speed of administration can at least be estimated. In contrast to this, the evaluation of the fraction absorbed after oral administration can be problematic. With the normal formulations, namely tablets, coated tablets, etc., the fraction present in dissolved form, but not yet absorbed (availments – DOST 1972, 1975) is influenced by a large number of factors (ZATHURECKY 1972). The pKa value of the antituberculotic and the pH value of the gastro-intestinal contents, as well as the intestinal motility (SCHANKER 1961; GOTHONI et al. 1972), determine the rate of absorption and the proportion absorbed. Moreover, the drugs with longer half-lives, such as RMP, reach parts of the intestine with a lower absorption capacity before they have been completely absorbed. The relationship between the dose and the serum concentration follows an S-shaped course (Fig. 7). In this case the increase ceases to be proportional at doses in excess of 1000 mg, which is attributed to a limited RMP-absorption capacity of the small intestine (KÖHLER and WINSEL 1982).

The mean quantity absorbed and the absorption half-life can be calculated with the aid of absorption constants or of the law of corresponding areas (WAGNER and NELSON 1963; CARPENTER et al. 1966; GIBALDI 1967; DOST 1972).

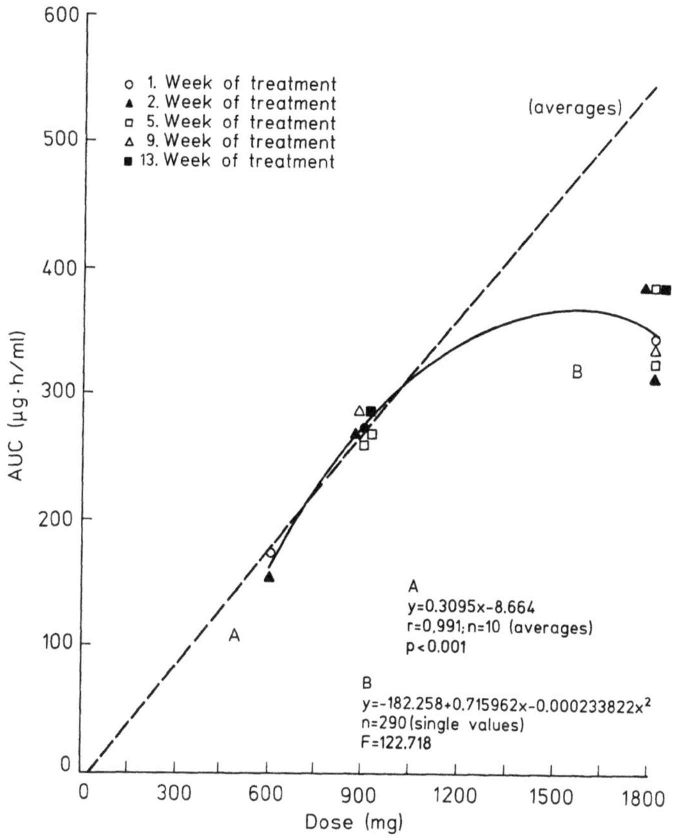

Fig. 7. Relationships between the RMP dose and AUC values in patients with pulmonary tuberculosis (KÖHLER and WINSEL 1982)

SM, KM, VM, and CM are absorbed in active form only to a very small extent after oral administration (SUREAU 1963; WELLES et al. 1966). Most antituberculosis drugs (SM, PAS, INH, KM, VM, ETH, CM, and RMP) – provided that an optimal mode of administration is used – are absorbed very rapidly (it takes 1 h to 2 h to reach the absorption elimination equilibrium = maximum of the serum concentration). With TSC, PZA, CS, TC, and EMB the absorption takes longer – up to 4 h (TATARINOVA et al. 1974). Very diverse time data are cited for DATC (LARKIN 1960; TACQUET et al. 1963; MEISSNER 1965; GUBLER et al. 1966; ROBINSON and HUNTER 1966; STEFFEN 1971).

In the case of the tetracyclines, if the quantity excreted with the urine is taken as a measure of absorption, the quantity absorbed depends on the distribution coefficient of the tetracycline in question, which is in turn determined by its structure. Thus, tetracycline is absorbed fastest and to the greatest extent, oxytetracycline and chlortetracycline less quickly, and demeclocycline least rapidly (see Table 2). The compounds developed later on, metacycline, doxycycline, and minocycline, on the other hand, are once again absorbed more rapidly and more

Table 2. Absorption of tetracyclines (measured on the basis of their urinary excretion – WALTER and HEILMEYER 1969)

Mode of administration	Excretion in 96 h (% of the administered dose)				
	Tetra-cycline	Oxytetra-cycline	Chlortetra-cycline	Demeclo-cycline	Rolitetra-cycline
p.o.	20–35	10–30	10–25	9–40	–
i.m.	40–60	40–60	–	–	40–60
i.v.	60	70	18	39	50–60

completely than oxytetracycline (ROBSON and SULLIVAN 1963; WALTER and HEILMEYER 1969; SENECA 1971; FOURTILLAN and SAUX 1978).

2. Factors Influencing the Absorption

a) Changes in Absorption due to a Different Mode of Administration

The mode of administration can influence both the pharmacokinetics and, in the event of bypass of the liver, the biotransformation rate as a result of the consequently diminished first-pass effect. It thus also has an influence on the biological activity and ultimately on the incidence of concentration-dependent side effects. In the treatment of tuberculosis an intravenous infusion of PAS and ETH helps to relieve the gastro-intestinal tract. Besides short-term infusion, prolonged infusion of higher doses of PAS is recommended. As expected, if this is done the antituberculotic concentrations are higher in the first few hours after the start of the infusion than in the case of oral administration (Fig. 8). At the end of the infusion, on the other hand, the concentration falls off more rapidly than after oral administration, since after i.v. administration the curve represents pure excretion whereas in oral administration we see the resultant absorption plus excretion (TACQUET et al. 1961; IWAINSKY et al. 1963; ORLOWSKI 1965; KUNTZ 1966; JUNGBLUTH and URBANCZIK 1974). Intravenous administration of RMP has only be-

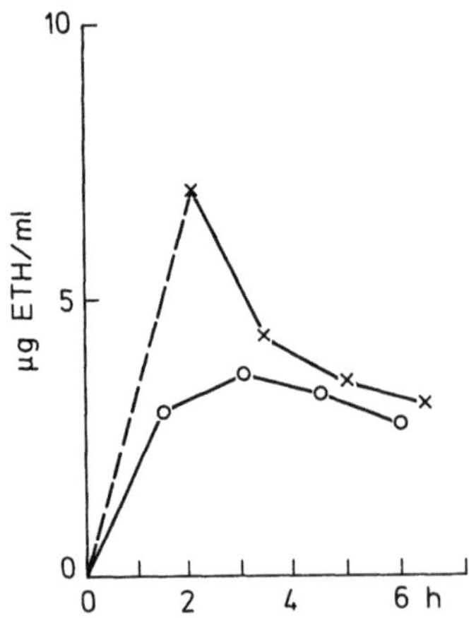

Fig. 8. Differences between serum ETH concentrations after intravenous infusion and oral administration. ×——×, 500 mg ETH i.v.; o——o, 500 mg ETH p.o. (IWAINSKY et al. 1965)

come possible in the last years as a result of special formulations and is normally used only in seriously ill patients (NILSSON and BOMAN 1981; WATTEL et al. 1981; NITTI et al. 1981).

Rectal administration generally gives rise to lower concentrations in the serum and, in the case of ETH, also to a change in the biotransformation process (HAEGI 1961; PÜTTER 1961; SIMÁNE and KRAUS 1962, 1963; GAJEWSKA 1967). In rectal administration of PZA or CS the reduced excretion of both these antituberculotics with the urine compared with that after oral administration indicates the occurrence of reduced absorption (SIMÁNE et al. 1964). Rectal administration is therefore recommended only for patients with serious gastro-intestinal disorders (MIKHAILOVA et al. 1974).

b) Influence of Structural Modifications of Drugs on Their Absorption

Modifications in the structure of antituberculosis drugs are made for two reasons. In the case of the rapidly absorbed compounds the aim of derivative formation is to achieve a slower absorption, avoiding the potentially risky concentration peaks and making the concentration curve run in the active region, i.e. above the MIC, for a longer time. With this aim SM derivatives, substituted PAS compounds, numerous hydrazones of INH and PZA derivatives have been tested and brought onto the market (FELDER et al. 1964; BARONTI and MANFREDI 1968; SMIRNOW 1972; SZABO and KISFALYDY 1973).

The second aim is to improve the absorption capacity of compounds or products and their pharmacokinetics i.e., to increase the efficacy without raising the dose, as e.g., with KM compounds (KUNIN 1966; FINLAND 1966) or TC derivatives (HIRSCH and FINLAND 1960; SCHACH VON WITTENAU et al. 1962; KNOTHE 1963; DIMMLING 1967; FEDORKO et al. 1968; KLASTERSKY and DANEAU 1972; DÜRCKHEIMER 1975). Starting from rifamicin, whose pharmacokinetics were very unfavourable for clinical application, and going through injectable rifamicin SV, it has been found possible by appropriate substitution (SCHIATTI and MAFFII 1967; SCHIATTI et al. 1967; HAEGI and MÜLLER 1967) to synthesize rifampicin with a half-life of 5 h to 6 h, FCE 22250 (semisynthetic rifamycin) with a half-life of 19 h in mice (O'BRIEN and SNIDER 1985) and finally cyclopentyl-rifamicin [3-(4-cyclopentyl-1-piperazinyl)iminomethylrifamicin SV] with a half-life of 24 h (TRUFFOT-PERNOT et al. 1983).

The SM-derivatives developed at the start of the 'seventies (WAGNER et al. 1971) have not been marketed. In the case of PAS and INH derivatives the hoped-for effects could not be achieved. Either – as is observed with most of the products – the quantity absorbed is substantially smaller than the quantity of the unchanged substance or the substituent is so loosely bound that the pharmacokinetics largely correspond to those of the original compound (MATSUZAKI and SAITO 1961; SHORT 1962; IWAINSKY et al. 1975; MYDLAK and VOLKMANN 1965). In addition, the slowly released unchanged compound undergoes greater biotransformation than after the administration of the original substance. This effect is manifested particularly clearly with PAS because of the high doses used (LEHMANN 1961). On intravenous administration of INH derivatives, it is difficult to determine the INH concentration in the serum and thus to evaluate the compound in question. Even when subtle determination methods are used it is very difficult to determine the INH exactly in the presence of a relatively large proportion of INH derivative (SCHWABE 1971; SAUERESSIG 1972). The results obtained with CS derivatives and tetracycline are more favourable. Terizidone [4,4'-phenylene-bis-(methyleneamino)-bis-3-isoazolidinone] is absorbed more rapidly and to a greater extent than CS (GAIDOV 1971; ZITKOVA and TOUŠEK 1973). The absorption of tetracycline is improved by the addition of chelating agents (ALTMAN et al. 1968).

c) Influence of Galenic Processing on the Absorption of Antituberculosis Drugs

By means of in-vitro studies the release of a drug from its pharmaceutical preparation can be clarified and optimized. In the last 15 years considerable methodological advances have been made in this sphere (JALSENJA et al. 1980; THOMA 1981; DE ZEEUW 1981). Thus, with justifiable expenditure, one can detect and possibly prevent the loss of biological efficacy due to activity-alternating interactions with inactive ingredients by degradation or modification of the drug itself (TC or CS, REGOSZ and ZUK 1980). The processes taking place in the inactive ingredients as a result of storage and influencing the bio-availability and release of the active substance can be likewise identified and prevented (GELBER et al. 1969; CIESZYNSKI 1971; Barr et al. 1972; ASKER et al. 1973a, b; TOMASSINI and NAPLATANOVA 1973; THOMA 1981).

PAS products, such as PAS bound to ion exchangers, tablets with an intestinal-juice-soluble coating (enteric-coated tablets), PAS granulate and the like have acquired clinical importance. The highest serum concentrations are achieved most rapidly with the dissolved PAS-Na salt (Fig. 9, WAGNER et al. 1973; PENTIKAINEN et al. 1973; SAVULA 1973). With most of the PAS preparations the absorp-

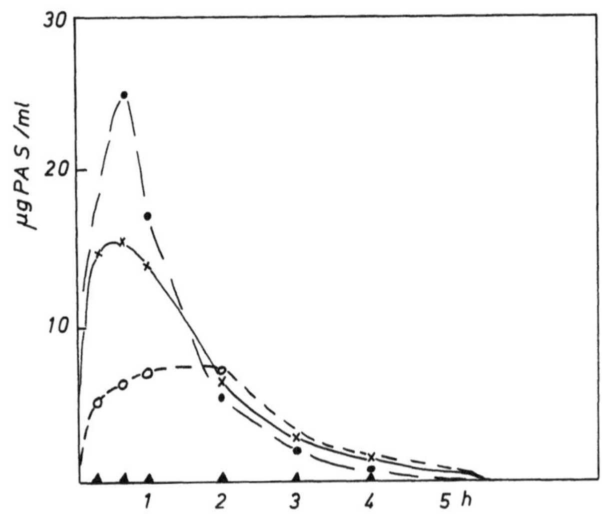

Fig. 9. Variation of serum PAS concentration after administration of various PAS preparations (WAGNER et al. 1973). ●---●, Solution of PAS-Na; ○---○, PAS tablets; ×——×, Suspension of PAS; ▲, PAS in enteric-coated tablets

tion is slower. The maximal serum concentrations are reached only after 4 h to 8 h (PAUL 1960; FROSTADT 1961; SELROSS 1961; HORNUNG et al. 1967; NIKODEMOWICZ et al. 1971). The very low, practically negligible, absorption of certain enteric-coated PAS tablets is surprising. Further-reaching interactions of PAS granulate were found by BOMAN et al. (1975). The bentonite used as an auxiliary agent adsorbed the RMP dose – given at the same time – very rapidly, and to such an extent that the bioavailability of the RMP was distinctly reduced.

In correspondence with a general trend, attempts have been made, especially with INH, to increase the efficacy while simultaneously reducing side effects by using retard preparations or liposomes (ABSHAGEN and DEMMER 1981; GREGORIADIS 1981). In animal experiments the administration of liposomes resulted in concentrations at the site of action 3 to 7 times higher than those after the administration of the dissolved drug (VLADIMIRSKY et al. 1980).

Slowly absorbable INH products with longer half-lives have been developed for the intermittent treatment of rapid inactivators (e.g., matrix INH, $t_{50\%}$ 4.5 h). As mentioned above, with these it is possible to increase the dose and at the same time to bring about a course of serum concentration that corresponds to that in slow inactivators (see Special Part, INH, Fig. 12; ELLARD et al. 1972; MITCHISON 1972; ELLARD et al. 1973; JEANES et al. 1973; EIDUS and HODGKIN 1975; KLEEBERG et al. 1975; ELLARD 1976).

The effects of antacids or of citric acid on the bio-availability of tetracycline under in-vitro conditions have already been revealed. However, in such investigations it is not always possible to predict the behaviour in-vivo (KHALIL et al. 1977; KORNER et al. 1978; MIYAZAKI et al. 1981). In animal experiments the absorption of tetracyclines is reduced in the presence of Ca^{++} and Fe^{++} ions but increased in the presence of Ca^{++} and salicylate, respectively by chelate formers such as ethylenediaminetetraacetic acid (POIGER and SCHLATTER 1979). The tetracycline concentration in the serum can be increased by combining chlortetracycline with tetracycline or by the use of rolitetracycline (VAN MARWYCK and GÄNGEL 1961; KNOTHE 1963; DIMMLING and WAGNER 1965).

All the attempts to improve the absorption of DATC (micronized powder, suspension of DATC in olive oil, etc.) have failed to give the desired result (MOODIE et al. 1964; EULE and WERNER 1966). The manufacture of enteric-coated ETH is evidently also problematic. In a comparison of products made by various companies different release and absorption rates were found (the latter determined on the basis of the serum concentration). The highest concentrations were attained with ETH hydrochloride or ETH dissolved in weak acids, the lowest with enteric-coated ETH (SIMÁNE and KRAUS 1963; GRÖNROOS and TOIVANEN 1964; VERBIST and DUTOIT 1966; MATTILA et al. 1967, 1968 b).

d) Influence of Food Consumption on the Absorption of Antituberculosis Drugs

The absorption of antituberculosis drugs is obviously impaired neither by other drugs nor by a reduction of the absorption area itself (experiments with INH and RMP); in the case of CS the absorption is accelerated. Only after repeated subtotal or total gastrectomy is the otherwise good absorption of EMB reduced by between 40% and 60% (KOB 1967; HAGELUND et al. 1977; KLEBER 1979). Gastric ulcers in the stage of exacerbation, on the other hand, give rise to a reduced absorption of INH (MIKHAILOVA et al. 1974). The water transfer through the intestine is only affected at toxic concentrations of ETH (MATTILA et al. 1968a).

Little is known about whether eating has any influence on the absorption of PAS. The process is unaffected by aluminium hydroxide (LANSDOWN and RADZIN 1963a, b). With INH and CS simultaneous or preceding (by up to an hour and a half) food consumption brings about slower and lower absorption; an aluminium hydroxide gel administered as an antacid has a similar effect (IWAINSKY and SIEGEL 1961; KOROTAEV and TATARINOVA 1972; HURWITZ and SCHLOZMAN 1974; MELANDER et al. 1976; KLEBER 1979) the absorption of EMB is not affected to any significant extent by simultaneous food consumption (PLACE et al. 1966).

Considerable individual differences and the alterations of the pharmacokinetics caused by induction are probably the reasons for the different assessments of the effect of food consumption on the absorption of RMP. Some authors have failed to find any differences caused by consumption of food or they only did so on the first day (BEEUWKES et al. 1969; HUSSELS 1969). Sex-linked and individual differences are manifested more strongly than those due to food intake (PORVEN and CANETTI 1968; HAGELUND et al. 1977). According to other investigations RMP is absorbed faster and to a greater extent on an empty stomach, with simultaneous shift of the peak serum concentration by 2 h (FURESZ et al. 1967; VERBIST and GYSELEN 1968; TSUKAMURA et al. 1972; SIEGLER et al. 1974; ZWOLSKA-KWIEK et al. 1975). Clinical observations also indicate that this is the case (GILL 1976). In extreme cases simultaneous consumption of food can largely prevent absorption (BEGG 1967).

3. Binding of Antituberculosis Drugs to Proteins and Blood Cells

Because of the important part it plays in the transport of substances to other compartments, in renal excretion, and in the decrease of concentration that can occur as a result of dialysis, the binding of antituberculotics to the serum proteins has been extensively studied by a variety of methods (SCHOLTAN 1964; FÜSGEN et al. 1977). The process is also important for the evaluation of the stability of antituberculotics and for their microbiological assay on protein-containing nutrient media. Studies on these special problems have been done with PZA, TC, VM, ETH, and RMP (PÜTTER 1961; PALLANZA et al. 1967; GRUNERT et al. 1968; CHOJKOWSKI 1971; KIVMAN and GEITMAN 1971, 1972; TOMCSÁNYI and JUHÁSZ 1973).

As can be seen from Table 3, TSC, CS, and KM are not bound by the serum proteins (SCHOLTAN 1964; KUNIN 1966; PINDELL 1966; PISSIOTIS et al. 1972; LEROY et al. 1978). SM is bound to the extent of 20%–34% (KUNIN 1967), PAS to between 58% and 73%, acetyl-PAS to more than 60%, and glycine-PAS to between 30% and 35% (JENNE 1964; KUNIN 1967).

Despite distinct interindividual scatter a correlation can be discerned between the bound fraction of PAS and the albumin concentration and a negative correlation between this magnitude and the bound fraction of acetyl-PAS (AOYAGI 1977). INH and acetyl-INH are bound little if at all, though binding is not ex-

Table 3. Binding of antituberculosis drugs to the serum proteins

Compound or biotransformation product	Bound fraction (%)	Compound or biotransformation product	Bound fraction (%)
TSC	Not bound		
SM	30–34	CS	Not bound
PAS	58–73	KM	Not bound
Acetyl-PAS	>60	DATC	Bound to erythrocytes? To the lipoprotein fraction?
Glycine-PAS	30–35	EMB	Bound to erythrocytes
INH	Small fractions	RMP	75–98
Acetyl-INH	Not bound		

Table 4. Binding of tetracyclines to the serum proteins

Compound	Bound fraction (%)	Authors
Tetracycline	20–28	Fabre et al. (1966)
	80	Fabre et al. (1967)
	55	Winkler andWeih (1967); Modr and Dvoracek 1976
	70	Benazet et al. (1968)
Oxytetracycline	23–42	Fabre et al. (1966)
	27	Fabre et al. (1967)
	34	Winkler and Weih (1967)
	20	Modr and Dvoracek (1966)
	10–15	Whelton (1974)
Chlortetracycline	42–54	Fabre et al. (1966)
	55	Fabre et al. (1967)
	87	Benazet et al. (1968)
	40–50	Whelton (1974)
Demeclocycline	34–48	Fabre et al. (1966)
	75	Fabre et al. (1967)
	68–91	Winkler and Weih (1967)
	89	Benazet et al. (1968)
Metacycline	84	Winkler and Weih (1967)
Doxycycline	25–31	Fabre et al. (1966)
	82	Fabre et al. (1967)
	82–93	Winkler and Weih (1967)
	Up to 90	Modr and Dvoracek (1976)
	80–95	Whelton (1974)

cluded for other biotransformation products of INH (MAHER and HANSEN 1960; CLAUNCH et al. 1963; JENNE 1964; KUNIN 1967). DATC may possibly be bound to erythrocytes or to the lipoprotein fraction (EMERSON and NICHOLSON 1965), whereas only small amounts of EMB are bound to proteins but considerable amounts to erythrocytes (PEETS and BUYSKE 1962; PLACE et al. 1966; PUJET and PUJET 1972; AOYAGI 1977).

Irrespective of the concentration in serum, between 75% and 98% of RMP is present in a bound form, the corresponding percentage at 5 °C being 65%. All the serum fractions are involved, half of the bound RMP being adsorbed on albumin (BEEUWKES et al. 1969; BINDA et al. 1971; BOMAN 1974; BOMAN and RINGBERGER 1974; AOYAGI 1977; ABAI and TOMCSANYI 1979).

By contrast, the binding of the tetracyclines depends on the serum concentration and on the pH value (DÜRCKHEIMER 1975). In studies on several samples relatively wide variation of the measurements was observed (BENNET et al. 1965; FABRE et al. 1966; BENAZET et al. 1968). Within the tetracycline group correlations are evident between the distribution coefficient (lipophilic/hydrophilic phase) and the strength of the binding; the more lipophilic the derivative, the more strongly is it bound to proteins (SCHACH VON WITTENAU and DELAHUNT 1966; SCHOLTAN 1968). The diketoenol system at C_{11}–C_{12} is principally responsible for the reaction with albumins. Among the tetracycline derivatives there are three groups with different binding strengths (Table 4 – PERENYI et al. 1971). According to studies on man, dogs, and rats, chlortetracycline is fixed most strongly, followed by demeclocycline and then by tetracycline and oxytetracycline (KUNIN and FINLAND 1961; SCHOLTAN 1968).

4. Distribution of Antituberculosis Drugs in the Body

The processes of permeation through cell membranes are important for the efficiency of antituberculotic drugs. Between the effect in vitro – directly estimated with the aid of radiolabelled antituberculotics (PLACE et al. 1966) or with phage-infected mycobacteria (STOTTMEIER et al. 1968; KONNO et al. 1970) and indirectly by the determination of the MIC for extra- and intracellularly growing mycobacteria (Table 5) – and the therapeutical efficiency exist clear differences for several antituberculotics (URBANCZIK and PETERSEN 1985). Therefore in the last years the problems of extra- and intracellular action and with it also of the type of action have been investigated under conditions comparable with those of the therapy of human tuberculosis, partially with a test model "human macrophages infected with virulent *Mycobacterium tuberculosis*" (CROWLE et al. 1984, 1985a, 1985b, 1986; HAND et al. 1984; ACOCELLA et al. 1985; CARLONE et al. 1985). The processes of permeation – in the case of RMP, PZA, and pyrazinoic acid of a passive nature (ACOCELLA et al. 1985) – can be probably influenced by several factors. Beside the known influence of the pH-value, the state of activation of the macrophages used in these experiments (BARTMANN et al. 1985) and also the quantity and the composition of the surfactant material surrounding the macrophages can be important (O'NEILL et al. 1984). A finally judging of the single components is only possible after systematic investigations considering all factors and exactly defining the experimental conditions (BARTMANN et al. 1985).

Table 5. Effect of antituberculosis drugs on extracellularly or intracellularly growing mycobacteria (WALTER and HEILMEYER 1969; CLINI and GRASSI 1970; KONNO et al. 1970; EULE et al. 1973; PAVLOV et al. 1974; KHEIFETS and KOZLOVA 1975)

Intra- and extracellular effects equal	Intracellular effect weaker	Stronger effect in monocytes	Ratio of extracellularly to intracellularly active concentration
–	TSC?	–	–
–	SM	–	1:20–100
–	PAS	–	1:50–100
INH	–	–	1:1
–	–	PZA	–
CS	–	–	1:1
TC	–	–	1:1
–	KM	–	1:15–60
–	DATC?	–	–
–	VM	–	1:10–500
ETH/PTH	–	–	1:1
EMB	–	–	?
–	CM	–	–
RMP	–	–	1:1

Table 6. Relative distribution volumes of antituberculosis drugs

Antituberculosis drug	Relative distribution volume (% of body weight)	Authors
EMB	119	PEETS and BUYSKE (1962)
ETH/PTH	86	GREENBERG and EIDUS (1962)
INH	61 ± 11	JENNE (1960, 1964)
KM	22–23	LEROY et al. (1978)
PAS	24 ± 3	JENNE (1964)
RMP	160	BINDA et al. (1971)
TC	100	CHULSKI et al. (1963)

On the other hand, pharmacokinetical investigations have shown, that for INH, PZA, CS, TC, ETH/PTH, EMB and RMP distribution throughout the entire body fluid must be reckoned with, largely in agreement with the relative distribution volume (Table 6) determined in another way (CHULSKI et al. 1963; ROBSON and SULLIVAN 1963). SM, PAS, KM and VM are distributed predominantly in the extracellular fluid, SM, for example, in 30% of the body fluid. A dose-dependent distribution volume is assumed for KM (SØRENEN et al. 1967). The distributions of TSC, DATC, and CM have not yet been definitively clarified.

The course of the concentrations in a non-vascularized region can be calculated from the invasion and elimination constants and the distribution volume (DETTLI and STAUB 1960; DETTLI 1961). Rises in concentrations in the tissue on simultaneous administration of hyaluronidase or trypsin (INH – WISNIEWSKY 1972), of insulin (INH – LUKJAN et al. 1969), or of cholinesterase inhibitors (SM

– GREEN 1963) have been confirmed experimentally. Because of the already discussed dose-dependent biotransformation, high PAS doses are required for adequate diffusion into the tissue (LEHMANN 1969). For INH it seems to have been confirmed that periodic administration gives higher intracellular concentrations than a largely constant concentration in the serum (VIVIEN et al. 1972; JENNE and BEGGS 1973).

a) Distribution of Antituberculosis Drugs in the Body Fluids and Organs – Autoradiographic Studies in Animals

The distribution of radiolabelled antituberculotics can be studied in animals autoradiographically on whole-body sections. If the individual investigations are carried out at intervals, the variation of the concentration can also be estimated. This technique has been used for SM, INH, CS, TC, and RMP (HANNGREN and ANDRÉ 1964; TOYOHARA and SHIGEMATSU 1969; BOMAN 1974, 1975; LICHEY et al. 1979; LISS et al. 1981).

b) Antituberculotically Active Fraction of Antituberculosis Drugs in Individual Organs

An exact measurement of the active (i.e., as a rule nonbiotransformed) fraction not bound to tissue constituents in organs is a laborious process. There is no doubt that the blood remaining in the tissue or the methods used to remove it were overestimated in the 1950's as sources of error; however, there are other problems. Stable labelling is the prerequisite for the use of radiolabelled drugs, i.e. the labelled group must not take part in exchange processes (KÖHLER and WINSEL 1982). After the passage through the body separation into biologically active and biologically inactive biotransformation products is necessary before the activity can be measured. In view of the concentrations to be determined, a selective chemical determination must be very sensitive. It is possible that tissue fractions interfere (POIGER and SCHLATTER 1976). As has been shown by carefully planned and executed studies on the INH concentration in the tissue, several interfering factors can also appear in microbiological determinations (BARTMANN and FREISE 1963; FABRE et al. 1977).

In animal-experimental distribution studies, e.g., with TSC (DRABKINA and GINZBURG 1977), besides the disease focus the organs that determine biotransformation and excretion are of major relevance. Attempts have been made by aimed concentration measurements on certain organs to clarify the causes of the occurrence of specific side effects (SOLOVIEV et al. 1977, 1978; FEDERSPIL 1979). In studies on resected material the disease focus with the surrounding tissue was used to substantiate the results of the animal experiments, to evaluate the penetration capacity, and to establish whether the dose had been sufficiently high (KHEINY et al. 1977; RADU et al. 1977; SILVOLA and OTTELIN 1977; KISLITSYNA and KOTOVA 1977, 1980; SIMON et al. 1978; KOCHANOVA et al. 1981; KOLACHEVSKAYA and GURYAN 1981). Besides this, the distribution of antituberculosis drugs into specific compartments relevant to their effect and above all for their side effects is a subject of increasing interest (ROCKER 1977). As regards the activity, the concentration of an antituberculosis drug in the cerebrospinal fluid is a matter of

Table 7. Antituberculosis concentration in the CSF (WALTER and HEILMEYER 1969; supplemented)

Antituberculosis drug	Concentration	
	In normal CSF	During meningitis
	(% of the serum concentration)	
SM	2–3	10–50
TSC	Insufficient	
PAS	5–30 dose-dependent	30–50
INH		55–90
PZA	$\leqq 50$	$\leqq 100$[a]
CS	50	
TC	5–10	15–25
KM	Insufficient	30
VM	$\leqq 10$	25–50
ETH/PTH	30–60	50 and more
EMB		25–40
RMP	$\leqq 10$	$\leqq 20$

[a] Forgan-Smith et al. (1973).

primary importance in view of the limited possibilities for the treatment of meningitis tuberculosa (FORGAN-SMITH et al. 1973, Table 7). Just as important is the permeation of antituberculotics into the tuberculous kidney (KÖHLER and WINSEL 1982) and, with respect to side effects, the variation of the concentration between the mother and foetus or, in the case of the ototoxic antibiotics, between the serum and the perilymph of the inner ear.

5. Excretion of Antituberculosis Drugs

a) Routes of Excretion

By far the majority of antituberculosis drugs and their corresponding biotransformation products are excreted via the kidneys (Table 8), namely TSC, SM, PAS, INH, PZA, CS, KM, VM, ETH/PTH, EMB, and CM. With TC and RMP enterohepatic circulation with biliary excretion is in the foreground, and in the case of DATC this route is predominant. The possibility of direct excretion into the lumen of the small intestine is also discussed for TC (SCHACH VON WITTENAU et al. 1972).

b) Influence of the Patient's Age on the Excretion of Antituberculosis Drugs

As with other drugs, the dose of a particular antituberculotic to be given in early infancy presents a difficult problem. For example, care is advised in the administration of tetracyclines, since a direct correlation is discernible between the renal function and the half-life of the tetracyclines (KUNIN 1967; SØRENEN et al. 1967). Furthermore, tetracyclines are contra-indicated in early infancy owing to their incorporation in the teeth of the first and second dentition.

Table 8. Excretion of antituberculosis drugs

Antituberculosis drug	Mode of excretion	Quantity excreted: In the urine (% of the administered dose)	Quantity excreted: With the faeces (% of the administered dose)
SM	Glomerular filtration	70	2
TSC			4–12
PAS	Glomerular filtration, tubular secretion	80	1–3
Acetyl-PAS, Glycine-PAS	Tubular secretion		
INH	Glomerular filtration, tubular reabsorption	85–98	0.5–10
PZA	Glomerular filtration, tubular reabsorption	≦35%	–
CS	Glomerular filtration,	≦38%	–
TC	Glomerular filtration, tubular absorption	60	20–50
KM	Glomerular filtration,	75–90	Small fractions
DATC	Biliary excretion	0–2	Main fraction
VM	Glomerular filtration,		?
ETH/PTH	Kidneys	?	–
EMB	Glomerular filtration, tubular secretion	80–90	≦20
Products of biotransformation	Glomerular filtration		
CM	Glomerular filtration	55–80%	
RMP	Largely biliary excretion	10–15	?

As studies from the last decade have shown, discernible changes in excretion are important in patients over the age of 50. If the elimination half-life of a drug correlates directly with its clearance (Table 9), it is likely that the half-life will increase in the presence of an age-determined reduction in this magnitude. To date an age-dependent reduced excretion of this kind has been observed for CS and terizidone (MATTILA et al. 1969; ZITKOVA and TOUSEK 1973), for KM (SIMON and AXLINE 1966; SØRENEN et al. 1967; HOLDINESS 1984), and for RMP (EULE et al. 1974a; ZWOLSKA-KWIECK 1974; WINSEL et al. 1985). The result is an elevated concentration in the serum or an increased $t_{50\%}$, provided that other routes of excretion are largely excluded.

c) Influence of Kidney-Function Disorders on the Excretion of Antituberculosis Drugs

Even in patients with healthy kidneys the serum SM concentration, which varies from patient to patient, is attributed to correspondingly individual differences in the renal clearance (LEVY et al. 1960). There are also close correlations between the excretion of PAS and the kidney function (KAMINSKAYA and KARACHUNSKY 1975). When the kidney function is impaired CS is excreted more slowly, with a

Table 9. Clearance of antituberculosis drugs

Antituberculosis drug	Clearance	Author
CM	44.4 ml/min	BLACK et al. (1966)
CS	?	
DATC	?	
EMB	?	
ETH/PTH	48 ml/min	GREENBERG and EIDUS (1962)
INH	35–49 ml/min	JENNE (1960)
	41 ml/min	JENNE (1964)
	25 ml/min	GREENBERG and EIDUS (1962)
KM	76% of the insulin clearance	
	60% of the creatinine clearance	
	0.8–1.6 × creatinine clearance	KUNIN (1967)
PAS	140 ml/min	JENNE (1960, 1964)
PZA	?	
RMP	15–45 ml/min	NAKAGAWA and SUNAHARA (1973)
SM	49.9 ml/min	BLACK et al. (1966)
	30–70 ml/min	KUNIN (1967)
TC	31–35 ml/min	FABRE et al. (1967)
Oxy TC	73 ml/min	
Demethylchlortetracycline	98 ml/min	
Desoxyoxytetracycline	35 ml/min	FABRE et al. (1966)
Chlortetracycline	22–33 ml/min	
Desoxyoxytetracycline	31–35 ml/min	WINKLER and WEIH (1967)
TSC	36.6–181.2 ml/min	WARESKA and SIEKIERZYNSKA (1967)
VM	?	

simultaneous rise of the CS concentration in the serum (WARESKA et al. 1963; KOROTAEV and TATARINOVA 1972).

The excretion of tetracycline is adversely affected by kidney disorders, and appropriate dosage schemes have been developed for such patients suffering from kidney disorders (PITTON and ROCH 1966; KUNIN 1967; MANNHARDT et al. 1971; JUNGBLUTH 1973). On the other hand, in insufficient glomerular filtration without oliguria the tetracycline-elimination process is unaffected (FABRE et al. 1967), nor is there any accumulation of doxycycline in patients with renal disease. The excretion of this compound is evidently less dependent on the kidney function than the excretion of the other tetracycline derivatives (STEIN et al. 1969; MANNHARDT et al. 1971; SCHACH VON WITTENAU et al. 1972). If the kidney function is impaired the excretion with the faeces may be increased (SCHACH VON WITTENAU and TWOMEY 1971).

Table 10. Dosage of antituberculosis drugs in renal insufficiency (HÖFFLER 1981)

Substance	Renal excretion of the unchanged substance	Accumulation of active substance likely in the presence of renal insufficiency	Dosage for patients with renal insufficiency	Main adverse reactions
SM	90%	+	GFR 90–50:0,5 g/day GFR 10–50:0,5–0,3 g/day GFR <10: 0,3–0,25 g/day	Ototoxicity, nephrotoxicity
INH	Up to 20%	∅	Unchanged	Liver-cell damage, peripheral-neuritis. Cave: slow inactivators!
PZA	Glomerular filtration	+	Reduced, extent unclear	Liver-cell damage
CS	50%	+	Reduced, extent unclear	CNS phenomena
VM	63–100%	+	Reduced, extent unclear	Ototoxicity, nephrotoxicity
ETH/PTH	5%	∅	Unchanged	Liver-cell damage, central nervous phenomena
EMB	45–65%	+	GFR 90–50:25 mg/kg/day GFR 10–50:15 mg/kg/day GFR <10: 10–15 mg/kg/day or every other day	Peripheral neuritis, atrophy of the optic nerve, retina defects
RMP	Up to 10%	∅	Unchanged	Thrombocytopenia, liver-cell damage, acute kidney failure

GFR, glomerular filtration rate.

The excretion of SM and KM is limited by the kidney function, making it necessary to adapt the dose to the clearance capacity (KUNTZ 1962; FUJII 1966; KUNIN 1966; QUINN et al. 1966; SØRENEN et al. 1967;; WHELTON 1974; LEROY et al. 1978; HOLDINESS 1984). A slight impairment of the kidney function does not have any far-reaching consequences for the elimination of EMB (STRAUSS and EHRHARDT 1970; ZELLER and RÓKA 1973). If a considerable restriction of the kidney function is present, and in nephrectomized patients, however, the half-life of EMB too is increased and the excretion is accordingly reduced (KROENING 1974; ZITKOVA and TOUSEK 1978). Measurement of the EMB concentration in the whole blood 12 h after administration of the drug seems to offer the best way of evaluating the risk of accumulation: if this value rises after 5 days on EMB therapy it appears to be necessary to determine in full the variation of the EMB concentration in the whole blood (KROENING 1974).

On the basis of these results it is proposed for the treatment of tuberculosis that INH, chlortetracycline, ETH or PTH and RMP be administered irrespective of the kidney function, whereas SM, PZA, CS, TC, KM, VM, EMB, and CM must be given in doses adapted to the kidney function, if the use of these agents is absolutely necessary (Table 10, SIEGENTHALER et al. 1968; JUNGBLUTH 1971; REIDENBERG et al. 1973; WHELTON 1974; HÖFFLER 1976, 1981; LEROY et al. 1978; TITARENKO et al. 1983; HOLDINESS 1984). For intermittent therapy with RMP it is recommended that to reduce the risk of immune reaction the age-determined reduction of the clearance should be taken into account and to reduce the RMP dose by 10% to 15% in patients over 55 (EULE et al. 1974a).

d) Influence of Liver Diseases on the Pharmacokinetics of Antituberculosis Drugs

The expected effects of liver disorders on the pharmacokinetics of individual drugs were determined about 20 years ago in experimental clinical studies. Since then fundamental problems have been recognized by improving the patients' selection with regard to the nature and duration of the disease and specific modifications have been made to certain drugs. For a number of drugs there are already suggested doses or possibilities of correcting the alterations caused by the liver disease (e.g., induction by other drugs) and warnings against the use of certain drugs in specific stages (e.g., barbiturates, prothazin, phenylbutazone, methohexital, theophylline, and others – SCHOENE et al. 1972; PIAFSKY et al. 1975; RICHTER et al. 1979; ZILLY 1979; HELD 1980; BAUMGARTEN 1983).

As a rule kidney damage results in a delayed excretion, the extent of which can be definitively determined on the basis of established clinico-chemical parameters, so that the dose can be appropriately adjusted if this proves necessary (Table 9, p. 425; Table 10, p. 426). However, liver disease affects at least 3 mutually independent processes: 1) the liver circulation, 2) the binding of drugs to serum proteins, and 3) the biotransformation capacity of the liver. These alterations, the intensity of which can vary, naturally have a considerable bearing on the pharmacokinetics of drugs that, because of their interrelationships, are difficult to predict.

So far it has not been possible to identify disease-determined alterations of this type. There is a lack of satisfactory correlations between the clinico-chemical parameters and the half-life or clearance regarding certain drug groups of apparently specific test substances. The galactosamine elimination test, the bromsulphalein retention test, and the indocyanine green test have all proved unsuitable. The aminopyrine test has failed to fulfill expectations (PAUMGARTNER 1980; HELD 1980; BAUMGARTEN 1983), nor does a determination of the biotransformation capacity permit any general statements to be made. Thus, the extent of a change in the pharmacokinetics of drugs due to liver disease cannot for the time being be reliably determined. Dose adaptation with the aid of a risk classification has been suggested to enhance the insight in the use of the drugs, but this requires constant monitoring and adjustment of the dose (ZYSSET and BIRCHER 1983).

Changes in the liver function, e.g., elevations of the aminotransferase, are relatively common in tuberculosis patients (ROTTACH 1979; EULE and IWAINSKY 1981). After a confirmation of the diagnosis immediate chemotherapy is absolutely necessary for several reasons. Regarding the antituberculosis drugs to be used in patients suffering simultaneously from a liver disease, the situation is clearer than for other groups of drugs.

1. It can be said with confidence that the active compound is not first formed as a result of biotransformation in the case of any of the 14 drugs considered here.
2. Since with CM, DATC, EMB, KM, SM, TSC, and VM biotransformation processes are only of secondary importance, any disease-determined changes in the liver's biotransformation capacity do not affect the pharmacokinetics of these compounds.
3. The pharmacokinetics of EMB and ETH are determined to a very substantial degree by the deep compartments of these antituberculotics, erythrocytes in the case of EMB and gastric juice in the case of ETH. The influence of liver diseases on the pharmacokinetics is therefore relatively weak.
4. If it is necessary to use PAS in the chemotherapy of tuberculosis patients it is recommended to neglect dose reduction in favor of a PAS concentration definitely known to be sufficient (HELD and FRIED 1977).
5. Care must be exercised with the tetracyclines. If their use is unavoidable, the therapy should be made intermittent because of the risk of accumulation (PITTON and ROCH 1966; KUNIN 1967).
6. In contrast to other drugs, INH is biotransformed by a non-microsomal acetylase. The presence of liver disease results in a prolonged half-life (+110% according to ACOCELLA et al. 1972). These alterations correlate with the bilirubin concentration in the serum. Modifications by as much as 30% have been observed in acute hepatitis. The genetically determined variability is more important. Liver disease is not regarded as a contra-indication for INH (LEVI et al. 1968; BAUMGARTEN 1983).
7. Liver diseases impair the biliary excretion of RMP, the disturbance not being compensated by an increased excretion with the urine, as a result of which the $t_{50\%}$ increases in such patients and the serum RMP concentration rises accordingly (BINDA et al. 1971; ACOCELLA et al. 1972; ACOCELLA 1978). In the course of longer treatment these alterations are largely eliminated by the induction process (pp 409–411). Only if this effect does not appear (which can be deduced from constant staining of the urine by RMP) should care be exercised in the use of RMP.

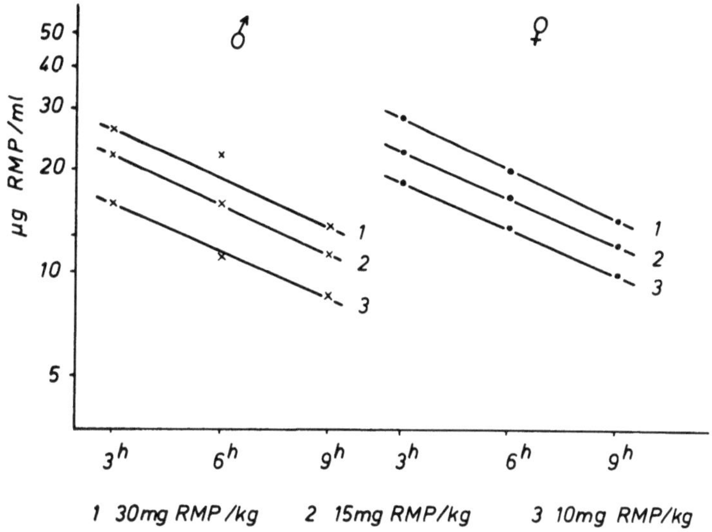

Fig. 10. Influence of sex on the course of the serum RMP concentration (after IWAINSKY et al. 1976)

6. Factors Influencing the Pharmacokinetics of Antituberculosis Drugs

a) Influence of Sex and Age

Sex-dependent differences have so far been observed only with RMP and TC, as is unanimously agreed by several authors (Fig. 10, IWAINSKY et al. 1974; OCHS and VERBURG-OCHS 1983; WINSEL et al. 1985). According to BOMAN (1974), in the case of RMP the causes lie not so much in sex-specific differences in biotransformation or excretion as in the corresponding differences in absorption and distribution into the tissue; this is also indicated by the fact that $t_{50\%}$ is practically the same in women and men (KÖHLER and WINSEL 1982). The reported differences between the serum PTH concentrations in men and women still require confirmation on larger numbers of patients (FRANZ et al. 1974).

In a classification based on age, different pharmacokinetics of certain drugs can be found in children and in patients over 50 in comparison with other patients. In children dosage referred to the body surface area is more correct than dosage referred to the body weight, since in children the extravasal space is larger in comparison with the body weight. Thus, the values for INH, EMB, and RMP in the serum are lower in children than in adults after equivalent doses based on the body weight (BARTMANN and MASSMANN 1960b; HUSSELS and OTTO 1971; HUSSELS et al. 1973; BENKERT et al. 1974; SIMON 1975; HOLDINESS 1984).

The doses of antibiotics and antituberculosis drugs must be established with some care. As mentioned above, the reduction of the renal clearance due to age is in itself sufficient to reduce the renal clearance of CS, KM, RMP and, at higher dose (50 mg/kg) of EMB as well, associated in most cases with an increased serum concentration or a prolonged half-life. With doxycycline and KM prolongations of the $t_{50\%}$ from 15 h–16.2 h to 20.6 h respectively from 2 h–4 h to 8.9 h have been observed, with correspondingly higher concentrations in the serum (SIMON and AXLINE 1966; WINKLER and WEIH 1967; ZITKOVA et al. 1976; ZITKOVA and TOUSEK 1978).

b) Influence of the Administration Intervals and the Dose

Any value measured in the course of intermittent therapy reflects the conditions to be expected at that time during treatment with sufficient accuracy. For daily administration this statement is not as reliable. For example, with TC derivatives and EMB after the start of the treatment a slight elevation of the serum concentration, lasting several days or weeks, is observed before the values settle at a constant level (PITTON and ROCH 1966; DOLUISIO and DITTERT 1969; MANNHARDT et al. 1971; SCHWABE et al. 1973; BENKERT et al. 1974; OMER 1978). The earlier requirement of withdrawing the therapy 2 days to 3 days before a serum concentration determination is neither necessary nor expedient. After a 24-h drug-free period the concentration as a rule falls off to values that can no longer be measured or to values irrelevant for the determination.

The ever more strongly emphasized recommendation of intermittent treatment has given new topicality to the question of a dose-proportional rise of the biologically active fraction in the serum. With SM, CS, and RMP the serum concentration on increasing the dose is subproportional, especially at 30 mg RMP/kg (HAAPANEN et al. 1960; LEVY et al. 1961; IWAINSKY et al. 1974; KÖHLER and WINSEL 1982). The EMB concentration in the serum rises proportionally up to a dose of 75 mg/kg (EULE and WERNER 1970). Other authors have observed an overproportional increase at doses above 2 g (STRAUSS and EHRHARDT 1970).

A dose-dependence of the biotransformation rate has been postulated for INH (ELLARD et al. 1973). In 1962 SHORT established that the biotransformation is independent on the dose up to 1600 mg of INH, whereas at higher doses (over 2 g, suicide attempts) an extremely high fraction of non-biotransformed INH was measured in 1965, probably as a result of saturation of the corresponding enzymes. In studies on larger groups of patients, in correspondence with the dependence postulated above, a greater-than-proportional increase of the serum INH concentration or of the excretion of non-biotransformed INH with the urine was found at doses as low as 15 mg INH/kg (SUNAHARA et al. 1963; IWAINSKY et al. 1977).

c) Influence of Combination Therapy on the Pharmacokinetics of Antituberculosis Drugs

Treatment of tuberculosis with several antituberculotics simultaneously is known to be superior to monotherapy, above all because of the resulting prevention of the development of resistance (PÖCH 1981). The relevant therapeutic recommendations therefore suggest the use of at least 2 and in the initial phase of 3 or 4 antituberculotic agents. In this form of therapy interference between the different drugs cannot be ruled out, be it in the binding to the serum proteins or in the biotransformation or excretion.

Questions of this kind have mostly been studied only on combinations of two drugs, in contrast to actual practice, because of the methodological difficulties involved. The drugs that have been studied are SM, PAS, INH, PZA, CS, KM, ETH, EMB, and RMP.

The influence of PAS and of structurally related compounds on the biotransformation of INH was a focal point of interest in the 1950's (see Special Part p. 491, INH, Fig. 13). The INH concentration in the serum is raised further by ETH, while CS, EMB, and RMP seem without effect. Diverse opinions are held about the effect of PZA, a statistically significant reduction of acetyl-INH formation being observed only in slow inactivators (JOHNSON et al. 1961; SCHMIDT 1966; MATTILA et al. 1969; VENHO and KOSKINEN 1971; SAUERESSIG 1972; VIVIEN et al. 1972; DUDCHIK and BILYK 1975). By contrast, the PZA concentration in the serum falls off with a simultaneous shift of the maximum if the drug is given in combination with INH or RMP. The PZA-concentration-lowering effect is at its strongest when 3 antituberculosis drugs are administered simultaneously (PZA + INH + RMP – BOULAHBAL et al. 1979). INH appears to increase the PTH concentration in the serum (FRANZ et al. 1974).

If PAS is given in combination with CS, the serum PAS concentrations fall off more quickly than after its administration on its own (MATTILA et al. 1969). In contrast to this, PAS slows down the excretion of KM when these two agents are administered together (KUNTZ 1962). The pharmacokinetic parameters of EMB and RMP are unaffected by INH (SCHMIDT 1966; BOMAN et al. 1970; CANETTI et al. 1970; ACOCELLA 1971). But with a triple drug combination INH + RMP + EMB there is a decrease of Ka as well as Ke, an increase of $t_{50\%}$, t_{max} and Vd for all the three antituberculotic drugs (ZITKOVA et al. 1983). However, when EMB + INH + RMP or EMB + INH + PTH are administered in combination, higher EMB concentrations are found in the serum than after EMB + RMP + PTH (TATARINOVA and CHUKANOV 1978). Lower RMP concentrations are measured when PAS granulate or EMB is given at the same time. In the case of PAS granulate RMP is adsorbed on the bentonite added to the granulate (BOMAN et al. 1971; BOMAN et al. 1975).

In view of the different parameters and reference magnitudes used, it is difficult to give a reliable order of magnitude for the changes observed. No conclusions have been drawn about the doses of the individual antituberculotics in combination therapy. With the exception of the PAS-RMP-bentonite example, these changes are evidently not very significant.

7. Antituberculotic Concentration in the Serum as a Parameter of Treatment Efficacy

The concentration of an antituberculosis drug prevailing at its site of action and its variation with time are determined by the drugs's uptake, distribution, biotransformation, and excretion. The concentration in diseased tissue can be determined only in exceptional cases, and with some difficulty, while the serum level can be determined in a sufficient number of patients by a very wide range of microbiological and chemical methods. By special investigations it has been possible to clear up some of the uncertainties about the relationship between drug concentrations in the tissue and serum and their variation as a function of time, controlled therapeutic studies having contributed further to this end. In a global determination of the antituberculotic activity in the serum after the administration of several drugs, however, conclusions about the tissue concentration can only be drawn if the specific distribution and elimination rates of the individual combination partners are known.

In general, the following parameters are derived from the course of the serum concentration: coverage, $t_{50\%}$, and exposure (the AUC).

Coverage: In the early days of chemotherapy the duration of persistence of an antituberculotic concentration above the MIC for the given pathogenic strain was regarded as decisive. Nowadays the term "coverage" refers to the period in which the concentration of an antituberculosis drug is more than 10 times the MIC (ELLARD 1976; TRIPATHY 1976; URBANCZIK and PETERSEN 1985), corresponding to the "safety factor" used by KRÜGER-THIEMER in connection with the dosage of bacteriostatically active compounds (KRÜGER-THIEMER and BÜNGER 1965/66).

$t_{50\%}$: In the early 'sixties the serum half-life of INH was introduced as a basis for evaluation (JENNE 1960). Since with the majority of antituberculosis drugs the fall in the serum concentration is likewise exponential, the determination of the half-life became a generally accepted practice. In the case of the rapidly eliminated antituberculotics with a short absorption phase the determination of the $t_{50\%}$ does not present any problems. If distribution into other compartments dependent on other factors takes place (e.g., ETH into the stomach – IWAINSKY et al. 1964, 1965; GRUNERT and IWAINSKY 1967), or the excretion is largely by the biliary route, the determination of the $t_{50\%}$ becomes problematic owing to the observed discontinuities (GIBALDI 1967), as can be demonstrated on the example of TC (SCHACH VON WITTENAU and CHIAINI 1968).

AUC: The maximum concentration attained and the course of the concentration with time are equally important for antimycobacterial efficacy. The area under the concentration-time curve (AUC) constitutes a more comprehensive exposure factor, also denoted as exposure time or as exposure factor (MITCHISON 1972; JENNE and BEGGS 1973; ELLARD 1976).

If, irrespective of the actual variation of their serum concentration, the antituberculotic drugs are arranged in order of their mean $t_{50\%}$, three groups can be recognized (Table 11). The first group is that of rapidly absorbed and rapidly

Table 11. Biological half-lives ($t_{50\%}$, β-phase) of antituberculotics

Antituberculosis drug	$t_{50\%}$	Authors
SM	132–162 min	KUNIN (1967)
	130–190 min	WALTER and HEILMEYER (1969)
	150 min	MODR and DVORACEK (1976)
	162±24 min	RONCORONI et al. (1981)
TSC	8–12 h	WALTER and HEILMEYER (1969)
PAS	45 min, 48 min	JENNE (1964)
	45 min	KUNIN (1967)
	35 min (17–64 min)	WAGNER et al. (1973)

Table 11 (continued)

Antituberculosis drug	$t_{50\%}$	Authors
INH	59 min (45–80 min)	JENNE (1960, 1964)
Rapid inactivation	66 min	KUNIN (1967)
	89 ± 3 min	MATTILA and TIITINEN (1967)
Slow inactivation	140–200 min	JENNE (1960, 1964)
	216 min	KUNIN (1967)
	187 ± 7 min	MATTILA and TIITINEN (1967)
PZA	14 h	SIMÁNE et al. (1964)
	12 ± 2.5 h	ELLARD (1969)
CS	10 h	KUNIN (1967)
	11–12 h	ZITKOVA and TOUSEK (1973)
Tetracycline	7.9 h	CHULSKI et al. (1963)
	8.5 h	KUNIN (1967); MODR and DVORACEK (1976)
	8.2 h	WINKLER and WEIH (1967)
Chlortetracycline	5.6 h	FABRE et al. (1966); Kunin (1967) WINKLER and WEIH (1967)
Oxytetracycline	9.2 h	FABRE et al. (1966); Winkler and WEIH (1967)
	9.6 h	KUNIN (1967)
	9 h	MODR and DVORACEK (1976)
Doxycycline	22.2 h	FABRE et al. (1966)
	15–16.2 h	WINKLER and WEIH (1967)
	15–21.5 h	SCHACH VON WITTENAU and CHIAINI (1968)
	22.2 h	STEIN et al. (1969)
	17 h	MODR and DVORACEK (1976)
KM	3.6 h	EICHENWALD (1966)
	2 h	SIMON and AXLINE (1966)
	3 h	KUNIN (1967)
	3.5–5 h	SØRENEN et al. (1967)
	4 h	MODR and DVORACEK (1976)
DACT	?	
VM	3–4 h	WALTER and HEILMEYER (1969)
ETH/PTH	120–132 min	GREENBERG and EIDUS (1962)
	112–143 min	PÜTTER (1964)
EMB	2.8 h	PLACE and THOMAS (1963)
	3.15–3.5 h	EULE and WERNER (1970)
	2.5–3.6 h	LEE et al. (1980) (multiple course)
CM	3–5 h	WALTER and HEILMEYER (1969)
	3–6 h	BLACK et al. (1966)
RMP	2–7.3 h	FURESZ et al. (1967)
	dependent on dose	ACOCELLA et al. (1972)
	and test strain	VERBIST et al. (1972)
	6.75 h	SUNAHARA and NAKAGAWA (1972) (chemical determination)
600 mg	5.79 ± 2.04 h	KÖHLER and WINSEL (1982)
900 mg	6.20 ± 1.71 h	M. tuberculosis as test strain
1800 mg	5.28 ± 1.31 h	

eliminated antituberculotics ($t_{50\%}$ up to 190 min) and includes PAS, INH (rapid inactivation), SM, INH (slow inactivation), and ETH or PTH. The $t_{50\%}$ of SM more or less corresponds to that of slow INH inactivation (LEVY et al. 1960). In the case of PAS, the course of the concentration can be influenced to a particularly great extent by the dose, the galenic formulation, and the form of administration (FROSTADT 1961; KUNTZ 1966; HORNUNG et al. 1967; LEHMANN 1969; NIKODEMOWICZ et al. 1971). The $t_{50\%}$ or AUC differences caused by the polymorphism of INH biotransformation amount to factors of 2.4 to 3 (MITCHISON 1972; VIVIEN et al. 1972). The extremes of the INH concentration in the serum differ by a factor of about 40 (BARTMANN and MASSMANN 1960). The use of slowly absorbable INH preparations (matrix INH, Tebesium – KLEEBERG et al. 1975; ELLARD 1976) is only useful for intermittent therapy of rapid inactivators. Since the serum ETH or PTH concentrations fluctuate strongly in one and the same individual from one test to the next (IWAINSKY et al. 1964, 1965; GRUNERT 1969; KALABUKHA 1971), correlations between the dose and the form of administration, the serum concentration, and activity can only be derived from studies on large groups of patients.

The second group of antituberculotic drugs, with half-lives of 3 h to 8 h, includes CM, EMB, KM, VM, and RMP (see Table 11), although, as mentioned above, in the case of EMB the erythrocytes are an additional compartment resulting in a multiphase course of the plasma concentration (JUNGBLUTH and URBANCZIK 1974; KROENING 1974; LEE et al. 1980). The $t_{50\%}$ of RMP is dose-dependent within certain ranges (ACOCELLA et al. 1971; CURCI et al. 1972; KÖHLER and WINSEL 1982), and furthermore, the test strain used is important for the results of microbiological determinations (PORVEN and CANETTI 1968; CANETTI et al. 1970). In studies on larger groups a relatively wide scatter of the individual $t_{50\%}$ values of RMP is reported, as a result of which two or more patient groups with different pharmacokinetics are presumed (CONSTANS et al. 1968; BABA et al. 1971; DE RAUTLIN DE LA ROY et al. 1971; VERBIST 1971; NAKAGAWA and SUNAHARA 1973; PAWLOWSKA and PNIEWSKI 1975; WINSEL et al. 1976).

Because of the effects on the frequency of side effects in intermittent treatment with RMP, the differences discernible between men and women regarding the serum RMP concentration (PORVEN and CANETTI 1968; IWAINSKY et al. 1974, 1976; BOMAN 1974; ZWOLSKA-KWIECK 1974) are important. During the induction phase the antimycobacterial activity in the serum falls off by around 10%, the $t_{50\%}$ decreases by about 1 h, and the RMP concentration in urine or the excretion rate by about 30% (BROUET et al. 1969; HAKIM et al. 1971; VERBIST 1971; VERBIST et al. 1972; CURCI et al. 1972; NITTI 1972; SUNAHARA and NAKAGAWA 1972; BOMAN 1974; IWAINSKY et al. 1974; KÖHLER and WINSEL 1982). In patients with cirrhosis of the liver no change in the mentioned parameters can be established. The deacetyl-RMP fraction is in such cases higher than in patients with healthy livers (CONSTANS et al. 1968; ACOCELLA 1971; ACOCELLA et al. 1972; DECROIX and DJUROVIC 1972). However, in a determination of the antituberculotic activity no clinically relevant changes caused by the induction were found (see p. 437).

The third group includes CS, TSC, PZA, and TC derivatives with half-lives between 7 h and 22 h. DATC probably belongs to this group as well, though no useful data are available on its $t_{50\%}$. Because of its relatively long absorption, which can be influenced in various ways by physiological factors, considerable scatter of the individual values is observed in studies on large groups of patients (MATTILA et al. 1969).

The antituberculotic concentration in the serum is a good basis for evaluation of the efficacy, being regarded as unsatisfactory by only a few authors (BENAZET et al. 1968). The following concentrations have proved adequate: a level 10 times the MIC 6 h after administration for SM, PAS, INH, KM, and ETH/PTH (KASS 1966) or after 6 h a concentration of 20 μg of SM and 0.4 μg of INH/ml serum or after 8 h to 12 h a concentration of 1 μg and 2 μg of EMB and 1 μg of RMP/ml serum (LEVY et al. 1961; SCHMIDT 1966; CONSTANS et al. 1968). In the case of TC a concentration 4 to 5 times the MIC is regarded as sufficient (OLON and HOLVEY 1968).

It is more difficult to analyse the relationship between the concentration of an antituberculosis drug in the serum and the occurrence of side effects. Apart from the antituberculotic concentration, a number of other generally or temporarily active factors, such as the inhibition of the renal elimination of uric acid by pyrazinoic acid and the resulting arthralgias (AKINOSHO 1979; JENNER et al. 1981), can give rise to side effects. It is therefore not surprising that in a synoptic comparison of the SM, TSC, and INH concentrations produced by the usual dosage no differences can be found between patients with and without side effects, although in this case the drugs are held responsible (VIRSIK et al. 1971). As far as CS is concerned, a relationship between the serum concentration and the appearance of side effects is on the one hand stated (ROZEWSKA et al. 1969) and on the other hand denied (KOROTAEV and TATARINOVA 1972). In intermittent therapy with RMP (once a week) it is possible with the aid of pharmacokinetic parameters to delimit risk groups in which side effects are likely to occur. The sex- and age-dependent elevation of the serum RMP concentration evidently acts additively with respect to side effects. Female patients over the age of 55 are affected by side effects more frequently than men of the same age group or than younger women. No side effects are encountered in men under 35 (EULE et al. 1974a).

IV. General Medical Relevance of the Results Obtained in the Field of Tuberculosis

The extensive experimental and clinical research carried out on tuberculosis in the last few decades has been favoured by a particular set of external circumstances. To counter the threatening development of tuberculosis after the second world war a number of tuberculosis research institutes were founded by affiliating appropriate research establishments to tuberculosis hospitals. Moreover bacteriological units active in the field of tuberculosis had the possibility to work on diagnostic and experimental problems by the same methods (IWAINSKY et al. 1975). Patients were available in sufficient numbers for clinicopharmacological studies. In the 'fifties and 'sixties they were normally hospitalized for several months.

The preliminary investigations served to establish effective chemotherapy, i.e., to maintain a sufficiently antituberculotic concentration in the serum. In the next phase it was necessary to delineate the range of insufficient drugs or derivates (INH- and PAS-derivatives, DATC, etc.) and studies on the relationships between the dose of an antituberculosis drug and its effects and side effects. Finally, the experimental basis for intermittent therapy was worked out (MITCHISON 1979) before optimization of the chemotherapy could be tackled. At present questions relating to short-term therapy are at the focus of interest (GROSSET 1978, 1981; ACOCELLA 1984; GIRLING 1984; BARTMANN et al. 1985; EULE et al. 1985; O'BRIEN et al. 1985).

A number of problems relating to the drugs' action mechanism, biotransformation, and pharmacokinetics were dealt with within the framework of these studies, in some cases for the first time, the relevance of which goes beyond the field of tuberculosis.

1. Studies on the Mode of Action

In addition to the supplementation and deepening of the knowledge already available on the mode of action of chemotherapeutic agents, starting points were worked out for improving the concept of active-substance research, the hitherto customary "active substance-pathogen" test model being replaced by the more informative "active substance-cell culture" model with pathogens or receptors. As a result of this modification, problems of permeability, stability to enzymes and the like could already be identified at this stage. The practice, common in the 1950's, of testing numerous derivatives that could be synthesized without great expense is being replaced by testing a smaller number of derivatives obtained by an aimed modification of the original molecule with simultaneous determination of the pharmacokinetic parameters. In this way it is largely becoming unnecessary to carry out corrections to the range later on, such as were necessary, for example, for a number of INH derivatives. At that time some part of these products were believed to have a better tolerability compared with the original drug before a determination of the total excretion revealed a lower absorption rate to be the reason for the ostensibly better tolerability.

It was thus that a specific branch of drug research took shape, resulting in recent years, in some very successful work, optimizing more than just chemotherapy of tuberculosis by the development – sometimes lasting several years – of derivatives of known drugs with a long $t_{50\%}$.

2. Studies on Biotransformation Processes

Comprehensive studies on the treatment of experimental tuberculosis have shown that one of the essential difficulties encountered in extrapolating the results of such studies with animals to man lies in the different biotransformation rates and patterns in the animal species used. The systematic investigation of biotransformation processes of antituberculosis drugs in various animal species that has since been performed means that an appropriate choice can now be made for subsequently initiated studies, i.e., that we can select an animal species that biotransforms the relevant substance in a manner largely corresponding to the situation in man.

Moreover studies on man and on animals extend our knowledge of the relationships between the drug structure and its biotransformation. INH was the first drug for which a hereditary polymorphism of biotransformation was established, a finding that simultaneously laid the foundations for pharmacogenetics. Only certain aspects of the biological function and the effects of this polymorphism in healthy people are known (CHAILLEUX et al. 1980), whereas the biochemical mechanism has been largely clarified. The different degrees of biotransformation of INH are caused by corresponding acetylation. In subsequent years a number of other drugs biotransformed in accordance with the same polymorphism were studied and problems relating to the determination of the inactivator type and to the effects and side effects of the non-biotransformed and therefore still active fraction of the same dose have been successfully solved. Finally, different degrees of drug interaction have been determined, caused by the biotransformation of the causative drug corresponding to the INH polymorphism.

Further-reaching investigations have in the meantime been started. It is known that a number of xenobiotics are converted in the body into biotransformation products having a stronger carcinogenic activity. Cytochrome P_{450}, aryl-hydrocarbon hydroxylase, and acetylase are involved in these processes. In contrast to the genetically fixed activity of acetylase, the first two enzyme complexes can be induced to different extents (IWAINSKY and WINSEL 1981; PFEIL et al. 1983). Similarly to the determination of the activity of aryl-hydrocarbon hydroxylase, the determination of the INH-inactivator type is now also used to distinguish genetically predisposed groups with an increased risk of cancer, e.g. in cancer of the bladder (CARTWRIGHT et al. 1982; MILLER 1982; MOMMSEN et al. 1982). The results obtained so far do not yet permit any reliable conclusions. If progress is to be made, both methodological difficulties and the uncertainties within the selection of patients and control groups must be eliminated.

Given a satisfactory tolerability of a drug, the active (i.e. as a rule the non-biotransformed) fraction can be increased over-proportionally to the administered dose if the biotransformation capacity of the prevailing process can be overcharged. This method has been tried out experimentally with PAS and is clinically practised with good results in a number of countries. Provided that certain prerequisites have been satisfied, it can serve as a model case for the optimization of chemotherapy.

In the use of RMP the problems of long-term therapy with inducing drugs with daily and intermittent administration constitute the focal point of interest. The appearance of differences in the biological activity of certain biotransformation products from one test strain to the next is a characteristic feature specific to RMP, and the therapy must be planned accordingly. All the biotransformation products exhibit much the same activity against mycobacteria. Problems related to induction thus reduce in the treatment of tuberculosis to problems of the inductor effect of RMP with respect to other drugs. In this context, for example, the interaction of RMP with steroids has had undesired effects (BOLT et al. 1975, 1976; BUFFINGTON et al. 1976). For the desired and in some cases already initiated use of RMP for treatment or prophylaxis of non-tuberculous diseases (ACOCELLA et al. 1977, 1980; NITTI et al. 1981; LLORENS-TEROL et al. 1981; WATTEL et al. 1981; OCKLITZ 1981; EULE et al. 1985) the studies performed with other test microorganisms than used in the tuberculosis sector play an important role. On the other hand, our knowledge of drugs for the treatment of non-specific infections and tuberculosis, such as the tetracyclines, SM, etc., has been determined to a very substantial extent by studies on patients not suffering from tuberculosis.

3. Studies on Pharmacokinetics

With regard to the relationships between drug structure, biotransformation, and pharmacokinetics, our previous knowledge was supplemented in particular by studies on INH and PAS derivatives, tetracyclines, and RMP derivatives. A differentiated picture of the pharmacokinetics of antituberculotic agents has thus emerged. As a result of detailed investigations on their serum concentrations, a number of deep compartments were discovered, such as the stomach ETH compartment controlled by the pH of the gastric juice, the EMB compartment in the erythrocytes, and the ototoxic aminoglycosides compartment in the perilymph of the inner ear. The reducing effect of the first two compartments on the serum concentration and hence on activity and the close correlations between the perilymph and side effects were recognized at an early stage. In addition, our knowledge of the correlations between the drug concentration in the maternal and foetal blood and between the serum level and that in the CSF has been broadened by studies on antituberculotics. Methodological development aims at obtaining differentiated statements about the distribution of antituberculosis drugs, especially at the focus of the disease (ALLEN et al. 1975; KÖHLER and WINSEL 1982; BODDINGIUS and STOLZ 1981).

Efforts are also under way at improving the cooperation of patients, most of whom are treated on an out-patient basis, by controlling the drug intake. Attempts are made here to use easily determinable drugs such as INH or RMP for detecting not only these drugs themselves but also for controlling the intake of other antituberculotics, especially when given in fixed combinations (KILBURN et al. 1972; STARK et al. 1975; TATARINOVA et al. 1979; BURKHARDT and NEL 1980; ELLARD et al. 1980; ROOTS 1986).

Studies performed in recent years on the renal excretion of drugs have revealed that their excretion can be slowed down not only in the presence of kidney damage but also as a result of an age-determined reduction of clearance. In this context it seems that for the time being studies on elderly people are necessary for every drug intended to be prescribed over a long period, so that the requisite dose reduction can be undertaken if necessary (RAMEIS et al. 1980; OCHS and VERBURG-OCHS 1983).

References

Mainly papers published after 1960 are included into the list of references. Publications to which one of the letters M, B or Ph is attached are reviews with the respective main topic: M = mode of action, B = biotransformation, Ph = pharmakokinetics.

Abai AM, Tomchani A (1979) Rifampicin binding by the blood serum proteins. Probl Tuberk 67 issue 1: 54–59

Abshagen U, Demmer F (1981) Vorteile und Probleme von Retardpräparaten. Med Klin 76:484–490

Acocella G (1971) A metabolic and kinetic study on the association rifampicin-isoniazid. Respiration 28 Suppl: 1–6

Acocella G (1978) Clinical pharmacokinetics of rifampicin. Clin Pharmacokinet 3:108–127
Acocella G (1984) La farmacocinetica dei farmaci antitubercolari nell' uomo. Minerva Med 75:561–563
Acocella G, Conti R (1980) Interaction of rifampicin with other drugs. Tubercle 61:171–177
Acocella G, Pagani V, Marchetti M, Baroni GC, Nicolis FB (1971) Kinetic studies on rifampicin. I. Serum concentration analysis in subjects treated with different oral doses over a period of two weeks. Chemotherapy 16:356–370
Acocella G, Bonollo L, Garimoldi M, Mainhardi M, Tenconi LT, Nicolis FB (1972) Kinetics of rifampicin and isoniazid administered alone and in combination to normal subjects and patients with liver disease. GUT 13:47–53
Acocella G, Hamilton-Miller JMT, Brumfitt W (1977) Can rifampicin use be safely extended? Lancet I:740–741
Acocella G, Brumfitt W, Hamilton-Miller JM (1980) Evidence that rifampicin can be used safely for nontuberculous diseases. Thorax 35:788
Acocella G, Carlone UA, Cuffini AM, Cavallo G (1985) The penetration of rifampicin, pyrazinamide and pyrazinoic acid into mouse macrophages. Amer Rev Respir Dis 132:1268–1273
Ahmad D, Mathur P, Ahuja S, Henderson R, Carruthers G (1979) Rifampicin-quinidine interaction. Br J Dis Chest 73:409–411
Akinosho BOO (1979) Pyrazinamide in the treatment of tuberculosis. A world review. Actes d'un Symposium tenu à Alger. Laboratoires Bracco, Milan, pp 25–29
Allen BW, Ellard GA, Gammon PT (1975) The penetration of dapsone, rifampicin, isoniazid and pyrazinamide into peripheral nerves. Br J Pharmacol 55:151–155
Altmann AE, Beeuwkes H, Brombacher PJ, Buytendijk HJ, Gijzen AHJ, Maesen FPV (1968) Serum levels of tetracycline after different administration forms. Clin Chim Acta 20:185–188
Aoyagi T (1977) Clinical problems on the binding of protein to antituberculous drugs. Kekkaku 52:459–468
Arima K, Izaki K (1963) Accumulation of oxytetracycline relevant to its bactericidal action in the cells of Escherichia coli. Nature 200:192–193
Asker A, El-Nakeeb M, Motawi M, El-Gindy N (1973a) Effect of certain tablet formulation factors on the antimicrobial activity of tetracycline hydrochloride and chloramphenicol. Part 2: effect of disintegrants. Pharmazie 28:474–476
Asker A, El-Nakeeb M, Motawi M, El-Gindy N (1973b) Effect of certain tablet formulation factors on the antimicrobial activity of tetracycline hydrochloride and chloramphenicol. Part 3: effect of lubricants. Pharmazie 28:476–478
Awaness AM, Mitchison DA (1973) Cumulative effects of pulsed exposures of Mycobacterium tuberculosis to isoniazid. Tubercle 54:153–158
Baba II, Takahashi R, Azuma Y (1971) Rifampicin in the retreatment of severe cavitary pulmonary tuberculosis. 2nd part: drug resistance, drug concentration in blood and side effects. Kekkaku 46:481–489
Baronti A, Manfredi N (1968) Blood levels of isoniazid and of its methane sulphonate derivative in rapid and slow inactivators after oral administration. Tubercle 49:104–109
Barr WH, Gerbracht LM, Letcher K, Plaut M, Strahl N (1972) Assessment of the biologic availability of tetracycline products in man. Clin Pharmacol Ther 13:97–108
Bartmann K (1960) Langfristige Einwirkung von Isonicotinsäurehydrazid und Streptomycin auf ruhende Tuberkelbakterien in vitro. Beitr Klin Tuberk 122:94–113
Bartmann K, Freise G (1963) Mikrobiologisch bestimmte Isoniazid-Konzentrationen im Gewebe von Tier und Mensch. Beitr Klin Tuberk 127:546–560
Bartmann K, Massmann W (1960) Der Blutspiegel des INH bei Erwachsenen und Kindern. Beitr Klin Tuberk 122:239–250
Bartmann K, Radenbach KL, Zierski M (1985) Wandlungen in den Auffassungen und der Durchführung der antituberkulösen Chemotherapie. Prax Klin Pulmol 39:397–420
Baumgarten R (1983) Arzneimittelnebenwirkungen – vorhersehbare Gefahr für Leberkranke? Z Ärztl Fortbild 77:373–375

Beeuwkes H, Buytendijk HJ, Maesen FPV (1969) Der Wert des Rifampicin bei der Behandlung von Patienten mit bronchopulmonären Affektionen. Arzneimittelforsch 19:1283–1285
Begg KJ (1967) The susceptibility of mycobacteria to rifamide and rifampicin. Addendum on serum levels. Tubercle 48:149–150
Beggs WH, Andrews FA (1973 a) Uptake of ethambutol by Mycobacterium smegmatis and its relation to growth inhibition. Am Rev Respir Dis 108:691–693
Beggs WH, Andrews FA (1973 b) Primary binding of ethambutol by Mycobacterium smegmatis. Am Rev Respir Dis 108:983–984
Beggs WH, Auran NE (1972) Uptake and binding of ^{14}C-ethambutol by tubercle bacilli and the relation of binding to growth inhibition. Antimicrob Agents Chemother 2:390–394
Beggs WH, Jenne JW (1969) Isoniazid uptake and growth inhibition of Mycobacterium tuberculosis in relation to time and concentration of pulsed drug exposures. Tubercle 50:377–385
Benazet F, Dubost M, Jolles G, Leau O, Pascal C, Preud'homme J, Terlain B (1968) Liaisons et modifications des antibiotiques in vivo (sang et foyer infectieux). Biologie Médicale 57:376–401
Bending MR, Skacel PO (1977) Rifampicin and methadone withdrawal. Lancet I:1211
Benkert K, Blaha H, Petersen KF, Schmid PCh (1974) Tagesprofile und Profilverlaufskontrollen von Ethambutol bei Kindern. Med Klin 69:1808–1813
Binda G, Domenichini E, Gottardi A, Orlandi B, Ortelli E, Pacini B, Foust G (1971) Rifampicin, a general review. Arzneimittelforsch 21:1907–1977 (W, B, Ph)
Black HR, Griffith RS, Peabody AM (1966) Absorption, excretion and metabolism of capreomycin in normal and diseased states. Ann NY Acad Sci 135:974–982
Boddingius J, Stolz E (1981) Do anti-leprosy drugs reach Mycobacterium leprae in peripheral nerves? Lancet I:774–775
Bolt HM, Kappus H, Bolt M (1974) Rifampicin and oral contraception. Lancet I:1280–1281
Bolt HM, Kappus H, Bolt M (1975) Effect of rifampicin treatment on the metabolism of oestradiol and 17-α-ethinyloestradiol by human liver microsomes. Eur J Clin Pharmacol 8:301–307
Bolt HM, Kappus H, Bolt M (1976) Interaction of rifampicin with estrogen metabolism. Naunyn-Schmiedebergs Arch Pharmacol 294 Suppl: R 8
Boman G (1974) Clinical and experimental studies on rifampicin: distribution, kinetics and drug interactions. Thesis, Stockholm
Boman G (1975) Autoradiographic studies of the distribution of rifampicin. Scand J Respir Dis Suppl 93:3
Boman G, Ringberger V-A (1974) Binding of rifampicin by human plasma proteins. Eur J Clin Pharmacol 7:369–373
Boman G, Borga O, Hanngren A, Malmborg A-St, Sjöqvist E (1970) Pharmakokinetische und genetische Gesichtspunkte über den Metabolismus von Isoniazid, p-Aminosalicylsäure und Rifampicin. Pneumonologie, Suppl 15–20
Boman G, Hanngren A, Malmborg A-St, Borga O, Sjöqvist F (1971) Drug interaction: decreased serum concentrations of RMP when given with PAS. Lancet I:800
Boman G, Lundgren P, Stjernström G (1975) Mechanism of the inhibitory effect of PAS granules on the absorption of rifampicin: adsorption of rifampicin by an excipient, bentonite. Eur J Clin Pharmacol 8:293–299
Bondarev IM, Bolgaya TM (1980) Effect of various isoniazid concentrations on a highly resistant variant of Mycobacterium tuberculosis. Probl Tuberk 58 issue 8: 65–69
Boulahbal F, Khaled S, Bouhassen H, Larbaoui D (1979) Étude de l'absorption et de l'élimination urinaire du pyrazinamide administré seul ou en association avec l'isoniazide et la rifampicine. Actes d'un Symposium „Le Pyrazinamide 25 ans après" tenu à Alger, Laboratoires Bracco, Milan, pp 35–42
Brouet G, Modai J, Vergez P (1969) Clinical trial of rifampin alone. A study of serum concentrations. Rev Tuberc Pneumol 33:27–42
Buffington GA, Dominguez JH, Piering WF, Hebert LA, Kauffman HM, Lemann J (1976) Interaction of rifampin and glucocorticoids. JAMA 236:1958–1960

Burkhardt KR, Nel EE (1980) Monitoring regularity of drug intake in tuberculous patients by means of simple urine tests. S Afr Med J 57:981–985
Canetti G, Djurovic V, Le Lirzin M, Thibier R, Lepeuple A (1970) Étude comparative de l' évolution des taux sanguins de rifampicine chez l' homme par deux méthodes microbiologiques différentes. Rev Tuberc Pneumol 34:93–106
Carlone NA, Acocella G, Cuffini AM, Forno-Pizzoglio MN (1985) Killing of macrophage-ingested mycobacteria by rifampicin, pyrazinamide and pyrazinoic acid alone and in combination. Am Rev Respir Dis 132:1274–1277
Carpenter OS, Northam JI, Wagner JG (1966) Use of kinetic models in the study of antibiotic absorption, metabolism and excretion. In: Herold M, Gabriel Z (eds) Antibiotics – Advances in research, production and clinical use. Butterworths, London, Prague: Czechoslowak Medical Press, pp 165–172
Cartwright RA, Rogers HJ, Barham-Hall D, Glashan RW, Ahmad RA, Higgins E, Kahn MA (1982) Role of N-acetyltransferase phenotypes in bladder carcinogenesis: a pharmacogenetic epidemiological approach to bladder cancer. Lancet II:842–845
Chailleux E, Moigneteau Ch, Ordronneau J, Le Normand Y, Kergueris MF, Veyrac MJ, Larousse C (1980) Étude simultanée de l' effet inducteur de la rifampicine et du phénotype d'acetylation de l'isoniazide, chez 21 tuberculeux soumis à un traitement mixte. Rev Fr Mal Respir 8:169–171
Chojkowski W (1971) Studies on binding of β-hydroxyethylpiperazinomethyl-tetracycline, phenoxymethylpenicillinate (PTP), phenoxymethylpenicillin (PV), cloxacillin (CL), erythromycin lactobionate (EL), lincomycin (LCM) and tetracycline (TC) by human blood albumins. Acta Pol Pharm 28:545–549
Chulski T, Johnson RH, Schlagel CA, Wagner JG (1963) Direct proportionality of urinary excretion rate and serum level of tetracycline in human subjects. Nature 198:450–453
Cieszýnski T (1971) Investigation of stability of therapeutics in lipophylic suppository bases. II. Determination of degradation degree of cyclovegantine, ethionamide and euphylline in suppositories. Acta Pol Pharm 28:374–384
Claunch BC, Castro V, Barnes WMT (1963) Studies on the binding of INH by serum proteins. Trans 22nd Res Conf Pulm Dis VAAF:37–42
Clini V, Grassi G (1970) The action of new antituberculous drugs on intracellular tubercle bacilli. Antibiot Chemother 16:20–26
Constans P, Saint-Paul M, Morin Y, Bonnaud G, Bariety M (1968) Rifampin: first study of plasma concentrations during prolonged treatment in pulmonary tuberculosis. Rev Tuberc Pneumol 32:991–1005
Crowle AJ, Sbarbaro JA, Judson FN, Douves GS, May MH (1984) Inhibition by streptomycin of tubercle bacilli within cultured human macrophages. Am Rev Respir Dis 130:839–844
Crowle AJ, Sbarbaro JA, Judson FN, May MH (1985a) The effect of ethambutol on tubercle bacilli within cultured human macrophages. Am Rev Respir Dis 132:742–745
Crowle AJ, Sbarbaro JA, Judson FN, Iseman M (1985b) The antimycobacterial activity of chemotherapic agents within the human macrophage – a new test model. Am Rev Respir Dis 131 Suppl: A 232
Crowle AJ, Sbarbaro JA, Iseman MD, May MH (1986) Effect of isoniazid and ceforanide against virulent tubercle bacilli in cultured human macrophages. Am Rev Respir Dis 133 issue 4, part 2: A 40
Curci G, Bergamini N, Veneri FD, Ninni A, Nitti V (1972) Half-life of rifampicin after repeated administration of different doses in humans. Chemotherapy 17:373–381
Darnis F (1976) Leberstoffwechsel von Arzneimitteln. MMW 118:805–810
Decroix G, Djurovic V (1972) Taux sanguin de rifampicine chez les tuberculeux cirrhotiques. Rev Tuberc Pneumol 36:1003–1008
Dettli L (1961) Zur pharmakotherapeutischen Beeinflussung gefäßloser Bezirke im Organismus. II. Mitt. Konzentrationsverläufe im Inneren gefäßloser Bezirke. Schweiz Med Wochenschr 91:921–927
Dettli L, Staub H (1960) Zur pharmakotherapeutischen Beeinflussung gefäßloser Bezirke im Organismus. Schweiz Med Wochenschr 90:924–929

Devereux TR, Serabjit-Singh CJ, Slaughter SR, Wolf CR, Philpot RM, Fouts JR (1981) Identification of cytochrome P-450 isozymes in nonciliated bronchiolar epithelial (Clara) and alveolar type II cells isolated from rabbit lung. Experimental Lung Res 2:221–230

Dickinson JM, Mitchison DA (1981) Experimental models to explain the high sterilizing activity of rifampin in the chemotherapy of tuberculosis. Am Rev Respir Dis 123:367–371

Dickinson JM, Mitchison DA (1985) Activity of the combination of fludalanine and cycloserine against mycobacteria in vitro. Tubercle 66:109–115

Dimmling Th (1967) Bakteriologische Untersuchungen über Resorption und Excretion sowie über das Wirkungsspektrum von Alpha-6-Desoxyoxytetracyclin (Doxycyclin). Med Klin 62:1269–1276

Dimmling Th, Wagner WH (1965) Konzentration von Tetracyclinen im Serum nach oraler und intravenöser Gabe. Arzneimittelforsch 15:1288–1292

Doluisio JT, Dittert LW (1969) Influence of repetitive dosing of tetracyclines on biologic half-life in serum. Clin Pharmacol Ther 10:690–701

Dost FH (1972) Absorption, Transit, Occupancy und Availments als neue Begriffe in der Biopharmazeutik. Klin Wochenschr 50:410–412

Dost FH (1975) Definition der Begriffe Availments und Availability. Klin Wochenschr 53:145–146

Drabkina RO, Ginzburg TS (1977) Antituberculous action and pharmacokinetics of thioacetazone. Probl Tuberk 55 issue 4: 69–71

Dubinin UP (1965) Molekulargenetik. Fischer, Jena

Dudchik GKh, Bilyk MA (1975) Mechanism of the excretion of the hina metabolites by the kidneys in patients with pulmonary tuberculosis. Probl Tuberk 53 issue 5: 57–61

Dürckheimer W (1975) Tetracycline: Chemie, Biochemie und Struktur-Wirkungs-Beziehungen. Angew Chem 87:751–784

Eda T (1963a) Studies on the action of isoniazid to tubercle bacilli and the mechanism of the isoniazid-resistance in mycobacteria. I. Kekkaku 38:37–41

Eda T (1963b) Studies on the action of isoniazid to tubercle bacilli and the mechanism of the isoniazid-resistance in mycobacteria. III. Kekkaku 38:395–398

Edwards OM, Courtenay-Evans RJ, Galley JM, Hunter J, Tait AD (1974) Changes in cortisol metabolism following rifampicin therapy. Lancet II:549–551

Eichenwald HF (1966) Some observations on dosage and toxicity of kanamycin in premature and full-term infants. Ann NY Acad Sci 132:984–991

Eidus L, Hodgkin MM (1975) A new isoniazid preparation designed for moderately fast and "fast" metabolizers of the drug. Arzneimittelforsch 25:1077–1080

Ellard GA (1969) Absorption, metabolism and excretion of pyrazinamide in man. Tubercle 50:144–158

Ellard GA (1976) A slow-release preparation of isoniazid: pharmacological aspects. Bull Int Union Tuberc 51:143–154

Ellard GA, Gammon PT, Lakshminarayan S, Fox W, Aber VR, Mitchison DA, Citron KM, Tall R (1972) Pharmacology of some slow-release preparations of isoniazid of potential use in intermittent treatment of tuberculosis. Lancet I:340–343

Ellard GA, Jenner PJ, Downs PA (1980) An evaluation of the potential use of isoniazid, acetylisoniazid and isonicotinic acid for monitoring the self-administration of drugs. Br J Clin Pharmacol 10:369–381

Ellard GA, Gammon PT, Polansky F, Viznerova A, Havlik I, Fox W (1973) Further studies on the pharmacology of a slow-release matrix preparation of isoniazid (Smith & Nephew HS82) of potential use in the intermittent treatment of tuberculosis. Tubercle 54:57–66

Emerson PA, Nicholson JP (1965) The absorption of 4,4-diisoamyloxythiocarbanilide (Isoxyl) using radioactive material (S^{35} tagged). Trans 24th Res Conf Pulm Dis VAAF:44–45

Eule H, Iwainsky H (1981) Zum Einfluß therapeutischer und biologischer Parameter auf das Auftreten von Nebenwirkungen und Beschwerden bei intermittierender Chemotherapie der Lungentuberkulose. Prax Pneumol 35:347–353

Eule H, Werner E (1966) Thiocarlide (4'4-diisoamyloxythiocarbanilide) blood levels in patients suffering from tuberculosis. Tubercle 47:214–220

Eule H, Werner E (1970) Ethambutol-Serumspiegel bei unterschiedlicher Dosierung: Vergleich von vier verschiedenen Bestimmungsmethoden. Z Erkr Atmungsorgane 133:443–448

Eule H, Krebs A, Iwainsky H (1973) Therapie der Tuberkulose. Übersicht über den erreichten Wissensstand, Entwicklungstendenzen und noch offene Probleme. Z Erkr Atmungsorgane 138:78–100

Eule H, Werner E, Winsel K, Iwainsky H (1974a) Intermittent chemotherapy of pulmonary tuberculosis using rifampicin and isoniazid for primary treatment: the influence of various factors on the frequency of side-effects. Tubercle 55:81–89

Eule H, Iwainsky H, Kärnbach E, Kaluza P, Werner E (1974b) Möglichkeiten einer weiteren Optimierung der Tuberkulosetherapie-Ergebnisse einer kontrollierten klinischen Studie. Z Erkr Atmungsorgane 141:233–249

Eule H, Werner E, Winsel K, Iwainsky H (1985) Zur Pharmakokinetik des RMP bei intermittierender Behandlung von Patienten mit Lungentuberkulose. 2. Mitt. Zum Einfluß des RMP auf die Entwicklung der Therapie von Mykobakteriosen und nichttuberkulösen Infektionskrankheiten. Pharmazie 40:276–277

Fabre J, Pitton JS, Kunz JP (1966) Distribution and excretion of doxycycline in man. Chemotherapia 11:73–85

Fabre J, Pitton JS, Vivieux C, Laurencet FL, Bernhardt JP, Godel JC (1967) Absorption, distribution et excrétion d'un nouvel antibiotique à large spectre chez l'homme. Schweiz Med Wochenschr 97:915–924

Fabre J, Blanchard P, Rudhardt M (1977) Über die Pharmakokinetik von Ampicillin, Cephalotin und Doxycyclin in den Geweben der Ratte. Med Klin Sondernummer:17–24

Fedorko J, Katz S, Allnoch H (1968) In vitro activity of minocycline, a new tetracycline. Am J Med Sci 255:252–258

Federspil P (1979) Antibiotikaschäden des Ohres, dargestellt am Beispiel des Gentamycins. Hals-, Nasen- und Ohrenheilkunde, Bd 28. Barth, Leipzig

Felder E, Pitré D, Tiepolo U (1964) Hydrolyse und Bildung von Morpholinomethylpyrazinamid. 2. Mitt. Über latente Formen chemotherapeutischer Wirkungsprinzipien. Arzneimittelforsch 14:1227–1230

Finland M (1966) Summary of the conference on kanamycin: appraisal after eigth years of clinical application. Ann NY Acad Sci 132:1045–1090

Forgan-Smith R, Ellard GA, Newton D, Mitchison DA (1973) Pyrazinamide and other drugs in tuberculous meningitis. Lancet II:374

Fourtillan J-B, Saux M-Cl (1978) Intérêt des tétracyclines de deuxième génération. Compartement pharmacocinétique. Sem Hôp Paris 54:224–230

Franz H, Urbanczik R, Stoll K, Müller U (1974) Prothionamid-Blutspiegel nach oraler Verabreichung von Prothionamid allein oder kombiniert mit Isoniazid und/oder mit Diamino-Difenylsulfon. Prax Pneumol 28:605–612

Frostadt S (1961) Continued studies in concentrations of para-amino-salicylic acid (PAS) in the blood. Acta Tuberc Scand 41:68–82

Füsgen I, Summa J-D, Weih H (1977) Verhalten der Serumspiegel von Oxytetracyclin und Doxycyclin unter der forcierten Diurese bei schweren Schlafmittelvergiftungen. Med Klin 72:1645–1648

Fujii R (1966) Postcript to the panel discussion: proper dosage of kanamycin for premature babies. Ann NY Acad Sci 132:1031–1036

Furesz S, Scotti R, Pallanza R, Mapelli E (1967) Rifampicin: A new rifamycin. III. Absorption, distribution and elimination in man. Arzneimittelforsch 17:534–537

Gaidov N (1971) Terisidon – A new synthetic tuberculosis-suppressing antibiotic. Probl Tuberk 49 issue 12: 19–22

Gajewska E (1967) Comparative determinations of concentration of ethionamide in the blood and urine. Gruzlica 35:573–576

Gassen HG (1982) Das bakterielle Ribosom: ein programmierbares Enzym. Angew Chem 94:15–27

Gelber R, Jacobsen P, Levy L (1969) A study of the availability of six commercial formulations of isoniazid. Clin Pharmacol Ther 10:841–848
Gibaldi M (1967) Pharmacokinetics of absorption and elimination of doxycycline in man. Chemotherapia 12:265–271
Gill GV (1976) Rifampicin and breakfast. Lancet II:1135
Girling DJ (1984) The role of pyrazinamide in primary chemotherapy for pulmonary tuberculosis Tubercle 65:1–4
Goldberg IH (1965) Mode of action of antibiotics. Am J Med 39:722–752
Goldshtein VD, Ioffe RA, Kryukov VL (1977) On the rifampicin pharmacokinetics in patients with pulmonary tuberculosis. Probl Tuberk 55 issue 4: 61–66
Gothoni G, Pentikäinen P, Vapaatalo HI, Hackman R, Björksten K (1972) Absorption of antibiotics: influence of metoclopramide and atropine on serum levels of pivampicillin and tetracycline. Ann Clin Res 4:228–232
Grassi GG (1971) Aspetti dell' attività antimicobatterica della rifampicina. Giorn Ital Mal Tor 25:77–88
Green VA (1963) Effect of neostigmine on the tissue concentration of antibiotic in streptomycin treated rats.
Greenberg L, Eidus L (1962) Antituberculous drugs (Th 1314 and INH) in the host organism. Br J Dis Chest 56:124–130
Gregoriadis G (1981) Targeting of drugs: implications in medicine. Lancet II:241–247
Grönroos JA, Toivanen A (1964) Blood ethionamide levels after administration of enteric-coated and uncoated tablets. Curr Ther Res 6:105–114
Gros L, Ringsdorf H, Schupp H (1981) Polymere Antitumormittel auf molekularer und zellulärer Basis? Angew Chemie 93:311–332
Grosset J (1978) The sterilizing value of rifampicin and pyrazinamide in experimental short course chemotherapy. Tubercle 59:287–297
Grosset J (1981) Studies in short-course chemotherapy for tuberculosis. Chest 80:719–720
Grunert M (1969) Untersuchungen zum Verhalten des α-Äthylisonicotinsäurethioamides und seines Sulfoxydes in vitro und in vivo. Dissertation, Sektion Chemie der Humboldt-Universität Berlin
Grunert M, Iwainsky H (1967) Zum Stoffwechsel des Äthionamids und seines Sulfoxydes im Makroorganismus. Arzneimittelforsch 17:411–415
Grunert M, Werner E, Iwainsky H, Eule H (1968) Veränderungen des Äthionamides und seines Sulfoxydes in vitro. Beitr Klin Tuberk 138:68–82
Gubler HU, Favez G, Bergier N, Maillard J-M, Friedrich T (1966) Beitrag zur Resorption von Thiocarlid beim Menschen. Beitr Klin Tuberk 133:126–139
Haapanen J, Gill R, Russell WF, Kass I (1960) Re-treatment of pulmonary tuberculosis. Experiences with various combinations of pyrazinamide, cycloserine and kanamycin in patients excreting tubercle bacilli resistant to both streptomycin and isoniazid. Am Rev Respir Dis 82:843–852
Haar F von der, Gabius H-J, Cramer F (1981) Aminoacyl-tRNA-Synthetasen als Zielenzyme für eine rationale Arzneimittelentwicklung. Angew Chem 93:250–256
Haegi V (1961) Zur Behandlung der Lungentuberkulose mit Ethionamid (Trécator). Schweiz Z Tuberk 18:218–226
Haegi V, Müller G (1967) Zur Tuberkulosebehandlung mit Rifamycin. Schweiz Med Wochenschr 97:1011–1014
Hagelund C-HH, Wåhlén P, Eidsaunet W (1977) Absorption of rifampicin in gastrectomized patients. Effect of meals. Scand J Respir Dis 58:241–246
Hakim J, Feldmann G, Boucherot J, Boivin P, Guibout P, Kreis B (1971) Effect of rifampicin, isoniazid and streptomycin on the human liver: a problem of enzyme induction. GUT 12:761
Hamacher H (1981) Möglichkeiten und Probleme organselektiver Wirkstoffe und Arzneiformen. Pharmazie 36:391–399
Hand WL, Sorwin RW, Steinberg Th H, Grossmann GD (1984) Uptake of antibiotics by human alveolar macrophages. Am Rev Respir Dis 129:933–937
Hanngren Ä, André T (1964) Distribution of ^{3}H-dihydrostreptomycin in tuberculous guinea-pigs. Acta Tuberc Scand 35:14–20

Hartmann G, Behr W, Beissner K-A, Honikel K, Sippel A (1968) Antibiotica als Hemmstoffe der Nukleinsäure- und Proteinsynthese. Angew Chem 80:710–718
Held H (1979) Interaktion von Rifampicin mit Phenprocoumon. Dtsch Med Wochenschr 104:1311–1314
Held H (1980) Verordnung von Arzneimitteln bei Leberkrankheiten. Internist (Berlin) 21:724–734
Held H, Fried F (1977) Elimination of para-aminosalicylic acid in patients with liver disease and renal insufficiency. Chemotherapy 23:405–415
Hendrickse W, McKiernan J, Pickup M, Lowe J (1979) Rifampicin – induced non responsiveness to corticosteroid treatment in nephrotic syndroms. Brit Med J I:306
Herken H, Gross R (1982) Praktisch wichtige Grundbegriffe der Pharmakokinetik. Internist (Berlin) 23:593–600
Hirsch HA, Finland M (1960) Comparative activity of four tetracycline analogues against pathogenic bacteria in vitro. Am J Med Sci 239:288–294
Höffler D (1976) Antibiotikatherapie bei Niereninsuffizienz. Dtsch Med Wochenschr 101:829–834
Höffler D (1981) Die Dosierung wichtiger Antibiotika und Tuberkulostatika bei Niereninsuffizienz. Internist (Berlin) 22:601–606
Holdiness MR (1984) Clinical pharmacokinetics of the antituberculosis drugs. Clin Pharmacokinet 9:511–544
Honikel K, Sippel A, Hartmann G (1968) Mode of action of antibiotics on DNA-directed polymerase reactions. Hoppe-Seylers Z Physiol Chem 349:957
Hornung St, Nikodemowicz E, Owsínski J, Rapf T (1967) Investigation into the metabolism of para-aminosalicyclic acid in the body. Gruzlica 35:657–664
Hurwitz Ch, Rosano CL (1962) Accumulation of label from ^{14}C-streptomycin by Escherichia coli. J Bacteriol 83:1193–1201
Hurwitz A, Schlozman DL (1974) Effects of antacids on gastrointestinal absorption of isoniazid in rat and man. Am Rev Respir Dis 109:41–47
Hussels H-J (1969) Zur Methodik der Serum-Konzentrationsbestimmungen des neuen Antibiotikums Rifampicin. Med-Lab 22:195–203
Hussels H-J, Otto HS (1971) Ethambutol-Serumkonzentrationen im Kindesalter. Pneumonologie 145:392–396
Hussels H-J, Kroening U, Magdorf K (1973) Ethambutol and rifampicin serum levels in children: second report on the combined administration of ethambutol and rifampicin. Pneumonologie 149:31–38
Ioffe RA (1973) Rifampicin passage with urine during treatment of tuberculous patients. Probl Tuberk 51 issue 12: 43–46
Iseman MD, Heifets L, Gangadharam PRJ (1986) Combination drug effects in the chemotherapy of M. avium-intracellulare: in vitro and in vivo observations. Am Rev Respir Dis 133 issue 4, part 2: A 41
Iwainsky H (1970) Der Ansatzpunkt der verschiedenen Therapeutica im Stoffwechsel des Tuberkelbakteriums. Pneumonologie, Suppl 1–14 (M)
Iwainsky H, Siegel D (1961) Über den Einfluß qualitativer Ernährungsfaktoren auf den INH-Stoffwechsel im Makroorganismus. Beitr Klin Tuberk 123:166–170
Iwainsky H, Käppler W (1974) Mykobakterien, Biochemie und biochemische Differenzierung, Bibliothek für das Gesamtgebiet der Lungenkrankheiten, Band 103. Barth, Leipzig
Iwainsky H, Winsel K (1981) Schadstoffe im Tabak und Tabakrauch. Z Erkr Atmungsorgane 157:90–102
Iwainsky H, Rogowski J, Grunert M (1963) Zur intravenösen Verabreichung von Ätina. Mschr Tbk-Bekpfg 6:146–153
Iwainsky H, Sehrt I, Grunert M (1964) Zum Stoffwechsel der Äthionamids. Naturwissenschaften 51:316
Iwainsky H, Sehrt I, Grunert M (1965) Zum Stoffwechsel des Äthionamids nach intravenöser Verabreichung. Arzneimittelforsch 15:193–197
Iwainsky H, Winsel K, Werner E, Eule H (1974) On the pharmacokinetics of rifampicin I: Influence of dosage and duration of treatment with intermittent administration. Scand J Respir Dis 55:229–236

Iwainsky H, Eule H, Werner E, Käppler W (1975) Messung der Antituberkulotikakonzentration in Körperflüssigkeiten und Organen mittels Mykobakterien. In: Meissner G, Schmiedel A (†), Nelles A (†) (Hrsg) Infektionskrankheiten und ihre Erreger, Bd 4, Teil III. Fischer, Jena, pp 159–181

Iwainsky H, Winsel K, Werner E, Eule H (1976) On the pharmacokinetics of rifampicin (RMP) during treatment with intermittent administration II. Influence of age and sex of the patients. Scand J Respir Dis 57:5–11

Iwainsky H, Eule H, Fischer P, Werner E, Winsel K, Franke H (1977) Die unterschiedliche INH-Inaktivierung bei intermittierender Chemotherapie. Z Erkr Atmungsorgane 147:41–50

Izaki K, Arima K (1965) Effect of various conditions on accumulation of oxytetracycline in Escherichia coli. J Bacteriol 89:1335–1339

Jalsenja I, Nixon JR, Senjkovic R, Stivic I (1980) Sustained-release dosage forms of microencapsulated isoniazid. J Pharm Pharmacol 32:678–680

Jeanes CWL, Schaefer O, Eidus L (1973) Comparative blood levels and metabolism of INH and an INH-matrix preparation in fast and slow inactivators. Can Med Assoc J 109:483–487

Jenne JW (1960) Studies of human patterns of isoniazid metabolism using an intravenous fall-off technique with a chemical method. Am Rev Respir Dis 81:1–9

Jenne JW (1964) Pharmacokinetics and the dose of isoniazid and para-aminosalicyclic acid in the treatment of tuberculosis. Antibiot Chemother 12:407–432

Jenne JW, Beggs WH (1973) Correlation of in vitro and in vivo kinetics with clinical use of isoniazid, ethambutol and rifampin. Am Rev Respir Dis 107:1013–1021

Jenner PJ, Ellard GA, Allan WGL, Singh D, Girling DJ, Nunn AJ (1981) Serum uric acid concentrations and arthralgia among patients treated with pyrazinamide-containing regimens in Hong Kong and Singapore. Tubercle 62:175–179

Jezequel AM, Orlandi F, Tenconi LT (1971) Changes of the smooth endoplasmic reticulum induced by rifampicin in human and guinea-pig hepatocytes. GUT 12:984–987

Johnson W, Mankiewicz E, Jasmin R, Corte G (1961) The effect of 5-bromsalicylhydroxamic acid on the acetalytion of isoniazid and its concentration in the blood. Am Rev Respir Dis 84:872–875

Jones WD Jr, David HL (1971) Inhibition by rifampin of mycobacteriophage D29 replication in its drug-resistant host, Mycobacterium smegmatis ATCC 607. Am Rev Respir Dis 103:618–624

Jungbluth H (1971) Isoniazid-Dosierung bei Niereninsuffizienz. Pneumonologie 145:383–384

Jungbluth H (1973) Tuberkulose-Chemotherapie bei Kranken mit vorgeschädigter Niere. Prax Pneumol 27:175–182

Jungbluth H, Urbanczik R (1974) Ethambutol-Serumspiegel nach oraler und intravenöser Verabreichung. Prax Pneumol 28:499–504

Käppler W (1986) Persönliche Mitteilung

Kalabukha AV (1971) Protionamide concentration in the blood of tuberculous patients. Probl Tuberk 49 issue 12: 26–29

Kaminskaya GO, Karachunsky MA (1975) Changes in the function of the liver and elimination of antituberculous drugs producing side-effects in patients with tuberculosis of the lungs. Probl Tuberk 53 issue 6: 47–51

Karlson P (1984) Kurzes Lehrbuch der Biochemie für Mediziner und Naturwissenschaftler. 12. Aufl. Thieme, Stuttgart

Kass I (1966) Kanamycin in the therapy of pulmonary tuberculosis in the United States. Ann N J Acad Sci 132:892–900

Khalil SA, Daabis NA, Naggar VF, Wafik M (1977) Effect of magnesium trisilicate and citric acid on the bioavailability of tetracycline in man. Pharmazie 32:519–522

Kheifets LB, Kozlova NE (1975) The effect of cycloserine and Terisidone on the intracellular multiplication of mycobacteria. Probl Tuberk 53 issue 1: 71–73

Kheiny I, Zagorska T, Yanik M, Melikher I (1977) Rifampicin concentration in the tissues of the locomotor system. Probl Tuberk 55 issue 4: 67–69

Kilburn JO, Beam RE, David HL, Sanchez E, Corpe RF, Dunn W (1972) Reagent-impregnated paper strip for detection of metabolic products of isoniazid in urine. Am Rev Respir Dis 106:923–924
Kislitsyna NA, Kotova NI (1977) Concentration of some antituberculous agents in the blood and resected sectors of the lungs in tuberculous patients. Probl Tuberk 55 issue 8: 72–75
Kislitsina NA, Kotova NI (1980) Rifampicin and isoniazid levels in blood and resected lungs of tuberculous patients treated with drug combinations. Probl Tuberk 58 issue 8: 63–65
Kivman GY, Geitman I Y (1971) Comparative studies on antibiotic levels in human blood and serum with the use of the agar-diffusion method. Antibiotiki 16:929–933
Kivman GY, Geitman IY (1972) Interaction of antibiotics with individual blood sera of humans and animals. Antibiotiki 17:467–471
Klastersky J, Daneau D (1972) Bacteriological evaluation of minocycline. A new tetracycline. Chemotherapy 17:51–58
Kleber FX (1979) Zur Resorption von Antituberkulotika bei magenresezierten, tuberkulosekranken Patienten. Prax Pneumol 33:38–44
Kleeberg H, Gärtig D, Glatthaar E, Nel E, Stander M (1975) Isoniazid metabolism in black patients. S Afr Med J 49:1503
Knothe H (1963) Neue Tetracyclinderivate. Antibiot Chemother (Basel) 11:97–117
Kob D (1967) Über die Resorption von D-Cycloserin und Isonikotinsäurehydrazid (INH) nach peroraler Verabreichung bei Magenresezierten und Normalpersonen, Dissertation, Friedrich-Schiller-Universität Jena
Kochanova NK, Mazaev MB, Tverdokhlebova NG (1981) Isoniazid levels in blood, urine and kidney tissue of rabbits with cavernous tuberculosis of single kidney. Probl Tuberk 58 issue 2: 64–67
Köhler H, Winsel K (1982) Klinische und experimentelle Untersuchungen zur Optimierung der Chemotherapie der Lungen- und Nierentuberkulose. Promotion B-Arbeit, Friedrich-Schiller-Universität, Jena
König H (1980) Pharmachemie im Wandel – Probleme und Chancen. Angew Chem 92:802–815
Kolachevskaya EN, Guryan IE (1981) Isoniazid levels in tissues of female patients with genital tuberculosis. Probl Tuberk 59 issue 9: 59–61
Konno K, Oizumi K, Hayashi I, Oka S (1970) Experimental and clinical studies of rifampicin in tuberculosis. Sci Rep Res Inst Tohoku Univ (Med). S 17:110–120
Korner I, Voigt R, Keipert S, Kalich R (1978) Wechselwirkungen zwischen makromolekularen Hilfsstoffen und Arzneistoffen. 11. Mitt. Einfluß von Makromolekülen auf die mikrobiologische Aktivität von Tetracyclinantibiotika. Pharmazie 33:72–73
Korotaev GA, Tatarinova NV (1972) Content of cycloserine in the blood serum and its discharge with the urine in patients with tuberculosis. Therap Arch 44:81–84
Kroening U (1974) Die Konzentrationsbestimmung von Ethambutol im Vollblut und ihre Bedeutung für den Nachweis der Kumulation des Medikamentes. Pneumonologie 151:135–146
Kroker R, Hegner D (1980) Interaction of rifamycin SV with hepatobiliary transport of taurocholic acid. Naunyn-Schmiedebergs Arch Pharmacol 313:Suppl R 63, Nr. 250
Krüger-Thiemer E, Bünger P (1965/66) The role of the therapeutic regimen in dosage design. Part I. Chemotherapia 10:61–73
Krüger-Thiemer E †, Kröger H, Nestler HJ, Seydel JK (1975) Wirkungsmodi antituberkulöser Chemotherapeutika: Pyridincarbonsäurethioamide, Thiocarbanilide und Thiosemicarbazone – Isoniazid – Inositanaloga – Tetracycline. In: Meissner G, Schmiedel A †, Nelles A † (Hrsg) Infektionskrankheiten und ihre Erreger, Band 4, Teil III, Fischer Jena pp 289–298, 257–288, 337–352, 353–357
Küchler E (1976) Chemische Methoden zur Untersuchung der Ribosomenstruktur. Angew Chem 88:555–564
Kunin CM (1966) Absorption, distribution, excretion and fate of kanamycin. Ann NY Acad Sci 132:811–818

Kunin CM (1967) A guide to use of antibiotics in patients with renal disease. Ann Intern Med 67:151–158
Kunin CM, Finland M (1961) Clinical pharmacology of the tetracycline antibiotics. Clin Pharmacol Ther 2:51–69
Kuntz E (1962) Kanamycin-Konzentrationen im Blut, Liquor und Pleuraexsudat. Klin Wochenschr 40:1107–1111
Kuntz E (1966) Untersuchungen über die Blutspiegelwerte und die Ausscheidung von p-Aminosalicylsäure (PAS-Natrium) bei i.v. Infusionsbehandlung. Beitr Klin Tuberk 133:12–24
Lampe J, Lampe H, Butschak G (1981) Klinische Aspekte der Enzyminduktion. Dtsch Gesundh-Wesen 36:1081–1086
Landsdown FS, Radzin I (1963a) Effect of aluminium hydroxide gel on blood concentrations of para-aminosalicyclic acid. Am Rev Respir Dis 88:721–724
Landsdown FS, Radzin I (1963b) Effect of aluminium hydroxide gel on blood level of para-aminosalicyclic acid. Trans 22nd Res Conf Pulm Dis VAAF:33–37
Larkin JC Jr (1960) Results of therapy with thiocarbanidin used with isoniazid or streptomycin. Am Rev Respir Dis 81:235–240
Lee CS, Brater DC, Gambertoglio JG, Benet LZ (1980) Disposition kinetics of ethambutol in man. J Pharmacokinet Biopharm 8:335–346
Lehmann J (1961) Chemische und experimentelle Grundlagen der PAS-Therapie. Wien Med Wochenschr 111:803–805
Lehmann J (1969) The role of the metabolism of p-aminosalicylic acid (PAS) in the treatment of tuberculosis. Scand J Respir Dis 50:169–185
Leroy A, Humbert G, Oksenhendler G, Fillastre JP (1978) Pharmacokinetics of aminoglycosides in subjects with normal and impaired renal function. Antibiot Chemother 25:163–180
Levi AJ, Sherlock S, Walker D (1968) Phenylbutazone and isoniazid metabolism in patients with liver disease in relation to previous drug therapy. Lancet I:1275–1279
Levy D, Russell WF Jr, Middlebrook G (1960) Dosages of isoniazid and streptomycin for routine chemotherapy of tuberculosis. Tubercle 41:23–31
Levy D, Russell WF Jr, Ninio S, Middlebrook G (1961) Effect of increasing dosage of streptomycinsulfate on serum levels of antimicrobially active drug. Dis Chest 39:161–164
Lichey J, Charissis G, Braunsdorf M, Franke J, Hahn W (1979) Accumulation of 99^{m}TC-tetracycline in lung infarction area. Respiration 37:220–223
Liss RH, Letourneau RJ, Schepis JP (1981) Distribution of ethambutol in primate tissues and cells. Am Rev Respir Dis 123:529–532
Llorens-Terol J, Martinez-Roig A, Busquets RM (1981) Rifampin for brucellosis treatment in children. In: Periti P, Grassi GG (eds) Current chemotherapy and immunotherapy. 12th International Congress of Chemotherapy (1981, Florence, Italy) Vol II. American Society for Microbiology, Washington, pp 975–977
Loos U, Musch E, Jensen JC, Mikus G, Schwabe HK, Eichelbaum M (1985) Pharmacokinetics of oral and intravenous rifampicin during chronic administration. Klin Wochenschr 63:1205–1211
Lukjan Z, Rogowski F, Olenski J (1969) The level of isoniazid labeled with C^{14} in the tissues of animals infected with tuberculosis and given insulin. Gruzlica 37:893–899
Madsen L, Goble M, Iseman M (1986) Ansamycin (LM 427) in the retreatment of drug-resistant tuberculosis. Am Rev Respir Dis 133: Issue 4, part 2, A 206
Maher JR, Hansen JD (1960) Paper electrophoresis separation and elution of some antituberculous drugs and their metabolites. Am Rev Respir Dis 81:373–381
Mannhart M, Dettli L, Spring P (1971) Die Elimination des Doxyzyklins und ihre Beeinflussung durch die Hämodialyse bei anurischen Patienten. Schweiz Med Wochenschr 101:123–127
Marwyck C Van, Gängel G (1961) Blutspiegelerhöhung durch Kombination von Tetracyclin und Chlortetracyclin nach oraler Verabreichung. Arzneimittelforsch 11:769–771
Matsuzaki Y, Saito C (1961) Studies on the blood concentrations of biologically active isoniazid and its derivatives and on the metabolic patterns of isoniazid. Kekkaku 36:61–62

Mattila MJ, Tiitinen H (1967) The rate of isoniazid inactivation in Finnish diabetic and non-diabetic patients. Ann Med Exp Fenn 45:423–427
Mattila MJ, Ronkanen A, Widnäs M (1967) Comparison of the serum concentrations of ethionamide and prothionamide. Scand J Clin Lab Invest 19 Suppl 95: 62
Mattila MJ, Takki S, Holsti LR (1968 a) Transfer of water and drugs by the isolated intestine of the X-irradiated rat. Arzneimittelforsch 18:889–890
Mattila MJ, Koskinen R, Takki S (1968 b) Absorption of ethionamide and prothionamide in vitro and in vivo. Ann Med Int Fenn 57:75–79
Mattila MJ, Nieminen E, Tiitinen H (1969) Serum levels, urinary excretion, and side-effects of cycloserine in the presence of isoniazid and p-aminosalicyclic acid. Scand J Resp Dis 50:291–300
McAllister WAC, Thompson PJ, Al-Habet SM, Rogers HJ (1983) Rifampicin reduces effectiveness and bioavailability of prednisolone. Br Med J 286:923–925
McCarthy CM (1981) Variation in isoniazid susceptibility of Mycobacterium avium during the cell cycle. Am Rev Respir Dis 123:450–453
Meissner J (1965) Verteilungsstudien mit radioaktiv markiertem Isoxyl. Beitr Klin Tuberk 132:322–324
Melander A, Danielson K, Hanson A, Jansson L, Rerup C, Schersten B, Thulin T, Wahlin E (1976) Reduction of isoniazid bioavailability in normal men by concomitant intake of food. Acta Med Scand 200:93–97
Mikhailova ES, Samtsov VS, Kartashov GV, Kanevskaya SS (1974) Treatment of patients with pulmonary tuberculosis and peptic ulcer through rectal introduction of tuberculostatics. Probl Tuberk 52 issue 12: 30–34
Miller ME (1982) Acetylator phenotype in bladder cancer. Lancet II:1348
Mišoň P, Trnka L (1973) Zum Wirkungsmechanismus von Rifampicin. Mschr Lungenkrkh Tbk-Bekpf 16:259–264
Mitchell JR, Thorgeirsson PU, Black M, Timbrell JA, Snodgrass WR, Potter WZ, Joliow DJ, Keiser HR (1975) Increased incidence of isoniazid hepatitis in rapid acetylators: possible relation to hydrazine metabolites. Clin Pharmacol Ther 18:70–79
Mitchison DA (1972) Current problems in the chemotherapy of tuberculosis: laboratory aspects. Trans 31th Pulm Dis Res Conf VAAF:23–29
Mitchison DA (1979) Basic mechanisms of chemotherapy. Chest 76 Suppl: 771–781
Miyazaki S, Inoue H, Nadai T (1981) Effect of antacids on the dissolution of minocycline and demethylchlortetracycline from capsules. Pharmazie 36:482–484
Modr Z, Dvoracek K (1976) Pharmakokinetik der Antibiotika. Dtsch Gesundh-Wesen 31:145–154
Mommsen S, Sell A, Barfod U (1982) N-Acetyltransferase phenotypes of bladder cancer patients in a low-risk population. Lancet II:1228
Moodie AS, Aquinas M, Foord RD (1964) Controlled clinical trial of 4,4′-diisoamyloxycarbanilide in the treatment of pulmonary tuberculosis. Tubercle 45:192–200
Mydlak G, Volkmann W (1965) Die Bedeutung der INH-Stoffwechselanalyse für die Therapie. Z Tuberk 124:44–48
Nakagawa H, Sunahara S (1973) Metabolism of rifampicin in the human body. 1st report. Kekkaku 48:167–176
Nakagawa H, Umene Z, Sunahara S (1981) Increased desacetylation of rifampicin and an adverse reaction. Kekkaku 56:577–586
Nikodemowicz E, Owsinski J, Kaminska M, Ostrowska A, Rapf T (1971) Investigation into the metabolism of para-aminosalicylic acid in the body. Gruzlica 34:1113–1121
Nilsson BS, Boman G (1981) Intravenous use of rifampicin. Eur J Respir Dis 62:212–214
Nitti V (1972) Antituberculosis activity of rifampin. Chest 61:589–598
Nitti V, Marmo E, Virgilio R, Delli Veneri F, Giordano L, Valentino B (1981) Pharmacokinetics of rifampin after single and repeated intravenous administration in patients with normal or impaired liver function. In: Periti P, Grassi GG (eds) Current chemotherapy and immunotherapy. 12th International Congress of Chemotherapy (1981, Florence, Italy) Vol II. American Society for Microbiology, Washington, pp 980–982
Nocke-Finck L, Breuer H, Reimers D (1973) Wirkung von Rifampicin auf den Menstruationszyklus und die Östrogenausscheidung bei Einnahme oraler Kontrazeptiva. Dtsch Med Wochenschr 98:1521–1523

Nodzu R, Watanabe H (1961) Die Beziehungen zwischen den physikalisch-chemischen Eigenschaften von Alkyl-Verbindungen und ihren bakteriostatischen Wirkungen gegen das *Mycobacterium tuberculosis*. Arzneimittelforsch 11:538–544

Oberti J, Najar I, Caravano R, Roux J (1981) In vitro concentration of tetracycline and rifampin in macrophages of normal mice and mice infected by brucella: influence on intracellular multiplication of bacteria. In: Periti P, Grassi GG (eds) Current chemotherapy and immunotherapy. 12th International Congress of Chemotherapy (1981, Florence, Italy) Vol II. American Society for Microbiology, Washington, pp 971–973

O'Brien RJ, Snider DE (1985) Tuberculosis drugs – old and new. Am Rev Respir Dis 131:309–311

Ochs HR, Verburg-Ochs B (1983) Einfluß von Alter, Gewicht, Geschlecht und Rauchgewohnheiten auf die Medikamentendosierung. Internist (Berlin) 24:167–181

Ocklitz HW (1981) Chemoprophylaxe bei Auftreten einer Meningokokken-Meningitis. Dtsch Gesundheitswes 36:2016–2018

Okolicsanyi L, Lirussi F, Nassuato G, Orlando R, Bussolon R, Dal Brun G (1980) Influence of rifamycin SV on bile acid metabolism in rats. Naunyn-Schmiedeberg's Arch Pharmacol 313:171–174

Olon LP, Holvey DN (1968) Evaluation of tetracycline phosphate complex, demethylchlortetracycline-HCl, and methacycline-HCl. Clin Med 75:33–44

Omer LMO (1978) Tagesprofile und Profilverlaufskontrollen von Ethambutol bei älteren Tuberkulosekranken. Prax Pneumol 32:252–256

O'Neill S, Lesperance E, Klass DJ (1984) Rat lung lavage surfactant enhances bacterial phagocytosis and intracellular killing by alveolar macrophages. Am Rev Respir Dis 130:225–230

Orlowski E-H (1965) Blutspiegelbestimmung bei oraler und intravenöser Therapie mit Aethionamid (Iridocin). Beitr Klin Tuberk 132:314–318

Otani G, Remmer H (1975) Participation of microsomal NADPH-cytochrome C reductase in the metabolism of rifampicin. Naunyn-Schmiedeberg's Arch Pharmacol 287:R76

Pallanza R, Arioli V, Furesz S, Bolzoni G (1967) Rifampicin: a new rifamycin. II. Laboratory studies on the antituberculous activity and preliminary clinical observations. Arzneimittelforsch 17:529–534

Paul K (1960) Beitrag zum heutigen Stand der Chemotherapie der Lungentuberkulose. II. Mitt. PAS-Blutspiegel bei verschiedener Applikation. Acta Tuberc Scand 38:82–90

Paumgartner G (1980) Der Einfluß von Lebererkrankungen auf Bioverfügbarkeit und Clearance von Medikamenten. Internist (Berlin) 21:718–723

Pavlov EP, Tushov EG, Kotlyarov LM (1974) The action of rifampicin on the extra- and intracellularly located *myco. tuberculosis*. Probl Tuberk 52 issue 12: 64–67

Pawlowska I, Pniewski T (1975) Studies on rifampicin (RMP) metabolism in patients with pulmonary tuberculosis. Gruzlica 43:977–986

Peets EA, Buyske DA (1962) Studies of the metabolism in the dog of ethambutol C^{14}, a drug having antituberculosis activity. Pharmacologist 4:171

Pentikainen P, Wan SH, Azarnoff DL (1973) Bioavailability studies on p-aminosalicylic and its various salts in man. Am Rev Respir Dis 108:1340–1347

Perenyi T, Biro L, Arr M, Novak EK, Szöke S, Feuer L (1971) Untersuchung der Albuminbindung der Tetracyclinderivate. I. Die Bedeutung der Bindung. Zusammenhänge zwischen der Struktur der Derivate und dem Ausmaß der Albuminbindung. Acta Pharm Hung 41:247–258

Perry W, Jenkins MV, Brown J, Erooga MA, Setchell KDR, Stamp TCB (1981) Metabolic consequences of rifampin-mediated enzyme induction during treatment for tuberculosis. In: Periti P, Grassi GG (eds) Current chemotherapy and immunotherapy. 12th International Congress of Chemotherapy (1981, Florence, Italy) Vol II. American Society for Microbiology, Washington, pp 987–990

Perumal VK, Gangadharam PRJ, Heifets LB, Iseman MD (1985) Dynamic aspects of the *in vitro* chemotherapeutic activity of ansamycin (rifabutine) on *M. intracellulare*. Am Rev Respir Dis 132:1278–1280

Peters U, Hausamen T-U, Grosse Brockhoff F (1974) Einfluß von Tuberkulostatika auf die Pharmakokinetik des Digitoxins. Dtsch Med Wochenschr 99:2381–2386

Pfeifer S, Borchert H-H (1978) Arzneimittel und Organismus – Einführung in Pharmakokinetik und Biotransformation. Pharmazie 33:128–174
Pfeil D, Friedrich J, Lampe J, Ruckpaul K (1983) Die Bedeutung der Aryl-Hydrocarbon-Hydroxylase-Aktivität bei der prospektiven Untersuchung schadstoffexponierter Personen. Dtsch Gesundh-Wesen 38:281–285
Piafsky KM, Sitar DS, Ragno RE, Ogilvie RI (1975) Disposition of theophylline in chronic liver disease. Clin Pharmacol Ther 17:241
Pindell MH (1966) The pharmacology of kanamycin – a review and new developments. Ann NY Acad Sci 132:805–810
Pissiotis CA, Nichols RL, Condon RE (1972) Absorption and excretion of intraperitoneally administered kanamycin sulfate. Surg Gynecol Obstet 134:995–998
Pitton JS, Roch P (1966) Serum levels of methacycline. Chemotherapia 11:331–337
Place VA, Thomas JP (1963) Clinical pharmacology of ethambutol. Am Rev Respir Dis 87:901–904
Place VA, Peets EA, Buyske DA (1966) Metabolic and special studies of ethambutol in normal volunteers and tuberculosis patients. Ann NY Acad Sci 135:775–795
Pöch G (1981) Potenzierung von Arzneimittel-Kombinationen. Med Klin 76:222–225
Poiger H, Schlatter Ch (1976) Fluorimetric determination of tetracyclines in biological materials. EXPEAM 32:781
Poiger H, Schlatter Ch (1979) Interaction of cations and chelators with the intestinal absorption of tetracycline. Naunyn-Schmiedeberg's Arch Pharmacol 306:89–92
Porven G, Canetti G (1968) Les taux de rifampicine dans le sérum de l'homme. Rev Tuberc 32:707–716
Powell-Jackson PR, Gray BJ, Heaton RW, Costello JF, Williams R, English J (1982) Adverse effect of rifampicin administration on steroid-dependent asthma. Am Rev Respir Dis 128:307–310
Pütter J (1961) Chemische Bestimmung des 2-Äthyl-isothionicotinsäureamids im Blut. Arzneimittelforsch 11:808–809
Pütter J (1964) Photometrische Bestimmung des 2-Äthyl-isothio-nicotinylamid in Organen und Körperflüssigkeiten. Arzneimittelforsch 14:1198–1203
Pujet J-C, Pujet C (1972) Dosages sanguine et humoraux de l'éthambutol administré par perfusion intraveineuse. Bordeaux Méd:1215–1222
Quinn EL, McHenry MC, Truant JP, Cox F (1966) The use of kanamycin in selected patients with serious infections caused by gram-negative bacilli: serum concentration and inhibition studies in patients with azotemia given reduced doses. Ann NY Acad Sci 132:850–853
Radu D, Huljic P, Hewel Th, Knetsch E (1977) Gewebespiegel nach intravenöser Anwendung von Tetracyclinen. Med Klin Sondernummer:25–28
Rameis H, Hitzenberger G, Jaschek I, Graninger W (1980) Ist die endogene Kreatinin-Clearance eine geeignete Basis für die Berechnung von Eliminationshalbwertszeiten des Gentamicins? Dtsch Med Wochenschr 105:1650–1654
Rapoport SM (1985) Medizinische Biochemie. 8. Auflage. Volk und Gesundheit, Berlin
Ratledge C (1977) The Mycobacteria. In: Cook JG (ed) Pattern of Progress. Meadowfield Press Ltd, Durham, England
De Rautlin de la Roy Y, Patte F, Morichau-Beauchant G (1971) Taux sériques de rifampicine avec des posologies réduites (300 mg/jour). Rev Tuberc Pneumol 35:342–350
Regosz A, Zuk G (1980) Studies on spectrophotometric determination of tetracycline and its degradation products. Pharmazie 35:24–26
Reichert D (1981) Giftung körperfremder Stoffe durch Konjugationsreaktionen. Angew Chem 93:135–142
Reidenberg MM, Shear L, Cohen RV (1973) Elimination of isoniazid in patients with impaired renal function. Am Rev Respir Dis 108:1426–1428
Reutgen H (1975) Wirkungsmodi antituberkulöser Chemotherapeutika: p-Aminosalizylsäure (PAS) – Ethambutol. In: Meissner G, Schmiedel A †, Nelles A † (Hrsg) Infektionskrankheiten und ihre Erreger, Band 4, Teil III. Fischer, Jena, pp 319–336; 299–318
Richardson JP (1975) Biosynthese der Ribonucleinsäuren. Angew Chem 87:497–504
Richter E, Gallenkamp H, Heusler H, Zilly W, Breimer DD (1979) Plasmaclearance von Methohexital bei akuter Hepatitis. Med Klin 74:1584–1588

Robinson OPW, Hunter PA (1966) Absorption and excretion studies with thiocarlide (4,4′-diisoamyloxythiocarbanilide) in man. Tubercle 47:207–213
Robson JM, Sullivan FM (1963) Antituberculosis drugs. Pharmacol Rev 15:169–223 (B, Ph)
Rocker I (1977) Rifampicin in early pregnancy. Lancet II:48
Roncoroni AJ Jr, Huchon GJ, Manuel C (1981) Pharmacokinetics of streptomycin (SM) in patients with pulmonary tuberculosis. Amer Rev Respir Dis 123 No 4, part 2: p 254
Roots I (1982) Genetische Ursachen für die Variabilität der Wirkungen und Nebenwirkungen von Arzneimitteln. Internist 23:601–609
Roots I (1986) Wann ist die Bestimmung von Arzneimittel-Konzentrationen im Plasma nützlich oder notwendig? – Gründe der Variabilität von Arzneimitteln. Internist 27:40–52
Rottach H (1979) Das Verhalten von sogenannten Leberparametern im Rahmen der medikamentösen Tuberkulosebehandlung. Prax Pneumol 33:603–608
Rozewska M, Gajewska E, Graczyk J (1969) Effect of cycloserin on the human body. Gruzlica 37:523–526
Rüger W (1972) Die Transkription der genetischen Information und ihre Regulation durch Proteinfaktoren. Angew Chem 84:961–972
Sarma GR, Kailasam S, Nair NGK, Narayana ASL, Tripathy SP (1980) Effect of prednisolone and rifampin on isoniazid metabolism in slow and rapid inactivators of isoniazid. Antimicrob Agents Chemother 18:661–666
Saueressig G (1972) Untersuchungen zur Harnausscheidung von INH bei intravenöser Na-Gluronazid-Therapie. Inaugural-Dissertation, Med Fakultät der Rheinischen Friedrich-Wilhelms-Universität zu Bonn
Savula MM (1973) Blood concentration and excretion of para-amino-salicylic acid and its metabolites following administration of the BEPAS preparation. Probl Tuberk 51 issue 10: 44–47
Schach von Wittenau M, Chiaini J (1968) A pharmacokinetic analysis of the absorption and elimination of doxycycline in man. Chemotherapy 13:249–251
Schach von Wittenau M, Delahunt CS (1966) The distribution of tetracyclines in tissues of dogs after repeated oral administration. J Pharmacol Exp Ther 152:164–169
Schach von Wittenau M, Twomey TM (1971) The disposition of doxycycline by man and dog. Chemotherapy 16:217–228
Schach von Wittenau M, Beereboom JJ, Blackwood RK, Stephens CR (1962) 6-Deoxytetracyclines. II. Stereochemistry at C 6. J Am Chem Soc 84:2645–2647
Schach von Wittenau M, Twomey TM, Swindell AC (1972) The disposition of doxycycline by the rat. Chemotherapy 17:26–39
Schanker LS (1961) Mechanisms of drug absorption and distribution. Annu Rev Pharmacol 1:29–44
Schiatti P, Maffii G (1967) Studies on distribution of dimethylhydrazone of 3-formyl rifamycin SV, a new antibiotic substance. Chemotherapia 12:234–246
Schiatti P, Dezultan VM, Serralunga MG, Maffii G (1967) Distribution, excretion and toxicity of rifazine, a new semisynthetic rifamycin. Chemotherapia 12:247–260
Schmidt LH (1966) Studies on the antituberculous activity of ethambutol in monkeys. Ann NY Acad Sci 135:747–758
Schoene B, Fleischmann RA, Remmer H, v. Oldershausen HF (1972) Induction of drug-metabolizing enzymes in human liver. Naunyn-Schmiedebergs Arch Pharmacol 274 Suppl: R101
Scholtan W (1964) Bestimmungsmethoden und Gesetzmäßigkeiten der Eiweißbindung von Sulfonamiden und Penicillinen. Antibiot Chemother 12:103–134
Scholtan W (1968) Die hydrophobe Bindung der Pharmaka an Humanalbumin und Ribonucleinsäure. Arzneimittelforsch 18:505–517
Schwabe HK (1971) Intravenöse Gluronazidgaben in Kombination mit kontinuierlicher Ethambutolmedikation per os. Pneumonologie 145:385–388
Schwabe HK, Thiesen GJ, Rausch R (1973) Myambutol-Serumspiegel bei kontinuierlicher Medikation. Prax Pneumol 27:44–46
Self TH (1980) Interaction of rifampin and chlorpropamide. Chest 77:800–801

Self TH, Mann RB (1975) Interaction of rifampin and warfarin. Chest 67:490–491
Selroos O (1961) Absorption and tolerance of large single doses of Kabipastin, a para-aminosalicyclic acid ion exchange resin combination. Acta Tuberc Scand 40:222–236
Seneca H (1971) Biological basis of chemotherapy of infections and infestations. Davis Company, Philadelphia (Ph)
Serabjit-Singh CJ, Wolf CR, Philpot RM, Plopper CG (1980) Cytochrome P-450: localization in rabbit lung. Science 207:1469–1470
Short EI (1962) Studies on the inactivation of isonicotinyl acid hydrazide in normal subjects and tuberculous patients. Tubercle 43:33–42
Siegenthaler W, Siegenthaler G, Beck D, Weidmann P (1968) Neue Antibiotica mit Ausnahme von Penicillinen, Streptomycin, Tetracyclinen und Chloramphenicol. Antibiot Chemother 14:253–280
Siegler DI, Bryant M, Burley DM, Citron KM, Standen SM (1974) Effect of meals on rifampicin absorption. Lancet II:197–198
Silvola H, Ottelin J (1977) Doxycyclin-Konzentrationen in Serum und Lungengewebe. Med Klin Sondernummer:29–32
Simáne Z, Kraus P (1962) Ethionamide (1314 Th) serum levels and its urinary excretion. Rozhl Tbk Praha 22:289–293
Simáne Z, Kraus P (1963) Variation in ethionamide serum levels after its administration in both tablet form and in solution. Rozhl Tbk Praha 23:262–264
Simáne Z, Kraus P, Spousta J (1964) Pharmacodynamics of cycloserine and pyrazinamide after rectal application. Rozhl Tbk Praha 24:483–485
Simon K (1975) Rifampicinbehandlung der Tuberkulose im Kindesalter. Med Klin 70:1095–1097
Simon HJ, Axline SG (1966) Clinical pharmacology of kanamycin in premature infants. Ann NY Acad Sci 132:1020–1025
Simon C, Sommerwerck D, Friehoff J (1978) Der Wert von Doxycyclin bei Atemwegsinfektionen (Serum-, Speichel-, Sputum-, Lungen- und Pleuraexsudatspiegel). Prax Pneumol 32:266–270
Smirnov GA (1972) Criteria and methods of determining inactivation of the hina preparations. Probl Tuberk 50 issue 4: 54–61
Sørenen AWS, Szabo L, Pedersen A, Scharff A (1967) Correlation between renal function and serum half-life of kanamycin and its application to dosage adjustement. Postgrad Med J Suppl: 37–43
Soloviev VN, Firsov AA, Dolgova GV, Berezhinskaya VV, Fishman VM (1977) Relationship between the neuromuscular blocking effect of gentamycin and streptomycin and their concentration in blood. Acta Biol Med Germ 36:1307–1314
Soloviev VN, Firsov AA, Berezhinskaya VV (1978) Relationship between the blood concentration of the drug and its cumulative effect: a pharmacokinetic analysis of the nephrotoxic action of gentamycin and streptomycin. Pharmazie 33:113–116
Stark JE, Ellard GA, Gammon PT, Fox W (1975) The use of isoniazid as a marker to monitor the self-administration of medicaments. Br J Clin Pharmacol 2:355–358
Steffen J (1971) Ist Isoxyl in den bisher angegebenen Dosierungen als Tuberkuloseheilmittel zu verwenden? Prax Pneumol 25:263–277
Stein W, Schoog M, Franz HE (1969) Doxycyclin-Serumspiegel bei niereninsuffizienten Patienten. Arzneimittelforsch 19:827–828
Stoltz M (1981) Short term induction by rifampicin and rifampicin quinone in mice. Naunyn-Schmiedebergs Arch Pharmacol 316 Suppl: R6 (No 23)
Stottmeier KD, Beam RE, Kubica GP (1968) The absorption and excretion of pyrazinamide (PZA) in rabbits and tuberculous patients. Trans 27th Pulm Res Conf VAAF:16
Strauss I, Erhardt F (1970) Ethambutol absorption, excretion and dosage in patients with renal tuberculosis. Chemotherapy 15:148–157
Strominger JL, Tipper DJ (1965) Bacterial cell wall synthesis and structure in relation to the mechanism of action of penicillins and other antibacterial agents. Am J Med 39:708–721
Sunahara S, Nakagawa H (1972) Metabolic study and controlled clinical trials of rifampin. Chest 61:526–532

Sunahara S, Mukoyama H, Ogawa M, Kawai K (1963) Urinary excretion of metabolites of INH and inactivation of sulfonamide in rapid, intermediate and slow inactivators of INH. Kekkaku 38:1–7

Sureau B (1963) Variations des taux sanguins dépendant d'introduction et du véhicule. Rev Fr Études Clin Biol 8:292–302

Syvälathti EKG, Pihlajamäki KK, Iisalo EI (1974) Half-life of tolbutamide in patients receiving tuberculostatic agents. Abstracts of the XXVII Nordic Congress of Pneumonology. Scand J Respir Dis Suppl 88:17

Szabo I, Kisfaludy L (1973) Ein neues, wirksames Antituberkulotikum. Tuberkulózis 24:140–142

Tacquet A, Macquet V, Gernez-Rieux C (1961) Sur un nouveau procédé d'administration de l'éthionamide. Rev Tuberc 25:339–353

Tacquet A, Guillaume J, Macquet V (1963) Étude expérimentale du métabolisme de la 4,4'-diisoamyl-oxythiocarbanilide marquée au soufre radioactif. Acta Tuberc Belg 54:59–65

Tatarinova NV, Chukanov VI (1978) Blood serum ethambutol concentration in tuberculous patients with different patterns of treatment. Probl Tuberk 56 issue 12: 62–65

Tatarinova NV, Kozulitsina GI, Korotaev GA (1974) Analysis of ethambutol concentration in the blood of tuberculous patients. Probl Tuberk 52 issue 10: 39–43

Tatarinova NV, Zhuk NA, Chukanov VI (1979) Qualitative reaction for determination of urine rifampicin with a purpose of control of the drug intake by patients. Probl Tuberk 57 issue 8: 62–65

Teunissen MWE, Bakker W (1984) Influence of rifampicin treatment on antipyrine clearance and metabolite formation in patients with tuberculosis. Br J Clin Pharmacol 18:701–706

Thoma K (1981) Biopharmazeutische Aspekte der pharmazeutischen Technologie. Pharmazie 36:185–193

Titarenko OT, Vakhmistrova TI, Perova TL (1983) Rifampicin excretion with urine in patients with renal insufficiency treated with rifampicin alone or in combination with isoniazid. Antibiotiki 28:698–702

Tomassini L, Naplatanova D (1973) Einfluß einiger Faktoren auf die in-vitro-Abgabegeschwindigkeit der Wirkstoffe aus Depottabletten. Pharmazie 28:447–449

Tomcsányi A, Juhász P (1973) Rifampicin-Blutspiegelbestimmung unter Verwendung von B. Subtilis Test-Organismus. Tuberkulózis 24:118–121

Toyohara M, Shigematsu A (1969) A study on the distribution of ^{14}C-labelled INH in whole body section of frozen mice by use of autoradiography and film scintillation counter. Kekkaku 44:357–360

Tripathy SP (1976) A slow-release preparation of isoniazid: therapeutic efficacy and adverse side-effects. Bull Int Union Tuberc 51:133–141

Truffot-Pernot Ch, Grosset J, Bismuth R, Lecoeur H (1983) Activité de la rifampicine administrée de manière intermittente et de la cyclopentyl rifamycine (ou DL 473) sur la tuberculose expérimentale de la souris. Rev Fr Mal Resp 11:875–882

Tsukamura M (1985a) *In vitro* antituberculosis activity of a new antibacterial substance ofloxacin (DL 8280). Am Rev Respir Dis 131:348–351

Tsukamura M (1985b) Antituberculosis activity of ofloxacin (DL 8280) on experimental tuberculosis in mice. Am Rev Respir Dis 132:915

Tsukamura M, Tsukamura S, Nakano E (1963) The uptake of isoniazid by mycobacteria and its relation to isoniazid susceptibility. Am Rev Respir Dis 87:269–275

Tsukamura M, Yokouchi J, Miwa T, Koike K (1972) Comparison of blood concentration of rifampicin between administration before and after breakfast. Kekkaku 47:69–73

Tsukamura M, Nakamura E, Yoshil S, Amano H (1985) Therapeutic effect of a new antibacterial substance ofloxacin (DL 8280) on pulmonary tuberculosis. Am Rev Respir Dis 131:352–356

Tsukamura M, Yoshil S, Yasuda Y, Saito H (1986) Antituberculosis chemotherapy including ofloxacin in patients with pulmonary tuberculosis not treated previously. Kekkaku 61:15–17

Tytor YN (1976) Liver function and metabolism of isoniazid and PAS in adolescents with intrathoracic tuberculosis. Probl Tuberk 54 issue 7: 29–32

Udou T, Mizuguchi Y, Yamada T (1986) Presence of beta-lactamase and aminoglycoside-acetyltransferase and possible participation of altered drug transport on the resistance mechanism. Am Rev Respir Dis 133:653–657

Ungheri D, Della Torre P, Della Bruna C (1986) Activity of rifabutine (LM 427) against Mycobacterium fortuitum in mice. Am Rev Respir Dis 133 issue 4, part 2: A 41

Urbanczik R, Petersen KF (1985) Überlegungen zur Entwicklung der Bakteriologie und der experimentellen Chemotherapie von Mycobakteriosen. Prax Klin Pneumol 39:421–430

Venho VMK, Koskinen R (1971) The effect of pyrazinamide, rifampicin and cycloserine on the blood levels and urinary excretion of isoniazid. Ann Clin Res 3:277–280

Verbist L (1971) Pharmacological study of rifampicin after repeated high dosage during intermittent combined therapy. I. Variation of the rifampicin serum levels (947 determinations). Respiration 28 Suppl: 7–16

Verbist L, Dutoit M (1966) Ethionamide blood levels after administration of the drug under various pharmaceutical forms. Arzneimittelforsch 16:773–778

Verbist L, Gyselen A (1968) Antituberculous activity of rifampin in vitro and in vivo and the concentrations attained in human blood. Am Rev Respir Dis 98:923–932

Verbist L, Mbete S, Van Landuyt H, Darras Th, Gyselen A (1972) Intermittent therapy with rifampin once a week in advanced pulmonary tuberculosis. Chest 61:555–563

Vesell ES (1972) Introduction: genetic and environmental factors affecting drug response in man. Fed Proc 31:1253–1269

Vesell ES (1981) Der Einfluß von Wirtsfaktoren auf die Wirkung von Medikamenten. II. Alter. Internist (Berlin) 22:99–105

Videau D (1968) Pénétration, site et mode d' action des antibiotiques chez la bactérie. Biol Méd 57:449–470

Virsik K, Bajan A, Havelka C, Badalik L, Schwartz E, Molnár L (1971) Serum levels of streptomycin, isoniazid and thiacetazone correlated to side-effects produced in patients with active pulmonary tuberculosis. Stud Pneumol Phtiseol Cechoslov 31:390–395

Vivien JN, Thibier R, Lepeuple A (1972) Recent studies on isoniazid. Adv Tuberc Res 18:148–230 (B, Ph)

Vladimirsky MA, Streltsov VP, Stepanov VM, Braude VI (1980) Liposomes as carriers of antituberculous drugs: a new approach to experimental chemotherapy of tuberculosis. Probl Tuberk 58 issue 7: 53–56

Wagner JG, Nelson E (1963) Per cent absorbed time plots derived from blood level and/or urinary excretion data. J Pharmac Sci 52:610–611

Wagner JG, Holmes PD, Wilkinson PK, Blair DC, Stoll RG (1973) Importance of the type of dosage form and saturable acetylation in determining the bioactivity of p-aminosalicylic acid. Am Rev Respir Dis 108:536–546

Wagner WH, Chou JTY, Ilberg v. C, Ritter R, Vosteen KH (1971) Untersuchungen zur Pharmakokinetik von Streptomycin. Arzneimittelforsch 21:2006–2016

Walter AM, Heilmeyer L (1969) Antibiotika-Fibel. 3. Auflage. Heilmeyer L, Otten H, Plempel M (Hrsg) Thieme Verlag, Stuttgart

Wareska W, Siekierzynska A (1967) Studies of the blood serum level and urinary excretion of Tebamine. Gruzlica 35:1265–1269

Wareska W, Klott M, Izdebska-Makosa (1963) Cycloserine excretion in cases of renal diseases. Gruzlica 31:664–668

Wattel F, Voisin C, Martin G, Courcol R, Durocher A, Duquesne B, Babry M (1981) Use of parenteral rifampin in patients with severe tuberculosis and severe nontubercular infections. In: Periti P, Grassi GP (eds) Current chemotherapy and immunotherapy. 12th International Congress of Chemotherapy (1981, Florence, Italy.) Vol II American Society for Microbiology, Washington, pp 982–984

Weidel W (1964) Ein neuer Typ von Makromolekülen. Angew Chem 76:801–807

Welles JS, Harris PU, Small RM, Worth HM, Anderson RC (1966) The toxicity of capreomycin in laboratory animals. Ann NY Acad Sci 135:960–973

Whelton A (1974) Antibacterial chemotherapy in renal insufficiency. Antibiot Chemother 18:1–48

White RJ (1975) Wirkungsmodi antituberkulöser Chemotherapeutika: Rifampicin. In: Meissner G, Schmiedel A †, Nelles A † (Hrsg) Infektionskrankheiten und ihre Erreger, Band 4, Teil III. Fischer, Jena, pp 365–381

White RJ, Lancini GC, Silvestri LG (1971) Mechanism of action of rifampin on Mycobacterium smegmatis. J Bacteriol 108:737–741

Winder FG (1982) Mode of action of the antimycobacterial agents. In: Ratledge C, Stanford J (eds) The Biology of Mycobacteria Vol 1. Academic Press, London New York Paris San Diago San Francisco Sao Paulo Sydney Tokyo Toronto, pp 354–422

Winkler E, Weih H (1967) Doxycyclin. Ergebnisse von Basisuntersuchungen. Med Klin 62:1257–1262

Winsel K, Iwainsky H, Werner E, Eule H (1976) Trennung, Bestimmung und Pharmakokinetik von Rifampicin und seinen Biotransformationsprodukten. Pharmazie 31:95–99

Winsel K, Eule H, Werner E, Iwainsky H (1985) Zur Pharmakokinetik des Rifampicins (RMP) bei intermittierender Behandlung von Patienten mit Lungentuberkulose. Pharmazie 40:253–256

Wisniewsky K (1972) The effect of trypsin on the absorption and distribution of isonicotinic acid hydrazide (INH) in tissues. Acta Physiol Pol 23:167–173

Youatt J (1969) A review of the action of isoniazid. Am Rev Respir Dis 99:729–749 (M)

Youatt J, Tham SH (1969a) An enzyme system of *Mycobacterium tuberculosis* that reacts specifically with isoniazid. II. Correlation of this reaction with the binding and metabolism of isoniazid. Am Rev Respir Dis 100:31–37

Youatt J, Tham SH (1969b) Radioactive content of *Mycobacterium tuberculosis* after exposure to ^{14}C-isoniazid. Am Rev Respir Dis 100:77–78

Zähner H (1977) Einige Aspekte der Antibiotica-Forschung. Angew Chem 89:696–703

Zathurecký L (1972) Beeinflussung der Arzneimittelwirkung durch die Arzneiform. Pharmazie 27:686–693

Zeeuw RA de (1981) Potentials of chromatographic methods in assessing the bioavailability and the pharmacokinetics of drugs. Pharmazie 36:178–184

Zeller F, Róka L (1973) Ethambutolausscheidung bei Tuberkulosepatienten mit mäßig eingeschränkter Nierenfunktion. Prax Pneumol 27:36–43

Zeyer J, Hurni H, Fischer R, Lauber E, Schönholzer G, Aebi H (1960) Versuche mit verschieden ^{14}C-markierter Benzoyl-p-aminosalicylsäure (B-PAS) in Kulturen von *Mycobacterium tuberculosis*. Z Naturforschung 15b:694–701

Zierski M (1981) Pharmakologie, Toxikologie und klinische Anwendung von Pyrazinamid. Prax Klin Pneumol 35:1075–1105

Zilly W (1979) Arzneimitteltherapie bei Lebererkrankungen. Med Klin 74:1575–1580

Zilly W, Breimer DD, Richter E (1977) Stimulation of drug metabolism by rifampicin in patients with cirrhosis or cholestasis measured by increased hexobarbital and tolbutamide clearance. Eur J Clin Pharmacol 11:287–293

Zilly W, Bopp E, Bürkl B, Richter E (1974) Der Einfluß von Rifampicin auf die Pharmakokinetik von Tolbutamid bei Gesunden. Verh Dtsch Ges Inn Med 80:1538–1540

Zitkova L, Tousek J (1973) Resorption and elimination of terizidone (Bracco) compared with cycloserine (Spofa). Stud Pneumol Phtiseol Cechoslov 33:37–43

Zitkova L, Tousek J (1978) Pharmacokinetics of cycloserine and ethambutol. Probl Tuberk 56 issue 3: 23–25

Zitkova L, Tousek J, Stastna J (1976) Pharmacokinetics of ethambutol after different single doses. Stud Pneumol Phtiseol Cechoslov 36:297–304

Zitkova L, Janko I, Tousek J (1983) Pharmacokinetics of antituberculosis drugs after oral isolated and simultaneous administration in triple combination. Czech Med 6:202–217

Zwolska-Kwiek Z (1974) Variability in rifampicin concentrations in the serum of patients with tuberculosis. Gruzlica 42:65–73

Zwolska-Kwiek Z, Lawicka E, Wasowska H (1975) Comparison of rifampicin serum levels after the administration before breakfast and 3 hours after breakfast. Gruzlica 43:151–156

Zysset T, Bircher J (1983) Dosisanpassung von Medikamenten für Leberpatienten mit Hilfe einer einfachen Risiko-Klassifikation. Internist (Berlin) 24:151–161

B. Special Part – The Antituberculosis Drugs

I. PAS

1. Mode of Action

a) Incorporation of PAS in Mycobacteria Sensitive or Resistant to the Drug

In the case of *M. smegmatis*, PAS is actively transported into the cells. Cyanide, iodoacetate, or formaldehyde all inhibit this transport system, which may possibly also be the one used by p-aminobenzoate. By contrast, salicylate is incorporated in a manner independent of the above (BROWN and RATLEDGE 1975a). The PAS-specific system is evidently already exhausted at concentrations of 1 μg PAS/ml (REUTGEN 1975). In older studies with PAS derivatives, it has been demonstrated by various methods that hydrolysis takes place before incorporation (ABRAHAM 1965), only benzoyl-PAS being taken up by the microorganisms as a whole molecule (ZEYER et al. 1960).

As with SM, the development of PAS resistance does not cause any change in the uptake of PAS. However, because of the greater affinity of p-aminobenzoate to enzymes detectable in PAS-resistant mycobacteria, higher PAS concentrations are necessary to bring about an inhibitory effect (HEDGECOCK 1965).

b) Mode of Action of PAS

The compound was developed by Lehmann as an antituberculotic on the basis of enzyme-theory (LEHMANN 1961). Already at the experimental stage, p-aminobenzoate proved the most effective PAS antagonist, as could be supposed from theoretical considerations (HEDGECOCK 1965). Only the absence of cross-resistance to sulphonamides was not in accord with the original preconceptions. On the basis of the available investigations, Seydel, Krüger-Thiemer and Wempe (KRÜGER-THIEMER 1963) suspected an intervention in the folic acid synthesis (Fig. 1). Via several intermediate stages 6-hydroxymethyl-2-amino-4-hydroxy-7,8-dihydropteridine is formed from a pyridine derivative and ribose-5-P. With the participation of ATP, Mg^{2+} ions, and p-aminobenzoyl-L-glutamate, this compound is converted into dihydropteroylglutamate. This is the most PAS-sensitive reaction of the synthesis pathway. Although no definite proof of this point of attack has been found in mycobacteria, some findings do indicate that this is the case. For example, compounds such as methionine, biotin and others, requiring an intact folic acid system that transfers C_1 fragments for their synthesis, do non-competitively compensate PAS activity (HEDGECOCK 1965). Other interventions in this synthetic pathway, occurring above all through the formation of Schiff bases, are only conceivable at high PAS concentrations.

However, the very specific effect on mycobacteria cannot be explained solely by a disturbance of the C_1-transfer reactions. Recently, certain regulation processes of the mycobacterial metabolism were found to be at least secondary points of attack (Fig. 2, RATLEDGE 1971). This simultaneously provides an explanation for the interaction between PAS and salicylate (REUTGEN 1975). So far as can be deduced from the metabolism of Fe, which is, however, still incompletely under-

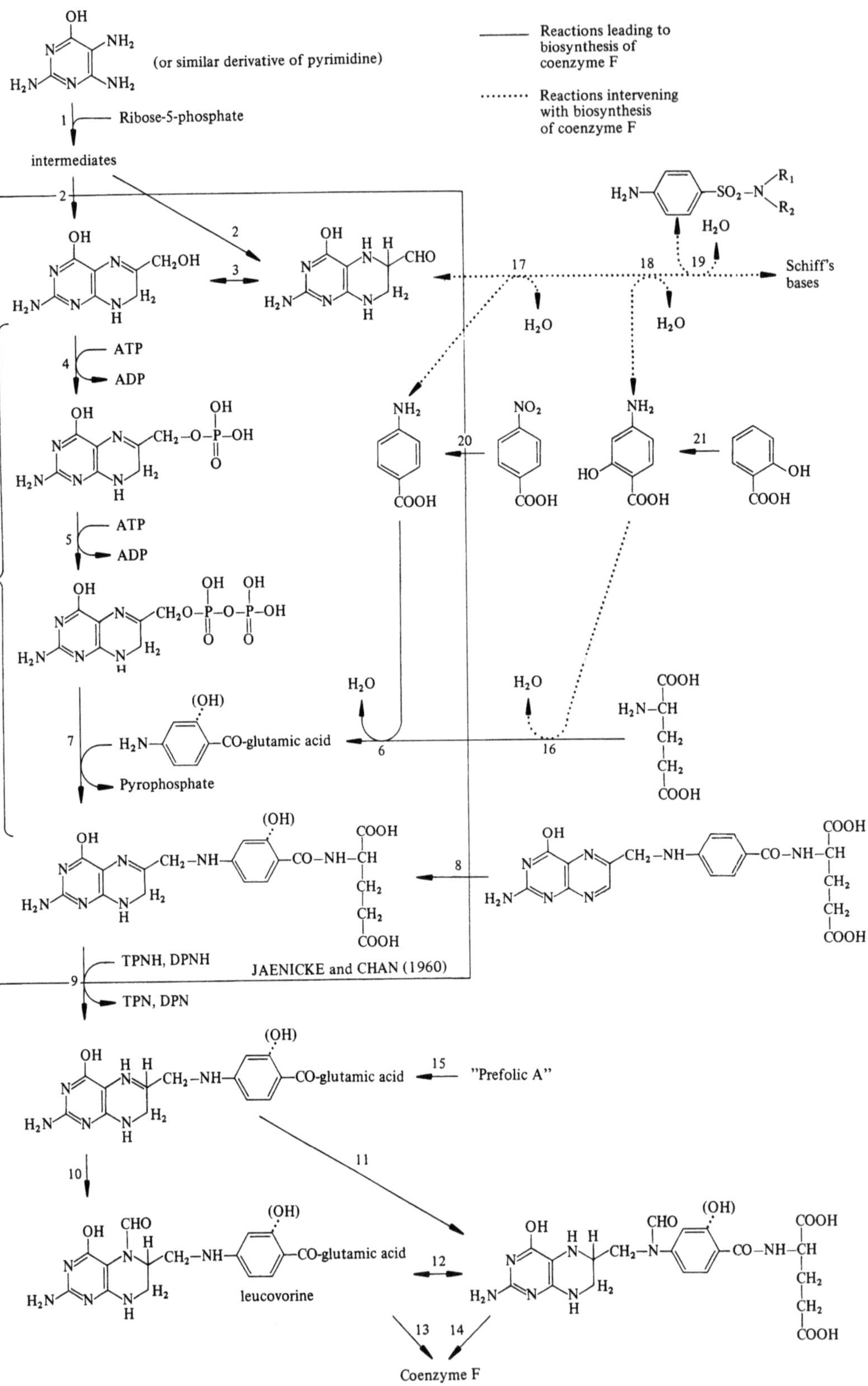

(or similar derivative of pyrimidine)
Reactions leading to biosynthesis of coenzyme F
Reactions intervening with biosynthesis of coenzyme F
Ribose-5-phosphate
intermediates
ATP
ADP
enzyme + ATP + Mg2+
CO-glutamic acid
Pyrophosphate
Schiff's bases
TPNH, DPNH
TPN, DPN
JAENICKE and CHAN (1960)
"Prefolic A"
leucovorine
Coenzyme F

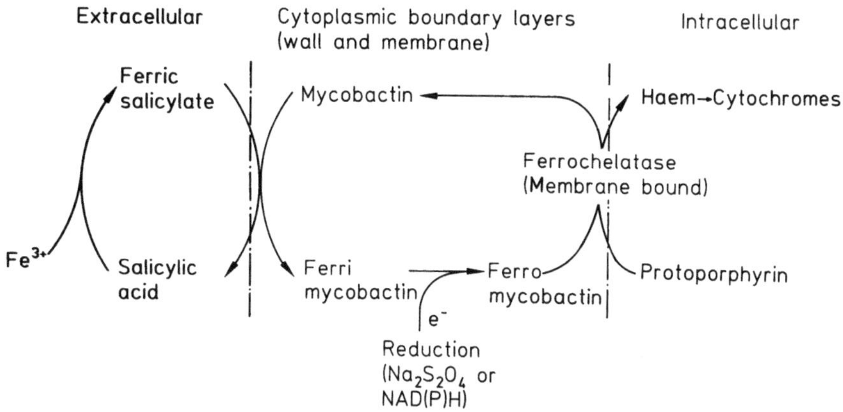

Fig. 2. Regulation of the iron metabolism in Mycobacteria (RATLEDGE 1971)

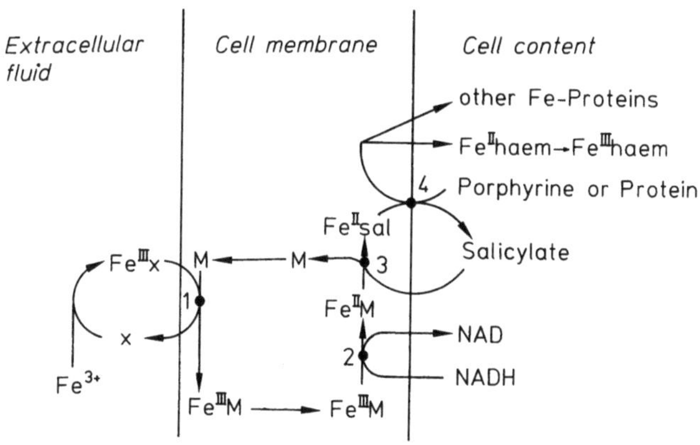

Fig. 3. Possible sites of attack of PAS in the iron metabolism in mycobacteria (RATLEDGE 1971). *1* Inhibition of the uptake of salicylate and iron ions into the cells; *2* Interference with mycobactin reductase; *3* Interference with the transport of Fe^{2+} salicylate; *4* Acts as a salicylate analog; *M*, desferrimycobactin; *x*, extracellular iron solubilizer

stood, PAS interferes at several points in these processes (RATLEDGE et al. 1974; BROWN and RATLEDGE 1975a, b; MACHAM and RATLEDGE 1975; MACHAM et al. 1975). PAS inhibits the uptake of FE^{2+} ions and of salicylate from the nutrient medium, interferes with the synthesis of mycobactin necessary for the Fe transport and thus, in the final analysis, reduces the activity of enzymes that require Fe ions (Fig. 3, RATLEDGE and BROWN 1972; BROWN and RATLEDGE 1975b).

Fig. 1. Sites of attack of PAS and other 4-aminobenzoic acid antagonists in the biosynthesis of folic acid (KRÜGER-THIEMER 1963)

2. Biotransformation

a) Biotransformation Pattern of PAS in Man and Animals

Acetylation of the free amino group and conjugation at the carboxyl group are the most important steps in the biotransformation process. In man, glycine-PAS represents the principal conjugation product, only traces of the corresponding sulphate and glucuronate compounds being found (Fig. 4, LEHMANN 1969). The hydroxyl group remains practically unchanged. Decarboxylation also takes place to a small extent (up to 4% of $^{14}CO_2$ from ^{14}C-PAS). The decarboxylation product excreted with the urine under normal conditions – m-aminophenol – originates mostly from the substance and is formed non-enzymatically during storage.

Biotransformation patterns corresponding to those in man have also been found in animals. PAS and glycine-PAS have been identified as well as acetyl-PAS and glucuronyl-acetyl-PAS. After the use of radiolabelled benzoyl-PAS, two other biotransformation products considered to be glucuronides were found besides PAS and acetyl-PAS (JEUNET et al. 1961, 1962). In animals, the decarboxylation of PAS is still less pronounced than in man. The formation determined in vivo corresponds to the release of CO_2 measured in the liver in vitro ($5–7 \times 10^{-3}$ µmol/g liver/h – JEUNET et al. 1962).

b) Influence of the Dose on the Biotransformation Rate

Among the biotransformation products formed, glycine-PAS in the plasma may possibly have a slight antituberculotic activity, whereas acetyl-PAS is inactive (SCHMIEDEL 1955; LEHMANN 1969).

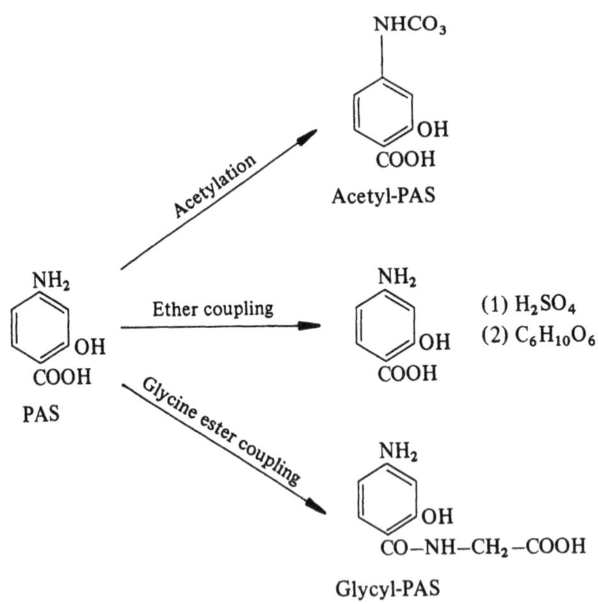

Fig. 4. Biotransformation products of PAS in man (LEHMANN, 1969)

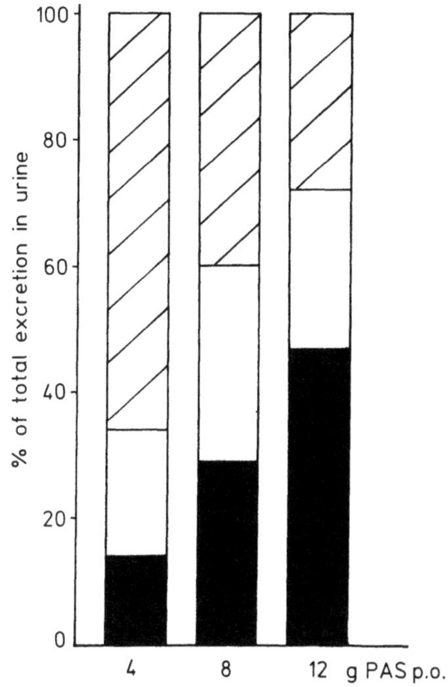

Fig. 5. Dependence of the biotransformation rate on the PAS dose administered (LEHMANN 1969). ■ Biologically active PAS; □ Glycine-PAS; ▨ Acetyl-PAS

In man the proportion of glycine-PAS is proportional to the dose of PAS; the situation with acetyl-PAS is more complicated. It seems that the acetylation already commences in the intestinal mucosa, since after oral administration of 12 g PAS 45% to 67% of the excreted quantity is acetylated, while after intravenous administration of the same dose only up to 25% undergoes acetylation (WAGNER et al. 1960). Furthermore, the rate of acetylation is influenced by the dose administered and the interval between individual administrations. In low doses, PAS is acetylated almost completely whereas at higher doses the fraction of acetyl-PAS falls off (Fig. 5, LEHMANN 1969). These findings have been interpreted as an exhaustion of the acetylation capacity. Evidently the organism can mobilize only a limited quantity of acetyl-coenzyme A in a unit of time (LEHMANN 1969; PENTIKAINEN et al. 1973). In correspondence with these findings, the administration of

Table 1. PAS concentrations in the serum (μg/ml) of tuberculosis patients after the infusion of PAS sodium (SCHMIEDEL 1955)

n	Dose	Infusion		Blood sample taken after the end of infusion (h)				
		30 min	2 h (end)	2	4	5	8	12
6	20 g PAS-Na	200	372	160	–	88	–	–
6	40 g PAS-Na	–	–	500	300		145	65

Table 2. PAS concentrations in the plasma (μg/ml) of tuberculosis patients after an intravenous infusion of 24 and 27 g of PAS (KUNTZ 1966)

Dose	Lenght of infusion (h)	*n*	Blood sample taken (h after start of infusion)							
			2	4	6	8	10	12	14 (16)	24
27 g	2	3	51.0± 8.9	24.0±10.2	13.6± 9.1	3.9± 3.5	0.9+ 2.0	0.3		
	4	4	29.9±17.3	34.9± 5.1	24.8± 9.9	9.7± 7.4	3.4± 3.5	1.8		
	6	3	23.3± 3.2	16.4± 1.2	18.0± 2.1	6.5± 1.7	0.7± 0.8	0.9±0.8		
	8	12	12.6± 4.4	15.2± 4.2	26.5±11.5	41.3±12.0	21.5±11.0	7.8±5.7	2.0±0.5	1.0
	10	5	9.1± 3.7	14.2± 3.0	18.7± 4.1	34.7±11.7	36.7±10.4	23.9±9.5	2.9±1.9	1.5
24 g	4	3	26.6± 2.9	26.6± 1.5	11.4± 0.3	3.7± 1.4	0.9	0.2		
	8	5	3.9± 2.7	10.9± 3.4	15.8± 7.7	38.1±26.6	21.3±11.3	8.3±4.1	2.2±1.1	0.3±1.1

Table 3. PAS concentration in the serum (μg/ml) of tuberculosis patients after an oral administration of PAS compounds (BANG et al. 1962; FROSTADT 1962; NIKODEMOWICZ et al. 1971)

n	Compound	Dose	Blood sample taken after hours											Authors
			1	2	3	4	6	7	8	9	10	12	14	
1	Na-PAS (Solution)	12 g PAS	13.3	26.1	–	17.3	–	6.2	–	2.8	–	1.2	–	BANG et al. (1962)
5	Granulate	12 g PAS	13.2	22.0	17.5	11.7	5.2	3.2	–	–	1.9	–	–	FROSTADT (1962)
11	Double-coated tablet	12 g PAS +0.43 g INH	15.4	30.3	–	26.4	–	–	14.8		–	6.5	3.5	NIKODEMOWICZ et al. (1971)

high doses of PAS or of equivalent compounds or long-term infusion of high doses of PAS in different galenic preparations (up to 27 g/day or more) is regarded as necessary for expedient clinical therapy (SCHMIEDEL 1955; FROSTADT 1962; BANG et al. 1962; KUNTZ 1966; NIKODEMOWICZ et al. 1971, Tables 1–3).

3. Pharmacokinetics

a) Absorption and Distribution of PAS

Like SM, INH, ETH, and RMP, PAS is absorbed very rapidly. 58%–73% of the PAS, more than 60% of acetyl-PAS, and 30%–35% of glycine-PAS are bound to serum proteins (see Table 3, p. 419). PAS is distributed in the extracellular space (see Table 6, p. 421). After the diffusion equilibrium has set in (15 min to 30 min, JENNE et al. 1961), the PAS concentration in the organs and tissue (apart from the kidney and the intestines) corresponds to that in the blood (LEHMANN 1969). PAS diffuses into caseous tissue, where concentrations of around half of those in the serum are found. In pregnant women, passage of the PAS into the foetal circulation is thought to be a possibility (JENNE 1964; MORDASINI and EULENBERGER 1971). The mean $t_{50\%}$ is 45 minutes. Largely similar results are obtained after the administration of ^{14}C-benzoyl-PAS (JEUNET et al. 1961).

b) Excretion of PAS

Some 80% of an administered dose is excreted by glomerular filtration and tubular secretion (PORTWICH 1964, see Table 8, p. 424). The acetylation of PAS ceases in the kidney. Thus, the PAS concentration in the serum can also be deduced from the ratio of acetyl-PAS + glycine/urinary PAS (LEHMANN 1969). After 2 h the maximal urinary PAS concentrations are reached, the bulk being excreted after only 6 h (SHENDEROVA and TERTERYAN 1973). By contrast, the elimination of acetyl-PAS commences only after 3 h (WAGNER et al. 1960), causing in some organs a shift in the ratio of the biotransformation products to PAS compared with the situation in the serum (LEHMANN 1969).

A two-way transport mechanism has been detected in the dog. The tubular reabsorption is influenced by the pH of the urine. The secretion can be blocked by probenecid (HUANG et al. 1960). It may well be that such processes are also relevant in man. Considerable biliary excretion and excretion via the intestines has been observed after the administration of certain PAS derivatives (JEUNET et al. 1961).

Further pharmacokinetic data are given in Tables 7, 9 and 11 in the General Part (pp. 423, 425, 432).

References

Abraham EP (1965) The chemistry of new antibiotics. Am J Med 39:692–707

Bang HO, Kramer Jacobsen L, Strandgaard E, Yde H (1962) Metabolism of isoniazid and para-amino-salicylic acid (PAS) in the organism and its therapeutic significance. Acta Tuberc Scand 41:237–251

Brown KA, Ratledge C (1975a) The effect of p-aminosalicylic acid on iron transport and assimilation in mycobacteria. Biochim Biophys Acta 385:207–220

Brown KA, Ratledge C (1975 b) Iron transport in Mycobacterium smegmatis: ferrimycobactin reductase (NAD(P)H: mycobactin oxidoreductase), the enzyme releasing iron from its carrier. Febs Letters 53:262–266
Frostadt S (1962) Continued studies in concentrations of para-amino-salicylic acid (PAS) in the blood. Acta Tuberc Scand 41:68–82
Hedgecock LW (1965) Comparative study of the mode of action of para-aminosalicylic acid on *Mycobacterium kansasii* and *Mycobacterium tuberculosis*. Am Rev Respir Dis 91:719–727
Huang KC, Moore KB, Campbell PC Jr (1960) Renal excretion of para-aminosalicylic acid: a two-way transport system in the dog. Am J Physiol 199:5–8
Jenne JW (1964) Pharmacokinetics and the dose of isoniazid and para-aminosalicylic acid in the treatment of tuberculosis. Antibiot Chemother 12:407–432
Jenne JW, MacDonald FM, Mendoza E (1961) A study of the renal clearance, metabolic inactivation rates, and serum fall-off interaction of isoniazid and para-aminosalicylic acid in man. Am Rev Respir Dis 84:371–378
Jeunet F, Lauber E, Aebi H (1961) Verteilung und Umsatz von ^{14}C-Benzoyl-p-Aminosalicylsäure bei der Maus. Naunyn-Schmiedebergs Arch Pharmacol 242:353–369
Jeunet F, Lauber E, Aebi H (1962) Bildung von Metaboliten der Benzoyl-para-amino-salicylsäure (C^{14}-B-PAS) in der Rattenleber und deren Ausscheidung in Harn und Galle. Naunyn-Schmiedebergs Arch Pharmacol 242:564–575
Krüger-Thiemer E (1965) Wirkungsweise der Sulfanilamide und der p-Aminosalicylsäure. In: Käppler W, Iwainsky H, Grunert M, Sehrt I, Reutgen H (Hrsg) Bericht über das II. Internationale Symposium „Bakteriologie und Biochemie der Mykobakterien". 20.–24.10.1963 Berlin-Buch, pp 386–414
Kuntz E (1966) Untersuchungen über die Blutspiegelwerte und die Ausscheidung von p-Aminosalicylsäure (PAS-Natrium) bei i.v. Infusionsbehandlung. Beitr Klin Tuberk 133:12–24
Lehmann J (1961) Chemische und experimentelle Grundlagen der PAS-Therapie. Wien Med Wochenschr 111:803–805
Lehmann J (1969) The role of the metabolism of p-aminosalicylic acid (PAS) in the treatment of tuberculosis. Scand J Respir Dis 50:169–185
Macham LP, Ratledge C (1975) A new group of water-soluble iron-binding compounds from mycobacteria: The exochelins. J Gen Microbiol 89:379–382
Macham LP, Ratledge C, Nocton JC (1975) Extracellular iron acquisition by mycobacteria: role of the exocholins and evidence against the participation of mycobactin. Infect Immun 12:1242–1251
Mordasini ER, Eulenberger J (1971) Tuberkulostatika, Teil 2, Spezifische Chemotherapeutika. Int J Clin Pharmacol Ther Toxicol 5:70–95
Nikodemowicz E, Owsinski J, Kaminska M, Ostrowska A, Rapf T (1971) Investigation into the metabolism of para-aminosalicylic acid in the body. Gruzlica 39:1113–1121
Pentikainen P, Wan SH, Azarnoff DL (1973) Bioavailability studies on p-aminosalicylic acid and its various salts in man. Am Rev Respir Dis 108:1340–1347
Portwich F (1964) Untersuchung des Mechanismus der Nierenausscheidung von Arzneimitteln. Antibiot Chemother 12:41–52
Ratledge C (1961) Transport of iron by mycobactin in *Mycobacterium smegmatis*. Biochem Biophys Res Commun 45:856–862
Ratledge C, Brown KA (1972) Inhibition of mycobactin formation in *Mycobacterium smegmatis* by p-aminosalicylate. A new proposal for the mode of action of p-aminosalicylate. Am Rev Respir Dis 106:774–776
Ratledge C, Macham LP, Brown KA, Marshall BJ (1974) Iron transport in *Mycobacterium smegmatis;* A restricted role for salicylic acid in the extracellular environment. Biochim Biophys Acta 372:39–51
Reutgen H (1975) Zum Wirkungsmechanismus der p-Aminosalicylsäure. In: Meissner G, Schmiedel A †, Nelles A † (Hrsg) Infektionskrankheiten und ihre Erreger, Band 4, Teil III. Fischer, Jena, pp 319–336
Schmiedel A (1955) Zur Frage der biologischen Wertigkeit chemisch nachgewiesener p-Aminosalicylsäure in Körperflüssigkeiten. Zentralbl Bakteriol Mikrobiol Hyg (A) 164:576–587

Shenderova RI, Terteryan EA (1973) Inactivation of PAS and Hina in tuberculous children. Probl Tuberk 51 issue 5: 67–71
Wagner J, Fajkošová D, Šimáne Z (1960) A comparative study on acetylation of para-aminosalicylic acid (PAS after oral and intravenous administration). Acta Tuberc Scand 38:339–346
Zeyer J, Hurni H, Fischer R, Lauber E, Schönholzer G, Aebi H (1960) Versuche mit verschieden ^{14}C-markierter Benzoyl-p-aminosalicylsäure (B-PAS) in Kulturen von *Mycobacterium tuberculosis*. Z Naturforschung 15 b:694–701

II. SM

1. Mode of Action

a) Uptake and Biotransformation of SM by Microorganisms Sensitive or Resistant to SM

In mycobacteria, the binding of SM at the cell surface is carried on by a second step that can be inhibited by cyanide or chloramphenicol (BEGGS and WILLIAMS 1971). The effect of chloramphenicol can also be observed in *E. coli*. In the case of this species at least induction of the already mentioned permease (p. 404, General Part) is considered likely (HURWITZ and ROSANO 1962, 1966; KOGUT and HARRIS 1969).

Adenyl-SM, a compound isolated from *E. coli*, and other SM biotransformation products found in other microorganisms (KLEIN and PRAMER 1961, 1962) have not so far been found in mycobacteria.

The development of resistance to SM does not change the latter's incorporation (HURWITZ and ROSANO 1962). Of the mycobacterial species studied only *M. fortuitum* possesses an enzyme capable of destroying SM, and so processes other than intensified degradation must be mainly responsible for the development of resistance (MORAVEK and TRNKA 1973).

b) Mode of Action of SM

The effect of SM depends on the growth intensity and thus on the supply of nutrients (KOGUT and HARRIS 1969). Within the cells, there is an SM "pool" of the SM fraction causing the inhibition (KOGUT and LIGHTBOWN 1966). The DNA and RNA synthesis remains unaffected (GAUZE et al. 1971), so that on the basis of structure-effect relationships, a competitive displacement of polyamines from their binding sites on the ribosomes is assumed to be the action principle (TANAKA et al. 1967; MASUKAWA and TANAKA 1968).

Attempts at hybridization with 30-S and 50-S ribosomes of SM-sensitive and SM-resistant bacteria have revealed that a 30-S ribosome subunit, namely the P_{10} protein or the S_{12} protein, constitutes the SM-sensitive site of the microorganism (COX et al. 1964; DAVIES 1964; DAVIES et al. 1964; PESTKA 1966; HAHN 1971; KRÜGER-THIEMER et al. 1975; MICHEL-BRIAND 1978). Before the attachment of the m-RNA, SM is bound irreversibly to a lysine group of the 30-S ribosome subunit, leading to a change in the configuration of the ribosome-m-RNA-t-RNA ternary complex (GOLDBERG 1965; QUESNEL et al. 1971; MICHEL-BRIAND 1978). This results in an erroneous reading in around half of the 64 possible codons. Only the 2 pyrimidine bases are wrongly read, the 5-terminal cytosine being read as uracil and vice versa, while the middle-position pyrimidines are read as pyrimidine or purine bases (DAVIES et al. 1966). Guanine is never read erroneously and also prevents an erroneous reading of the corresponding codon. Erroneous readings of this type can be recognized indirectly by the formation of abnormal proteins, e.g. without enzyme activity (PINKETT and BROWNSTEIN 1974). In addition, an inhibition of the incorporation of amino acids into proteins is discernible (DAVIES 1964; DAVIES et al. 1966; HAHN 1971).

2. Biotransformation of SM in the Macroorganism

So far, despite intensive searches, no biotransformation products of this antibiotic have been found. The SM concentration in the serum of 501 patients displays a single-peak distribution (LEVY et al. 1960; HANSSON et al. 1966).

3. Pharmacokinetics

a) Distribution of SM in the Macroorganism

Like most antituberculotics, SM is absorbed very rapidly on its parenteral administration (1 h–2 h to a state of absorption/elimination equilibrium). Twenty – 34% of the dose is bound to the serum proteins (see Table 3, p. 419; KUNIN 1967). SM is distributed almost exclusively in the extracellular fluid. The antibiotic has an affinity to tissues of mesenchymal origin. The SM concentrations in the liver and kidney are high, as are those in the thyroid and muscle, while the concentrations in the spleen and the lungs are low. Therapeutically active concentration are rarely measured in the lymph nodes or in bone. SM permeates serous effusions only slowly, reaching concentrations about one-quarter of those in the serum. The rate of diffusion into abscesses depends on the thickness of the fibrotic wall. The concentration maximum appears later than that in the serum and is considerably lower (Fig. 1, HEVÉR and RISKÓ 1960; AROSENIUS et al. 1961; MORDASINI and EULENBERGER 1971).

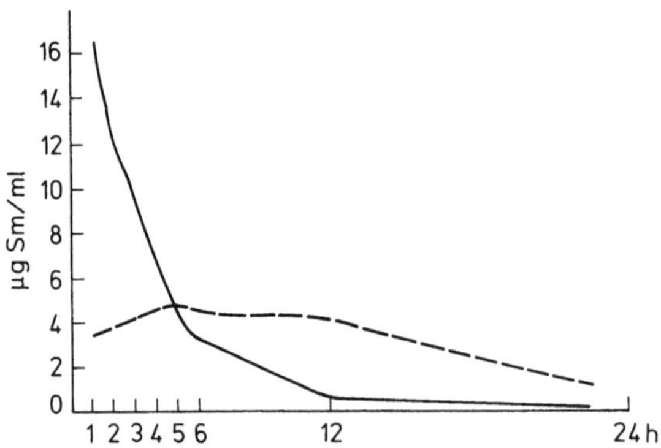

Fig. 1. SM concentration in the serum and in an abscess (HEVÉR and RISKÓ 1960). —— Serum concentration; ---- Abscess concentration

b) Passage of SM into Specific Compartments

Since damage to the foetus is a possibility, and in the case of ototoxic antituberculotic drugs has, in fact, been confirmed (VARPELA 1964; PODVINEC et al. 1966; RASMUSSEN 1969; GANGUIN 1971), the passage of antituberculotic drugs and, in this case, of SM and other ototoxic antituberculotics into the placenta and foetus has attracted particular interest. Compared with the maternal serum a dose-dependent reduction of the concentrations of the antituberculotic by 50% and more is observed (PODVINEC et al. 1966; TOYOHARA 1974).

The SM levels measured in the CSF are very much lower than those in the serum (see Table 7, p. 423), so that parenteral administration of this antibiotic alone is questionable in meningitis tuberculosa.

In patients with kidney damage, i.e., with the likelihood of impaired excretion and correspondingly elevated antituberculotic concentration in the serum, an intensified ototoxicity of SM, KM, VM, and CM has been observed. Correlations were therefore thought to exist between the drug concentration and its ototoxicity. Studies on the metabolism of the inner ear have revealed that perilymph, evidently formed directly from the serum is responsible for feeding the hair cells (FERNÁNDEZ 1967; GERHARDT et al. 1973; KELLERHALS 1973). The four antibiotics thus enter this perilymph by passive transport, as does penicillin. However, in contrast to penicillin, tetracyclines, or RMP, on repeated administration progressive accumulation for a limited period was observed first in guinea pigs and cats and later in man as well. Apart from the first few hours, the antibiotic concentration is higher than the serum values and has a longer half-life (Fig. 2, VOLDŘICH 1965; VRABEC et al. 1965; STUPP et al. 1967; FELGENHAUER and LAGLER 1970; CADA 1971; WATANABE et al. 1971; FEDERSPIL 1979). This is due to membrane

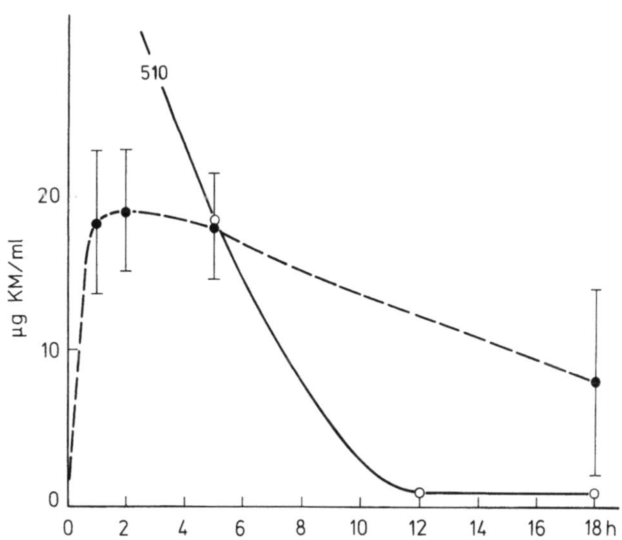

Fig. 2. KM concentration in serum and perilymph of guinea pig (KELLERHALS 1973). Dose: 250 mg KM/kg. o—o KM concentration in serum; ●- - -● KM concentration in perilymph

Table 1. SM concentration in the serum (μg/ml) of tuberculosis patients after i.m. administration of 0.75-lg of SM (VIRSIK et al. 1971)

n	Blood sample taken after				
	40 min	1 h	2 h	3 h	6 h
28	16.7	24.8	20.1	18.9	6.8

damage induced by the ototoxic antibiotics that subsequently also affects the transport of K^+ ions (MENDELSOHN and KATZENBERG 1972). The result is that invasion of the antibiotics is facilitated and their elimination disturbed (STUPP and RAUCH 1966). The extent of the invasion depends on the peak concentration appearing in the serum after the injection of the antibiotics (the ototoxic concentration of KM is 30 μg/ml). This peak (and thus ototoxic damage) can be largely prevented by the adoption of suitable dosage schemes or by using an intravenous drip (FEDERSPIL 1979). A favorable concentration course has also been observed for the SM derivatives developed in the early 1970's (WAGNER 1971; WAGNER et al. 1971; KELLERHALS 1973). Doubt has recently been cast on these ideas, which have been replaced by the following hypothesis: Instead of this being an accumulation in the inner ear, there is an electrostatic adsorption of the antibiotics on the negatively charged component of the outer plasma membrane. This leads to a reversible competitive displacement of the Ca^{2+}ions. Aminoglycosides, after being actively transported into the cell, bond to phosphatidylinosite phosphate. This prevents hydrolysis of the latter and the consequent reactions as well as disturbs the integrity and structure of the membrane. In vitro studies provide some evidence of the first step (23rd Workshop on Inner Ear Biology, Berlin 1986).

c) Excretion of SM

The antibiotic undergoes glomerular filtration, 70% of the dose being excreted in unchanged form with the urine. Inter-individual differences in the SM concentrations, already evident in patients without kidney damage, are attributed to individual variations of the renal clearance (LEVY et al. 1961). Therefore, in the presence of kidney damage SM should be given in doses adapted to the residual renal function (HÖFFLER 1981; see Table 10, p. 426). The course of the SM concentration in the serum after i.m. administration is reproduced in Table 1.

Further pharmacokinetic parameters are shown in Tables 8, 9, and 11 of the General Part, pp. 424, 425, 432.

References

Arosenius KD, Björk VO, Laurell G (1961) The streptomycin-concentration in tuberculosis cavities. Thorax 16:361–363

Beggs WH, Williams NE (1971) Streptomycin uptake by *Mycobacterium tuberculosis*. Appl Microbiol 21:751–753

Cada K (1971) The ototoxic action mechanism of streptomycin and kanamycin. Stud Pneumol Phtiseol Cechoslov 31:405–410

Cox EC, White JR, Flaks JG (1964) Streptomycin action and the ribosome. Proc NY Acad Sci 51:703–709
Davies JE (1964) Studies on the ribosomes of streptomycin-sensitive and resistant strains of Escherichia coli. Proc NY Acad Sci 51:659–664
Davies J, Gilbert W, Gorini L (1964) Streptomycin, suppression and the code. Proc NY Acad Sci 51:883–890
Davies J, Jones DS, Khorana HG (1966) A further study of misreading of codons induced by streptomycin and neomycin using ribopolynucleotides containing two nucleotides in alternating sequence as templates. J Mol Biol 18:48–57
Federspil P (1979) Antibiotikaschäden des Ohres, dargestellt am Beispiel des Gentamycins. Hals-, Nasen- und Ohrenheilkunde, Band 28. Barth, Leipzig
Felgenhauer F, Lagler F (1970) Experimental animal investigations with rifampicin on the question of its influence on the vestibular system and its period of retention in the perilymph of the inner ear. Antibiotics Chemother 16:361–368
Fernández C (1967) Biochemistry of labyrinthine fluids. Inorganic substances. Arch Otolaryng 86:116–127
Ganguin G (1971) Auswirkungen einer antituberkulösen Chemotherapie bei tuberkulösen Schwangeren auf die Frucht. Z Erkr Atmungsorgane 134:95–103
Gauze GG, Fatkullina LG, Dolgilevich SM (1971) Effect of antibiotics with different mechanisms of action on incorporation of labeled desoxynucleoside triphosphates to DNA of isolated rat liver mitochondria. Antibiotiki 17:296–301
Gerhardt H-J, Scheibe F, Berndt H (1973) Biochemische Aspekte und Möglichkeiten in der Lärmschadenforschung des Innenohres. Z Gesamte Hyg 19:21–24
Goldberg IH (1965) Mode of action of antibiotics. Am J Med 39:722–752
Hahn FE (1971) Streptomycin. Antibiot Chemother 17:29–51 (M)
Hansson E, Hanngren Ä, Ullberg S (1966) Autoradiographic distribution studies with labelled penicillin, streptomycin, tetracycline and cycloserine. In: Herold M, Gabriel Z (eds) Antibiotics – Advances in research, production and clinical use. London: Butterworths, Prague: Czechoslovak Medical Press, pp 156–164
Hevér E, Riskó T (1960) Studies on streptomycin levels of blood and abscess. Acta Tuberc Scand 38:40–50
Höffler D (1981) Die Dosierung wichtiger Antibiotika und Tuberkulostatika bei Niereninsuffizienz. Internist (Berlin) 22:601–606
Hurwitz C, Rosano CL (1962) Accumulation of label from ^{14}C-streptomycin by Escherichia coli. J Bacteriol 83:1193–1201
Hurwitz C, Rosano CL (1966) Further evidence for a streptomycin permease. In: Herold M, Gabriel Z (eds) Antibiotics – Advances in research, production and clinical use. London: Butterworths, Prague: Czechoslovak Medical Press, pp 668–671
Kellerhals B (1973) Zur Ototoxizität der Aminoglykosid-Antibiotika. MMW 115:1667–1672
Kibirige MS, Jones PM, Williams F, Burn JL (1986) Serum streptomycin levels in tuberculosis meningitis in an infant. Lancet I:806–807
Klein D, Pramer D (1961) Bacterial dissimilation of streptomycin. J Bacteriol 82:505–510
Klein D, Pramer D (1962) Some products of the bacterial dissimilation of streptomycin. J Bacteriol 83:309–313
Kogut M, Harris M (1969) Effects of streptomycin in bacterial cultures growing at different rates; interaction with bacterial ribosomes in vivo. Eur J Biochem 9:42–49
Kogut M, Lightbown JW (1966) The mode of action of streptomycin: effects of the intracellular antibiotic on the growth of Escherichia coli. In: Herold M, Gabriel Z (eds) Antibiotics – Advances in research, production and clinical use. London: Butterworths, Prague: Czechoslovak Medical Press, pp 32–37
Krüger-Thiemer E †, Kröger H, Nestler HJ, Seydel JK (1975) Wirkungsmodi antituberkulöser Chemotherapeutika: Inositanaloga. In: Meissner G, Schmiedel A †, Nelles A † (Hrsg) Infektionskrankheiten und ihre Erreger, Band 4, Teil III. Fischer, Jena, pp 337–352
Kunin CM (1967) A guide to use of antibiotics in patients with renal disease. Ann Intern Med 67:151–158

Levy D, Russell WF Jr, Middlebrook G (1960) Dosages of isoniazid and streptomycin for routine chemotherapy of tuberculosis. Tubercle 41:23–31
Levy D, Russell WF Jr, Ninio S, Middlebrook G (1961) Effect of increasing dosage of streptomycinsulfate on serum levels of antimicrobially active drug. Dis Chest 39:161–164
Masukawa H, Tanaka N (1968) Miscoding activity of amino-sugars. J Antibiotics 21:70–72
Mendelsohn M, Katzenberg I (1972) The effect of kanamycin on the cation content of the endolymph. Laryngoscope 82:397–403
Michel-Briand Y (1978) Mécanismes d'action des antibiotiques, à propos de quelques exemples. CR Soc Biol 172:609–627
Moravek J, Trnka L (1973) Enzymatic inactivation of streptomycin in mycobacteria. Stud Pneumol Phtiseol Cechoslov 33:346–351
Mordasini ER, Eulenberger J (1971) Tuberkulostatika, Teil 1. Int J Clin Pharmacol Ther Toxicol 4:467–486
Pestka S (1966) Studies on the formation of transfer ribonucleic acid-ribosome complexes. I. The effect of streptomycin and ribosomal dissoziation on ^{14}C-aminoacyl transfer ribonucleic acid binding to ribosomes. J Biol Chem 241:367–372
Pinkett MO, Brownstein BL (1974) Streptomycin-induced synthesis of abnormal protein in an Escherichia coli mutant. J Bacteriol 119:345–350
Podvinec S, Mihaljevic B, Marcetic A, Simonovic M (1966) Experimental investigations into the passage of streptomycin through the placenta in white rats. In: Herold M, Gabriel Z (eds) Antibiotics – Advances in research, production and clinical use. London: Butterworths, Prague: Czechoslovak Medical Press pp 198–202
Quesnel LB, York P, Skinner VM (1971) Drug dependence and phenotypic masking in streptomycin dependent and paromomycin dependent mutants of Escherichia coli. Microbios 4:97–107
Rasmussen F (1969) The oto-toxic effect of streptomycin and dihydrostreptomycin on the foetus. Scand J Resp Dis 50:61–67
Stupp H, Rauch S (1966) Anreicherungsvorgänge im Innenohr – ihre klinische und physiologische Bedeutung. Arch Ohrenheilkunde 187:636–642
Stupp H, Rauch S, Sous H, Brun JP, Lagler F (1967) Kanamycin dosage and levels in ear and other organs. Arch Otolaryng 86:515–521
Tanaka N, Masukawa H, Umezawa H (1967) Structural basis of kanamycin for miscoding activity. Biochem Biophys Res Commun 26:544–549
Toyohara M (1974) The experimental study on the transmission of the antituberculous drugs to fetuses. Kekkaku 49:97–99
Varpela E (1964) On the effect exerted by first-line tuberculosis medicines on the foetus. Acta Tubercul Scand 35:53–69
Voldřich L (1965) The kinetics of streptomycin, kanamycin and neomycin in the inner ear. Acta Oto-Laryng 60:243–248
Virsik K, Bajan A, Havelka C, Schwartz E, Molnar L (1971) Serum levels of streptomycin, isoniazid and thiacetazone correlated to side-effects in patients with active pulmonary tuberculosis. Stud Pneumol Phtiseol Cechoslov 31:3–8
Vrabec DP, Cody DTR, Ulrich JA (1965) A study of the relative concentrations of antibiotics in the blood, spinal fluid, and perilymph in animals. Ann Otol Rhinol Laryngol 74:688–705
Wagner WH (1971) The pharmacokinetics of streptomycin. Stud Pneumol Phtiseol Cechoslov 31:276–279
Wagner WH, Chou JTY, Ilberg C v, Ritter R, Vosteen KH (1971) Untersuchungen zur Pharmakokinetik von Streptomycin. Arzneimittelforsch 21:2006–2016
Watanabe Y, Nakajina R, Oda R, Uno M, Naito T (1971) Experimental study on the transfer of kanamycin to the inner ear fluids. Med J Osaka Univ 21:257–263

III. TSC

1. Mode of Action

The processes that possibly occur during the uptake or biotransformation of TSC by mycobacteria have hitherto been investigated only superficially in relation to the clinical importance of this antituberculotic and the relative insensitivity of the methods available for determining TSC concentrations (Svinchuk et al. 1978).

In view of the cross-resistance demonstrated between TSC, DATC, and ETH/PTH (Trnka et al. 1966), common points of attack or ones situated close to one another in the metabolic process are assumed to exist. They could be related to the group common to the thiosemicarbazones, thiocarbanilides, and carbothionamides, namely the $-\underset{\underset{\displaystyle S-}{\|}}{C}-N$-group.

Because of the loss of stability to acid observed in this group of antituberculotics only in the case of ETH/PTH, and the specific influence of ETH on growth in the depth of agar media (Schmiedel et al. 1964), however, it is believed that the carbothionamides may have an additional point of attack (Kakimoto et al. 1961, 1962; Seydel 1963; Krüger-Thiemer et al. 1975). Intracellular conversion into an active compound (release of H_2S) cannot be ruled out. Under the conditions of endogenous respiration, the acid-soluble fraction constitutes one site of attack of these three antituberculotics, the incorporation of ^{32}P into the polyphosphates being prevented (Reutgen and Iwainsky 1968). The passage of other radiolabelled compounds into the remaining fractions is partly inhibited (Tsukamura et al. 1964) and an influence on the pyridoxal system is assumed (Kakimoto et al. 1961).

2. Biotransformation

Nothing is known certainly about the biotransformation of TSC in the macroorganism, probably for the reason discussed above.

Table 1. TSC concentrations in the blood of tuberculosis patients (Drabkina and Ginzburg 1977)

TSC concentration in the blood after administration of					
50 mg TSC			100 mg TSC		
Blood sample taken after hours	n	µg/ml	Blood sample taken after hours	n	µg/ml
2	8	2.8±0.4	2	12	5.2±0.7
4	9	2.5±1.1	4	8	4.1±0.9
6	15	0.37±0.1	6	12	3.6±0.5
8	8	0	8	5	2.7±0.5
10			10	3	2.5
12			12	2	1.8

3. Pharmacokinetics

TSC is absorbed very rapidly. It does not bind to serum proteins. Its distribution volume has not yet been definitively established. In animal experiments, the maximum TSC concentration in serum is reached after 2 h, falling by about 50% after 3 h. After 5 h TSC is no longer detectable in the serum. The following values have been measured in man after 2 h: lungs 2 μg/ml, liver 14.9 μg/ml, kidneys 3.7 μg/ml (DRABKINA and GINZBURG 1977). The TSC concentration in the blood is shown in Table 1.

The concentration of TSC in human adrenals is high. In the skin and mucosae too the concentrations are far above those in the other organs, which are largely similar. Determinations on several days in the course of treatment in one and the same patient reveal considerable fluctuations in the TSC concentration (MORDASINI and EULENBERGER 1971). The drug is said to have a half-life of 8^{h}–12^{h}. TSC is excreted renally, 4%–12% of the administered quantity being recovered in the faeces. Data on the TSC concentration in the CSF and relating to pharmacokinetic parameters will be found in Tables 7–9 and 11 of the General Part (pp. 423, 424, 433).

References

Drabkina RO, Ginzburg TS (1977) Antituberculous action and pharmacokinetics of thioacetazone. Probl Tuberk 55 issue 4: 69–71
Kakimoto S, Seydel J, Wempe E (1961) Struktur und Wirkung von Carbothionamiden. Jber Borstel 5:240–281
Kakimoto S, Seydel J, Wempe E (1962) Zusammenhänge zwischen Struktur und Wirkung bei Carbothionamiden. Arzneimittelforsch 12:127–133
Krüger-Thiemer E †, Kröger H, Nestler HJ, Seydel JK (1975) Wirkungsmodi antituberkulöser Chemotherapeutika: Pyridincarbonsäureethioamide, Thiocarbanilide und Thiosemicarbazone. In: Meissner G, Schmiedel A †, Nelles A † (Hrsg) Infektionskrankheiten und ihre Erreger, Band 4, Teil III. Fischer, Jena, pp 289–298
Mordasini ER, Eulenberger J (1971) Tuberkulostatika, Teil 2, Spezifische Chemotherapeutika. Int J Clin Pharmacol Ther Toxicol 5:70–95
Reutgen H, Iwainsky H (1968) Untersuchungen zum endogenen Stoffwechsel von Mykobakterien. 4. Mitt. Über den Einfluß von Äthionamid auf den endogenen Stoffwechsel von *Myc. smegm.* Z Naturforschung 23b:976–982
Schmiedel A, Lawonn H, Gerloff W (1964) Über die Wirkungsweise des α-Äthyl-thioisonicotinsäureamid (Ethionamid) auf Tuberkulosebakterien in der Agar-Hohe-Schicht-Kultur. Beitr Klin Tuberk 129:317–325
Seydel J (1965) Struktur und Wirkung von Pyridincarbonsäurethioamiden und Pyridincarbonsäurehydraziden. In: Käppler W, Iwainsky H, Grunert M, Sehrt I, Reutgen H (Hrsg) Bericht über das II. Internationale Symposium „Bakteriologie und Biochemie der Mykobakterien" 20.–24.10.1963. Berlin-Buch, pp 414–427
Svinchuk VS, Kramarenko VF, Orlinsky MM (1978) Determination of thioacetazone in the urine. Probl Tuberk 56 issue 7: 74–76
Trnka L, Havel A, Urbanczik R (1966) Neueste Tuberkulostatika, ihre Bedeutung und Möglichkeiten der Wertbestimmung im Reagenzglas. Chemotherapia 11:121–134
Tsukamura M, Tsukamura S, Mizuno S, Nakano E (1964) The mechanism of action of ethionamide. Am Rev Respir Dis 89:933–935

IV. PZA

1. Mode of Action

A worth mentioning antituberculotic effect of PZA can only be detected in monocyte – cultures or on nutrient media with a pH of less than 5.6 (at best pH 4.9). Such pH is evidently optimal for permeation of PZA but not for the growth of mycobacteria. Therefore, largely for methodological reasons, problems relating to the uptake and biotransformation of PZA in mycobacteria and to the effects of PZA resistance on these processes have been studied only sporadically.

On the basis of comparative studies on *M. tuberculosis* and *M. bovis*, Konno formulated a hypothesis about the action mechanism of PZA. In both species, the nicotinamidase is identical with the PZAase (KONNO et al. 1967; BRANDER 1972). *M. tuberculosis* is sensitive to PZA while having a relatively high nicotinamidase-PZAase activity, whereas in qualitative tests *M. bovis* shows no nicotinamidase-PZAase and is resistant to PZA. In *M. tuberculosis*, the development of resistance to PZA goes hand in hand with a loss of the amidase activity.

Evidently, compared with pyrazinoic acid, PZA is the substrate that permeates more readily (like INS/INA). Inside the mycobacterial cells pyrazinoic acid is formed by enzymatic release of the amide group, in high concentrations inhibiting the metabolic processes in *M. tuberculosis* and only to a slight extent, insufficient to effect inhibition, in *M. bovis*. However, other mycobacterial species such as *M. avium* or *M. smegmatis* do not conform to this hypothesis. They are only slightly sensitive to PZA and exhibit high nicotinamidase activity.

2. Biotransformation

Pyrazinoic acid can be separated from unchanged PZA by selective extraction and identified. By contrast, no appreciable amounts of other biotransformation products, especially conjugates, could be isolated even by the use of specific chromatographic techniques and counter-current distribution. According to ELLARD (1969), the PZA concentration in the serum is substantially higher than that of the acid, whilst according to GIALDRONI-GRASSI (1979), the PZA levels are only about half the levels of pyrazinoic acid. However, only 4% of the administered dose is excreted as unchanged PZA in the 24-h urine, whereas ~ 30% is excreted in the form of the pyrazinoic acid (Fig. 1, ELLARD 1969). Since complete absorption from the intestinal tract can be assumed from studies of the faeces, even taking into account excretion lasting more than 24 h, about 60% must be converted into non-determinable biotransformation products of still unknown structures.

In studies on larger numbers of healthy volunteers and patients, considerable scatter of the individual values is observed. As the values in an individual patient are relatively constant (patient-specific $t_{50\%}$), the interindividual $t_{50\%}$ differences are attributed to differences in the extent of the biotransformation (ELLARD 1969; GURUMURTHY et al. 1981). A low rate of biotransformation could mean a greater risk of side effects (GRASSI 1979).

The duration of PZA therapy has no bearing on the activity of the host-organism's pyrazinamide-desamidase involved in the biotransformation. The enzyme has been detected in various tissues of mouse, rat, guinea pig, and rabbit; the bulk

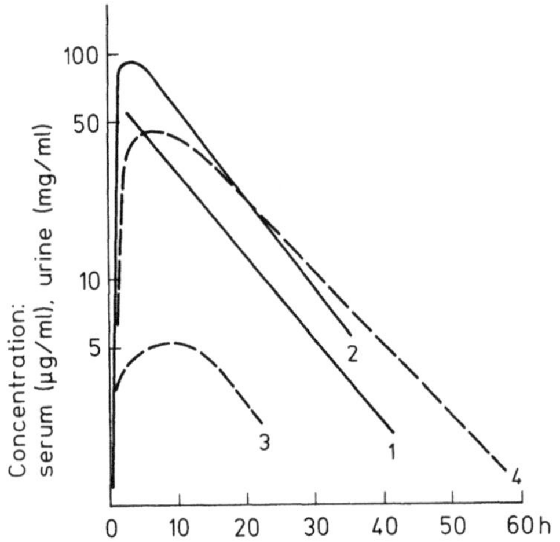

Fig. 1. Course of the concentrations of PZA and of its biotransformation product pyrazinoic acid in the serum and their excretion with the urine (ELLARD 1969). *1* PZA concentration in the serum; *2* PZA concentration in the urine; *3* Pyrazinoic acid concentration in the serum; *4* Pyrazinoic acid concentration in the urine

of it is localized in the microsomal fraction of the liver. There may possibly be some connections between the NADase activity and the efficacy of PZA in various animal species (TOIDA 1973; GRASSI 1979; GURUMURTHY et al. 1981).

3. Pharmacokinetics

PZA is absorbed more slowly than INH and PAS, the maximal serum concentration only being reached after 2 h (Fig. 1). Up to 3 g the value increases in proportion to the dose (Tables 1 and 2). PZA is distributed over all the body water. Both in man and in animals, the diffusion into organs is relatively slow. Accordingly, the PZA concentrations in the lungs, liver, and kidneys are lower than that in the serum. PZA cannot be detected in the spleen, brain, or the skeletal muscle (STOTTMEIER et al. 1968; ELLARD 1969). The question whether PZA passes into the foetus is still open. However, PZA concentrations have been detected in the CSF that appear to be sufficient for the treatment of meningitis tuberculosa (GIALDRONI-GRASSI 1979; LARBAOUI 1979, see Table 7, p. 423). The $t_{50\%}$ values

Table 1. Course of PZA concentration in serum (µg/ml) in healthy volunteers and in tuberculosis patients (ZIERSKI 1981)

Dose	Blood sample taken after h				
	1	2	3	6	24
20–22 mg/kg (0.5 g–1.5 g 3 × daily)	28.8 (7–60)	31.5 (10–50)	31.3 (7.5–52.5)	24.4 (10–45)	5.8 (3.3–11)
44 mg/kg (3.0 g every 2 days	50.5 (6–65.7)	54.8 (25–66)	56.1 (46–62)	44.8 (39–55)	10.2 (5.7–22)
66 mg/kg (4.5 g)	45.7 (29–60)	–	82.9 (48–109)	76.8 (54–112)	19.3 (16–21)

Table 2. Course of PZA concentration in serum (μg/ml) in healthy volunteers and in tuberculosis patients (SUBBAMMAL et al. 1968)

	n	Dose (mg/kg)	Blood sample taken after h			
			1	3	6	24
Volunteers	3	22	19	27	23	8
		44	24	52	46	14
		66	44	70	57	19
Patients	6	66		86	85	
		88		105	131	

are between 7 h and 14 h regardless of the dose administered (ELLARD 1969; GIALDRONI-GRASSI 1979; GURUMURTHY et al. 1981, see Table 11, p. 433).

Within the first 6 h, the excretion of PZA and pyrazinoic acid follows an exponential course (Fig. 1). There is a close correlation between the serum $t_{50\%}$ and the quantity of PZA excreted unchanged with the urine. PZA and pyrazinoic acid are subject to glomerular filtration; 98% of the PZA is reabsorbed, while pyrazinoic acid is not (ELLARD 1969, see Table 8, p. 424). Further data on pharmacokinetic parameters, doses to be given in the event of kidney damage, etc. are given in Tables 9–11 of the General Part (pp. 425, 426, 433).

References

Brander E (1972) A simple way of detecting pyrazinamide resistance. Tubercle 53:128–131

Ellard GA (1969) Absorption, metabolism and excretion of pyrazinamide in man. Tubercle 50:144–158

Gialdroni-Grassi G (1979) Caractéristiques pharmacologiques et métabolisme du pyrazinamide chez l'homme. Actes d' un Symposium „Le pyrazinamide 25 ans après", tenu à Alger. 1.–2. 4. 1979, Laboratoires Bracco, Milan, pp 31–34

Grassi C (1979) Considérations sur l'activité antimycobactérienne du pyrazinamide dans les conditions expérimentales différentes. Actes d' un Symposium „Le pyrazinamide 25 ans après", tenu à Alger. 1.–2. 4. 1979, Laboratoires Bracco, Milan, pp 45–47

Gurumurthy P, Krishnamurthy PV, Sarma GR (1981) Pyrazinamide deamidase activity in tuberculous disease. Am Rev Respir Dis 124:97

Konno K, Feldmann FM, McDermott W (1967) Pyrazinamide susceptibility and amidase activity of tubercle bacilli. Am Rev Respir Dis 95:461–469

Larbaoui D (1979) Le pyrazinamide, 25 ans après. Actes d' un Symposium tenu à Alger, 1.–2. 4. 1979. Laboratoires Bracco, Milan pp 15–23

Stottmeier KD, Beam RE, Kubica GP (1968) The absorption and excretion of pyrazinamide. I. Preliminary study in laboratory animals and in man. Am Rev Respir Dis 98:70–74

Subbammal S, Krishnamurthy DV, Tripathy SP, Venkataraman P (1968) Concentrations of pyrazinamide attained in serum with different doses of the drug. Bull WHO 39:771–774

Toida I (1973) Metabolism of pyrazinamide. Pyrazinamide deamidase of animal tissues. Am Rev Respir Dis 107:630–638

Zierski M (1981) Pharmakologie, Toxikologie und klinische Anwendung von Pyrazinamid. Prax Pneumol 35:1075–1105

V. INH

1. Mode of Action

a) Incorporation of INH in Mycobacteria

INH is incorporated in the cells by diffusion and by an aerobic process interpreted as active transport (TSUKAMURA et al. 1963; WIMPENNY 1967b). At 100 μg/ml–200 μg/ml, its saturation range is far above its MIC (YOUATT and THAM 1969c) and is rarely reached. As permeation advances, INH accumulates in the cells. The ratio of intracellular to extracellular INH increases in the first 8 h, only thereafter remaining more or less stable (Figs. 1 and 2, BEGGS and JENNE 1969, 1970; JENNE and BEGGS 1973). In the cells INH is hydrolyzed to isonicotinic acid, which at physiological pH is no longer capable of permeation, this acid is ultimately entering into other reactions. Since the accumulation does not take place in cell-free extracts and under conditions of endogenous respiration, essentially higher INH concentrations are required to inhibit the metabolic processes under these conditions (IWAINSKY and REUTGEN 1968; BEGGS and JENNE 1970).

The cells' capacity to bind INH can be saturated by concentrations that no longer exert any inhibitory activity in the culture filtrate (BEGGS et al. 1968; YOUATT and THAM 1969b). Like the PAS derivatives INH derivatives are hydrolyzed before their incorporation in the cells.

b) Biotransformation of INH by Mycobacteria

INH-sensitive mycobacteria (BCG) form, in addition to isonicotinic acid, 4-hydroxymethylpyridine and very probably the hydrazone of α-ketoglutaric acid (Fig. 3, YOUATT 1961, 1969; YOUATT and THAM 1969c). The parallels with the bio-

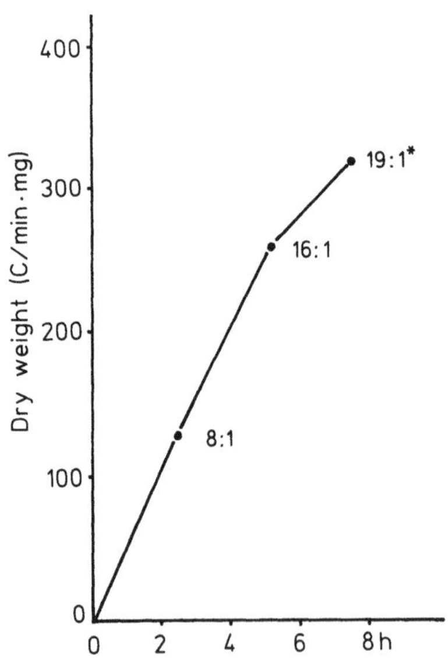

Fig. 1. Incorporation of ^{14}C-INH in *Mycobacterium tuberculosis* as a function of contact time (BEGGS and JENNE 1970, 0.1 μg ^{14}C-INH/ml). * Intracellular/extracellular INH ratio at the stated times

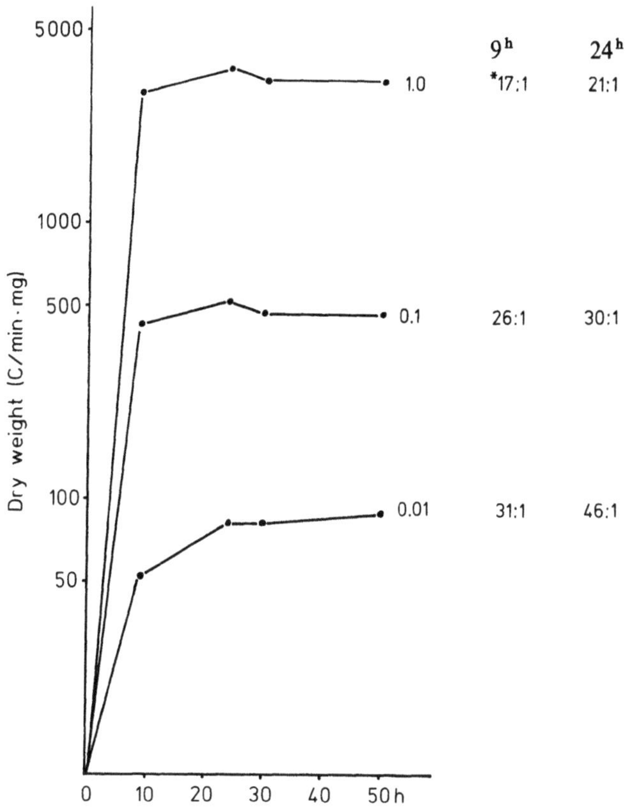

Fig. 2. Influence of the INH concentration and the contact time on the incorporation of ^{14}C-INH in *Mycobacterium tuberculosis* (BEGGS and JENNE 1970). 0.01/0.1/1.0 = μg INH/ml.* Intracellular/extracellular INH ratio at the stated times

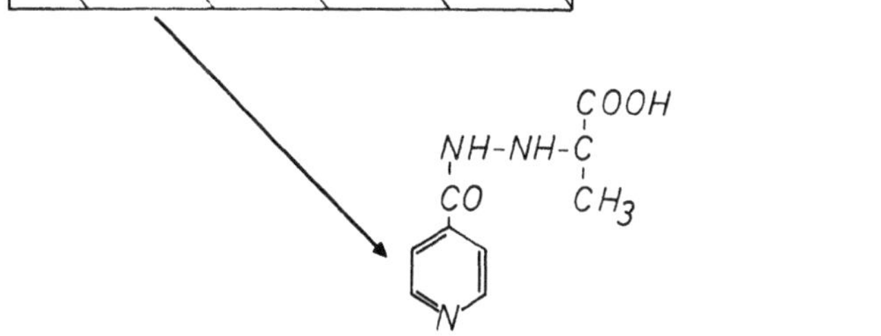

Fig. 3. Biotransformation of INH by INH-sensitive and INH-resistant mycobacteria. ▨ Biotransformation by INH-resistant populations

transformation of physiological nicotinic acid are remarkable; the analogous 3-hydroxymethylpyridine has likewise been found in mycobacteria (GROSS et al. 1967, 1968; ZURECK 1968).

INH can be converted merely in a shaken culture with phosphate buffer and ammonium chloride (YOUATT 1965). The different biotransformation rates that have been reported (WIMPENNY 1967b; YOUATT and THAM 1969a) can probably be explained by different experimental conditions. According to comprehensive studies, between about 50% and 60% is present as isonicotinic acid, 20% as 4-hydroxymethylpyridine, and 20% as a hydrazone. INH-resistant microorganisms form only isonicotinic acid. In the case of *M. smegmatis* hydrazine can also be detected after a lag phase of several hours (FISHBAIN et al. 1972).

c) Uptake of INH by INH-Resistant Mycobacteria

The rate of incorporation in INH-resistant populations remains more or less constant over a wide range of temperature (5 °C–37 °C, EDA 1963a), while the temperature-dependence of the INH uptake observed in the sensitive pathogens indicates that enzymatically regulated processes are at work. According to more recent investigations, it is the absence of the aforementioned aerobic process (see Section 1.a) and not, as was originally assumed, a change in permeation (EDA 1963a) that is responsible for the reduced INH-uptake in INH-resistant populations (YOUATT 1969). A reciprocal relationship exists between INH uptake and INH-resistance (Fig. 4, EDA 1963b; TSUKAMURA et al. 1963; BEGGS et al. 1968; SRIPRAKASH and RAMAKRISHNAN 1970; JENNE and BEGGS 1973).

In addition, the possibility of enzymatic destruction of INH is discussed and the existence of a so-called anti-INH factor has been confirmed by several

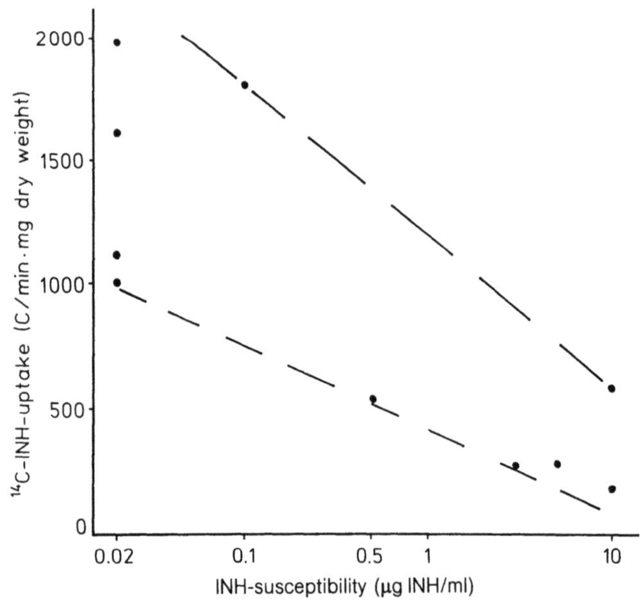

Fig. 4. Correlations between ^{14}C-INH uptake and the degree of resistance to INH of mycobacteria (TSUKAMURA et al. 1963)

authors. This factor is dialysable and re-extractable. However, no correlation has been found between the anti-INH factor and INH-resistance (YOUMANS and YOUMANS 1960; KRAUS et al. 1961). In addition, there is an enzyme that can be induced by INH, the so-called hydrazidase (TOIDA 1962a, b), whose formation is strongly dependent on the nitrogen sources present in the nutrient medium (TOIDA and SAITO 1962). The inductor- and substrate-specificity are not very pronounced, as a result of which the hydrazidase could also be a proteolytic enzyme or an amidase (TOIDA 1962c).

d) Mode of Action of INH

There is hardly any substance group essential for mycobacteria upon which INH has not been found to act. In 1957, KRÜGER-THIEMER reviewed the hypotheses that had hitherto been put forward, evaluated them critically, and hence derived his ideas on the mode of action of INH – "the isonicotinic acid hypothesis" (Fig. 5). A revision carried out by his colleagues in the years leading up to 1975 and taking account of studies that had since been published led fundamentally to the same hypothesis (KRÜGER-THIEMER et al. 1975), although it was a long time

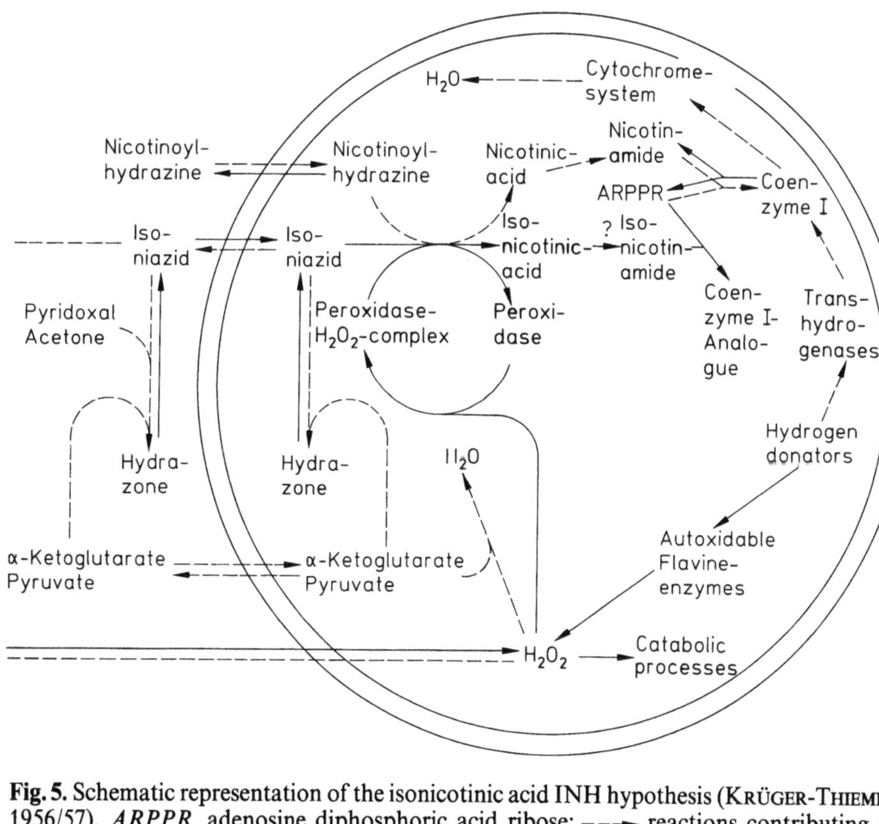

Fig. 5. Schematic representation of the isonicotinic acid INH hypothesis (KRÜGER-THIEMER 1956/57). *ARPPR,* adenosine diphosphoric acid ribose; ---► reactions contributing to damage to the bacteria by hydrogen peroxide; —► reactions counteracting damage to the bacteria by hydrogen peroxide; ⫽ cell membrane

before definite proof of it could be given (Robson and Sullivan 1963; Iwainsky 1970; Ramakrishnan et al. 1972; Zierski and Rotermund 1984).

However, by 1975 the following points had been clarified on the basis of the expanded information obtained in the previous 10 years regarding the biochemistry of mycobacteria (Iwainsky and Käppler 1974) and as a result of refinements in the experimental procedure:

1) A number of the changes observed are not caused solely by INH. For example, a yellow pigment that can be detected after exposure to INH is observed only when a *Sauton* nutrient medium is used and not with a *Proskauer-Beck* medium (Winder et al. 1967; Youatt 1969). Certain INH-antagonists are only active in the presence of asparagine (Youatt 1969). The accumulation of carbohydrates following contact with INH is reduced if ammonium ions are used as the source of nitrogen instead of asparagine and casein hydrolysate.

2) The effect of INH is already evident after 1 h (Bekierkunst and Bricker 1967; Winder et al. 1967; Youatt 1969; Winder and Collins 1970; Wang and Takayama 1972). A lag phase appears only in whole-cell experiments with a determination of terminal reactions of the metabolism or of cell growth. Intervention in transcription, translation, or protein synthesis can thus be excluded for reasons of time.

3) The exact relationships between intracellular INH (or isonicotinic acid, INA) concentration and activity are clarified by a simultaneous determination of the incorporation of INH (Youatt and Tham 1969b; Wang and Takayama 1972). The primary site of attack of INH lies definitely in the acid-soluble cell fraction (Eda 1963c).

4) In studies on the incorporation and oxidative degradation of certain nutrients an influence of INH on the nucleic acid fraction, enzymes of the tricarboxylic acid cycle, and aminotransferases was established (Tsukamura and Mizuno 1962; Wimpenny 1967a; McClatchy and Smith 1968; McClatchy 1971; Suryanarayana et al. 1973).

5) A rapid increase of the soluble carbohydrates and of acid-soluble phosphate has been observed in *M. tuberculosis*, *M. bovis* BCG, and *M. smegmatis*

Table 1. Influence of INH on the chain length of the fatty acids in the triglycerides of various BCG lipid fractions (Winder and Rooney 1968) (18 h of incubation with 10 µg INH/ml)

Lipid fraction	Control culture		INH culture	
	Chain length of the fatty acids			
	C_{12}–C_{16}	C_{16} and more	C_{12}–C_{16}	C_{16} and more
	Fraction (%)			
Ethanol-ether-soluble neutral fats	42	58	50	50
Wax A	35	65	51	49
Ethanol-ether-insoluble, chloroform-soluble fraction	35	65	45	55
Bound lipids	41	59	45	55

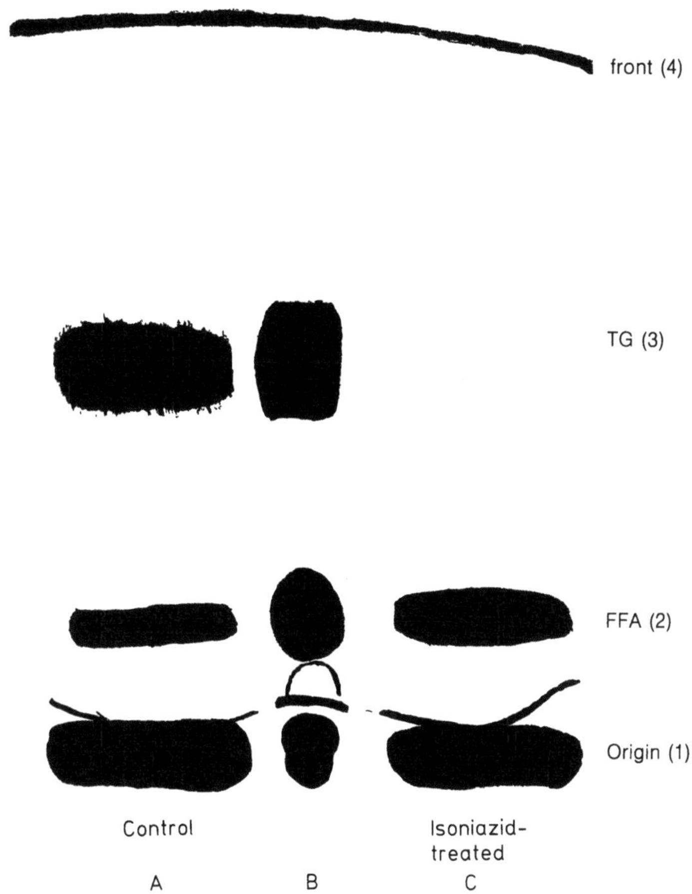

Fig. 6. Influence of INH on the composition of the wax-A fraction of BCG (WINDER and ROONEY 1968, thin-layer chromatogram, schematic representation). *A* Control; *B* test substances; *C* run with 10 μg INH/ml; *1* start; *2* free fatty acids; *3* triglycerides; *4* solvent front

after the addition of INH (WINDER 1964). α,α′-Trehalose, trehalose-6-(P), Glu-6-(P), and Glu-1-(P) were found in the carbohydrate fraction, as a result of which inhibition of the carbohydrate degradation was assumed (WINDER and BRENNAN 1964; WINDER et al. 1967). In addition, an increase of the inorganic phosphate and the formation of fluorescing and UV-absorbing substances and the already mentioned yellow pigment or its colourless precursor have been observed (WINDER 1964; YOUATT 1969; YOUATT and THAM 1969a).

6) Exposure to INH affects the lipid metabolism of mycobacteria (WINDER and ROONEY 1968; WINDER and COLLINS 1970), the fraction of short-chain fatty acids being increased while that of those with more than 16 C-atoms is decreased (Table 1, Fig. 6).

The mechanisms responsible for the lengthening of the fatty acid chains are evidently impaired by the INH. This also explains the inhibition of the mycolic acid synthesis, which proceeds in proportion to intracellular ^{14}C-INH activity (Wang and Takayama 1972). The inhibition is reversible if the exposure to INH is limited (Takayama et al. 1974). Ultimately this intervention in the bacterial metabolism can lead to changes in the cell membrane (Brennan et al. 1970; Winder and Rooney 1970) and to the loss of the stability to acid.

7) The effect of INH can be counteracted by nicotinic acid hydrazide even after 6 h of contact with INH, as is evident from the renewed onset of partial growth. Accordingly, the antagonistic effect of nicotinic acid hydrazide to INH cannot be due to a displacement mechanism acting at the cell surface. One important argument against the Krüger-Thiemer hypothesis is thus refuted.

8) In agreement with this hypothesis a reduction of the NAD concentration is found both under conditions of endogenous respiration and in proliferating mycobacteria after administration of INH (Iwainsky and Reutgen 1968; Winder and Collins 1968; Jackett et al. 1977). In the case of *M. tuberculosis* too a reduced NAD concentration can be established after only 4 h, whereas with *E. coli,* as one would expect in the case of insensitivity to INH, no change in the NAD concentration is discernible.

A number of objections to the Krüger-Thiemer hypothesis are thus countered and some points are found to agree with it. In 1976 it was possible with the aid of ^{3}H-INH to detect the INH-analog of NAD suggested by the hypothesis in *Mycobacterium tuberculosis,* thus confirming the validity of the Krüger-Thiemer hypothesis with regard to one essential point (Seydel et al. 1976).

The following sequence of events is postulated:

1. Rapid permeation of the INH into the mycobacterial cells.
2. Oxidation of the permeated fraction within the cells by peroxidase and catalase in the presence of endogenous hydrogen peroxide to form isonicotinic acid.
3. Accumulation of non-permeable INA in the bacterial cells.
4. INA disturbs the activity of NAD by the formation of enzymatically inactive NAD-analog.
5. Oxidation of the substrate hydrogen to water via the respiratory chain is thus partly or completely inhibited.
6. In compensation the substrate hydrogen is oxidized, by autoxidizable flavine enzymes, to hydrogen peroxide.
7. In consequence of the increased hydrogen peroxide production, catabolic processes are intensified.

The first three points are based on mutually confirming studies performed by several independent working groups. The formation of the NAD-analog of INA was demonstrated by Seydel et al. in 1976. The first steps of the action mechanism of INH thus appear to be largely clarified, while the subsequent reactions and their time sequence are still unknown. They apparently include the inhibition of mycolic acid synthesis detected by Winder et al. in comparative investigations on the action mechanisms of INH, ETH, DATC, and TSC, the first three of these compounds all being found to exert this effect. Since, owing to the absence of cross-resistance between INH on the one hand and ETH or DATC on the other, an intervention proceeding in the same way is unlikely, Winder presumes that ETH acts directly and does not exclude the possibility of INH acting via the route postulated by Krüger-Thiemer (Winder 1982). Thus, Winder probably means a disturbance of the mycobacterial metabolism, which is relatively non-specific with regard to the causative compound but which sets in rapidly and can be detected exactly, although the actual triggering steps are still unknown.

2. Biotransformation

a) Biotransformation Patterns of INH in Man and in Animals

In 1952 isonicotinic acid (INA, KELLY et al. 1952) and in 1953 the conjugation product of INA with glycine (isonicotinuric acid = INU, CUTHBERTSON et al. 1953) were identified as biotransformation products of INH. In 1953, with the aid of countercurrent distribution, acetyl-INH formed by a reaction with acetyl-coenzyme A was also isolated and identified (HUGHES 1953; WEBER et al. 1968). Subsequently in the determination of the unchanged INH by various chemical methods sometimes considerable differences have also been found, so that other biotransformation products determinable to different extents as "INH" were as-

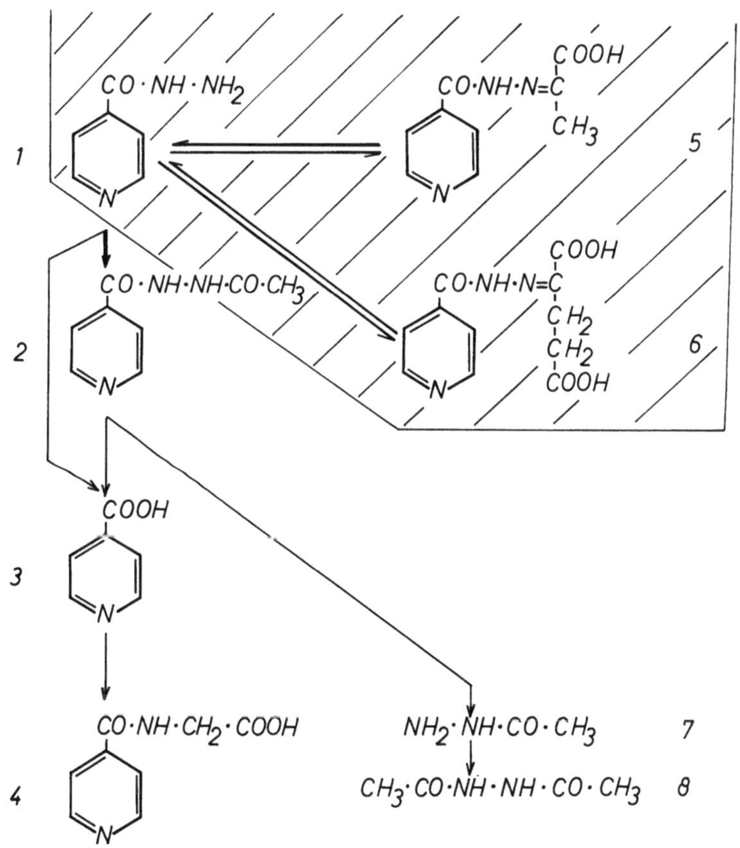

Fig. 7. Biotransformation of INH in vivo. ▨ biotransformation without loss of biological activity; *1* INH; *2* Acetyl-INH; *3* INA; *4* INU; *5* N-Isonicotinoyl-N'-pyruvic acid hydrazone; *6* N-Isonicotinoyl-N'-(α-ketoglutaric acid) hydrazone; *7* Monoacetylhydrazine; *8* Diacetylhydrazine

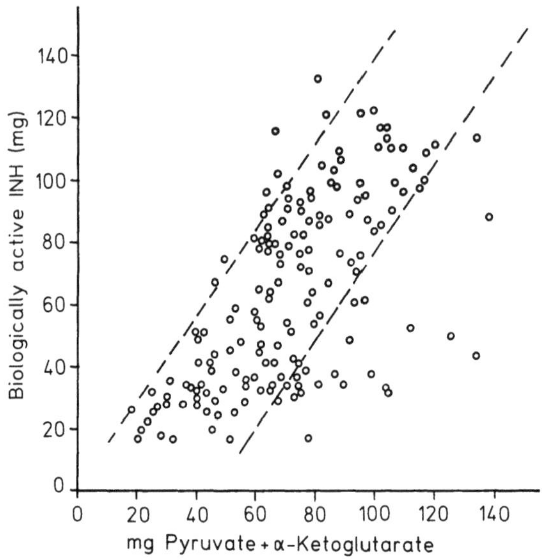

Fig. 8. Relationships between the excretion of biologically active INH and α-keto acids (PFAFFENBERG et al. 1960)

sumed to exist, and a search for them was initiated. In 1954 the hydrazone of pyruvic acid and of α-ketoglutaric acid were detected by ZAMBONI and DEFRANCESCHI. These are readily hydrolyzed back to the starting compounds (Fig. 7, IWAINSKY et al. 1965, 1967; RITTER 1973; ELLARD 1976). Further-reaching reactions of INH with endogenous carbonyl compounds can be demonstrated indirectly (increased excretion of α-keto acids, pyridoxine, loss of activity of pyridoxine-dependent enzymes, etc., Fig. 8, PFAFFENBERG et al. 1960; KRULIK and KOHOUT 1962; RAJTAR-LEONTIEW 1969; WOOD and PEESKER 1971).

The acetylhydrazine found as a biotransformation product of aroylhydrazines (TURNBULL et al. 1962) has only recently been isolated from INH (ELLARD 1976). In addition, conversion of the hydrazine formed as an intermediate into ammonium ions is assumed, since an increased level of these ions in the serum is observed after administration of INH (ZIPORIN et al. 1962; ZIPORIN 1964; SMIRNOV 1977).

It has not been possible to identify other presumed biotransformation products, such as isonicotinoyl-INH, isonicotinamide, INA oxide, methyl-N-INA, 4-hydroxymethylpyridine, the glucose hydrazone, or a condensation product of INA and glucuronate, in studies performed specifically for this purpose, largely by making use of column or paper chromatography (PFAFFENBERG et al. 1960; PETERS et al. 1965b, c).

In 1954 to 1955 ZAMBONI and DEFRANCESCHI found the same biotransformation products of INH in rats, guinea pigs, and rabbits as in man. The transfer of acetyl-coenzyme A to INH detected in man can also be observed in rhesus monkeys and in green monkeys (GOEDDE et al. 1966). A high rate of acetylation correlates with a low concentration of biologically active INH.

b) Biotransformation of INH and Antituberculotic Activity

In addition to the pyridine ring, the free hydrazine group is necessary for the biological activity of INH. Thus, conversion into INA or INU is always associated with a complete loss of biological activity. In the case of acetyl-INH, reactivation by retrogressive cleavage would be conceivable. However, it has been found consistently in very many studies that the INH is not released from acetyl-INH. Thus, apart from the hydrazone formation, all the remaining biotransformation processes also result in inactivation of the INH. Moreover, antagonism between INH and acetylhydrazine can be detected in vitro (ELLARD 1976).

c) Determination of INH and Its Biotransformation Products

The prerequisites for obtaining the results outlined above and for a determination of the rate of the biotransformation in patients were an improvement of the chromatographic techniques and the development of rapid sensitive, and specific methods for the determination of unchanged INH or of specific biotransformation products (cf. IWAINSKY et al. 1967). Specifically, depending on the available facilities, about 25 years ago this involved the fluorimetric determination of INH (PETERS 1960a; SCOTT and WRIGHT 1967; THENAULT et al. 1976), the ultramicromethod developed by NIELSCH and GIEFER in 1959 for determination of chromatographically separated INH biotransformation products (HELLER et al. 1961), microbiological procedures (EVANS et al. 1960; GANGADHARAM et al. 1961), and in particular the vertical diffusion test developed by SCHMIEDEL (SCHMIEDEL 1960; BARTMANN and MASSMANN 1960a, 1961; GRUMBACH et al. 1960; OKINAKA et al. 1961; DUFOUR et al. 1964; PIKORA et al. 1982) and ion-exchange chromatography (HELLER et al. 1961; PETERS et al. 1965b, c). In recent years more modern techniques such as gas chromatography, high-pressure liquid chromatography, polarography, and the like have been applied increasingly for the analysis of INH (FRÁTER-SCHRÖDER and ZBINDEN 1976; SUSHKIN and GUZEEVA 1978; STEPANOV 1981; v. SASSEN and CASTRO-PARVA 1981; MUSCH et al. 1981; LAUTERBURG et al. 1981; MEURICE et al. 1984). In most of the chemical and microbiological methods because of the readiness with which hydrazones are cleaved, it is impossible to differentiate between them and unchanged INH.

d) Genetically Fixed Polymorphism of INH and Other Drugs

In studies on larger groups of patients the values for "unchanged" INH (usually INH + hydrazones) do not have a normal distribution but exhibit a bimodal or trimodal course (Fig. 9), irrespective of whether the fall in the INH serum concentration is determined on the basis of the $t_{50\%}$ (JENNE 1960), the serum concentration 4 h–6 h after administration of the drug (LEVY et al. 1960), or the excretion of biologically active INH with the urine (IWAINSKY et al. 1960; PFAFFENBERG et al. 1963). Repetition of the tests, sometimes over several years, in healthy volunteers and in patients has revealed striking individual constancy of the biotransformation of INH. The assumed genetic fixing of the biotransformation rate was confirmed by studies on identical and non-identical twins (BÖNICKE and LISBOA 1957; OKINAKA et al. 1961). This phenomenon does not correlate with the ABO blood-group system (KASENOV and STAMBEKOW 1981). Autosomal-dominant

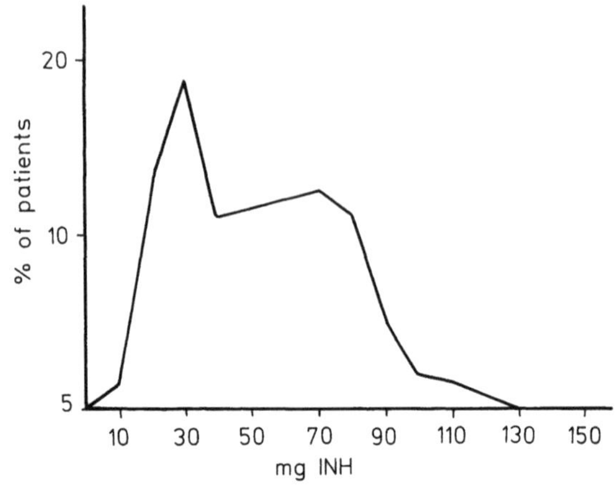

Fig. 9. Distribution curve of biologically active INH in the urine (oral administration of 300 mg to 203 patients

transmission is assumed to be the cause of a disposition for rapid biotransformation of INH (INH inactivation). SUNAHARA found that his results agreed more satisfactorily with the expected figures when transmission without dominance is assumed. He differentiated between homozygous slow inactivators (SI, genotype SS), a heterozygous middle group (genotype RS), and homozygous rapid inactivators (RI, genotype RR, SUNAHARA 1962; SUNAHARA et al. 1963 a; DUFOUR et al. 1964). The first of these transmission processes is, however, supported in later publications as well, chiefly among pharmacogeneticists (EVANS and WHITE 1964; LA DU 1972; GOEDDE 1974).

The mode of administration has no influence, bimodal or trimodal distribution also being detectable after intravenous or i.m. administration (JENNE 1964; TIITINEN 1969 b, c; VENKATARAMAN et al. 1972). The sum of all the biotransformation products (total INH) exhibits a normal distribution (Fig. 10). The individual values for INH and total INH show, moreover, that a low concentration of INH correlates with low absorption only in exceptional cases (IWAINSKY et al. 1965). Thus, absorption differences can be ruled out as the cause. Nor does the cause of the bimodal or trimodal distribution of the INH values lie in differences in INH binding to the serum proteins, in the renal clearance, or in the tubular reabsorption (JENNE et al. 1961; GOEDDE and SCHOPF 1964).

Intensive investigations performed on a few volunteers have failed to reveal any differences in the INA and INU formation correlating with the fraction of INH (PETERS et al. 1964). INU is probably formed from INA only secondarily, and has so far been detected only in the urine (VIVIEN et al. 1972). The decisive reaction for the different extents of the biotransformation is apparently acetylation (PETERS et al. 1964). In contrast to many other drugs, this occurs in the nonmicrosomal fraction of the liver (LEVI et al. 1968; ACKERMANN 1973; NOTTER and ROLAND 1978).

Investigation of the biotransformation of INH in liver homogenates has brought to light a close correlation between the acetylation capacity of the liver

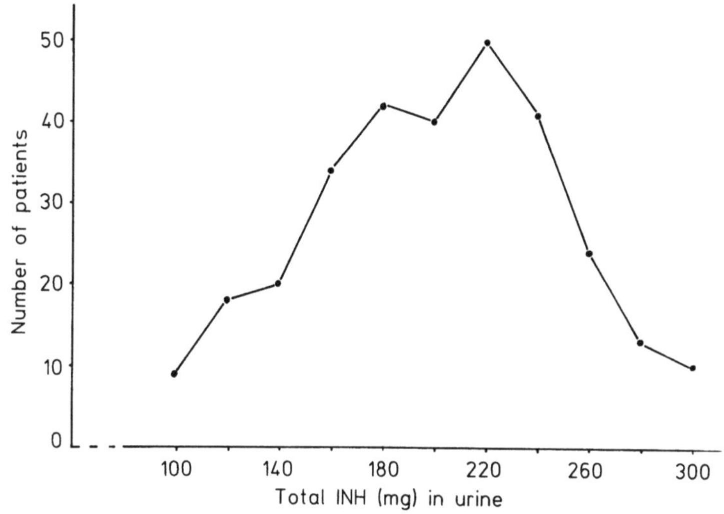

Fig. 10. Distribution of the total-INH values in 203 patients (dose 300 mg)

and the INH-biotransformation status previously determined in the same individual (JENNE and BOYER 1962; EVANS and WHITE 1964; JENNE 1965; JENNE et al. 1969). To clarify the situation further, the hepatic N-acetyl-transferase was isolated from previously typed liver samples and purified. The enzyme preparations thus obtained failed, however, to show any difference in the biotransformation of INH (JENNE 1965). The substrate affinities on the donor and acceptor side are likewise largely the same, and thus the differences in the biotransformation of INH were attributed to differences in the number of enzyme molecules formed (JENNE et al. 1969). It may be that extrahepatic N-acetyl-transferases also play a part, such enzymes having been detected in the intestinal mucosa in man (JENNE 1965; NAKAGAWA and SUNAHARA 1967). In rabbits with rapid INH biotransformation the activity of the extrahepatic enzymes is negligible, whereas in the case of a slow biotransformation these enzymes, which differ in respect to the optimal pH value and the stability of hepatic N-acetyl transferase, do play a part (HEARSE and WEBER 1970; KERGUERIS et al. 1983).

Acetylation corresponding with the INH biotransformation has been detected for hydralazine, dapsone, sulphafurazole, sulphapyridine, and sulphadimidine (JENNE et al. 1961; JENNE and BOYER 1962; FRYMOYER and JACOX 1963 a, b; MUKOYAMA et al. 1963; SUNAHARA et al. 1963 b; JENNE 1965; PETERS et al. 1965 a; TIITINEN 1969 c; RAO et al. 1970; SCHRÖDER 1972; VIZNEROVA et al. 1973; BEIGUELMAN et al. 1974). By contrast, p-aminobenzoic acid, PAS, and sulphanilamide are acetylated by a different enzyme that produces a single-peaked distribution curve of the relevant concentration values (JENNE and BOYER 1962; JENNE 1964; EVANS and WHITE 1964; GOEDDE and SCHOPF 1964; PETERS et al. 1965 a; JENNE et al. 1969; TIITINEN 1969 c). Accordingly, polymorphism corresponding to the INH biotransformation can only be detected in compounds with a free hydrazine group on the ring system or in sulphanilic acid derivatives with a second ring system (Fig. 11).

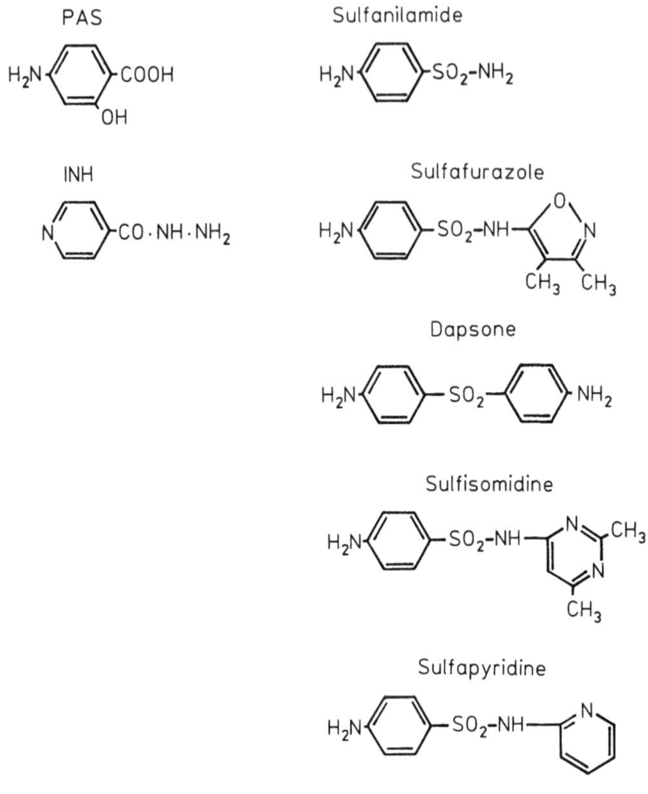

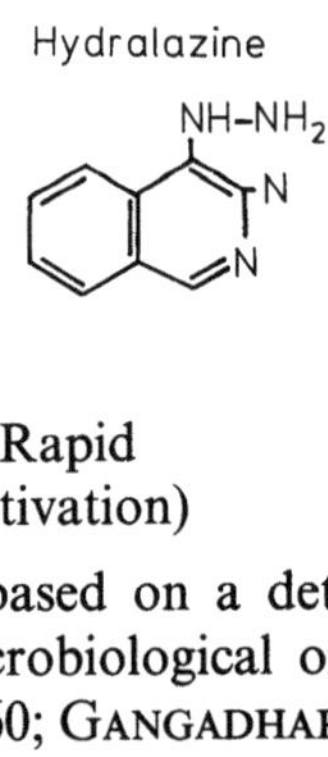

Fig. 11. Influence of the structure of drugs on their biotransformation pattern

e) Possible Ways of Differentiating Between Rapid and Slow INH Biotransformation (INH Inactivation)

The first attempts at differentiation were based on a determination of "unchanged" INH (INH + hydrazones) by microbiological or chemical methods (EVANS et al. 1960; GROSSET and CANETTI 1960; GANGADHARAM et al. 1961). The vertical diffusion test (SCHMIEDEL 1960; IWAINSKY et al. 1961; SUNAHARA et al. 1963a), the determination of the $t_{50\%}$ using two or three measurements (JENNE 1960; SCOTT et al. 1969; TIITINEN 1969a) and the fluorimetric method (PETERS 1960a; KAGAMIJAMA and MAJIMA 1961) proved of particular importance for this purpose. 6 h to 10 h after the administration of INH the biotransformation difference become particularly clear (SCHMIEDEL 1961; IWAINSKY et al. 1965).

A satisfactory correlation exists between the INH concentration in the serum and the fraction excreted with the urine (PFAFFENBERG et al. 1960; IWAINSKY et al. 1961; SHORT 1962b; ROZNIECKI 1968). Therefore, after this discovery had been made, patients were increasingly assigned to one of two or three INH-inactivation types on the basis of the assay of "unchanged" INH in the urine (JEANES et al. 1972; SMIRNOV 1972; SHENDEROVA and TERTERYAN 1973). However, the outcome of the test obviously depends on the urine being collected quantitatively. To eliminate the uncertainty involved when the patient's cooperation is relied on, recourse was made to the possibility, proposed by SHORT in 1962, of improving the determination of the acetyl-INH/INH ratio (ROZNIECKI 1968; MASON and RUSSELL 1971; RUSSELL 1972; VENKATARAMAN et al. 1972), especially since in the meantime a relatively simple and specific method for acetyl-INH had been developed (EIDUS and HAMILTON 1964; COURTY et al. 1981). With the aid of this method a urine sample collected within a prespecified period is sufficient.

Because of the problems of storage and transportation of such samples for analysis (at normal ambient temperature the concentration of acetyl-INH tends to fall off, especially in the blood), in recent times dapsone, sulphadimidine, or other drugs metabolized by the same N-acetyl-transferase as INH have been used as test substances and the concentration of the monoacetylated compound or the $t_{50\%}$ has been measured (FRYMOYER and JACOX 1963a, b; EVANS 1969; RAO et al. 1970; EZE and EVANS 1972; SCHRÖDER 1972; SEN et al. 1972; VIZNEROVA et al. 1973; ELLARD and GAMMON 1978; HANSON et al. 1981; KERGUERIS et al. 1983; GUPTA et al. 1984). The usefulness of the individual procedures and the possibilities of automating them are currently under investigation (EIDUS et al. 1973; HODGKIN et al. 1973, 1974; JESSAMINE et al. 1974; VARUGHESE et al. 1974).

f) Biotransformation of INH after the Administration of INH Derivatives and INH Retard Preparations

In the 1950's many INH derivatives, predominantly hydrazones, were tested in experimental and clinical studies in the hope that their use would result in improved tolerance and in a potentiation of activity as a result of suppression of the biotransformation.

It is assumed for all the tested compounds that after oral administration hydrolysis precedes absorption, this having been demonstrated for a number of hydrazones. In consequence of the hydrolysis the absorption phase is prolonged, while the amount absorbed is reduced – on average to about 30%. Accordingly, the maximum serum concentration is substantially lower and appears at a later time. This means that when the derivative is administered a higher serum concentration is measured after 5 h than after the administration of INH itself (MATSUZAKI and SAITO 1961; SHORT 1962a; IWAINSKY et al. 1965; BARONTI and MANFREDI 1968). After intravenous infusion of gluconazide (hydrazone from INH and glucuronate) a classification into rapid and slow inactivators is no longer possible for methodological reasons (SAUERESSIG 1972). All in all, none of the products came up to expectations. The differences in the biotransformation of INH could thus be only partly balanced out. The dose increase necessary because of the reduced absorption resulted in an increase in costs unacceptable for the chemotherapy of tuberculosis.

Intermittent treatment, which is more and more used, has given new life to the discussions on the different modes of INH biotransformation. The side effects of INH appear more frequently after the dose of 10 mg/kg usually selected for this form of treatment than after daily administration of 5 mg/kg. A prolongation of

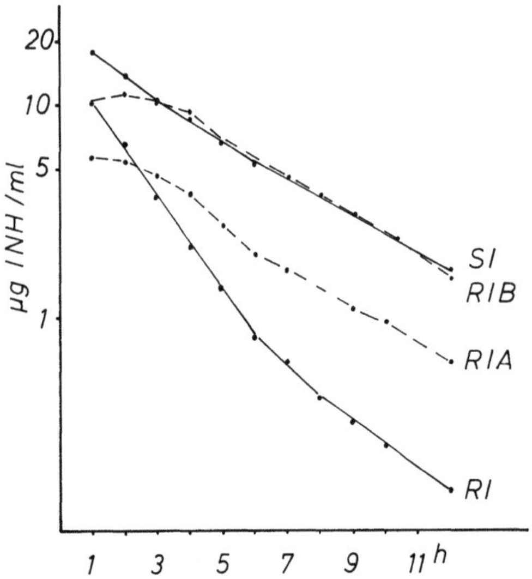

Fig. 12. Influence of pharmaceutical formulation on the INH concentration in serum (JEANES et al. 1973). *SI* Slow INH inactivation, 10 mg INH/kg; *RI* Rapid INH inactivation, 10 mg INH/kg; *RIA* Rapid INH inactivation, 20 mg matrix INH/kg; *RIB* Rapid INH inactivation, 30 mg matrix INH/kg

the $t_{50\%}$, attempted in the presence of rapid biotransformation of INH by means of sulphamethazine or acetyl-INH, was unsuccessful. Slowly absorbable INH formulations such as matrix INH, enteric INH, tebesium, or their mixtures have been studied in trials (ELLARD 1976; ELLARD et al. 1972, 1973; EIDUS and HODGKIN 1975; KLEEBERG et al. 1975; TRIPATHY 1976). After correspondingly elevated doses in rapid INH inactivators serum INH values corresponding to the concentration course after normal doses in slow inactivators are achieved (Fig. 12, JEANES et al. 1973; EIDUS et al. 1974a).

g) Influence of Other Antituberculosis Drugs, Biological Factors and Secondary Diseases on the Biotransformation of INH

The chemotherapy of tuberculosis takes the form of a combined treatment, at least in the initial phase. The influence of the products making up the combination on the biotransformation of INH was therefore studied early on. In pigeon liver homogenates the acetylation of INH is competitively inhibited by PAS (JENNE and BOYER 1962). According to the preliminary reports PAS also seemingly suppresses the biotransformation of INH in man, at least in part. Extensive studies, some taking account of the INH-inactivation types, have yielded contradictory results (BARTMANN and MASSMANN 1960b; PETERS 1960b; DES PREZ and BOONE 1961; SHENDEROVA and TERTERYAN 1973; TYTOR 1975). The different doses of PAS and unsatisfactory techniques used must be help responsible for these discrepancies, because only the non-biotransformed fraction of PAS can have a decisive effect on the biotransformation of INH. Evaluation of all the studies reveals an increase of the mean INH concentration in the serum as a result of simultaneous administration of PAS (KAGAMIJAMA and MAJIMA 1961; VIVIEN et

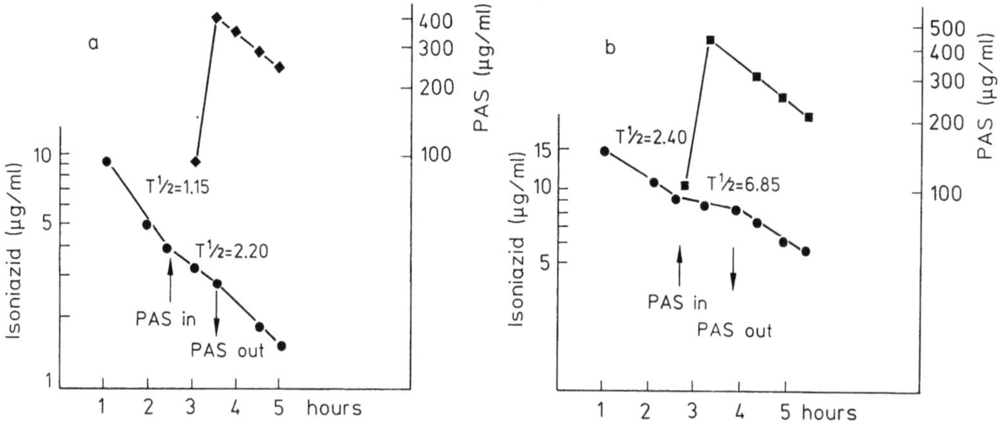

Fig. 13a, b. Influence of PAS (10 mg/kg i.v.) on the $t_{50\%}$ of INH for rapid (**a**) and slow (**b**) inactivation (BOMAN et al. 1970). ●——●: INH; ■——■: PAS

al. 1972), the effect being more strongly pronounced in rapid than in slow INH inactivators (BARTMANN and MASSMANN 1960a; ZDUŃCZYK-PAWELEK et al. 1965; KREUKNIET et al. 1967). Delayed absorption and acetylation were assumed to occur (TIITINEN and MATTILA 1968). In agreement with this an increase of the $t_{50\%}$ of INH can only be observed in the presence of high PAS concentrations in the serum (Fig. 13, BOMAN et al. 1970).

5-Bromosalicylhydroxamic acid, first studied by HORNUNG et al. 1957 (JOHNSON et al. 1961; ZDUŃCZYK-PAWELEK et al. 1965) exerts a far stronger influence on the biotransformation of INH. On the other hand, SM, ETH, CS, DATC, and RMP have no effect (SOKOLOWA et al. 1981). ETH/PTH increase the INH concentration, high doses of PZA suppress the formation of acetyl-INH, especially in slow INH inactivators (TIITINEN 1969c; BOMAN et al. 1970; VENHO and KOSKINEN 1971; FRANZ et al. 1974; DUDCHIK and BILYK 1975). Only in one case has a change in the acetylation rate of INH during treatment with INH, EMB, and RMP been reported, in which no liver damage was discernible (ALBENGRES et al. 1977).

The biotransformation of INH is not affected to any essential degree by the consumption of food, by sex, or by age, provided that the patient is over 15 years of age (BARTMANN and MASSMANN 1960b; IWAINSKY and SIEGEL 1961; TIITINEN 1969c; VIVIEN et al. 1972; FARAH et al. 1977; IWAINSKY and WINSEL 1977; GOBERT et al. 1980; PIKORA et al. 1980; GUPTA et al. 1984; PILHEU et al. 1985). In children the ratio of rapid to slow inactivators is 45 to 55%, the same as in adults. The $t_{50\%}$ values correspond as well. Because of a more strongly pronounced first pass effect and a higher liver/body weight ratio, INH is biotransformed more rapidly in children. Higher doses should be given, with a higher degree of adaptation to the inactivator status, than is necessary in adults (BARTMANN and MASSMANN 1961; ADVENIER et al. 1981). Secondary diseases have only small effects. Infectious hepatitis does not give rise to a shift in the normal distribution of the inactivator types (FUXA 1967), nor does manifest diabetes in adults (PFAFFENBERG et al. 1960; IWAINSKY et al. 1965). Among the juvenile diabetics the incidence of rapid inactivators is higher than among normal patients (MATTILA and TIITINEN 1967). In patients in diabetic coma acetyl-INH cannot be detected as a biotransformation product of INH. Acute and chronic liver diseases, especially those caused by alcohol abuse, can cause the $t_{50\%}$ to increase (LEVY et al. 1960; KLINGER 1981). Simultaneous consumption of alcohol results in a shortening of the $t_{50\%}$ of e.g. sulphadimidine in both inactivator types.

h) Influence of Race-Dependent Factors on the Biotransformation of INH

In accordance with the postulated types of inactivation (see Section 2.d), 3 types – rapid inactivators (RI), the middle group, and slow inactivators (SI) – can be distinguished in the countries of the Far East (KOIZUMI and OKAMOTO 1962; SUNAHARA et al. 1963a, b; DUFOUR et al. 1964). In Europe, North America, Africa, and India only 2 types (SI and RI) can be distinguished, owing to the composition of the population, which is more unfavourable for division into the individual types. The boundaries of the middle group cannot be clearly delimited. It seems that rapid inactivators and the middle group are together determined by the old, established test methods and the newly developed ones (SCOTT et al. 1969; ELLARD et al. 1981).

Among the Japanese, Eskimos, Laplanders, and Indians the proportion of rapid inactivators is relatively high, in extreme cases as high as 90% (see Table 2; ARMSTRONG and PEART 1960; TIITINEN et al. 1968; JEANES et al. 1972; EIDUS et al. 1974b). Among the white population of Europe and North America there is some 40% of rapid inactivators (BARTMANN and MASSMANN 1960a; LEVY et al. 1960; PFAFFENBERG et al. 1960; BERNARD et al. 1961; IWAINSKY et al. 1961; VIVIEN and GROSSET 1961; SHORT 1962b; MYDLAK and VOLKMANN 1965; VOLKMANN and MYDLAK 1965; MATTILA and TIITINEN 1967; TIITINEN 1969c; VIVIEN et al. 1972; FARHAT et al. 1973; VIVIEN et al. 1973; SZCZAWINSKA et al. 1976; HOUIN and TILLEMENT 1980). 60% of the native population of Africa constitutes rapid inactivators (GLATTHAAR et al. 1977; SALAKO and FADEKE ADEROUNMU 1977; BOUAYAD et al. 1982). On the other hand, among the black Africans of North America the incidence of allelomorphs is more or less evenly distributed. Among the black Africans living in Europe the proportion of slow inactivators is higher (DUFOUR et al. 1964; BERGOGNE-BEREZIN and MODAI 1975; BERGOGNE-BEREZIN et al. 1976). Egyptians too seem to have a relatively high proportion of slow inactivators (HASHEM et al. 1969) and among the Ethiopians, according to preliminary studies, the proportion is 50%.

i) Biotransformation of INH in Animals

It seems doubtful that the differences in INH inactivation encountered in different animal species should be due only to the different activities of the hepatic N-acetyl-transferase. For example, the activity of this enzyme extracted from the monkey spleen and kidney (Macaca irus) exhibits a two-peak distribution, while that from the liver has only one activity peak. There is no negative correlation between the rate of acetylation and the INH concentration in the serum (SUNAHARA et al. 1968). In rabbits the plasma INH concentration has a single-peak distribution, although INH and sulphadiazine are evidently metabolized by the same enzyme to different extents, corresponding to the situation in man (FRYMOYER and

Table 2. INH-inactivator status in various population groups

Country of origin	No. of patients	Proportion of:			Differentiation method	Authors
		Rapid inactivators (RI)	The middle group	Slow inactivators (SI)		
GDR	344	41%	–	59%	INH excretion with the urine	IWAINSKY et al. (1961)
	554	44%	–	56%	Serum concentration after 10 h	
	392	41%	–	59%	Visual test (INH in the urine)	
GDR	375	35%	–	65%	Serum concentration after 10 h (1963)	PFAFFENBERG et al. (1963)
	850 diabetics	38%	–	62%		
GDR	646	46%	–	54%	Serum concentration	MYDLAK and VOLKMANN (1965)
GDR	271	36%	–	64%	INH excretion in the urine	TEICHMANN and KÖHLER (1964)
GDR	50 with infectious hepatitis	46%	–	54%	Serum concentration after 1+6 h	FUXA (1967)
Japan	200	38%	42%	20%	Serum concentration after 6 h	NAKAGAWA and SUNAHARA (1967)
U.A.R.	50	18%	–	82%	Serum concentration after 6 h	HASHEM et al. (1969)
Finland	341	42%	–	58%	$t_{50\%}$	TIITINEN (1969a)
Finland	116	41%	–	58%	$t_{50\%}$	TIITINEN (1969b)
Sweden	130	32%	–	68%	$t_{50\%}$	BOMAN et al. (1970)
Canada	120	46%	10%	49%	Acetyl-INH/INH in the urine	MASON and RUSSEL (1971)
Canada						
Eskimos	26	100%	–	–	$t_{50\%}$	JEANES et al. (1972)
Indians	46	63%	–	37%	Acetyl-INH/INH in the urine	
U.S.A.	181	32%	–	68%	Sulphadimidine test in the urine	SMITH et al. (1972)
India	124	46%	–	54%	INH after 4.5 h	VENKATARAMAN et al. (1972)
		39%	–	61%	acetyl-INH/INH in the urine	
France	123	44%	–	56%	INH-inactivation index	VIVIEN et al. (1972)
	648	39%	–	61%		
C.S.S.R.	421					
Bohemia and Prague		39%	–	61%	Sulphadimidine test in the urine	VIZNEROVA et al. (1973)
Slovakia		45%	–	55%		

Table 3. Half-lives of antituberculosis drugs in various animal species

Antituber-culosis drug	Animal Species	$t_{50\%}$ (min)	Authors
INH	Mouse	40–50	BARTMANN and MASSMANN (1961)
	Rat	24–36	PETERS (1960a)
	Guinea pig	74	DICKINSON et al. (1968)
	Rabbit	55	GREENBERG and EIDUS (1962)
	Dog	150–240	PETERS (1960a)
	Monkey	54–72	PETERS (1960a)
CS	Mouse	25	
	Guinea-pig	60	IWAINSKY et al. (1967)
	Rabbit	150	
	Rhesus Monkey	7.75 h	
ETH	Rabbit	35	GREENBERG and EIDUS (1962)
EMB	Mouse	< 3.2 h	
	Monkey	~ 3.2 h	PLACE and THOMAS (1963)
RMP	Rabbit	4–4.2 h	NITTI (1972)
	Dog	8 h	FINKEL et al. (1971)
KM	Horse	87	
	Sheep	112	BAGGOT (1978)
	Dog	58	

JACOX 1963a, b; KERGUERIS et al. 1983). In-vitro tests reveal considerable differences in the acetylation capacity, while in in-vivo tests these are only slight. Accordingly, in the rabbit the acetylation capacity of the intestinal mucosa has a considerable effect on the biotransformation rate (HEARSE and WEBER 1970). This is also indicated by the essentially greater biotransformation of INH after oral administration compared to intramuscular administration (NAKAGAWA and SUNAHARA 1967).

Differences in INH biotransformation have been detected in the monkey, including the non-anthropoid primates (GOEDDE and SCHOPF 1964; GOEDDE et al. 1965, 1966; SCHLOOT et al. 1967; VIVIEN et al. 1972). Corresponding polymorphism has also been observed in rabbits and in rats. In both species tests on INH and sulphadiazine yield the same results (FRYMOYER and JACOX 1963a, b; JENNE 1964, 1965). The relatively weak activity of INH in rats is explained by the predominance of a type with rapid biotransformation of INH (GRUMBACH et al. 1960). Accordingly, the $t_{50\%}$ of INH is used as a reference parameter for selecting the animal species for experimental chemotherapy of tuberculosis (Table 3).

j) Influence of the Biotransformation of INH on the Effect and Side Effects of Chemotherapy

The influence of rapid inactivation of INH on the therapeutic outcome in the case of a daily treatment with 3 antituberculosis drugs was investigated early on. Initially it was reported that rapid inactivators are encountered more often among the chronic cases or among patients undergoing a considerable number of curative procedures, so that this inactivator type was regarded as a risk group for the long-term prognosis (TEICHMANN and KÖHLER 1964; MYDLAK and VOLKMANN 1965; VOLKMANN and MYDLAK 1965). A cure rate of practically 100% was achieved by improved therapeutic management, especially by strict monitoring of the drug intake and, in addition, a poorer recovery rate was not confirmed for the rapid inactivators (BANG et al. 1962; ZDUNCZYK-PAWELEK et al. 1962; GOW and EVANS 1964; TIITINEN 1969b, c; PARROT et al. 1983; ELLARD 1984; ZIERSKI and ROTERMUND 1984). With the nowadays customary intermittent therapy too no indications of failure of INH in consequence of its rapid biotransformation have been found. Only in therapeutic studies in which antituberculotics are used sparingly does the rapid inactivator come out worse than the SI with regard to the therapeutic results (BERNSTEIN 1981).

The connections between the biotransformation of INH and the occurrence of side effects are undisputed. Slow inactivators suffer from side effects more often than do fast inactivators (EVANS 1968; VIVIEN et al. 1972; SEHM and URBANCZIK 1974; MITCHELL et al. 1975; MUSCH et al. 1981; SOKOLOWA et al. 1984). Accordingly, INH is one of the factors responsible for stressing the organism and not acetyl-INH.

The relationships between liver toxicity and the biotransformation of INH have not been clarified in every detail. Slow inactivators are only at greater risk than rapid inactivators of contracting INH-induced hepatitis in the first 8 weeks of the treatment (BARTMANN 1977; GRÖNHAGEN-RISKA et al. 1978). There is evidently no distinct connection between the INH-inactivator type and an elevation of the concentration of aminotransferases or liver damage (SMITH et al. 1972; TYTOR 1976; ELLARD et al. 1981; BERNSTEIN 1981; ELLARD 1984; GURUMURTHY et al. 1984). Although the concentration of the hepatotoxic monoacetylhydrazine is higher in the rapid than in the slow inactivators, this compound is probably converted into diacetylhydrazine by the same enzyme that acetylates INH, and indeed to a greater extent in rapid inactivators than in slow inactivators, as a result of which the differences initially present in the monoacetylhydrazine concentration are largely equalized (TIMBRELL et al. 1977; BERNSTEIN 1981; von SASSEN et al. 1982). Newer investigations (administration of INH and ^{14}C-acetyl-INH, measuring the exhalation of $^{14}CO_2$) have shown that very slow acetylators are exposed to more acetylhydrazine than other acetylators (LAUTERBURG et al. 1985).

Furthermore, the different rates of INH inactivation are seemingly important for the pharmacokinetics of other drugs, and thus in some cases for their toxicity as well (MEYER and MEIER 1982). For example, the changes in the $t_{50\%}$ of antipyrine on simultaneous administration of INH are dependent on the INH-inactivator type (CHAILLEUX et al. 1980; MUSCH et al. 1981; GRECH BELANGER et al. 1983). On simultaneous treatment with procainamide the fraction of N-acetylprocainamide falls off drastically, with corresponding prolongation of the $t_{50\%}$ of the unchanged procainamide, as a result of competitive displacement. The causes of the interactions occurring on combination of INH, warfarin, bishydroxycoumarin, and phenytoin are still to be established. Whatever the case may be, it is necessary to adjust the dose of these drugs (ROSENTAL et al. 1977; SPROUSE et al. 1978; MILLER et al. 1979).

3. Pharmacokinetics

a) Distribution of INH in the Macroorganism

INH is absorbed very rapidly, the maximum concentration in the serum being reached 30 min to one hour after oral administration. Only a small fraction is bound to the serum proteins (see Table 3, p. 419). The substance is distributed throughout the body water. One hour after the administration of INH in therapeutic doses, the substance can be detected in all organs, in the subcutaneous tissue, and in the muscle. After 6 h, it remains only in the liver, lungs, stomach, brain, kidneys, and the bladder, and after 24 h only in the liver. It diffuses very rapidly into all the tissue and body fluids, a diffusion equilibrium between the serum and tissue setting in only 15 to 50 min after administration (Jenne et al. 1961; Greenberg and Eidus 1962; Frymoyer and Jacox 1963a). The concentration in the lungs corresponds to that in the serum, although, similarly to the case with SM – it is considerably lower in the focus wall and in caseous tissue (Fig. 14; Schmiedel et al. 1960; Bartmann and Freise 1963; Eule and Werner 1965). On local administration into cleaned out cavities, a distribution of the INH in the organism is detectable (Fig. 15; Kandt and Flach 1965). The transcapillary diffusion of INH takes place more rapidly than that of glucose in the lungs and depends on the temperature.

Between the mother and the foetus the serum concentration falls by 50% or more (Toyohara 1974), a fall in concentration similarly being observed between the serum and the CSF (Table 7, p. 423, Lamedica et al. 1983).

b) Excretion of INH by the Macroorganism

INH undergoes glomerular filtration and tubular reabsorption. Its excretion is unaffected by the age of the patient. The excretion of INH and of its biotransformation products (85%–98% of the total INH – Peters et al. 1965b; 10% as biologically active INH in rapid inactivators and 25%–30% in slow inactivators

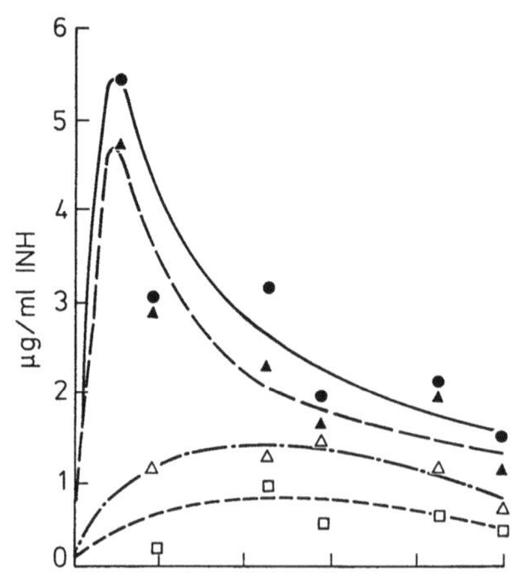

Fig. 14. INH concentration in serum and in the lung tissue of patients suffering from tuberculosis (Bartmann and Freise 1963, 5 mg INH/kg i.m.). ——— INH concentration in serum; —— INH concentration in normal lung tissue; —·— INH concentration in focus wall; ----- INH concentration in caseous mass

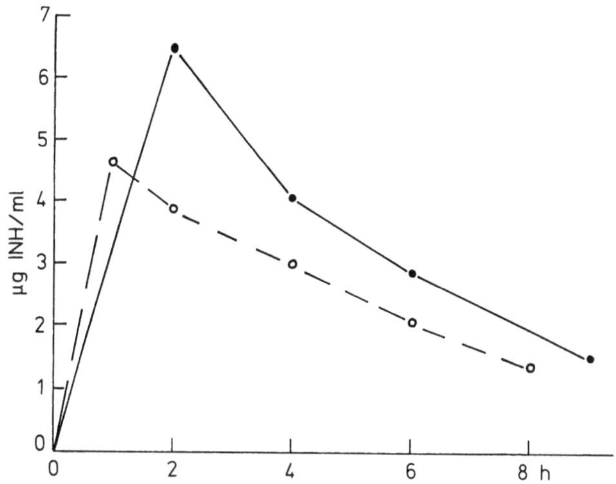

Fig. 15. INH concentration in serum after intracavitary and oral administration (KANDT and FLACH 1965, slow INH inactivation). o----o Local administration of 500 mg INH; •——• Oral administration of 420 mg INH

– IWAINSKY et al. 1965) reflects very precisely the extent of the biotransformation which determines the course of the INH concentration in the serum. The INH-polymorphism, the influence of PAS on acetylation of INH, the pharmacokinetics of slowly absorbable INH products, and other factors can therefore also be established by determining the excretion of antituberculotically active INH or the ratio of INH/total INH or acetyl-INH/INH in the urine. Renal function disorders do not impair the excretion of INH so that, as is the case with chlortetracycline, ETH/PTH, and RMP, an adjustment of the dose to the kidney function is unnecessary in the chemotherapy of tuberculosis with INH (JUNGBLUTH 1971, 1973; REIDENBERG et al. 1973; HÖFFLER 1976, 1981; TITARENKO et al. 1982, see Table 10, p. 426). Further data on pharmacokinetic parameters are given in Table 6 (distribution volume, p. 421), Table 8 (excretion, p. 424), Table 9 (clearance, p. 425), and Table 11 ($t_{50\%}$, p. 433). The course of the serum INH concentration after various doses is reproduced in Figs. 12, 14, and 15.

In the older studies, the proportion of rapid inactivators is usually given as considerably lower. In the first studies, the boundary between rapid and slow inactivators did not correspond to the biological limit, resulting in a depression in the distribution curve. According to Schmiedel (2nd study on differences in INH inactivation), some of the rapid inactivators were consequently assigned to a different group.

References

Ackermann E (1973) Der Arzneimittelmetabolismus beim Menschen und seine Bedeutung für die Pharmakotherapie und ihre Nebenwirkungen. Dtsch Ges Wesen 28:721–725

Advenier C, Saint-Aubin A, Scheinmann P, Paupe J (1981) Pharmacocinétique de l'isoniazide chez l'enfant. Rev Fr Mal Resp 9:365–374

Albengres E, Houin G, Breau J-L, Hirsch A (1977) Modification, en cours de traitement, de la vitesse d' acétylation de l'isoniazide sans atteinte hépatique decelable. Nouv Presse Méd 6:2869–2871

Armstrong AR, Peart HE (1960) A comparison between the behavior of Eskimos and non-Eskimos to the administration of isoniazid. Am Rev Respir Dis 81:588–594
Baggot JD (1978) Comparative pharmacokinetics of kanamycin. Abstracts of the 7th Int. Congress of Pharmacology, Pergamon Press, Paris, p. 787 Nr 2451
Bang HO, Kramer Jacobsen L, Strandgaard E, Yde H (1962) Metabolism of isoniazid and para-amino-salicylic acid (PAS) in the organism and its therapeutic significance. Acta Tuberc Scand 41:237–251
Baronti A, Manfredi N (1968) Blood levels of isoniazid and of its methane sulphonate derivative in rapid and slow inactivators after oral administration. Tubercle 49:104–109
Bartmann K (1977) Die Ermittlung von Nebenwirkungen bei chronischer Arzneitherapie am Beispiel der hepatotoxischen Wirkung von Isoniazid und Rifampicin. Verh Dtsch Ges Inn Med 83:1518–1529
Bartmann K, Massmann W (1960a) Über die mikrobiologische INH-Bestimmung nach Schmiedel. Beitr Klin Tuberk 122:192–197
Bartmann K, Massmann W (1960b) Der Blutspiegel des INH bei Erwachsenen und Kindern. Beitr Klin Tuberk 122:239–250
Bartmann K, Massmann W (1961) Experimentelle Untersuchungen zur Dosierung von INH. Beitr Klin Tuberk 124:310–319
Bartmann K, Freise G (1963) Mikrobiologisch bestimmte Isoniazid-Konzentrationen im Gewebe von Tier und Mensch. Beitr Klin Tuberk 127:546–560
Beggs WH, Jenne JW (1969) Isoniazid uptake and growth inhibition of *Mycobacterium tuberculosis* in relation to time and concentration of pulsed drug exposures. Tubercle 50:377–385
Beggs WH, Jenne JW (1970) Capacity of tubercle bacilli for isoniazid accumulation. Am Rev Respir Dis 102:94–96
Beggs WH, Jenne JW, Hall WH (1968) Isoniazid uptake in relation to growth inhibition of *Mycobacterium tuberculosis*. J Bacteriol 36:293–297
Beiguelman D, Pinto W Jr, El-Gusindy MM, Krieger H (1974) Factors influencing the level of dapsone in blood. Bull WHO 51:467–471
Bekierkunst A, Bricker A (1967) Studies on the mode of action of isoniazid on mycobacteria. Arch Biochem Biophys 122:385–392
Bergogne-Berezin E, Modai J (1975) Comparison of isoniazid inactivation in African Negroes and in Europeans. Rev Fr Mal Resp 3:397–412
Bergogne-Berezin E, Nouhouayi A, Modai J, Vivien JN (1976) Pharmacokinetic study of isoniazid in black African subjects. Rev Fr Mal Resp 4:399–408
Bernard E, Israël L, Pariente D, Sausy J (1961) Taux d' INH libre résiduel et résultats thérapeutiques chez 104 tuberculeux pulmonaires „neufs". Rev Tub Pneumol 25:319–338
Bernstein RE (1981) The hepatotoxicity of isoniazid among the three acetylator phenotypes. Am Rev Respir Dis 123:568–570
Bönicke R, Lisboa BP (1957) Über die Erbbedingtheit der intraindividuellen Konstanz der Isoniazidausscheidung beim Menschen (Untersuchungen an eineiigen und zweieiigen Zwillingen). Naturwissenschaften 44:314
Boman G, Borga O, Hanngren A, Malmborg A-ST, Sjöqvist E (1970) Pharmakokinetische und genetische Gesichtspunkte über den Metabolismus von Isoniazid, p-Aminosalicylsäure und Rifampicin. Pneumonologie, Suppl:15–20
Bouayad Z, Chevalier B, Maurin R, Bartal M (1982) Phénotype d'acétylation de l'isoniazide au Maroc. Rev Fr Mal Resp 10:401–407
Brennan PJ, Rooney SA, Winder FG (1970) The lipids of *Mycobacterium tuberculosis* BCG: Fractionation, composition, turnover and the effects of isoniazid. Ir J Med Sci 3:371–390
Chailleux E, Moigneteau Ch, Ordronneau J, Le Normand Y, Kergueris MF, Veyrac MJ, Larousse C (1980) Étude simultanée de l'effet inducteur de la rifampicine et du phénotype d'acétylation de l'isoniazide, chez 21 tuberculeux soumis a un traitement mixte. Rev Fr Mal Resp 8:169–171
Courty G, Tessier R, Neuzil E (1981) Le test d'Eidus dans la mesure du facteur d'acétylation de l'isoniazide, applications thérapeutiques. Bordeaux Méd 14:903–911

Cuthbertson WFJ, Ireland DM, Wolff W (1953) Detection and identification of some metabolites of isonicotinic acid hydrazide (isoniazid) in human urine. Biochem 55:669–671

Des Prez R, Boone IU (1961) Metabolism of C^{14}-isoniazid in humans. Am Rev Resp Dis 84:42–51

Dickinson JM, Ellard GA, Mitchison DA (1968) Suitability of isoniazid and ethambutol for intermittent administration in the treatment of tuberculosis. Tubercle 49:351–366

Dudchik GKh, Bilyk MA (1975) Mechanism of the excretion of the hina metabolites by the kidneys in patients with pulmonary tuberculosis. Probl Tuberk 53 issue 5: 57–61

Dufour AP, Knight RA, Harris HW (1964) Genetics of isoniazid metabolism in Caucasian, Negro and Japanese populations. Science 145:391

Eda T (1963a) Studies on the action of isoniazid to tubercle bacilli and the mechanism of the isoniazid-resistance in mycobacteria. I Kekkaku 38:37–41

Eda T (1963b) Studies on the action of isoniazid to tubercle bacilli and the mechanism of the isoniazid-resistance in mycobacteria. II Kekkaku 38:107–110

Eda T (1963c) Studies on the action of isoniazid to tubercle bacilli and the mechanism of the isoniazid-resistance in mycobacteria. III Kekkaku 38:395–398

Eidus L, Hamilton EJ (1964) A new method for the determination of N-acetyl-isoniazid in urine of ambulatory patients. Am Rev Respir Dis 89:587–588

Eidus L, Hodgkin MM (1975) A new isoniazid preparation designed for moderately fast and "fast" metabolizers of the drug. Arzneimittelforsch 25:1077–1080

Eidus L, Varughese P, Hodgkin MM, Hsu AHE, McRae KB (1973) Simplification of isoniazid phenotyping procedure to promote its application in the chemotherapy of tuberculosis. Bull WHO 49:507–516

Eidus L, Hodgkin MM, Hsu AHE, Schaefer O (1974a) Pharmacokinetic studies with an isoniazid slow-releasing matrix preparation. Am Rev Respir Dis 110:34–42

Eidus L, Hodgkin MM, Schaefer O, Jessamine AG (1974b) Distribution of isoniazid inactivators determined in Eskimos and Canadian college students. Rev Can Biol 33:117–123

Ellard GA (1976) A slow-release preparation of isoniazid: pharmacological aspects. Bull Int Union Tuberc 51:143–154

Ellard GA (1984) The potential clinical significance of the isoniazid acetylator phenotype in the treatment of pulmonary tuberculosis. Tubercle 65:211–217; Rev Mal Resp 1:207–219

Ellard GA, Gammon PT (1978) Acetylator phenotyping is important in TB patients. Curr Ther 19:130

Ellard GA, Gammon PT, Lakshminarayan S, Fox W, Aber VR, Mitchison DA, Citron KM, Tall R (1972) Pharmacology of some slow-release preparations of isoniazid of potential use in intermittent treatment of tuberculosis. Lancet I:340–343

Ellard GA, Gammon PT, Polansky F, Viznerova A, Havlik I, Fox W (1973) Further studies on the pharmacology of a slow-release matrix preparation of isoniazid (Smith and Nephew HS82) of potential use in the intermittent treatment of tuberculosis. Tubercle 54:57–66

Ellard GA, Girling DJ, Nunn AJ (1981) The hepatotoxicity of isoniazid among the three acetylator phenotypes. Am Rev Respir Dis 123:568

Eule H, Werner E (1965) Simultane INH- und Äthioniamid-Konzentrationsbestimmung in der Lunge. Z Tuberk 123:335–338

Evans DAP (1968) Genetic variations in the acetylation of isoniazid and other drugs. Ann NY Acad Sci 151:723–733

Evans DAP (1969) An improved and simplified method of detecting the acetylator phenotype. J Med Genet 6:405–407

Evans DAP, White TA (1964) Human acetylation polymorphism. J Lab Clin Med 63:394–403

Evans DAP, Storey PB, Wittstadt FB, Manley KA (1960) The determination of the isoniazid inactivator phenotype. Am Rev Respir Dis 82:853–861

Eze LC, Evans DAP (1972) The use of the auto-analyzer to determine the acetylator phenotype. J Med Genetics 9:57

Farah F, Taylor W, Rawlins MD, James O (1977) Hepatic drug acetylation and oxidation: effects of aging in man. Br Med J 2:155–156
Farhat S, Jordanoglou J, Pallikaris G, Lyberatos K, Hadjiidannou J, Gardikas C (1973) Slow and rapid inactivators of isoniazid among Greek patients. Am Rev Respir Dis 108:1242–1243
Finkel JM, Pittillo RF, Mellett LB (1971) Fluorometric and microbiological assays for rifampicin and the determination of serum levels in the dog. Chemotherapy 16:380–388
Fishbain D, Ling G, Kushner DJ (1972) Isoniazid metabolism and binding by sensitive and resistant strains of Mycobacterium smegmatis. Can J Microbiol 18:783–792
Franz H, Urbanczik R, Stoll K, Müller U (1974) Prothionamid-Blutspiegel nach oraler Verabreichung von Prothionamid allein oder kombiniert mit Isoniazid und/oder mit Diamino-Difenylsulfon. Prax Pneumol 28:605–612
Fráter-Schröder M, Zbinden G (1976) A gaschromatographic assay for the determination of isoniazid N-acetylation; observation in rats with induced constant urine flow. EXPEAM 32:767
Frymoyer JW, Jacox RF (1963a) Investigation of the genetic control of sulfadiazine and isoniazid metabolism in the rabbit. J Lab Clin Med 62:891–904
Frymoyer JW, Jacox RF (1963b) Studies of genetically controlled sulfadiazine acetylation in rabbit livers: possible identification of the heterozygous trait. J Lab Clin Med 62:905–909
Fuxa E (1967) Das Verhalten der Elimination von Isonikotinsäurehydrazid bei Patienten mit Hepatitis infectiosa. Dissertation, Med Akademie Erfurt
Gangadharam PRJ, Bathia AL, Radhakrishna S, Selkon JB (1961) Rate of inactivation of isoniazid in South Indian patients with pulmonary tuberculosis. 1.: Microbiological assay of isoniazid in serum following a standard intramuscular dose. Bull WHO 25:765–777
Glatthaar E, Gärtig D, Stander MF, Kleeberg HH (1977) Isoniazid levels in black patients dosed with a matrix preparation (Tebesium). Prax Pneumol 31:885–889
Gobert C, Saint-Aubin A, Houin G (1980) Metabolisme de l'isoniazide chez le vieillard. Consequences pratiques. Rev Geriat 5/5:211–216
Goedde HW (1974) Pharmakogenetik: Variabilität von Arzneimittelwirkung und Stoffwechselreaktionen. Internist (Berlin) 15:27–39
Goedde HW, Schopf E (1964) Pharmakogenetik (klinische Probleme und biochemisch-genetische Grundlagen). Med Klin 59:1849–1860
Goedde HW, Löhr GW, Waller HD (1965) Ergebnisse und Probleme der Pharmakogenetik. Arzneimittelforsch 15:1460–1468
Goedde HW, Schloot W, Valesky A (1966) Enzymatische Umsetzung von Isonicotinsäurehydrazid – ein pharmakogenetisches Problem. Arzneimittelforsch 16:1030–1034
Gow JG, Evans DAP (1964) A study of the influence of the isoniazid inactivation phenotype on reversion in genito-urinary tuberculosis. Tubercle 45:136–143
Grech Belanger O, Belanger PM, Lachance J (1983) Inhibitory effect of isoniazid on antipyrine clearance in man. J Clin Pharmacol 23:540–544
Greenberg L, Eidus L (1962) Antituberculous drugs (Th 1314 and INH) in the host organism. Br J Dis Chest 56:124–130
Grönhagen-Riska C, Hellstrom P-E, Fröseth B (1978) Predisposing factors in hepatitis induced by isoniazid-rifampin treatment of tuberculosis. Am Rev Respir Dis 118:461–466
Gross D, Feige A, Zureck A, Schütte H-R (1967) 3-Hydroxymethylpyridin, ein neues Stoffwechselprodukt der Mykobakterien. Z Naturforschung 22b:835–838
Gross D, Feige A, Zureck A, Schütte H-R (1968) Die Biosynthese von 3-Hydroxymethylpyridin bei Mycobacterium bovis Stamm BCG. Eur J Biochem 4:28–30
Grosset J, Canetti G (1960) Donnés complémentaires sur le dosage de l'isoniazide actif du sérum sanguin par la méthode de diffusion verticale. Dosage en présence de PAS. Rev Tub Pneumol 24:633–647
Grumbach F, Grosset J, Canetti G (1960) L'inactivation de l'isoniazide chez le rat. Son incidence sur les résultats de la chimiothérapie de la tuberculose dans cette espèce. Ann Inst Pasteur 98:642–656

Gupta RC, Nair CR, Jindal SK, Malik SK (1984) Incidence of isoniazid acetylation phenotypes in North Indians. Int J Clin Pharmacol Ther Toxicol 22:259–264
Gurumurthy P, Krishnamurthy MS, Nazareth O, Parthasarathy R, Sarma GR, Somasundaram PR, Tripathy SP, Ellard GA (1984) Lack of relationship between hepatic toxicity and acetylator phenotype in three thousand South Indian patients during treatment with isoniazid for tuberculosis. Am Rev Respir Dis 129:58–61
Hanson A, Melander A, Wåhlin-Boll E (1981) Acetylator phenotyping: a comparison of the isoniazid and dapsone tests. Eur J Clin Pharmacol 20:233–234
Hashem N, Khalifa S, Nour A (1969) The frequency of isoniazid acetylase enzyme deficiency among Egyptians. Am J Phys Anthrop 31:97–102
Hearse DJ, Weber WW (1970) Evidence for genetic and enzymatic heterogeneity in the „slow" isoniazid acetylator. Fed Proc 29:803 Abs
Heller A, Kasik JE, Clark L, Roth LJ (1961) Ion exchange method for determination of 1-isonicotinyl-2-acetylhydrazide (acetylated isoniazid) in biological fluids. Analytic Chem 33:1755–1757
Hodgkin MM, Hsu AHE, Varughese P, Eidus L (1973) Evaluation of a new method for phenotyping of slow and rapid acetylators. Int J Clin Pharmacol 7:355–362
Hodgkin MM, Eidus L, Hamilton EJ (1974) Screening of isoniazid inactivators by dilution test. Bull W.HO 51:428–430
Höffler D (1976) Antibiotikatherapie bei Niereninsuffizienz. Dtsch Med Wochenschr 101:829–834
Höffler D (1981) Die Dosierung wichtiger Antibiotika und Tuberkulostatika bei Niereninsuffizienz. Internist (Berlin) 22:601–606
Houin G, Tillement JP (1980) Conséquences thérapeutiques de la mesure de l'indice d'inactivation de l'isoniazide au cours du traitement antituberculeux. Thérapie 35:597–605
Hornung S, Malowicz F, Broda Z, Neciuk-Szczerbiński Z, Paryski E, Polończyk M, Rapf T (1957) Results of a team research on the effect of brom-salicyl-hydroxamic acid T_{40} on the drugresistance in tuberculosis. Gruzlica 25:701–708
Hughes HB (1953) On the metabolic fate of isoniazid. J Pharmacol Exper Ther 109:444–452
Iwainsky H (1970) Der Ansatzpunkt der verschiedenen Therapeutica im Stoffwechsel des Tuberkelbakteriums. Pneumonologie 143 (Suppl 1970):1–14 (M)
Iwainsky H, Siegel D (1961) Über den Einfluß qualitativer Ernährungsfaktoren auf den INH-Stoffwechsel im Makroorganismus. Beitr Klin Tuberk 123:166–170
Iwainsky H, Reutgen H (1968) Untersuchungen zum endogenen Stoffwechsel von Mykobakterien. 3. Mitt. Über den Einfluß von Isonikotinsäurehydrazid auf den endogenen Stoffwechsel von Mykobakterien. Z Naturforschung 23b:982–989
Iwainsky H, Käppler W (1974) Mykobakterien, Biochemie und biochemische Differenzierung. Bibliothek für das Gesamtgebiet der Lungenkrankheiten, Band 103. Barth, Leipzig
Iwainsky H, Winsel K (1977) Die Bedeutung der unterschiedlichen Azetylierung für Wirkung und Nebenwirkung des Isoniazids. Zentralbl Pharm 116:507–515
Iwainsky H, Gerloff W, Schmiedel A (1961) Die Differenzierung zwischen INH-Inaktivierern und normal abbauenden Patienten mit Hilfe eines einfachen Testes. Beitr Klin Tuberk 124:384–389
Iwainsky H, Schmiedel A, Kauffmann G-W (1965) Der unterschiedliche INH-Abbau und seine Bedeutung für den Verlauf der Lungentuberkulose. In: Steinbrück P (Hrsg) Die Therapie der Lungentuberkulose. Volk und Gesundheit, Jena, pp 159–175
Iwainsky H, Kauffmann G-W, Siegel D, Gerischer C (1960) Über den Einfluß des INH-Stoffwechsels auf die Behandlung der Lungentuberkulose. Beitr Klin Tuberk 122:324–332
Iwainsky H, Reutgen H, Sehrt I, Grunert M (1967) Über das Schicksal von Tuberkulostatika im Makro- und Mikroorganismus. Z Tuberk 126:106–130 (B, Ph)
Jackett PS, Aber VR, Mitchison DA (1977) The relationship between nicotinamide adenine dinucleotide concentration and antibacterial activity of isoniazid in *Mycobacterium tuberculosis*. Am Rev Respir Dis 115:601–607

Jeanes CWL, Schaefer O, Eidus L (1972) Inactivation of isoniazid by Canadian Eskimos and Indians. Can Med Assoc J 106:331–335
Jeanes CWL, Schaefer O, Eidus L (1973) Comparative blood levels and metabolism of INH and an INH-matrix preparation in fast and slow inactivators. Can Med Assoc J 109:483–487
Jenne JW (1960) Studies of human patterns of isoniazid metabolism using an intravenous fall-off technique with a chemical method. Am Rev Respir Dis 81:1–9
Jenne JW (1964) Pharmacokinetics and the dose of isoniazid and para-aminosalicylic acid in the treatment of tuberculosis. Antibiot Chemother 12:407–432
Jenne JW (1965) Partial purification and properties of the isoniazid transacetylase in human liver. Its relationship to the acetylation of para-aminosalicylic acid. J Clin Invest 44:1991–2002
Jenne JW, Beggs WH (1973) Correlation of in vitro and in vivo kinetics with clinical use of isoniazid, ethambutol and rifampin. Am Rev Respir Dis 107:1013–1021
Jenne JW, Boyer PD (1962) Kinetic characteristics of the acetylation of isoniazid and para-aminosalicylic acid by a liver-enzyme-preparation. Biochim Biophys Acta 65:121–127
Jenne JW, MacDonald FM, Mendoza E (1961) A study of the renal clearance, metabolic inactivation rates, and serum fall-off interaction of isoniazid and para-aminosalicylic acid in man. Am Rev Respir Dis 84:371–378
Jenne JW, White TA, Evans DAP (1969) Substrate affinities of the rapid and slow N-acetyltransferase from human liver. Trans 28th Pulm Dis Res Conf VAAF:47–49
Jessamine AG, Hodgkin MM, Eidus L (1974) Urine tests for phenotyping slow and fast acetylators. Can J Publ Hlth 65:119–123
Johnson W, Mankiewicz E, Jasmin R, Corte G (1961) The effect of 5-bromsalicylhydroxamic acid on the acetalytion of isoniazid and its concentration in the blood. Am Rev Respir Dis 84:872–875
Jungbluth H (1971) Isoniazid-Dosierung bei Niereninsuffizienz. Pneumonologie 145:383–384
Jungbluth H (1973) Tuberkulose-Chemotherapie bei Kranken mit vorgeschädigter Niere. Prax Pneumol 27:175–182
Kagamiyama M, Majima M (1961) Studies on the plasma concentration of INH (isoniazid) by Peters' fluorometric procedure. Kekkaku 36:770–775
Kandt D, Flach W (1965) Blut- und Harnspiegelmessungen bei intrakavitärer INH-Applikation. Ein Beitrag zur Prüfung der Resorptionsverhältnisse der Kavernenwand. Beitr Klin Tuberk 130:94–100
Kasenov KU, Stambekow AS (1981) Study on relation between isoniazid inactivation and genetic marker of blood (ABO). Probl Tuberk 59 issue 10:50–52
Kelly JM, Poet RB, Chesner LM (1952) Observations on the metabolic fate of nydrazid (isonicotinic acid hydrazide). Amer Chem Soc Abstr 122nd meeting, p 3C
Kergueris MF, Larousse C, Le Normand Y, Bourin M (1983) Acetylation character of isoniazid in the rabbit and in man. Eur J Drug Metab Pharmacokinet 8:133–136
Kleeberg H, Gärtig D, Glatthaar E, Nel E, Stander M (1975) Isoniazid metabolism in black patients. S Afr Med J 49:1503
Klinger W (1981) Alkohol und Arzneimittelbiotransformation. Z Gesamte Inn Med 36:543–547
Koizumi K, Okamoto R (1962) A study on the distribution of the plasma concentration of active INH in pulmonary tuberculous patients. Kekkaku 37:18–22
Kraus P, Urbančík R, Šimáně Z, Reil I (1961) A contribution to the problem of the anti-isoniazid factor. Am Rev Respir Dis 84:684–689
Kreukniet J, Blom van Assendelft PM, Mouton RP, Tasman A, Bangma PJ (1967) The influence of para-aminosalicylic acid on isonicotinic acid hydrazide blood levels after oral and intravenous administration. Scand J Respir Dis 47:236–243
Krüger-Thiemer E (1957) Biochemie des Isoniazids. I. Isoniazidmetabolismus. Jber Borstel 4:299–509 (M, B)
Krüger-Thiemer E †, Kröger H, Nestler HJ, Seydel JK (1975) Wirkungsmodi antituberkulöser Chemotherapeutika. Isoniazid. In: Meissner G, Schmiedel A †, Nelles A † (Hrsg) Infektionskrankheiten und ihre Erreger, Band 4, Teil III. Fischer Jena, pp 257–288

Krulik R, Kohout M (1962) Élimination des acides alpha cétoniques après l' administration de la pyrazinamide, de 1314 Th et de l' isoniazide. Acta Tuber Scand 41:298–303
La Du BN (1972) Isoniazid and pseudocholinesterase polymorphismus. Fed Proc 31:1276–1283
Lamedica G, Penco G, Spandonari MM, Jannuzzi C (1983) Clinical pharmacology of isoniazid in children. Usefulness of monitoring therapy. Chemiotherapia 2:410–416
Lauterburg BH, Smith CV, Mitchell JR (1981) Determination of isoniazid and its hydrazino metabolites, acetylisoniazid, acetylhydrazine, and diacetylhydrazine in human plasma by gas chromatography-mass spectrometry. J Chromatogr 224:431–438
Lauterburg BH, Smith CV, Todd EL, Mitchell JR (1985) Oxidation of hydrazine metabolites formed from isoniazid. Clin Pharmacol Ther 38:566–571
Levi AJ, Sherlock S, Walker D (1968) Phenylbutazone and isoniazid metabolism in patients with liver disease in relation to previous drug therapy. Lancet I:1275–1279
Levy D, Russel WP Jr, Middlebrook G (1960) Dosages of isoniazid and streptomycin for routine chemotherapy of tuberculosis. Tubercle 41:23–31
Mason E, Russell DW (1971) Isoniazid acetylation rates (phenotypes) of patients being treated for tuberculosis. Bull WHO 45:617–624
Matsuzaki Y, Saito C (1961) Studies on the blood concentrations of biologically active isoniazid and its derivatives and on the metabolic patterns of isoniazid. Kekkaku 36:61–62
Mattila MJ, Tiitinen H (1967) The rate of isoniazid inactivation in Finnish diabetic and non-diabetic patients. Ann Med Exp Fenn 45:423–427
McClatchy JK (1971) Mechanism of action of isoniazid on Mycobacterium bovis strain BCG. Infect Immun 3:530–534
McClatchy JK, Smith JA (1968) Inhibition of DNA synthesis in *Mycobacterium tuberculosis* BCG by isoniazid. Trans 27th Pulm Dis Res Conf, VAAF:15
Meurice JC, Castets AM, Ranger S, Fourtillan JB, Besson J, Boita F, Patte F (1984) Étude comparative de 2 méthodes de dosage de l'isoniazide sérique chez 413 patients: méthode microbiologique, chromatographie liquide à haute performance. Rev Pneumol Clin 40:233–236
Meyer UA, Meier PJ (1982) Klinisch bedeutsame vererbte Unterschiede in der Arzneimittelwirkung. Schweiz Med Wochenschr 112:666–669
Miller RR, Porter J, Greenblatt DJ (1979) Clinical importance of the interaction of phenytoin and isoniazid. Chest 75:356–358
Mitchell JR, Thorgeirsson PU, Black M, Timbrell JA, Snodgrass WR, Potter WZ, Joliow DJ, Keiser HR (1975) Increased incidence of isoniazid hepatitis in rapid acetylators: possible relation to hydrazine metabolites. Clin Pharm Ther 18:70–79
Mukoyama H, Sunahara M, Ogawa M, Kawai K (1963) Urinary excretion of metabolites of isoniazid and inactivation of sulfonamide in rapid, intermediate and slow inactivators of isoniazid. Kekkaku 38:1–7
Musch E, Wang JK, Dengler HJ (1981) Alterations of drug metabolism during tuberculostatic therapy. Naunyn-Schmiedebergs Arch Pharmacol 316 Suppl: R 79, No 313
Mydlak G, Volkmann W (1965) Die Bedeutung der INH-Stoffwechselanalyse für die Therapie. Z Tuberk 124:44–48
Nakagawa H, Sunahara Sh (1967) Studies on metabolism of isoniazid by a new chemical determination of isoniazid (2nd report). Trimodal distribution of blood levels, inactivation in intestine and combination of isoniazid with serum protein. Kekkaku 42:203–212
Nielsch W, Giefer L (1959) Photometrische Bestimmung von Isonikotinsäurehydrazid (INH), INH-Derivaten und ihren Metaboliten in biologischen Proben. Arzneimittel-Forsch 9:636–641; 700–707
Nitti V (1972) Antituberculosis activity of rifampin. Chest 61:589–598
Notter D, Roland E (1978) Localisation des N-acétyltransférases dans les cellules sinusoidales hépatiques. Influence du zymosan sur l' acétylation de la sulfaméthazine et de l'isoniazide chez le rat et dans le foie isolé perfusé. CR Soc Biol 172:531–533
Okinaka S, Yoshida S, Mikami R, Kira S (1961) A study on the plasma concentration of active isoniazid in twins. Kekkaku 36:27–60

Parrot R, Boval C, Grosset J, Gaillard JP (1983) Adapter ou ne pas adapter la posologie de l'isoniazide? Rev Fr Mal Respir 11:705–712

Peters JH (1960 a) Studies on the metabolism of isoniazid. I. Development and application of a fluorometric procedure for measuring isoniazid in blood plasma. Am Rev Respir Dis 81:485–497

Peters JH (1960 b) Studies on the metabolism of isoniazid. II. The influence of para-aminosalicylic acid on the metabolism of isoniazid by man. Am Rev Respir Dis 82:153–163

Peters JH, Miller KS, Brown P (1964) Acetylation as the genetic determinant of the metabolism of isoniazid by man. Fed Proc 23:280

Peters JH, Gordon GR, Brown P (1965 a) The relationship between the capacities of human subjects to acetylate isoniazid, sulfanilamide and sulfamethazine. Life Sci 4:99–107

Peters JH, Miller KS, Brown P (1965 b) The determination of isoniazid and its metabolites in human urine. Anal Biochem 12:379–394

Peters JH, Miller KS, Brown P (1965 c) Studies on the metabolic basis for the genetically determined capacities for isoniazid inactivation in man. J Pharmacol Exp Ther 150:298–304

Pfaffenberg R, Iwainsky H, Jähler H, Siegel D (1960) Über den Stoffwechsel des Isonicotinsäurehydrazid (INH) und der α-Ketosäuren bei tuberkulösen Diabetikern. Beitr Klin Tuberk 123:63–71

Pfaffenberg R, Iwainsky H, Jähler H (1963) INH-Stoffwechsel und Tuberkuloseverlauf bei Diabetikern. Tuberk-Arzt 17:299–313

Pikora T, Hejný J, Melicher J (1980) Serum levels of isoniazid after single doses of isoniazid of 14 mg/kg b.w. Stud Pneumol Phtiseol Cechoslov 40:398–403

Pikora T, Hejný J, Melicher J, Strmen J (1982) Serum INH levels in patients after doses of 5 mg/kg and 14 mg/kg of body weight. Stud Pneumol Phtiseol Cechoslov 42:156–161

Pilheu J, Fernandez JG, Mingolla L, Terren A, Barberis S, Altclas J, Montiel G, Kaler G (1985) Plasma concentration of isoniazid in the elderly. Am Rev Respir Dis 131 Suppl: A 229

Place VA, Thomas JP (1963) Clinical pharmacology of ethambutol. Am Rev Respir Dis 87:901–904

Rajtar-Leontiew Z (1969) The effect of isoniazid on the metabolism of pyridoxine in experimental tuberculosis in rats. Gruzlica 37:109–113

Ramakrishnan T, Suryanarayana Murthy P, Gopinathan KP (1972) Intermediary metabolism of mycobacteria. Bacteriol Rev 36:65–108

Rao KVN, Mitchison DA, Nair NGG, Prema K, Tripathy SP (1970) Sulphadimidine acetylation test for classification of patients as slow or rapid inactivators of isoniazid. Br Med J 3:495–497

Reidenberg MM, Shear L, Cohen RV (1973) Elimination of isoniazid in patients with impaired renal function. Am Rev Resp Dis 108:1426–1428

Ritter W (1973) Neue Ergebnisse über Biotransformation und Pharmakokinetik von Antituberkulotika. Prax Pneumol 27:139–145 (B, Ph)

Robson JM, Sullivan FM (1963) Antituberculosis drugs. Pharmacol Rev 15:169–223 (B, Ph)

Rosental AR, Self TH, Baker ED, Linden RA (1977) Interaction of isoniazid and warfarin. JAMA 238:2177

Rózniecki J (1968) Percentage ratio of free isoniazid and acetyl-isoniazid in the urine as a method of determination of the isoniazid inactivation pattern. Gruzlica 36:971–973

Russell DW (1972) Simplified isoniazid acetylator phenotyping. Can Med Assoc J 106:1155–1156

Salako LA, Fadeke Aderounmu A (1977) Determination of the isoniazid acetylator phenotype in a West African population. Tubercle 58:109–112

Sassen W v, Castro-Parva M (1981) HPLC-determination of isoniazid and isoniazid metabolites in biological fluids. Naunyn Schmiedebergs Arch Pharmacol 316 Suppl: R 78, No 312

Sassen W v., Musch E, Castro-Parva M, Eichelbaum M (1982) Pharmacokinetics and metabolism of isoniazid in relation to hepatotoxic side effects during antituberculous therapy. Naunyn Schmiedebergs Arch Pharmacol 319 Suppl: R 88, No 349

Saueressig G (1972) Untersuchungen zur Harnausscheidung von INH bei intravenöser Na-Gluronazid-Therapie. Inaugural-Dissertation, Med Fakultät der Rheinischen Friedrich-Wilhelms-Universität zu Bonn

Schloot W, Blume K-G, Goedde HW, Flatz G, Bhaibulaya M (1967) Studies on isoniazid conversion in Thailand. Humangenetik 4:274–279

Schmiedel A (1960) Weitere Untersuchungen über das Wesen und die klinische Bedeutung der hochgradigen Isoniazidinaktivierung im Körper. Beitr Klin Tuberk 122:232–238

Schmiedel A (1961) The problem of rapid isoniazid inactivation. Bull Int Union Tuberc 31:508–512

Schmiedel A, Ermisch U, Doerfel G (1960) Zur Chemotherapie der Lungentuberkulose mit Ultraschall-Aerosolen. Dtsch Ges Wesen 15:2430–2434

Schröder H (1972) Simplified method for determining acetylator phenotype. Br Med J 3:506–507

Scott EM, Wright RC (1967) Fluorometric determination of isonicotinic acid hydrazide in serum. J Lab Clin Med 70:355–360

Scott EM, Wright RC, Weaver DD (1969) The discrimination of phenotypes for rate of disappearance of isonicotinoyl hydrazide from serum. J Clin Invest 48:1173–1176

Sehm G, Urbanczik R (1974) Die Bedeutung der INH-Schnell- und Langsaminaktivierer für die Transaminasenanstiege bei der kombinierten INH-RMP-Therapie. Prax Pneumol 28:613–615

Sen PK, Saha JR, Chatterjee R (1972) Isoniazid inactivation in tuberculous patients. Indian J Med Res 60:19–27

Seydel JK, Tono-Oka S, Schaper K-J, Bock L, Wienke M (1976) Mode of action of isoniazid (INH). Arzneimittelforsch 26:477–478

Shenderova RI, Terteryan EA (1973) Inactivation of PAS and hina in tuberculous children. Probl Tuberk 51 issue 5: 67–71

Short EI (1962a) A comparative study of the metabolism and toxicity of isoniazid and isoniazone calcium pyruvate. Tubercle 43:22–32

Short EI (1962b) Studies on the inactivation of isonicotinyl acid hydrazide in normal subjects and tuberculous patients. Tubercle 43:33–42

Smirnov GA (1972) Criteria and methods of determining inactivation of the hina preparations. Probl Tuberk 50 issue 4: 54–61

Smirnov GA (1977) Decomposition of the hina and cycloserine preparations in the organism of patients with tuberculosis of the lungs. Probl Tuberk 55 issue 8: 63–66

Smith J, Tyrrell WF, Gow A, Allan GW, Lees AW (1972) Hepatotoxicity in rifampin-isoniazid treated patients related to their rate of isoniazid inactivation. Chest 61:587–588

Sokolowa GB, Vilenskaya RN, Ivleva AY, Galenko NN, Ziya AV (1981) On isoniazid pharmacokinetics in combined chemotherapy of tuberculosis. Probl Tuberk 59 issue 10: 24–28

Sokolova GB, Ivleva AY, Ziya AV, Zeliger LR, Suvorova VJ, Galenko NN (1984) Clinical pharmacology of isoniazid. Probl Tuberk 62 issue 9: 55–60

Sprouse JS, Schneck DW, Hayes AH Jr (1978) The effect of isoniazid and other drugs on the acetylation of procainamide in the intact rat. J Pharmacol Exp Ther 207:698–704

Sriprakash KS, Ramakrishnan T (1970) Isoniazid-resistant mutants of *Mycobacterium tuberculosis* H37Rv: Uptake of isoniazid and the properties of NADase inhibitor. J Gen Microbiol 60:125–132

Stepanov VM (1981) Kinetics of isoniazid distribution after intravenous administration. Probl Tuberk 59 issue 8: 66–69

Sunahara S (1962) Genetical, geographical and clinical studies on isoniazid metabolism. Bull Int Union Tuberc 32:513–540

Sunahara S, Urano M, Lin HT, Cheg TJ, Jarumilinda A (1963a) Further observations on trimodality of frequency distribution curve of biologically active isoniazid blood levels and "cline" in frequencies of alleles controlling isoniazid inactivation. Acta Tuberc Pneumol Scand 43:181–195

Sunahara S, Mukoyama H, Ogawa M, Kawai K (1963 b) Urinary excretion of metabolites of INH and inactivation of sulfonamide in rapid, intermediate and slow inactivators of INH. Kekkaku 38:1–7
Sunahara S, Urano M, Kawai K, Honjo S, Takasaki S, Fujiwara T (1968) The patterns of isoniazid inactivation in Macaca irus. Kekkaku 43:97–102
Suryanarayana Murthy P, Sirsi M, Ramakrishnan T (1973) Effect of isoniazid on the carbohydrate metabolism of isoniazid-susceptible and isoniazid-resistant *Mycobacterium tuberculosis* H37Rv. Am Rev Respir Dis 107:139–141
Sushkin AG, Guzeeva SA (1978) Polarographic determination of isoniazid in the urine. Probl Tuberk 56 issue 7: 76–79
Szczawinska K, Chodera A, Cenajek D, Szczawinski R (1976) Pharmacokinetics of isoniazid (INH) in slow and rapid inactivators during combined treatment. I. Symposium für Klinische Pharmakologie, 7. 12. 1976, Dresden, DDR
Takayama K, Armstrong EL, David HL (1974) Restoration of mycolate synthetase activity in *Mycobacterium tuberculosis* exposed to isoniazid. Am Rev Respir Dis 110:43–48
Teichmann W, Köhler R (1964) Beitrag zur schnellen Differenzierung des individuellen INH-Stoffwechsels. Prax Pneumol 18:535–541
Thénault D, Saltiel JC, Houin G, Vivien JN, Tillement JP, Chretien J (1976) Comparative study of two procedures for measuring isoniazid levels in serum. Rev Fr Mal Resp 4:565–566
Tiitinen H (1969 a) Isoniazid and ethionamide serum levels and inactivation in Finnish subjects. Scand J Respir Dis 50:110–124
Tiitinen H (1969 b) Isoniazid inactivation status and the development of chronic tuberculosis. Scand J Respir Dis 50:227–234
Tiitinen H (1969 c) Modification by para-aminosalicylic acid and sulfamethazine of the isoniazid inactivation in man. Scand J Respir Dis 50:281–290
Tiitinen H, Mattila MJ (1968) Modification of the serum isoniazid levels by different preparations of para-aminosalicylic acid. Arzneimittelforsch 18:623–625
Tiitinen H, Mattila MJ, Eriksson AW (1968) Comparison of the isoniazid inactivation in Finns and Lapps. Ann Med Int Fenn 57:161–166
Timbrell JA, Wright JM, Baillie TA (1977) Monoacetylhydrazine as a metabolite of isoniazid in man. Clin Pharmacol Ther 22/51:602–608
Titarenko OT, Vakhmistrova TI, Perova TL (1982) Time course of isoniazid excretion in chronic renal insufficiency. Probl Tuberk 60 issue 2: 48–52
Toida I (1962 a) Hydrazidase activity of isoniazid-resistant cells of mycobacteria grown on metal-supplemented media. Kekkaku 37:85–91
Toida I (1962 b) Induced formation of hydrazidase. Kekkaku 37:582–585
Toida I (1962 c) Isoniazid-hydrolyzing enzyme of mycobacteria. Am Rev Respir Dis 85:720–726
Toida I, Saito C (1962) Effect of nitrogen-source on hydrazidase activity. Kekkaku 37:287–290
Toyohara M (1974) The experimental study of the transmission of the antituberculous drugs to fetuses. Kekkaku 49:97–99
Tripathy SP (1976) A slow-release preparation of isoniazid: therapeutic efficacy and adverse side-effects. Bull Int Union Tuberc 51:133–141
Tsukamura M, Mizuno S (1962) Mode of action of isoniazid viewed from isotope incorporation studies. Kekkaku 37:29–35
Tsukamura M, Tsukamura S, Nakano E (1963) The uptake of isoniazid by mycobacteria and its relation to isoniazid susceptibility. Am Rev Respir Dis 87:269–275
Turnbull LB, Yard AS, McKennis H Jr (1962) Acetylhydrazine as an intermediate in the metabolism of aroylhydrazines. J Med Pharm Chem 5:1327–1334
Tytor YM (1975) Isoniazid and PAS metabolism and bacteriostatic activity of the blood in adolescents with intrathoracic tuberculosis. Probl Tuberk 53 issue 7: 51–54
Tytor Y N (1976) Liver function and metabolism of isoniazid and PAS in adolescents with intrathoracic tuberculosis. Probl Tuberk 54 issue 7: 29–32
Varughese P, Hamilton EJ, Eidus L (1974) Mass Phenotyping of isoniazid inactivators by automated determination of acetylisoniazid in urine. Clin Chem 20:639–641

Venho VMK, Koskinen R (1971) The effect of pyrazinamide, rifampicin and cycloserine on the blood levels and urinary excretion of isoniazid. Ann Clin Res 3:277–280
Venkataraman P, Menon NK, Nair NGK, Radhakrishna S, Ross CH, Tripathy SP (1972) Classification of subjects as slow or rapid inactivators of isoniazid, based on the ratio of the urinary excretion of acetylisoniazid to isoniazid. Tubercle 53:84–91
Vivien JN, Grosset J (1961) Le taux d' isoniazide actif dans le sérum sanguin. Adv Tuberc Res 11:45–125 (B, Ph)
Vivien JN, Thibier R, Lepeuple A (1972) Recent studies on isoniazid. Adv Tuberc Res 18:148–230 (B, Ph)
Vivien JN, Thibier R, Lepeuple A (1973) La pharmacocinétique de l'isoniazide dans la race blanche. Rev Fr Mal Resp 1:753–772
Víznerová A, Slavíková Z, Ellard GA (1973) The determination of the acetylator phenotype of tuberculosis patients in Czechoslovakia using sulphadimidine. Tubercle 54:67–71
Volkmann W, Mydlak G (1965) INH-Stoffwechsel und Resistenzentwicklung. Beitr Klin Tuberk 131:89–95
Wang L, Takayama K (1972) Relationship between the uptake of isoniazid and its action on in vivo mycolic acid synthesis in *Mycobacterium tuberculosis*. Antimicrob Agents Chemother 2:438–441
Weber WW, Cohen SN, Steinberg MS (1968) Purification and properties of N-acetyltransferase from mammalian liver. Ann NY Acad Sci 151:734–741
Wimpenny JWT (1967a) Effect of isoniazid on biosynthesis in *Mycobacterium tuberculosis* var. *bovis* BCG. J Gen Microbiol 47:379–388
Wimpenny JWT (1967b) The uptake and fate of isoniazid in *Mycobacterium tuberculosis* var. *bovis* BCG. J Gen Microbiol 47:389–403
Winder F (1964) Early changes by isoniazid in the composition of *Mycobacterium tuberculosis*. Biochim Biophys Acta 82:210–212
Winder FG (1982) Mode of action of the antimycobacterial agents and associated aspects of the molecular biology of the mycobacteria. In: Ratledge C, Stanford J (eds) The biology of the mycobacteria, Vol 1. Academic Press, London New York Paris San Diego San Francisco Sao Paulo Sydney Tokyo Toronto, pp 353–438
Winder F, Brennan P (1964) The accumulation of free trehalose by mycobacteria exposed to isoniazid. Biochim Biophys Acta 90:442–444
Winder F, Collins P (1968) The effect of isoniazid on nicotinamide nucleotide levels in *Mycobacterium bovis,* strain BCG. Am Rev Respir Dis 97:719–720
Winder F, Collins PB (1970) Inhibition by isoniazid of synthesis of mycolic acids in *Mycobacterium tuberculosis*. J Gen Microbiol 63:41–48
Winder FG, Rooney SA (1968) Effects of isoniazid on the triglycerides of BCG. Am Rev Respir Dis 97:938–940
Winder F, Rooney SA (1970) The effect of isoniazid on the carbohydrates of *M. tuberculosis* BCG. Biochem J 117:355–368
Winder F, Brennan PJ, McDonnell I (1967) Effects of isoniazid on the composition of mycobacteria, with particular reference to soluble carbohydrates and related substances. Biochem J 104:385–393
Wood JD, Peesker SJ (1971) Sequential lowering and raising of brain γ-aminobutyric acid levels by isonicotinic acid hydrazide. Can J Physiol Pharmacol 49:780–781
Youatt J (1961) The formation of 4-pyridine methanol from isonicotinic acid hydrazide (isoniazid) by mycobacteria. Aust J Chem 14:308–311
Youatt J (1965) Changes in the phosphate content of mycobacteria produced by isoniazid and ethambutol. Aust J Exp Biol Med Sci 43:305–314
Youatt J (1969) A review of the action of isoniazid. Am Rev Respir Dis 99:729–749 (M)
Youatt J, Tham SH (1969a) An enzyme system of *Mycobacterium tuberculosis* that reacts specifically with isoniazid. Am Rev Respir Dis 100:25–30
Youatt J, Tham SH (1969b) An enzyme system of *Mycobacterium tuberculosis* that reacts specifically with isoniazid. II. Correlation of this reaction with the binding and metabolism of isoniazid. Am Rev Respir Dis 100:31–37
Youatt J, Tham SH (1969c) Radioactive content of *Mycobacterium tuberculosis* after exposure to ^{14}C-isoniazid. Am Rev Respir Dis 100:77–78

Youmans AS, Youmans GP (1960) The production of "Anti-Isoniazid" substance by Isoniazid-susceptible, Isoniazid-resistant, and unclassified strains of mycobacteria. Am Rev Respir Dis 81:929–931
Zamboni V, Defranceschi A (1954) Identification of isonicotinoylhydrazones of pyruvic and α-ketoglutaric acid in rat urine after treatment with isonicotinic acid hydrazide (isoniazid). Biochem Biophys Acta 14:430–432
Zdunczyk-Pawelek H, Blitek-Golc D, Kostrzewska K (1962) The concentration of biologically active Isoniazid in patients' serum. Acta Tuberc Scand 42:138–148
Zdunczyk-Pawelek H, Otrzowsek N, Kostrzewska K (1965) Der Einfluß des gleichzeitigen Verabreichens von 5-Bromsalicylhydroxamid-Säure (T_{40}) und INH auf die Konzentration des freien INH im Harn des Tuberkulosekranken. Z Tbk 124:149–152
Zierski M, Rotermund CH (1984) Isoniazid – Wesentliches und Neues. Prax Klin Pneumol 38:201–216
Ziporin ZZ (1964) Effect of Isoniazid on blood ammonia concentrations. Am Rev Respir Dis 89:936–937
Ziporin ZZ, Chambers JS, Taylor RR, Wier JA (1962) The effect of Isoniazid administration on the blood ammonia in tuberculous patients. Am Rev Respir Dis 86:21–28
Zureck A (1968) 3-Hydroxymethyl-Pyridin im Stoffwechsel von Mykobakterien. Zentralbl Bakteriol Mikrobiol Hyg A 206:522–529

VI. Tetracyclines

1. Mode of Action

The extent of the incorporation inhibitable by so-called decouplers (e.g., 2.4-dinitrophenol, azide) depends on the nature of the energy source supplied by the nutrient medium. For example, glucose stimulates the incorporation of TC. In *E. coli* the accumulation of TC is stimulated by Mg^{2+} ions, probably as a result of chelation. In TC-resistant microorganisms (*E. coli*), the uptake of TC is reduced, but not so much as that of INH or CS (ARIMA and IZAKI 1963; IZAKI and ARIMA 1963, 1965; IZAKI et al. 1966; DÜRCKHEIMER 1975).

Similarly, the formation of an Mg^{2+}-chelate complex is seemingly necessary for TC to act inside the cell (VIDEAU 1968). It appears that a complex of this kind inhibits the binding of aminoacyl-t-RNA to the ribosomal A-adhesion site (LASKIN and LAST 1971) or the earlier step of the binding of lysine to the corresponding t-RNA and its attachment in ribosomes (GOTTESMAN 1967; ČERNÁ et al. 1969; DÜRCKHEIMER 1975; KRÜGER-THIEMER et al. 1975). Once formed, a ternary ribosome-m-RNA-t-RNA complex can no more be influenced by TC than can the puromycin-induced release of the peptide chain synthesized in the ribosomes (GOLDBERG 1965; CUNDLIFFE and MCQUILLEN 1967; ČERNÁ et al. 1969). On the other hand, no further reaching impairment of the incorporation of adenine into mitochondrial DNA can be observed (GOLDBERG 1965; GAUZE et al. 1971).

2. Biotransformation

The TC's appear to circulate as Ca^{2+} chelates and, in this form, are more protected against biotransformation processes than are other antituberculosis drugs The discoloration of the teeth, observed as a side effect under certain conditions after TC therapy, is due to analogous binding of TC to the Ca^{2+} ions present in bone and in teeth. Such binding can be prevented by the addition of substances that complex with Ca^{2+}, for example EDTA (KELLY and BUYSKE 1960; EISNER and WULF 1963; FINERMAN and MILCH 1963; BRAZDA 1964; BRAZDA et al. 1966; BENAZET et al. 1968). Epimerization associated with a loss of activity (EISNER and WULF 1963) can already occur during storage of samples or in the course of mild analytical procedures, e.g. during countercurrent distribution (KELLY and BUYSKE 1960; KELLY et al. 1961; SCHACH VON WITTENAU et al. 1972). It is therefore difficult to determine the extent of the biotransformation that takes place in vivo. It seems that, contrary to the former opinion, the tetracyclines of the older generation and doxycycline are biotransformed after all. Six biotransformation products of minocycline have been isolated from human urine, two of them with their biological activity at least partly intact (HANSSON et al. 1966; FABRE et al. 1966; NELIS and DE LEENHEER 1981; BÖCKER et al. 1982; BÖCKER and ESTLER 1983).

Thorough investigations with ^{14}C- and ^{3}H-labelled compounds yielded virtually the same results in the dog and the rat. Only in the case of chlortetracycline is a considerably higher proportion of the epimerization product found (4-epichlor-TC – KELLY and BUYSKE 1960; KELLY et al. 1961; EISNER and WULF 1963; SCHACH VON WITTENAU and TWOMEY 1971).

3. Pharmacokinetics

a) Absorption and Distribution

The TC's are absorbed relatively slowly; the process being strongly influenced by the distribution coefficient of the tetracycline. Chelate formers increase the degree of absorption, while Ca^{2+} and Fe^{3+} ions reduce it. The extent of the protein binding varies (between 20 and 80%), depending on the structure of the TC. Three groups with different degrees of binding can be distinguished (Table 4, p. 419).

TC's are distributed throughout the body water (Table 6, p. 421). They have a special affinity for the skeleton and the teeth, this property being apparently due to complexing with Ca^{2+} ions that is associated with other processes (BUYSKE et al. 1960; KELLY and BUYSKE 1960; FINERMAN and MILCH 1963; BRAZDA 1964; MALEK et al. 1966a). The incorporation of TC in the skeleton, detectable by fluorescence, corresponds in its intensity to the growth lines and is used for marking purposes (ANTALOVSKA and BERAN 1966; JOHNSON 1966; HAWKINS 1972). The deposited TC is not harmful to the individual and, in pregnant women, the foetus is not endangered (OKLUND et al. 1981).

In accordance with the affinity of the particular derivative, the TC concentration in the organs and tissues ranges from 0.3 to 3.1 times the serum concentration. The reticuloendothelial system has the highest concentrations, followed by the liver, kidneys, and intestines. TC cannot be detected in the brain. The ratios of the organ concentrations differ for the individual TC derivatives, the lipid solubility being a decisive factor for the distribution (KUNIN and FINLAND 1961; SCHACH VON WITTENAU and YEARY 1963; FABRE et al. 1967, 1977; WINKLER and WEIH 1967). Irregular distribution only becomes discernible in states of shock (MALEK et al. 1966b). In mice an age- and sex-dependence of the TC distribution has been demonstrated, the TC concentration in the liver being lower in older mice than in middle-aged animals (HOPF 1983).

Table 1. Tetracycline concentrations in the serum of patients after oral and intravenous administration

Dose	200 mg doxycycline 18.00 h + 100 mg doxycycline 7.00 h		200 mg doxycycline		200 mg minocycline		200 mg minocycline			600 mg doxycycline	
Mode of adminis- tration	i.v.		i.v.		i.v.		p.o.			p.o.	
Blood sample taken after hours	μg TC/ml	*n*	μg TC/ml	*n*	μg TC/ml	*n*	μg TC/ml	*n*	Blood sample taken after hours	μmol/l	*n*
1	9.3 (3.2–16)		5.01 ± 0.4		4.39 ± 0.94						
2	7.0 (5 – 8)	12	4.69 ± 0.23		3.35 ± 0.62		2.10 ± 0.16				
3	3.2 (1.8– 4)				2.64 ± 0.46		2.12 ± 0.16	19			
4			3.62 ± 0.26								
6			3.0 ± 0.25	10	1.60 ± 0.22	8	1.69 ± 0.1		6	25.5 ± 2.0	
8			2.79 ± 0.23						24	14.7 ± 2.1	
10			2.48 ± 0.22						48	4.5 ± 1.1	10
12			2.21 ± 0.19						72	2.3 ± 1.6	
25					0.74				96	1.2 ± 0.5	
1	8.0 (7 –9)										
2	4.8 (1.5–8)	6									
3	3.7 (1 –6)										
	THADEPALLI et al. (1980)		SIMON et al. (1978)		SOMMERWERCK et al. (1978)		SOMMERWERCK et al. (1978)			MARLIN et al. (1981)	

The TC concentration in pulmonary tissue is between 20% and 60% of the serum concentration and is particularly high in inflamed lung tissue. Penetration into the bronchial mucus is also dependent on the degree of inflammation. Thus, the concentration in purulent sputum can be 10 times as high as that in normal sputum, in which 5 to 42% of the serum concentration is found. All authors unanimously conclude from the measurements that TC concentrations above the MIC are also reached in normal sputum (HARTNETT and MARLIN 1976; KAHAN et al. 1977; ZIMMERMANN et al. 1977; BERGOGNE-BEREZIN et al. 1978; MARSCHANG et al. 1978; SOMMERWERCK et al. 1978; MAC ARTHUR et al. 1978; CLAUBERG 1979; MARLIN et al. 1981).

In necrotic tissue the TC concentrations are higher than those in normal tissue (KUNIN and FINLAND 1961; BENAZET et al. 1968). TC has also been detected in the synovial fluid with a delayed concentration peak and a half-life that depends on the degree of inflammation (POHL 1964; EHRLICH 1972), in the tonsils (BERRETINI 1968), and in the pleural fluid (ALBAUM et al. 1964). TC reaches the gall-bladder via the bloodstream (ONDRACEK and ZASTAVA 1966).

In the foetus a fall of the TC concentration by 50% and more, referred to the concentration in the maternal serum, must be borne in mind. The course of the TC concentration in the CSF corresponds to that in the serum and is influenced by the duration of treatment (Table 7, p. 423, TABER et al. 1967).

b) Excretion

TC's are excreted via the kidneys and via the intestinal tract. Some 60% of the initial dose is recovered in the urine and between 20% and 50% in the faeces (Table 8, p. 424, WINKLER and WEIH 1967; BENAZET et al. 1968; SCHACH VON WITTENAU et al. 1972). Between 69% and 75% of the glomerularly filtered fraction is reabsorbed in the tubules. The volume and the pH value of the urine have no effect on the glomerular filtration (KUNIN and FINLAND 1961; FABRE et al. 1966, 1967). There is a direct correlation between the $t_{50\%}$ of the TC's (Table 11, p. 433) and the renal function. The excretion of TC is affected by liver and kidney diseases and thus, in such patients, the dose should be reduced or derivatives less strongly influenced by the renal function, such as chlor-TC or doxy-TC, should be used. The latter's excretion is thought to be perhaps partly switched over to the faecal route, via the enterohepatic circulation. Direct excretion into the lumen of the small intestine is also considered as a possibility. Table 1 lists the TC concentrations in the serum of patients after oral and intravenous administration.

References

Albaum G, Konrad RM, Thum HJ (1964) Untersuchungen über den Antibiotika-Spiegel im Pleuraexsudat nach Thorax-Eingriffen und prophylaktischer intravenöser Applikation von Oxytetracyclin. Arzneimittelforsch 14:1137–1139

Antalovská Z, Beran J (1966) The fluorescence of tetracycline antibiotics (TA) in the hard dental tissues in an experiment. In: Herold M, Gabriel Z (eds) Antibiotics – Advances in research, production and clinical use. London: Butterworths, Prague: Czechoslovak Medical Press, pp 392–396

Arima K, Izaki K (1963) Accumulation of oxytetracycline relevant to its bacterial action in the cells of Escherichia coli. Nature 200:192–193

Benazet F, Dubost M, Jolles G, Leau O, Pascal C, Preudhomme J, Terlain B (1968) Liaisons et modifications des antibiotiques in vivo (sang et foyer infectieux). Biologie Médicale 57:376–401
Bergogne-Berezin E, Morel C, Even P, Benard Y, Kafe H, Berthelot G, Pierre J, Lambert-Zechovsky N (1978) Pharmacokinetic study of antibiotics in human respiratory tract. Nouv Presse Méd 7:2831–2836
Berrettini B (1968) Contents of ampicillin and doxycycline in the human tonsil. Chemotherapy 13:362–365
Böcker R, Estler C-J, Weber A (1982) Metabolism of doxycycline. Lancet II:1155
Böcker R, Estler C-J (1983) Formation and disposition of a metabolite of doxycycline. Naunyn-Schmiedebergs Arch Pharmacol 322 Suppl: R112
Brázda O (1964) Inkorporation von Tetrazyklinen in Zähnen. Dtsch Stomat 14:780–787
Brázda O, Kolc J, Zástava V (1966) The deposition of tetracyclines in hard dental tissues. In: Herold M, Gabriel Z (eds) Antibiotics – Advances in research, production and clinical use. London: Butterworths, Prague: Czechoslovak Medical Press, pp 397–400
Buyske DA, Eisner HJ, Kelly RG (1960) Concentration and persistence of tetracycline and chlortetracycline in bone. J Pharmacol Exp Ther 130:150–156
Černá J, Rychlík I, Pulkrábek P (1969) The effect of antibiotics on the coded binding of peptidyl-t-RNA to the ribosome and on the transfer of the peptidyl residue to puromycin. Eur J Biochem 9:27–35
Clauberg C (1979) Doxycyclin-Spiegel in Lungen- und Bronchialgewebe. MMW 121:1469–1470
Cundliffe E, McQuillen K (1967) Bacterial protein synthesis: The effect of antibiotics. J Mol Biol 30:137–146
Dürckheimer W (1975) Tetracycline: Chemie, Biochemie und Struktur-Wirkungs-Beziehungen. Angew Chem 87:751–784
Ehrlich GE (1972) Concentrations of tetracycline and minocycline in joint effusions following oral administration. Pennsylvania Med J 75:47–49
Eisner HJ, Wulf RJ (1963) The metabolic fate of chlortetracycline and some comparisons with other tetracyclines. J Pharmacol Exp Ther 142:122–131
Fabre J, Pitton JS, Kunz JP (1966) Distribution and excretion of doxycycline in man. Chemotherapia 11:73–85
Fabre J, Pitton JS, Vivieux C, Laurencet FL, Bernhardt JP, Godel JC (1967) Absorption, distribution et excrétion d'un nouvel antibiotique à large spectre chez l'homme. Schweiz Med Wochenschr 97:915–924
Finerman GAM, Milch RA (1963) *In vitro* binding of tetracyclines to calcium. Nature 198:486–487
Fabre J, Blanchard P, Rudhardt M (1977) Pharmacokinetics of ampicillin, cephalothin and doxycycline in various tissues of the rat. Chemotherapy 23:129–141
Gauze GG, Fatkullina IG, Dolgilevich SM (1971) Effect of antibiotics with different mechanisms of action on incorporation of labeled desoxynucleoside triphosphates to DNA of isolated rat liver mitochondria. Antibiotiki 17:296–301
Goldberg IH (1965) Mode of action of antibiotics. Am J Med 39:722–752
Gottesman ME (1967) Reaction of ribosome-bound peptidyl transfer ribonucleic acid with aminoacyl transfer ribonucleic acid or puromycin. J Biol Chem 242:5564–5571
Hansson E, Hanngren Ä, Ullberg S (1966) Autoradiographic distribution studies with labelled penicillin, streptomycin, tetracycline and cycloserine. In: Herold M, Gabriel Z (eds) Antibiotics – Advances in research, production and clinical use. London: Butterworths, Prague: Czechoslovak Medical Press, pp 156–164
Hartnett BJS, Marlin GE (1976) Doxycycline in serum and bronchial secretions. Thorax 31:144–148
Hawkins KI (1972) Fluorometric determination of demethylchlortetracycline and tetracycline in mammalian bone. Analytic Biochem 45:128–136
Hopf G (1963) Comparative evaluation of the hepatotoxicity of tetracycline in old and medium-aged female mice. Naunyn-Schmiedebergs Arch Pharmacol 322 Suppl: R118
Izaki K, Arima K (1963) Disappearance of oxytetracycline accumulation in the cells of multiple drug-resistant Escherichia coli. Nature 200:384–385

Izaki K, Arima K (1965) Effect of various conditions on accumulation of oxytetracycline in Escherichia coli. J Bacteriol 89:1335–1339
Izaki K, Kiuchi K, Arima K (1966) Specificity and mechanism of tetracycline resistance in a multiple drug resistant strain of Escherichia coli. J Bacteriol 91:628–633
Johnson NW (1966) The distribution and stability of tetracyclines in dental tissues. In: Herold M, Gabriel Z (eds) Antibiotics – Advances in research, production and clinical use. London: Butterworths, Prague: Czechoslovak Medical Press, pp 378–391
Kahán IL, Kulka F, Vigh E (1977) Klinische und experimentelle Erfahrungen bei intravenöser Verabreichung von Tri-doxycyclin. Pneumonol Hung 30:104–109
Kelly RG, Buyske DA (1960) Metabolism of tetracycline in the rat and the dog. J Pharmacol Exp Ther 130:144–149
Kelly RG, Kanegis LA, Buyske DA (1961) The metabolism and tissue distribution of radio-isotopically labeled demethylchlortetracycline. J Pharmacol 134:320–324
Krüger-Thiemer E †, Kröger H, Nestler HJ, Seydel JK (1975) Wirkungsmodi antituberkulöser Chemotherapeutika: Tetracycline. In: Meissner G, Schmiedel A †, Nelles A † (Hrsg) Infektionskrankheiten und ihre Erreger, Band 4, Teil III. Fischer, Jena, pp 353–357
Kunin CM, Finland M (1961) Clinical pharmacology of the tetracycline antibiotics. Clin Pharmacol Ther 2:51–69
Laskin AJ, Last JA (1971) Tetracycline. Antibiot Chemother 17:1–28 (M)
MacArthur CGC, Johnson AJ, Chadwick MV, Wingfield HJ (1978) The absorption and sputum penetration of doxycycline. Antimicrob Chemother 4:509–514
Malek P, Cervinka F, Zastava V, Demelova M, Kolc J (1966a) A method of ascertaining the biological activity of the fixed form of tetracycline antibiotics in tissues. In: Herold M, Gabriel Z (eds) Antibiotics – Advances in research, production and clinical use. London: Butterworths, Prague: Czechoslovak Medical Press, pp 131–136
Malek P, Zastava V, Kolc J (1966b) The distribution of tetracycline antibiotics in shock and in uremia. In: Herold M, Gabriel Z (eds) Antibiotics – Advances in research, production and clinical use. London: Butterworths, Prague: Czechoslovak Medical Press, pp 207–212
Marlin GE, Cheng S, Thompson PJ (1981) Sputum and plasma doxycycline concentrations after a single oral 600 mg doxycycline dose in patients with chronic bronchitis. Eur J Respir Dis 62:276–280
Marschang A, Diezel PB, Klein G (1978) Die Konzentrationen von Doxycyclin im Blutserum und Bronchialsekret. Prax Pneumol 32:271–273
Nelis HJCF, de Leenheer AP (1981) Unique metabolic fate of a tetracycline (minocycline). Lancet II:938
Oklund SA, Prolo DJ, Gutierrez RV (1981) The significance of yellow bone. Evidence for tetracycline in adult human bone. JAMA 246:761–763
Ondracek Z, Zastava V (1966) Gall bladder diseases and tetracycline antibiotics. In: Herold M, Gabriel Z (eds) Antibiotics – Advances in research, production and clinical use. London: Butterworths, Prague: Czechoslovak Medical Press, pp 127–130
Pohl W (1964) Demethylchlortetracyclin in Punktaten seröser Höhlen. Arzneimittelforsch 14:1058–1059
Schach von Wittenau M, Twomey TM (1971) The disposition of doxycycline by man and dog. Chemotherapy 16:217–228
Schach von Wittenau M, Yeary R (1963) The excretion and distribution in body fluids of tetracyclines after intravenous administration to dogs. J Pharmacol 140:258–266
Schach von Wittenau M, Twomey TM, Swindell AC (1972) The disposition of doxycycline by the rat. Chemotherapy 17:26–39
Simon C, Sommerwerck D, Friehoff J (1978) Der Wert von Doxycyclin bei Atemwegsinfektionen (Serum-, Speichel-, Sputum-, Lungen- und Pleuraexsudatspiegel). Prax Pneumol 32:266–270
Sommerwerck D, Simon C, Friehoff J (1978) Minocyclin zur Therapie von Atemwegsinfektionen. Dtsch Med Wschr 103:822–825
Taber LH, Yow MD, Nieberg FG (1967) The penetration of broad-spectrum antibiotics into the cerebrospinal fluid. Ann NY Acad Sci 145:473–481

Thadepalli H, Mandal AK, Bach VT, Oparah SS (1980) Tissue levels of doxycycline in the human lung and pleura. Chest 78:304–305
Videau D (1968) Pénétration, site et mode d'action des antibiotiques chez la bactérie. Biol Méd 57:449–470
Winkler E, Weih H (1967) Doxycyclin. Ergebnisse von Basisuntersuchungen. Med Klin 62:1257–1262
Zimmermann I, Ulmer WT, Ritzerfeld W (1977) Tetracyclin-Spiegel im Sputum bei chronisch-obstruktiver Bronchitis. MMW 119:845–848

VII. VM

1. Mode of Action

In the cross-resistance between VM, CM, SM, and KM (GILL HAN BAI and SUNG CHIN KIM 1980) particularly close relationships are discernible between VM and CM (TRNKA et al. 1964, 1966; TSUKAMURA 1969), and a common site of attack is therefore assumed for these two antibiotics. The incorporation of amino acids different from those in a control experiment was at first attributed to an erroneous reading of the genetic code (GOLDBERG 1965). However, according to the results of more recent studies, an inhibition of protein synthesis takes place primarily (TANAKA and IGURA 1968), either as a result of a disturbance in the formation of the initial complex from 30-S and 50-S ribosomes and m-RNA or of a hindered transport of peptidyl-RNA from the ribosomal A- to P-sites (LIOU and TANAKA 1976; WURMBACH and NIERHAUS 1979). In *M. smegmatis*, depending on the degree of resistance, VM causes modifications of the 30-S or 50-S ribosomes (YAMADA et al. 1972).

2. Biotransformation

After the passage through the macroorganism, 63%–100% of the administered dose is excreted with the urine (HÖFFLER 1981), but no biotransformation products have so far been detected.

3. Pharmacokinetics

VM is distributed very rapidly and solely in the extracellular space. No data are available on its binding to the serum proteins. Immediately after its intravenous infusion, 180 μg–200 μg VM/ml appear in the lungs. The concentrations may therefore correspond to those reached in the serum (KUGEL et al. 1965; see Table 1 for the serum concentrations after i.m. administration). VM diffuses only to a very small extent into serous cavities and other compartments, less than 40% of

Table 1. Concentration of viomycin in the serum of 9 healthy volunteers after intramuscular injection of 1 g of the active substance (BARTMANN et al. 1956)

Time after injection	1 h	2 h	4 h	6 h
Extremes μg/ml	66–20	66–25	33–10	33–5
Mean values μg/ml	40	42	20	15

the serum VM concentration being measured at such sites (MORDASINI and EULENBERGER 1971). Only very small fractions of VM reach the placenta and the foetus (ROBSON and SULLIVAN 1963; WALTER and HEILMEYER 1969; SENECA 1971). VM undergoes glomerular filtration; the dose given should be governed by the renal function (HÖFFLER 1981, Table 10, p. 426). Further pharmacokinetic parameters are given in Tables 7–9 and 11 of the General Part (pp. 423–425, 433).

References

Bartmann K, Blisse A, Zander J (1956) Bakteriologische Untersuchungen über die Wirkung von Viomycin auf Tuberkelbakterien. Beitr Klin Tuberk 115:211–222

Gill Han Bai, Sung Chin Kim (1980) Study on tuberactinomycin-N (TUM-N) (Part II). Crossresistance of tubercle bacilli to TUM N, VM, CPM, KM, and SM. Tuberc Respir Dis 27:19–26

Goldberg IH (1965) Mode of action of antibiotics. Am J Med 39:722–752

Höffler D (1981) Die Dosierung wichtiger Antibiotika und Tuberkulostatika bei Niereninsuffizienz. Internist (Berlin) 22:601–606

Kugel E, Polz E, Schmiedel A (1965) Erfahrungen über die Infusionsbehandlung mit Viocin. Beitr Klin Tuberk 131:291–299

Liou YF, Tanaka N (1976) Dual actions of viomycin on the ribosomal functions. Biochem Biophys Res Commun 71:477–483

Mordasini ER, Eulenberger J (1971) Tuberkulostatika, Teil 1. Int J Clin Pharmacol Ther Toxicol 4:467–486 (Ph)

Robson JM, Sullivan FM (1963) Antituberculosis drugs. Pharmacol Rev 15:169–223 (B, Ph)

Seneca H (1971) Biological basis of chemotherapy of infections and infestations. Davis, Philadelphia (Ph)

Tanaka N, Igura S (1968) Effects of viomycin and polymycin B on protein synthesis in vitro. J Antibiot (Tokyo) 21:239–240

Trnka L, Kuska J, Havel A (1964) Zur Problematik der antimykobakteriellen Wirkung und Kreuzresistenz von Capreomycin. Prax Pneumol 18:798–802

Trnka L, Havel A, Urbancik R (1966) Neueste Tuberkulostatika, ihre Bedeutung und Möglichkeiten der Wertbestimmung im Reagenzglas. Chemotherapia 11:121–134

Tsukamura M (1969) Cross-resistance relationship between capreomycin, kanamycin and viomycin resistance in tubercle bacilli from patients. Am Rev Respir Dis 99:780–782

Walter AM, Heilmeyer L (1969) Antibiotika-Fibel. 3. Auflage. Heilmeyer L, Otten H, Plempel M (Hrsg) Thieme, Stuttgart

Wurmbach P, Nierhaus KH (1979) Codon-anticodon interaction at the ribosomal P (peptidyl-t-RNA) site. Proc Natl Acad Sci USA 76:2143–2147

Yamada T, Masuda K, Shoji K, Hori M (1972) Analysis of ribosomes from viomycin-sensitive and -resistant strains of *Mycobacterium smegmatis*. J Bacteriol 112:1–6

VIII. CS

1. Mode of Action

D-CS is taken up by *E. coli* with a transport system specific to glycine and D-alanine, while L-alanine penetrates into the cell via another system inaccessible to CS. The reduced uptake of CS by resistant microorganisms, especially CS-resistant *E. coli*, is due to a drastic (up to 90%) reduction of the glycine-D-alanine transport system (WARGEL et al. 1970, 1971).

CS exerts a bacteriostatic activity when cell destruction by autolysins which become active immediately after contact with CS is prevented (ROGERS and

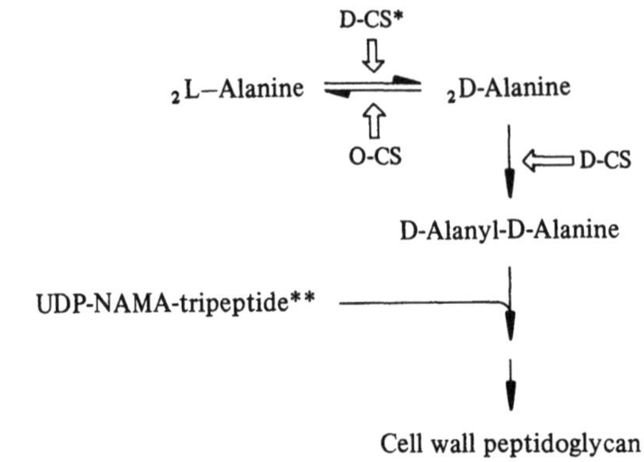

Fig. 1. Sites of attack of CS (D-CS) and o-carbamyl-D-serine (O-CS) in the mucopeptide synthesis of microorganisms (DAVID 1970b). * only at high concentrations of D-cycloserine (2.4×10^{-4} M or higher); ** Uridine diphosphate-*N*-acetyl muramyl-tripeptide in most bacteria. Uridin diphosphate -*N*-acetyl glycolyl muramyl-D-alanyl-D-glutamyl- meso diaminopimelic acid in *Mycobacterium tuberculosis*

FORSBERG 1971). Damage to the cell wall can be seen in the electron microscope (IMAEDA et al. 1968). The accumulation of amino sugars in the culture filtrate indicates the CS-induced disturbance of mucopeptide formation necessary for the synthesis of reticular mureine (see General Part, p. 408).

In mycobacteria this disturbance ultimately results in a loss of stability to acid.

CS inhibits the two enzymes necessary for the formation of the dipeptide D-alanyl-D-alanine (Fig. 1), the synthetase being inhibited more strongly than the racemase. At low concentrations the point of attack of CS is on the donor side of the enzyme. The binding is 100 times as strong as that of D-alanine. There is thus no difference from synthetases of other microorganisms, and the greater sensitivity of mycobacteria to CS must be determined by other factors (DAVID et al. 1969). Of the antagonists, D-alanine – as one would expect – has the strongest activity. For steric reasons L-CS is always inactive (ZYGMUNT 1963; STROMINGER and TIPPER 1965; CURTIS et al. 1965).

The racemase is also inhibited by o-carbamyl-D-serine; on combination of the latter compound with CS a synergistic effect can be observed (Fig. 1, DAVID 1970a, b). However, the inhibition of the racemase by o-carbamyl-D-serine cannot be eliminated by D-alanine.

Further-reaching disturbances, e.g. of the aminotransferase activity of *E. coli*, occur only at higher CS concentrations. The intervention in the protein spectrum of *Micrococcus lysodeikticus* established under similar conditions (GRULA and KING 1971) probably indicates incipient metabolic dysfunction.

2. Biotransformation

It is difficult to evaluate the results obtained previously on this problem by microbiological methods, since the tendency of CS to form biologically inactive dimerization products in aqueous solution even at normal temperature was only discovered relatively late (WARGEL et al. 1970).

A considerable proportion of the administered dose cannot be detected in the excyctions, neither by nitroprusside sodium – staining nor by microbiological methods. After parenteral administration the biologically active fraction is invariably higher than that after oral administration, so that the possibility of inactivation already setting in the gastrointestinal tract must be considered. For organ homogenates too the conclusion of a conversion of CS must be drawn, since, as in-vitro experiments, a reduced biological activity is found after the passage through the organism. However, the in-vitro and in-vivo degradations do not follow strictly parallel courses (FREERKSEN et al. 1959; CREMA and BERTE 1960; HANSSON et al. 1966). If ring cleavage, possibly occurring with the aid of a cycloamides, is assumed to be the cause of these activity losses (nitroprusside sodium test negative), the expected degradation product serine, ammonium ions, water, etc. can be reliably detected only after labelling of CS with radioactive or stable isotopes because of the ubiquitous nature of their occurrence. Increased excretion of ammonium ions has been established in 40 tuberculosis patient following CS therapy (SMIRNOV 1977).

In the urine of guinea pigs and mice a biotransformation product stainable with nitroprusside sodium and not consisting of acetyl-CS has been detected. The incidence of small quantities of this compound, whose structure is still unknown, was confirmed in subsequent investigations.

3. Pharmacokinetics of CS

CS is absorbed more slowly than INH or PAS. A CS derivative, terizidone (4,4′-phenylene-bis-(methylamine)-bis-3-isoazolidine) is absorbed more rapidly and more quantitatively than CS itself (GAIDOV 1971; ZITKOVA and TOUSEK 1973). As with INH, simultaneous consumption of food delays and reduces the absorption of CS (KOROTAEV and TATARINOVA 1972).

CS does not become bound to serum proteins. It is distributed throughout the body water. After oral administration to man the CS concentrations in most of the organs are higher than that in the serum (see Tables 1–3 for CS and teridizone concentrations in the blood or the serum). Particularly high concentrations are measured in the salivary glands, the testicles, the epididymis, and in serous cavities. About 50% of the serum concentration is localized in the CSF (Table 7, see p. 423). After subcutaneous administration to rats the concentration in the liver and lungs is about one-third of the concentration in the serum, while that in the

Table 1. CS concentrations in the blood of 385 tuberculosis patients (536 individual curves, KRACKHARDT 1960)

Administration of the drug	250 mg ↓		250 mg ↓		250 mg ↓		250 mg ↓		
Cs concentration, μg/ml		15,7		19,2		22,5			6–7
Time of blood sample withdrawal, h	0	3	6	9	12	15	18	21	24

Table 2. CS concentrations in the blood in dependence of the body weight after administration of a unifrom dose of 1 g (KRACKHARDT 1960)

Body weight, kg	<55	56–60	61–65	66–70	71–75	76–80	81–85	86–90
CS concentration, µg/ml	28,1	25,1	25,9	22,0	23,4	22,4	21,0	19,4
Daily dose, mg/kg body weight	>18,2	16,7	15,4	14,3	13,3	12,5	11,7	11,1

Table 3. Course of the concentrations of CS and terizidone in the serum (µg/ml) of tuberculosis patients after oral administration of 0.5 g (ZITKOVA and TOUSEK 1973)

Drug	*n*	Time of blood sample withdrawal (h)								
		1	2	3	4	6	8	9	12	24
500 mg										
CS	15	8,4	14,1	14,4	12,7	11,0	9,5	8,6	6,7	3,3
Terizidone	14	12,0	16,1	16,3	14,9	13,5	11,9	10,7	7,8	5,9

Table 4. Excretion of CS (% of the administered dose) in the 24-h urine after administration of 1 g of CS (KRACKHARDT 1960)

Patient	1st day	2nd day	3rd day	4th day	5th day	Individual means
K.H.	33,4	37,1	26,4	32,4	46,5	35,2
I.L.	32,1	33,7	37,1	38,7	46,0	37,5
S.H.	41,4	46,8	51,5	33,7	43,1	43,3
L.W.	40,8	49,3	43,6	67,7	48,5	50,0
M.K.	34,5	49,6	21,1	41,8	33,1	36,0
H.M.	33,9	47,0	47,5	49,3	51,5	45,8
W.J.	44,4	61,0	32,9	35,9	55,2	45,9
H.H.	51,8	48,8	45,1	29,7	51,9	45,5
W.A.	47,3	43,0	39,0	30,8	25,7	37,2
H.C.	26,1	48,7	52,2	39,2	28,1	38,9
Mean daily value	38,6	46,5	39,6	39,9	43,0	

kidneys is very much higher. Only small quantities are found in the brain. Repeated investigations on the same individual yield extensively consistent values (CREMA and BERTE 1960).

CS is excreted by the renal route (Table 8, p. 424), up to 47% of the administered dose being recovered in the urine (KRACKHARDT 1960; STEPANIANE et al. 1960, Table 4). In the dog the renal clearance corresponds to the glomerular filtration rate. The excretion is unaffected by probenecid (FREERKSEN et al. 1959).

Accordingly, in renal impairment CS is found to be eliminated more slowly. If treatment is necessary, the dose should be reduced corresponding to the kidney function (Table 10, p. 426 – WARESKA et al. 1963; KOROTAEV and TATARINOVA 1972; JUNGBLUTH 1973; HÖFFLER 1981).

The age-determined reduction of the renal clearance means that CS and terizidone are excreted less resulting in an increased CS level in the serum and a prolonged $t_{50\%}$ (MATTILA et al. 1969; ZITKOVA and TOUSEK 1973, 1978).

The wide variation of the $t_{50\%}$ among the individual species must likewise be attributed to a correspondingly modified elimination (elimination half-lives: mouse 0.6 h–3.7 h, rat 1.8 h, guinea pig 0.7 h–1.7 h, rhesus monkey 2.1 h–12.5 h, baboon 4.5 h, man 7 h–15 h, Table 3, p. 494). There is no correlation between the $t_{50\%}$ and the extent of the CS excretion with the urine. On the other hand, animal experiments have revealed the expected close correlation between the $t_{50\%}$ and the therapeutic activity. For further data on the pharmacokinetics see Tables 3, 9, and 11 of the General Part, pp. 419, 425, 433).

References

Crema A, Berté F (1960) Über die Verteilung und Stoffwechsel des Cycloserins bei der Ratte. Naunyn-Schmiedebergs Arch Pharmacol 239:475–480

Curtis R, Charamella LJ, Berg CM, Harris PE (1965) Kinetic and genetic analyses of D-cycloserine inhibition and resistance in Escherichia coli. J Bacteriol 90:1238–1250

David HL (1970a) Effect of o-carbamyl-D-serine on the growth of *Mycobacterium tuberculosis*. Am Rev Respir Dis 102:68–74

David HL (1970b) Susceptibility of Mycobacterium intracellulare to o-carbamyl-D-serine. Am Rev Respir Dis 102:105–106

David HL, Takayama K, Goldman DS (1969) Susceptibility of mycobacterial D-alanyl-D-alanine synthetase to D-cycloserine. Am Rev Respir Dis 100:579–581

Freerksen E, Krüger-Thiemer E, Rosenfeld M (1959) Cycloserin (D-4-Amino-isoxazolidin-3-on). Antibiot Chemother 6:303–396 (Ph)

Gaidov N (1971) Terisidon – a new synthetic tuberculosis-suppressing antibiotic. Probl Tuberk 49 issue 12: 19–22

Grula EA, King RD (1971) Changes in the cell membranes of dividing and nondividing cells of Micrococcus lysodeikticus disIIp^{+}. Biochem Biophys Res Commun 44:1356–1363

Hansson E, Hanngren Ä, Ullberg S (1966) Autoradiographic distribution studies with labelled penicillin, streptomycin, tetracycline and cycloserine. In: Herold M, Gabriel Z (eds) Antibiotics – Advances in research, production and clinical use. London: Butterworths, Prague: Czechoslovak Medical Press, pp 156–164

Höffler D (1981) Die Dosierung wichtiger Antibiotika und Tuberkulostatika bei Niereninsuffizienz. Internist (Berlin) 22:601–606

Imaeda T, Kanetsuna F, Rieber M (1968) In vitro effect of cycloserine on mycobacterial ultrastructure. Tubercle 49:385–396

Jungbluth H (1973) Tuberkulose-Chemotherapie bei Kranken mit vorgeschädigter Niere. Prax Pneumol 27:175–182

Korotaev GA, Tatarinova NV (1972) Content of cycloserine in the blood serum and its discharge with the urine in patients with tuberculosis. Therap Arch 44:81–84

Krackhardt H (1960) Blutspiegel und Ausscheidung des Cycloserins bei länger dauernder Medikation. Schweiz Z Tuberk 17:403–416

Mattila MJ, Nieminen E, Tiitinen H (1969) Serum levels, urinary excretion, and side-effects of cycloserine in the presence of isoniazid and p-aminosalicylic acid. Scand J Respir Dis 50:291–300

Rogers HJ, Forsberg CW (1971) Role of autolysins in the killing of bacteria by some bactericidal antibiotics. J Bacteriol 108:1235–1243

Smirnov GA (1977) Decomposition of the hina and cycloserine preparations in the organism of patients with tuberculosis of the lungs. Probl Tuberk 55 issue 8: 63–66
Stépaniane ES, Bréguer MA, Boligne IP (1960) Concentration de cyclosérine dans le sang et son excrétion. Probl Tuberk 38 issue 3: 89–94
Strominger JL, Tipper DJ (1965) Bacterial cell wall synthesis and structure in relation to the mechanism of action of penicillins and other antibacterial agents. Am J Med 39:708–721
Wareska W, Klott M, Izdebska-Makosa Z (1963) Cycloserine excretion in cases of renal diseases. Gruzlica 31:664–668
Wargel RJ, Shadur CA, Neuhaus FC (1970) Mechanism of D-cycloserine action: transport systems for D-alanine, D-cycloserine, L-alanine, and glycine. J Bacteriol 103:778–788
Wargel RJ, Shadur CA, Neuhaus FC (1971) Mechanism of D-cycloserine action: transport mutants for D-alanine, D-cycloserine and glycine. J Bacteriol 105:1028–1035
Zitkova L, Tousek J (1973) Resorption and elimination of terizidone (Bracco) compared with cycloserine (Spofa). Stud Pneumol Phtiseol Cechoslov 33:37–43
Zitkova L, Toushek I (1978) Pharmacokinetics of cycloserin and ethambutol. Probl Tuberk 56 issue 3: 23–25
Zygmunt WA (1963) Antagonism of D-cycloserine inhibition of mycobacterial growth by D-alanine. J Bacteriol 85:1217–1220

IX. ETH/PTH

1. Mode of Action

Because of its unpleasant side effects (smell and taste sensations, gastric and intestinal disturbances, and others), ETH/PTH has always been used only in patients with monoresistant or polyresistant mycobacteria. The interactions between these antituberculotics and mycobacteria have therefore aroused no more than limited interest. The mode of action probably corresponds largely to that of the thiosemicarbazones (TSC) and thiocarbanilides (DATC) (KRÜGER-THIEMER et al. 1975). In addition, inhibition of mycolic acid synthesis can be observed (WINDER 1982). This intervention probably results in the loss of stability to acids. The influence of ETH on mycobacterial growth in the depth of agar media indicates the questions still to be answered, as does the cross-resistance between ETH and TSC, which is believed to be based on a common process in the uptake of these antituberculotics into the mycobacterial cell (WINDER 1982).

2. Biotransformation

The biotransformation of ETH/PTH has been the subject of more thorough investigation in view of the close structural connections with INH, although considerable methodological difficulties have arisen.

a) Possibilities of Assay of ETH, PTH, and Their Biotransformation Products

In both compounds the ethyl or propyl group (in ETH and PTH respectively) localized in the α-position prevents cleavage of the pyridine ring such as takes place in INH or INA. e.g., in the course of the reaction with bromocyanogen. Thus, it is impossible to determine the total excretion of ETH or PTH. However, ETH and some of its biotransformation products can be determined spectrophotometrically or polarographically (SIMÁNE and KRAUS 1962; IWAINSKY et al. 1964, 1965; PÜTTER 1964; GRUNERT and IWAINSKY 1971 a; TIKHONOV et al 1976). If the renal excretion of ETH and its biotransformation products are investigated difficulties arise, some of them expected, in the spectrophotometric determinations of the mixtures present in the urine. The use of different methods gave different results for the same material; nor was it possible to eliminate the interference completely, even with improved techniques (GRUNERT and IWAINSKY 1971 b; PÜTTER 1972). So far only 7% of the administered dose has been quantitatively determined in urinary excretion. The proportion of other biotransformation products isolated by ion-exchange chromatography, such as the amide of ethylisonicotinic acid or ethylisonicotinic acid (JOHNSTON et al. 1967) can for the time being only be estimated, though it never exceeds 5% of the quantity administered.

b) Reversible Conversion of ETH and PTH into the Corresponding Sulphoxides

After the addition of hydrogen peroxide to a solution of ETH or PTH the solution turns deep yellow with the formation of the corresponding sulphoxide. These sulphoxides exhibit a specific absorption curve. After the administration of ETH the absorption curves of serum and urine samples are modified in an analogous fashion and thus indicate the formation of the sulphoxide as biotransformation product (Fig. 1). The unchanged ETH and its sulphoxide are evidently in equilibrium, the sulphoxide having a comparable biological activity and being separated off with the aid of thin-layer or paper chromatography (GRUNERT and IWAINSKY 1971 b; PÜTTER 1972). The sulphoxides are formed rapidly, being already detectable 15 min after administration of the drugs, and in mouse organs account for

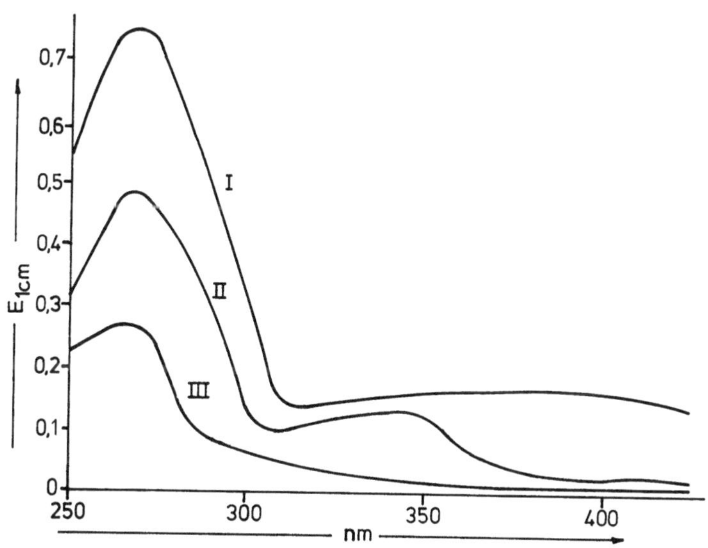

Fig. 1. Formation of the sulphoxide in the macroorganism after intravenous infusion of ETH (GRUNERT and IWAINSKY 1971c). Absorption curve of the urine extract. I:0–6 h after infusion; II:6–12 h after infusion; III:12–24 h after infusion

approximately 15% of the administered dose (GRUNERT and IWAINSKY 1967). Even in the case of thioacetamide, the simplest representative of this substance group, the respective sulphoxide is formed as a biotransformation product. The reaction is therefore regarded as the general route of the biotransformation of thioamides (AMMON et al. 1967).

As one would expect, the stability of a compound has a considerable bearing on its pharmacokinetics. After the administration of the sulphoxide, therefore, the ETH concentration in the organism is substantially lower than after the administration of ETH itself, owing to the low stability and the slower rate at which equilibrium sets in in the case of the former. Apart from the greater difficulties in manufacturing, this behaviour in the macroorganism was the reason why the sulphoxide is not used in therapeutic practice, even though it would have been better suited than ETH for infusion therapy (the usual procedure in the mid-1960's) owing to its water solubility.

c) Biotransformation Products of ETH and PTH

In addition to the sulphoxide, a number of other ETH biotransformation products have been detected by a wide variety of methods (Fig. 2). N-Methylpyridinium compounds are formed by methylation at the ring nitrogen. During hydroxylation of the ring nitrogen unstable 6-hydroxy compounds are formed, which re-

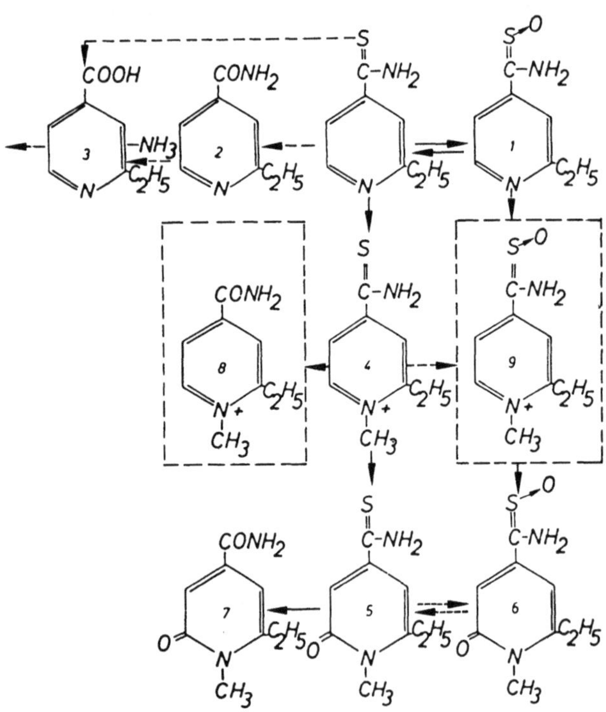

Fig. 2. Biotransformation products of ETH. *1* ETH sulphoxide; *2* amide of 2-ethylisonicotinic acid; *3* 2-ethylisonicotinic acid; *4, 8, 9* N-methylpyridinium compounds; *5, 6, 7* 6-oxodihydropyridine derivatives

arrange into 6-oxodihydropyridines. Each of these series of compounds is associated with other reactions known for ETH or PTH, namely with sulphoxide formation and conversion into the amide of the acid. Loss of the amide group has so far been observed only in the case of the amide of ethylisonicotinic acid (GRUNERT 1969; RITTER 1973). Some of these biotransformation products are fluorescent (BIEDER and MAZEAU 1964; JOHNSTON et al. 1967). This property is also used to check the ETH uptake (VENKATARAMAN et al. 1967), since a positive result is a reliable indicator of the passage of ETH through the organism.

d) Biotransformation of ETH and PTH in Man and in Animals

So far as many as 7 biotransformation products have been detected in the mouse, 4 only in low concentrations or only on occasion; 8 respectively 4 have been detected in the rat, 15 respectively 7 in the dog, and up to 7 in man. In contrast to other organs, only ETH, sulphoxide, and the amide of ethylisonicotinic acid can be determined in the gastric juice by thin-layer chromatography (JOHNSTON et al. 1967; GRUNERT 1969; GRUNERT and IWAINSKY 1971 b).

Three absorption maxima are evident in the chloroform extract of human urine after the administration of ETH. The maximum at 260 nm to 270 nm is due to ETH, the amide of ethylisonicotinic acid, and other substances. The maximum at 320 nm to 340 nm indicates the presence of oxomethylsulphoxide and three other fluorescing biotransformation products, while the maximum at 395 nm is caused by sulphoxide.

Studies on 156 urine samples of 0 h–6 h urine indicate the rapid onset of the biotransformation processes by the absence of the first maximum (Table 1). The majority of the urine samples exhibit a maximum at 320 nm to 340 nm, i.e., oxomethylsulphoxide and other compounds are present. A maximum indicating the presence of sulphoxide is only evident in one-third of the patients in the 0 h–6 h urine, thus emphasizing once again the low degree of stability of this biotransformation product. Methyl-ETH constitutes the main determinable excretion product (~65%, GRUNERT 1969; GRUNERT and IWAINSKY 1971 b, c). The constant position of the absorption maximum in 12 out of 13 patients, most of whom were studied on more than one occasion, could be indicative of the presence of specific biotransformation types.

Whereas the sulphoxide formation by ETH or PTH has no essential effect on their biological activity, no antimycobacterial activity has as yet been demon-

Table 1. Influence of the time of excretion on the position of the absorption maxima in the urine (infusion of 500 mg of ETH as the hydrochloride, measurement on the chloroform extract, GRUNERT and IWAINSKY 1971c)

Urine collection time	No. of samples with maximum		No maximum
	At 320 nm–340 nm	At 395 nm	
0 h– 6 h	33	16	3
6 h–12 h	45	0	7
12 h–24 h	35	0	17

strated for the other biotransformation products. Loss of the sulphur group in accordance with the postulated action mechanism is definitely always associated with a loss of biological activity.

3. Pharmacokinetics

Like INH, ETH and PTH are distributed rapidly and completely throughout the body water, the equilibrium setting in within 20 min. No signs of organ-specific accumulation or retention of ETH have been found (GREENBERG and EIDUS 1962; HAMILTON et al. 1962; PÜTTER 1964). The sulphoxide fraction detectable after the administration of ETH is between 15% and 20% in the individual organs and substantially lower only in the liver (GRUNERT and IWAINSKY 1967). In comparison with the serum, the ETH concentrations in the lungs are slightly lower and in tuberculous lesions some 80%–95% of the concentration in the serum (EULE and WERNER 1964; EULE 1965; TSUKAMURA 1972). The question whether ETH and PTH cross the placenta to pass into the foetus has not yet been answered. ETH and PTH diffuse into the CSF and, like INH and RMP, are still suitable for the therapy of meningitis tuberculosa (PILHEU 1975; Table 7, p. 423).

After intravenous infusion of ETH hydrochloride (see Table 2 for the serum concentrations), because of its pKa value ETH diffuses from the bloodstream into the gastric juice, where it reaches concentrations far above those determined in the serum (Fig. 3). There is a statistically significant correlation between the acidity of the gastric juice and the ETH concentration (Fig. 4; IWAINSKY et al. 1965; GRUNERT 1969; GRUNERT and IWAINSKY 1971 c). Because of the greater stability of ETH in gastric juice and the strong suppression of biotransformation that takes place there, the gastric juice represents a deep compartment for ETH and its sulphoxide. It is responsible for the non-exponential fall of the serum ETH concentration that varies from experiment to experiment in one and the same individual. Rectal administration in particular leads to considerable inconsistencies of the ETH concentration in the serum (EULE 1965, Table 3).

Only up to 5% of an administered dose can be detected as ETH or its biotransformation products in the urine on the basis of their specific absorption curves, 1% being in the form of the biologically active fraction (RIST 1960; GREENBERG and EIDUS 1962; IWAINSKY et al. 1963, 1965; PÜTTER 1964; EULE 1965; GRUNERT and IWAINSKY 1967; JOHNSTON et al. 1967). Excretion with the bile is considered as a possibility (GREENBERG and EIDUS 1962). However, despite intensive searches, no appreciable spectrophotometrically determinable fractions of ETH

Table 2. Course of ETH concentration in serum (μg/ml) of tuberculosis patients after intravenous infusion of 500 mg of ETH (GRUNERT (1969)

n	End of infusion	Blood sample taken thereafter at		
		1.5 h	3 h	4.5 h
26	7.0	3.4	2.6	1.9

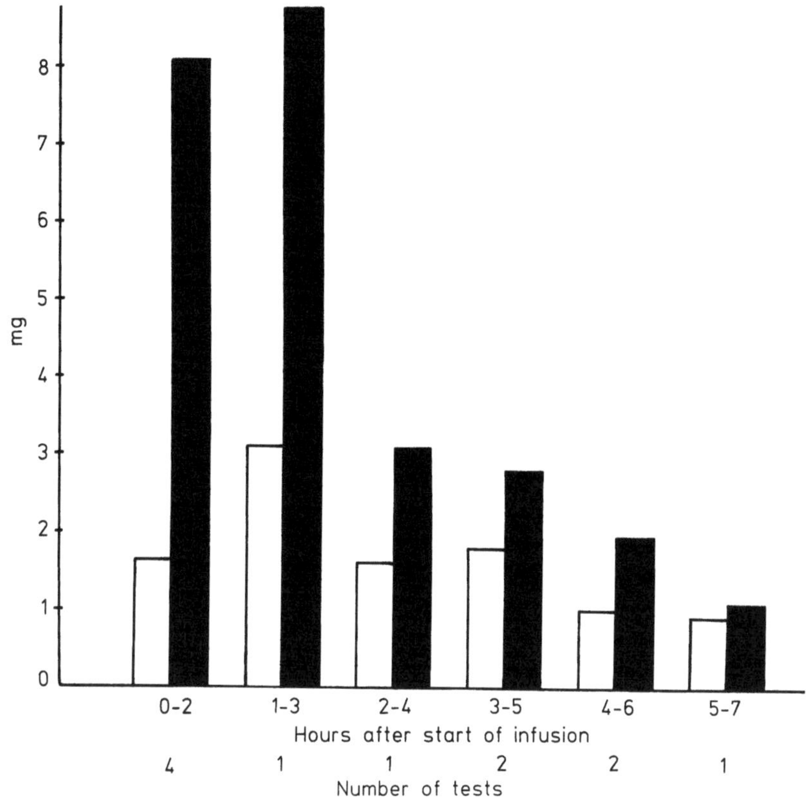

Fig. 3. Influence of the interval between the start of infusion and the removal of the gastric juice on concentrations of ETH and its sulphoxide in the gastric juice. (GRUNERT 1969; GRUNERT and IWAINSKY 1971 c, dose: 500 mg ETH i.v.). ■ ETH; □ Sulphoxide

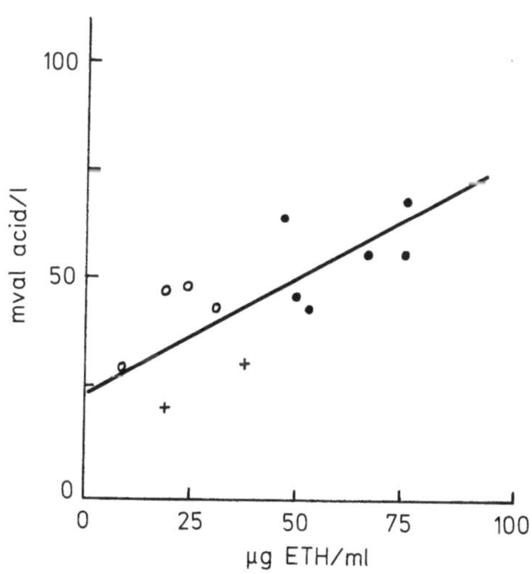

Fig. 4. Relationship between the acidity and the ETH concentration of the gastric juice after intravenous infusion of ETH (500 mg, GRUNERT 1969; GRUNERT and IWAINSKY 1971 c). Interval between the start of infusion and the removal of gastric juice. ● = 0–2 h; ○ = 2.5–3.5 h; + = 4–5 h. Correlation coefficient of the regression line r 0.68

Table 3. ETH concentration in serum (μg/ml) after rectal administration of 0.5 g of ETH in suppository form (EULE 1965)

Proportions of the individual groups referred to the total number of patients studied (%)				
11 "failures" always <2.1 μg ETH/ml	7.7 Always <3.0 μg ETH/ml	40.3 3 μg/ml– 3.85 μg/ml	36.5 Moderate ETH concentrations	4.5 High ETH concentrations

or its biotransformation products have been found in the faeces (IWAINSKY et al. 1963, 1965; PÜTTER 1964).

Further pharmacokinetic parameters relating to ETH/PTH are given in Tables 6 (distribution volume, p. 421), 8 (excretion, p. 424), 9 (clearance, p. 425), 10 (dose levels in the presence of kidney damage, p. 426), and 11 ($t_{50\%}$, p. 433) in the General Part of this review.

References

Ammon R, Berninger H, Haas HJ, Landsberg I (1967) Thioacetamid-sulfoxid, ein Stoffwechselprodukt des Thioacetamids. Arzneimittelforsch 17:521–523

Bieder A, Mazeau L (1964) Recherches sur le métabolisme de l'éthionamide chez l'homme. Séparation et identification de certains métabolites par chromatographie sur couche mince. Thérapie 19:897–907

Eule H (1965) Aethionamid-Konzentration im Blut, Harn, gesunder und kranker Lunge. Beitr Klin Tuberk 132:339–342

Eule H, Werner E (1964) Recherches sur la concentration de l' éthionamide dans le poumon humain sain et tuberculeux. Rev Tuberc 28:1301–1308

Greenberg L, Eidus L (1962) Antituberculous drugs (Th 1314 and INH) in the host organism. Br J Dis Chest 56:124–130

Grunert M (1969) Untersuchungen zum Verhalten des α-Äthylisonicotinsäurethioamides und seines Sulfoxydes in vitro und in vivo. Dissertation, Sektion Chemie der Humboldt-Universität Berlin

Grunert M, Iwainsky H (1967) Zum Stoffwechsel des Äthionamids und seines Sulfoxydes im Makroorganismus. Arzneimittelforsch 17:411–415

Grunert M, Iwainsky H (1971a) Pharmakokinetik und Biotransformation von Äthionamid. I. In vitro bestimmbare pharmakokinetisch bedeutsame Parameter. Z Erkr Atmungsorgane 134:83–93

Grunert M, Iwainsky H (1971b) Pharmakokinetik und Biotransformation von Äthionamid. II. Zur quantitativen Bestimmung von Äthionamid, Sulfoxyd und Methyl-Äthionamid in biologischem Material. Z Erkr Atmungsorgane 134:219–225

Grunert M, Iwainsky H (1971c) Pharmakokinetik und Biotransformation von Äthionamid. III. Zum Verhalten des Äthionamids im Makroorganismus. Z Erkr Atmungsorgane 134:227–233

Hamilton EJ, Eidus L, Little E (1962) A comparative study in vivo of isoniazid and alpha-ethylthioisonicotinamide. Am Rev Respir Dis 85:407–412

Iwainsky H, Rogowski J, Grunert M (1963) Zur intravenösen Verabreichung von Ätina. Mschr Tbk-Bekpfg 6:146–153

Iwainsky H, Sehrt I, Grunert M (1964) Zum Stoffwechsel des Äthionamids. Naturwissenschaften 51:316

Iwainsky H, Sehrt I, Grunert M (1965) Zum Stoffwechsel des Äthionamids nach intravenöser Verabreichung. Arzneimittelforsch 15:193–197

Johnston JP, Kane PO, Kibby MR (1967) The metabolism of ethionamide and its sulphoxide. J Pharm Pharmac 19:1–9
Krüger-Thiemer E †, Kröger H, Nestler HJ, Seydel JK (1975) Wirkungsmodi antituberkulöser Chemotherapeutika: Pyridincarbonsäurethioamide, Thiocarbanilide und Thiosemicarbazone. In: Meissner G, Schmiedel A †, Nelles A † (Hrsg) Infektionskrankheiten und ihre Erreger, Band 4, Teil III. Fischer, Jena, pp 289–298
Pilheu JA (1975) Rifampicin concentrations in cerebrospinal fluid of patients with tuberculous meningitis. Am Rev Respir Dis 111:240
Pütter J (1964) Photometrische Bestimmung des 2-Äthyl-isothio-nicotinylamid in Organen und Körperflüssigkeiten. Arzneimittelforsch 14:1198–1203
Pütter J (1972) Bestimmung von Prothionamid und Äthionamid sowie den entsprechenden Sulfoxiden im Blutplasma. Arzneimittelforsch 22:1027–1031
Rist N (1960) L' activité antituberculeuse de l' éthionamide (L'alpha-éthylthioisonicotinamide ou 1314 Th). Étude expérimentale et clinique. Adv Tuberc Res 10:69–126
Ritter W (1973) Neue Ergebnisse über Biotransformation und Pharmakokinetik von Antituberkulotika. Prax Pneumol 27:139–145 (B, Ph)
Simáne Z, Kraus P (1962) Ethionamide (1314 Th) serum levels and its urinary excretion. Rozhl Tbk (Praha) 22:289–293
Tikhonov VA, Grigalyunas AP, Guzeeva SA (1976) Polarographic investigation of the blood ethionamide and prothionamide concentration in patients with tuberculosis of the lungs. Probl Tuberk 54 issue 5: 75–78
Tsukamura M (1972) Permeability of tuberculous cavities to antituberculous drugs. Tubercle 53:47–52
Venkataraman P, Eidus L, Tripathy SP, Velu S (1967) Fluorescence test for the detection of ethionamide metabolites in urine. Tubercle 48:291–296
Winder FG (1982) Mode of action of the antimycobacterial agents and associated aspects of the molecular biology of the mycobacteria. In: Ratledge C, Stanford J (eds) The biology of the mycobacteria, Vol 1. Academic Press London New York Paris San Diego San Francisco Sao Paulo Sydney Tokyo Toronto, pp 353–438

X. KM

1. Mode of Action

In the light of the cross-resistance observed between SM and KM, it was assumed that the latter would also intervene in protein synthesis (Krüger-Thiemer et al. 1975). According to electron-microscopic investigations, exposure to KM results in modifications of the normal ribosome structure and in clumping of the cytoplasm. At the biochemical level, inhibition of polypeptide synthesis is evident in *Mycobacterium bovis* (BCG). The ribosome cycle breaks down. The polysomes disintegrate and the m-RNA breaks away from the ribosomes (Konno et al. 1973, 1977). In *Mycobacterium ranae* (*fortuitum*), the development of KM resistance goes hand in hand with intracellular enzymatic phosphorylation of aminoglycoside (Grange and Nordstrom 1974).

2. Biotransformation

Balance experiments on KM have revealed a certain difference between the quantity administered and the quantity excreted in an unchanged form (urinary excretion 75%–90%, small fractions with the faeces). However, so far it has been impossible to detect any biotransformation products of KM.

Table 1. Course of the KM serum concentration in patients with lung disease after intramuscular administration of lg of KM (FARAGÓ et al. 1974)

	n	Blood sample taken after		
		1 h–1.5 h	2 h–2.5 h	3 h–3.5 h
Mean value, µg/ml	16	26	29.7	35
Extremes, µg/ml		25–36.5	22–38.5	34–36

3. Pharmacokinetics

KM is distributed only in the extracellular space, equilibrium setting in rapidly, in accordance with a single-compartment model. The distribution volume is thought to be dependent on the dose (SØRENEN et al. 1967; ORME and CUTLER 1969). There is no binding to the serum proteins (Tables 3 and 6, pp. 419 and 421).

The concentrations of KM in the kidney and liver correspond to those in the serum (Table 1). In pulmonary tissue and in pleural exudation, the concentrations are about one-third of those measured in the serum. By contrast, only small quantities can be found in the myocardium and in bone. KM does not always penetrate fibrosclerotic tissue in sufficient concentration. It cannot be detected in the sputum (KUNTZ 1962; KUNIN 1966; TSUKAMURA 1972; FARAGO et al. 1974). Various figures are given for KM for its passage from the mother to the foetus (ROBSON and SULLIVAN 1963; WALTER and HEILMEYER 1969; SENECA 1971). The course of the KM concentration in the CSF resembles damped oscillation (Table 7, p. 423). The concentrations are substantially lower than in the serum, but they do remain above the MIC for a longer time in the CSF. The point of intersection between the serum and CSF concentrations occurs at 3.5 h. The small quantity of KM that passes into the CSF depends on the degree of inflammation and can be twice as high in inflamed tissue as in healthy tissue (KUNTZ 1962; EICHENWALD 1966; KUNIN 1966; PESNEL et al. 1973). The correlations between the concentration course in the serum and perilymph on the one side and ototoxicity on the other side are presented in greater detail in the section on SM.

In animals the fall of the KM concentration in the serum follows a biexponential course. The $t_{50\%}$ is relatively short – 87 min in the horse, 112 min in the sheep, and 58 min in the dog (BAGGOT 1978, Table 3, p. 494).

Excretion is almost exclusively via the kidneys (YOW and ABU-NASSAR 1963; KUNIN 1966; PINDELL 1966; SØRENEN et al. 1967; PISSIOTIS et al. 1972; Table 8, p. 424). Besides glomerular filtration, reabsorption and tubular filtration cannot be ruled out (KUNIN 1966). The excretion and the closely related $t_{50\%}$ of KM in the serum (Table 11, p. 433) correlate directly with the renal function (KUNTZ 1962; FUJII 1966; QUINN et al. 1966; SIMON and AXLINE 1966; SØRENEN et al. 1967; KNOWLES et al. 1971). Accordingly, an age-determined reduction of the excretion of KM is observed (SIMON and AXLINE 1966; SØRENEN et al. 1967).

References

Baggot JD (1978) Comparative pharmacokinetics of kanamycin. Abstracts 7th Int Congress Pharmacol Paris Pergamon Press, p 787 Nr 2451

Eichenwald HF (1966) Some observations on dosage and toxicity of kanamycin in premature and full-term infants. Ann NY Acad Sci 132:984–991

Faragó E, Kiss J, Fábián E, Molnár E (1974) Untersuchung des Kanamycin Serum- und Lungengewebespiegels im Menschen. Tuberkulózis (Budapest) 27:213–216

Fujii R (1966) Postcript to the panel discussion: proper dosage of kanamycin for premature babies. Ann NY Acad Sci 132:1031–1036

Grange JM, Nordstrom G (1974) Kanamycin and neomycin resistance in Mycobacterium ranae (fortuitum) associated with serological and biochemical markers. Zentralbl Bakteriol Mikrobiol 226:369–375

Knowles BR, Lucas SB, Mawer GE, Stirland RM, Tooth JA (1971) Use of a digital computer programme as a guide to the precribing of kanamycin in patients with renal insufficiency. Brit Pharm Soc 43:481P–482P

Konno K, Oizumi K, Kumano N, Oka S (1973) Mode of action of kanamycin on *Mycobacterium bovis* BCG. Am Rev Respir Dis 108:101–107

Konno K, Motomiya M, Oizumi K, Ariji F (1977) The 52nd Annual Meeting Special Lecture III. Mode of action of antituberculosis drugs on tubercle bacilli. Kekkaku 52:661–668

Krüger-Thiemer E †, Kröger H, Nestler HJ, Seydel JK (1975) Wirkungsmodi antituberkulöser Chemotherapeutika: Inositanaloga. In: Meissner G, Schmiedel A †, Nelles A † (Hrsg) Infektionskrankheiten und ihre Erreger, Band 4, Teil III. Fischer, Jena, pp 337–352

Kunin CM (1966) Absorption, distribution, excretion and fate of kanamycin. Ann NY Acad Sci 132:811–818

Kuntz E (1962) Kanamycin-Konzentrationen im Blut, Liquor und Pleuraexsudat. Klin Wochenschr 40:1107–1111

Orme BM, Cutler RE (1969) The relationship between kanamycin pharmacokinetics, distribution and renal function. Clin Pharmacol Ther 10:543–550

Pesnel G, Geslin P, Borderon J-C, Reinert P, Canet J, Farbe A, Bouhana A, Solle R, Lajouanine P (1973) Apport pratique d'un laboratoire spécialisé en antibiothérapie dans un service de pédiatrie générale. II. Rôle du laboratoire dans le contrôle du traitement antibiotique. Ann Pediat 20:245–262

Pindell MH (1966) The pharmacology of kanamycin – a review and new developments. Ann NY Acad Sci 132:805–810

Pissiotis CA, Nichols RL, Condon RE (1972) Absorption and excretion of intraperitoneally administered kanamycin sulfate. Surg Gynecol Obstet 134:995–998

Quinn EL, McHenry MC, Truant JP, Cox F (1966) The use of kanamycin in selected patients with serious infections caused by gram-negative bacilli: serum concentration and inhibition studies in patients with azotemia given reduced doses. Ann NY Acad Sci 132:850–853

Robson JM, Sullivan FM (1963) Antituberculosis drugs. Pharmacol Rev 15:169–223 (B, Ph)

Seneca H (1971) Biological basis of chemotherapy of infections and infestations. Davis Company, Philadelphia (Ph)

Simon HJ, Axline SG (1966) Clinical pharmacology of kanamycin in premature infants. Ann NY Acad Sci 132:1020–1025

Sørenen AWS, Szabo L, Pedersen A, Scharff A (1967) Correlation between renal function and serum half-life of kanamycin and its application to dosage adjustement. Postgrad Med J Suppl:37–43

Tsukamura M (1972) Permeability of tuberculous cavities to antituberculosis drugs. Tubercle 53:47–52

Walter AM, Heilmeyer L (1969) Antibiotika-Fibel. 3. Auflage. Heilmeyer L, Otten H, Plempel M (Hrsg) Thieme, Stuttgart

Yow EM, Abu-Nassar H (1963) Kanamycin: A re-evaluation after three years' experience. Antibiot Chemother 11:148–174

XI. DATC

1. Mode of Action

No definite results have been obtained regarding the incorporation and biotransformation of DATC by mycobacteria and about the influence of DATC resistance on these processes. Like INH and ETH, DATC inhibits the synthesis of mycolic acid (WINDER 1982; see INH p. 481, ETH/PTH p. 520, TSC p. 471). In view of the differences between these 3 agents with regard to cross resistance, loss of stability to acid, and the influence on mycobacterial growth in the depth of agar media, the question arises whether this inhibition of mycolic acid synthesis is to be regarded as indicative of a common step in the mode of action (KRÜGER-THIEMER et al. 1975) or whether it constitutes a sensitive "marker" for general metabolic disturbances.

2. Biotransformation

Because of the small proportion excreted with the urine, because of relatively insensitive, only group-specific, chemical detection methods, and because of the problems that arise when radiolabelled (preferably ^{35}S-labelled) DTAC is used, it is impossible to obtain exact data on the routes of biotransformation. However, the formation of several compounds of still unknown structure should not be ruled out (TACQUET et al. 1963; ROBINSON and HUNTER 1966).

3. Pharmacokinetics

All attempts to effect a decisive improvement in the absorption of DATC (use of micropowders, suspension of DATC in olive oil, etc.) have failed to produce the desired result (MOODIE et al. 1964; EULE and WERNER 1966). The concentration of DATC in the serum (Table 1) evidently exhibits considerable individual fluctuations owing to the prolonged nature of the incorporation (LARKIN 1960; TACQUET et al. 1963; MEISSNER 1965; GUBLER et al. 1966; ROBINSON and HUNTER 1966; STEFFEN 1971), binding to erythrocytes or to a lipoprotein fraction possibly is taking place (Table 3, p. 419; EMERSON and NICHOLSON 1965). The distribution space is yet to be clarified, as is the question of passage of DATC into the foetus and the CSF. In animal experiments ^{35}S-labelled DATC concentrates in the liver, lungs and spleen, values of nearly 10 μg DATC/g tissue being reached. The con-

Table 1. DATC concentrations in the serum (μg/ml) of 31 patients after oral administration of 2×3 g of DATC (2×6 tablets of 0.5 g with an interval of 6 h) or the same quantity (2×6 g) in fat granulate form (EULE and WERNER 1966)

Blood sample taken at	0 h	3 h	6 h	9 h	12 h	24 h
	After the first dose					
Tablets	0.2	4.4	4.8	5.5	4.8	0.5
Granulate	0.1	1.8	3.4	4.2	3.8	0.4

centrations in the lymph, brain, and subcutaneous fat are lower (MEISSNER 1965).

Small quantities of DATC are eliminated by the biliary route, the fraction eliminated with the urine (0%–2%) being negligible (Table 8, p. 424; EMERSON and NICHOLSON 1965; MEISSNER 1965; ROBINSON and HUNTER 1966). By far the bulk of the administered dose leaves the organism in an unchanged form with the faeces despite all attempts to improve the absorption.

The different therapeutic effects obtained experimentally depending on the animal species used (good effect in the mouse, guinea pig, and rabbit, scarcely any effect in the monkey) may possibly be due to differences in enteral absorption, although the available data on the absorption rate are not very reliable (FREERKSEN 1963; LUCCHESI 1963; SCHMIDT 1963; URBANCZIK and TRNKA 1963; MEISSNER 1965).

References

Emerson PA, Nicholson JP (1965) The absorption of 4,4-diisoamyloxythiocarbanilide (Isoxyl) using radioactive material (S^{35} tagged). Trans 24th Res Conf Pulm Dis VAAF:44–45

Eule H, Werner E (1966) Thiocarlide (4,4-diisoamyloxythiocarbanilide) blood levels in patients suffering from tuberculosis. Tubercle 47:214–220

Freerksen E (1963) Experimentelle Erfahrungen über 4,4′-Diisoamyloxythiocarbanilide (Isoxyl). Acta Tuberc Pneumol Belg 54:12–34

Gubler HU, Favez G, Bergier N, Mailard J-M, Friedrich T (1966) Beitrag zur Resorption von Thiocarlid beim Menschen. Beitr Klin Tuberk 133:126–139

Krüger-Thiemer E †, Kröger H, Nestler HJ, Seydel JK (1975) Wirkungsmodi antituberkulöser Chemotherapeutika: Pyridincarbonsäurethioamide, Thiocarbanilide und Thiosemicarbazone. In: Meissner G, Schmiedel A †, Nelles A † (Hrsg) Infektionskrankheiten und ihre Erreger, Band 4, Teil III. Fischer, Jena, pp 289–298

Larkin JC Jr (1960) Results of therapy with thiocarbanidin used with isoniazid or streptomycin. Am Rev Respir Dis 81:235–240

Lucchesi M (1963) Recherches expérimentales sur le 4,4′-diisoamyloxythiocarbanilide (Isoxyl). Acta Tuberc Pneumol Belg 54:42–58

Meissner J (1965) Verteilungsstudien mit radioaktiv markiertem Isoxyl. Beitr Klin Tuberk 132:322–324

Moodie AS, Aquinas M, Foord RD (1964) Controlled clinical trial of 4,4′-diisoamyloxycarbanilide in the treatment of pulmonary tuberculosis. Tubercle 45:192–200

Robinson OPW, Hunter PA (1966) Absorption and excretion studies with thiocarlide (4,4′ diisoamyloxythiocarbanilide) in man. Tubercle 47:207–213

Schmidt LH (1963) Discussion remark. Trans 22nd Res Conf Pulm Dis VAAF, p 254

Steffen J (1971) Ist Isoxyl in den bisher angegebenen Dosierungen als Tuberkuloseheilmittel zu verwenden? Prax Pneumol 25:263–277

Tacquet A, Guillaume J, Macquet V (1963) Étude expérimentale du métabolisme de la 4,4′-diisoamyloxythiocarbanilide marquée au saufre radioactif. Acta Tuberc Belg 54:59–65

Urbanczik R, Trnka L (1963) Report on the antimicrobial activity of Isoxyl on M. tuberculosis "in vitro" and "in vivo". Acta Tuberc Pneumol Belg 54:66–86

Winder FG (1982) Mode of action of the antimycobacterial agents and associated aspects of the molecular biology of the mycobacteria. In: Ratledge C, Stanford J (eds) The biology of the mycobacteria, Vol. 1. Academic Press London New York Paris San Diego San Francisco Sao Paulo Sydney Tokyo Toronto, pp 353–438

XII. CM

1. Mode of Action

CM is not a homogenous substance. Depending on the separation method selected for its preparation, 2, 4, or 8 fractions can be determined, half of them being biologically inactive (HERR 1962; JUNGE 1972; RITTER 1973). CM inhibits cellular protein synthesis, although the finer points of its mode of action are still largely unknown (VÄRE 1974).

2. Biotransformation

55%–80% of the administered dose are excreted in an unchanged form with the urine within 24 h. No biotransformation products can be detected by paper chromatography after the passage of CM through the macroorganism (BLACK et al. 1966).

3. Pharmacokinetics

CM is rapidly distributed. The distribution volume is still to be clarified. 2 h after its administration, when the distribution equilibrium is established the maximum of the concentration is reached in the serum. It falls off within 10 h to about 1/10 of the peak level (Table 1). Like SM, CM undergoes glomerular filtration. 55% –80% of the administered dose is excreted with the urine within 24 h (Table 2). CM does not diffuse into fibrosclerotic lesions to a sufficient extent (TSUKAMURA 1972). No accumulation takes place if the kidney function is normal. In the presence of kidney damage the dosage should be adjusted to the residual function. In animal experiments low-grade elimination with the bile has also been detected (BLACK et al. 1966; WELLES et al. 1966). Further data on the $t_{50\%}$ and on excretion are given in Tables 8, 9, and 11 of the General Part, see pp. 424, 425 and 433.

Table 1. CM concentration in the serum (µg/ml) of tuberculotic patients after i.m. administration of a dose of 1 g

n	Time of blood sample withdrawal (h)							Authors
	1	2	4	6	10	12	24	
10	29,1	32,7	19,8	12,1	–	3,2	1,0	BLACK et al. (1966)
28	–	29,4	–	10,4	4,0	–	–	MORSE et al. (1966)
10	–	24,5	15,1					Donomae (1966)

Table 2. Excretion of CM in the urine of tuberculotic patients after i.m. administration of a dose of 1 g (BLACK et al. 1966)

n	0–6	6–12	12–24	0–24
10	329 mg (33%)	193 mg (19%)	49 mg (5%)	571 mg (57%)

References

Black HR, Griffith RS, Peabody AM (1966) Absorption, excretion and metabolism of capreomycin in normal and diseased states. Ann NY Acad Sci 135:974–982

Donomae J (1966) Capreomycin in the treatment of pulmonary tuberculosis. Ann NY Acad Sci 135:1011–1038

Herr EB Jr (1963) Chemical and biological properties of capreomycin and other peptide antibiotics. Antimicrob Agents Chemother 1962:201–212

Junge O (1972) Dünnschichtchromatographische Auftrennung der Antibiotika Carbenicillin, Polymycin und Capreomycin. Int J Clin Pharmacol 6:67–76

Morse WC, Sproat EF, Arrington CW, Hawkins JA (1966) *M. tuberculosis* in vitro susceptibility and serum level experiences with capreomycin. Ann NY Acad Sci 135:983–988

Ritter W (1973) Neue Ergebnisse über Biotransformation und Pharmakokinetik von Antituberkulotika. Prax Pneumol 27:139–145 (B, Ph)

Tsukamura M (1972) Permeability of tuberculous cavities to antituberculous drugs. Tubercle 53:47–52

Väre T (1974) Rifampicin, ethambutol and capreomycin in the treatment of pulmonary tuberculosis. Scand J Respir Dis Suppl 87:6–57

Welles JS, Harris PU, Small RM, Worth HM, Anderson RC (1966) The toxicity of capreomycin in laboratory animals. Ann NY Acad Sci 135:960–973

XIII. EMB

1. Mode of Action

As with TC, the formation of a less polar chelate complex that is thus more suitable for permeation is postulated for EMB as the first stage before its uptake into mycobacteria (Shepherd et al. 1966). That this is the case is also indicated by the reduced incorporation in the presence of certain ions (Forbes et al. 1966). Uptake by the pathogens increases with increasing incubation time, in proportion to the EMB concentration introduced (Fig. 1). Neither accumulation against the concentration gradient nor inhibition of the incorporation by 2,4-dinitrophenol, azide, or chloramphenicol can be detected, i.e., the EMB is taken up into the microorganisms by diffusion (Beggs and Auran 1972; Jenne and Beggs 1973), the actual process differing depending on whether proliferating or non-proliferating pathogens are present.

In studies on the incorporation of radiolabelled compounds (^{14}C-acetate, ^{14}C-α-ketoglutarate, ^{14}C-glycine, ^{14}C-glutamate, ^{14}C-leucine, $^{32}PO_4^{3-}$, $^{35}SO_4^{2-}$, ^{35}S-methionine) EMB has been found to possess many means of influencing the metabolism (Youatt 1965; Tsukamura and Mizuno 1967). However, they probably tend more to represent the incipient breakdown of the metabolic process rather than the primary site of attack of EMB.

There are few findings relating to this point, although they have been confirmed by several working groups. The effect of EMB on cell growth is evident only after a lag phase lasting several hours and is reversible within certain exposure limits (Forbes et al. 1965, 1966). Accordingly, even when the EMB has been removed before the renewed onset of cell proliferation a lag phase dependent on the exposure time can be observed (Forbes et al. 1965). Processes that can be interpreted as compensation are evident; for example, after initial inhibition of the ^{32}P-uptake by EMB 4 h to 8 h after the beginning of contact the RNA fraction

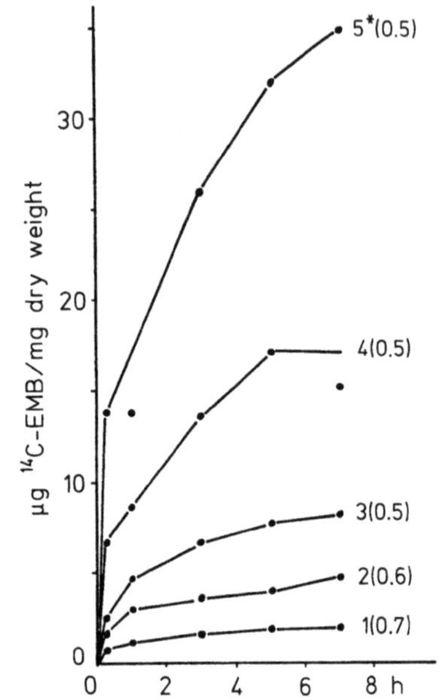

Fig. 1. Uptake of ^{14}C-EMB by *Mycobacterium tuberculosis* (BEGGS and AURAN 1972). *1* 0.2 µg EMB/ml; *2* 0.5 µg EMB/ml; *3* 1.0 µg EMB/ml; *4* 2.5 µg EMB/ml; *5* 5.0 µg EMB/ml; * In brackets: Ratio of intracellular/extracellular EMB after 5 h

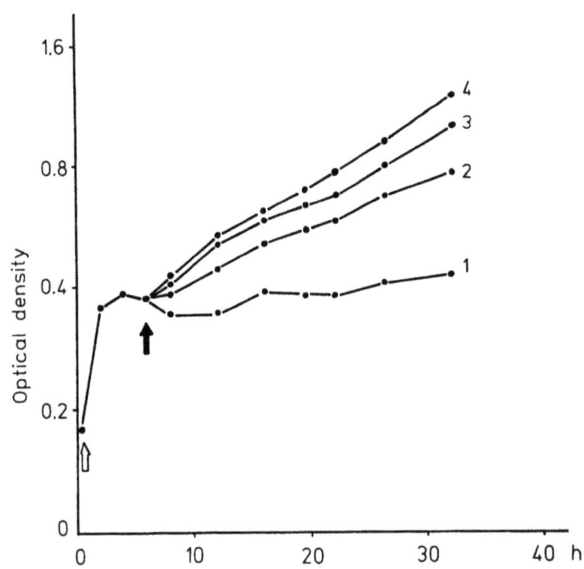

Fig. 2. Prevention of EMB-determined inhibition of the nucleic acid metabolism of *Mycobacterium smegmatis* by spermidine or Mg^{2+} ions (FORBES et al. 1965). *1* 13 µg EMB/ml; *2* 13 µg EMB/ml + 0.5 mmol spermidine/l; *3* 13 µg EMB/ml + 20 mmol Mg^{2+}/l; *4* 13 µg EMB/ml + 0.5 mmol spermidine/l + 20 mmol Mg^{2+}/l; ⇧ Addition of EMB; ⬆ Addition of spermidine or Mg^{2+}

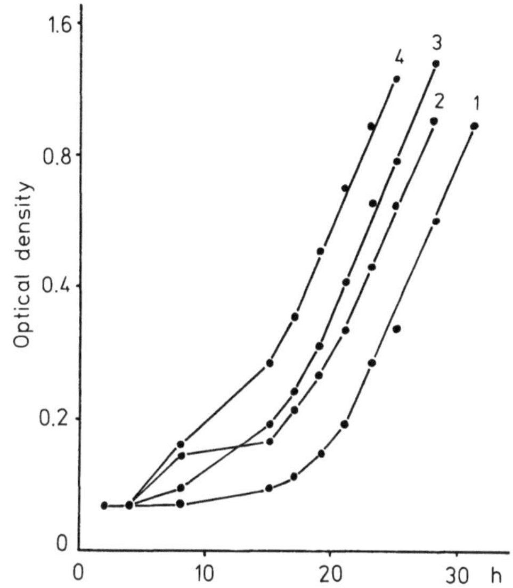

Fig. 3. Shortening of the lag phase before renewed growth following contact with EMB (*Mycobacterium smegmatis* incubated with 10 μg EMB/ml for 6 h at 37 °C, FORBES et al. 1965). *1* no addition; *2* 0.5 mmol spermidine/l; *3* 10 mmol Mg^{2+}/l; *4* 0.5 mmol spermidine/l + 10 mmol Mg^{2+}/l

exhibits values equal to or even higher than those in the control (REUTGEN and IWAINSKY 1972; BEMSKI 1973).

In the event of contact with EMB the degradation of RNA apparently takes place faster than its synthesis (FORBES et al. 1966). Another point is that the glycerol turnover is disturbed (KUCK et al. 1963; REUTGEN and IWAINSKY 1970). On the basis of the antagonistic effect of polyamines and Mg^{2+} ions on the effects of EMB (evaluation of the inhibitory concentration by simultaneous addition of antagonists, Fig. 2; shortening of the lag phase observed after the action of EMB by antagonists, Fig. 3, FORBES et al. 1965), and bearing in mind some more recent studies on the phosphate and nucleic acid metabolism, REUTGEN (1975) formulated the following hypothesis concerning the mode of action of EMB: cellular polyamines form stable complexes with transfer- and ribosomal RNA. These complexes are important for ribosomal function. EMB competes with the polyamines, inhibits the ribosomal RNA and protein synthesis, and thus ultimately inhibits growth.

EMB forms stable chelate complexes with metal ions, especially cellular Mg^{2+}. In this way the functional capacity of the ribosomes on the one hand and the function of enzymes activated by Mg^{2+} ions on the other hand is impaired, with consecutive disturbance of the phosphate, lipid, and protein metabolism.

2. Biotransformation

By countercurrent distribution and paper chromatography a dialdehyde, a dicarboxylic acid, and a glucuronide of EMB have been detected as biotransformation products in human and dog urine after the administration of ^{14}C-EMB (Figs. 4

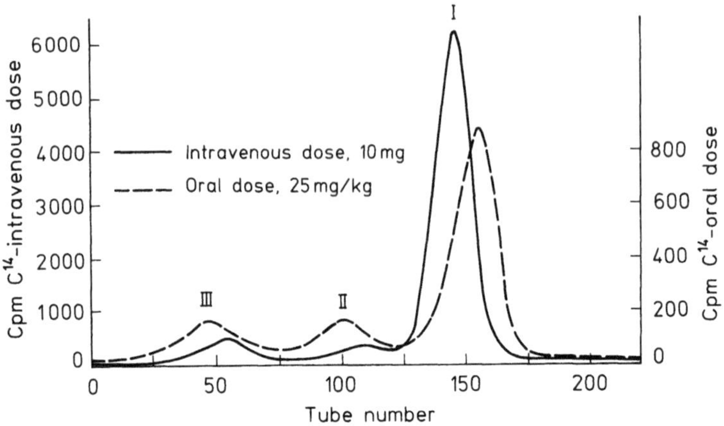

Fig. 4. Countercurrent distribution of biotransformation products of ^{14}C-EMB excreted with the urine (PEETS et al. 1965). ——— urinary excretion after 10 mg EMB/kg i.v.; ---- urinary excretion after 25 mg EMB/kg p.o.; *I* EMB; *II* Dialdehyde; *III* 2,2′-(Ethylenediimino) dibutyric acid

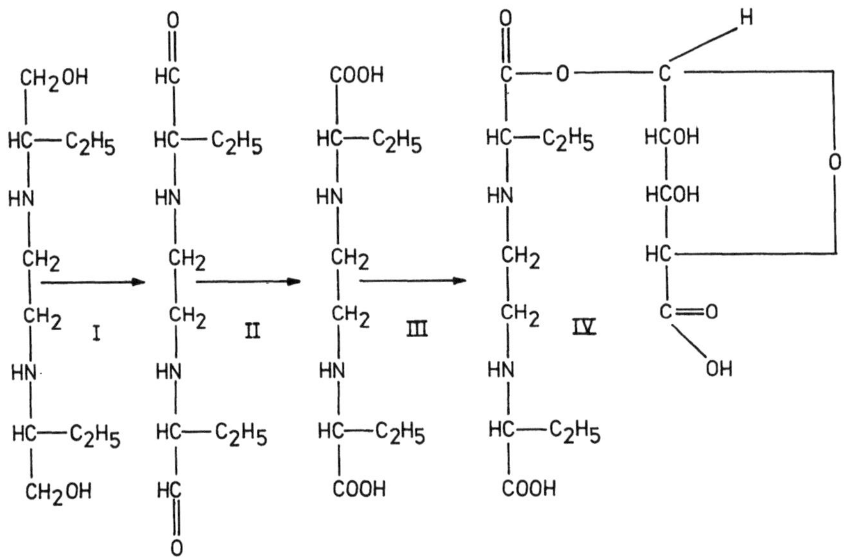

Fig. 5. Structural formulae of the biotransformation products of EMB (KANTHER 1970). *I* EMB; *II* Dialdehyde; *III* 2,2′-(Ethylenediimino)dibutyric acid; *IV* Glucuronide of 2,2′-(ethylenediimino)dibutyric acid

and 5, PEETS et al. 1965; PLACE et al. 1966; KANTHER 1970). On oral administration the proportion of unchanged EMB is higher than that after intravenous injection. In view of the relatively high individual scatter and the small number of patients studied, the authors consider the influence of the route of administration on the rate of oxidation of EMB to be slight. Some 10% to 15% of the quantity excreted with the urine is present in the form of the aforementioned, biologically inactive, biotransformation products of EMB (PEETS et al. 1965).

Table 1. Course of EMB concentration [μg/ml] in serum and plasma after administration of various doses

Dose and route adminis-tration	*n*	Time of taking blood sample after dosage 1	2	4	6	7	8	24 h	Authors
25 mg/kg oral	14[a]	–	4,5	3,1	1,8	–	–	–	JUNGBLUTH and URBANCZIK (1974)
	13[b]	1,8 ±1,5	2,6 ±1,9	2,4 ±1,0	–	1,3 ±0,5	–	0,3 ±0,0	OMER (1978)
	10[a]	3,0	5,0	3,0	1,5	–	0	–	EULE and WERNER (1970)
50 mg/kg oral	10[a]	4,0	8,0	5,2	3,3	–	2,1	–	EULE and WERNER (1970)
75 mg/kg oral	10[a]	5,5	11,2	8,1	5,0	–	3,2	–	

[a] Serum concentration,
[b] Plasma concentration; persons 60–78 years old

Table 2. Influence of the duration of treatment on the plasma EMB concentration in elderly patients (60–78 years of age, 2-h values, μg/ml, OMER 1978)

n	Age	1st day	1st week	2nd week	3rd week	4th week	5th week
13	67,5±2,0	2,6±1,9	2,8±1,8	2,9±1,5	3,7±1,4	3,8±1,3	3,7±1,7

3. Pharmacokinetics

EMB is probably protected, like TC, from greater biotransformation by chelate formation taking place in vivo. The release of certain heavy metal ions, especially Zn^{2+} and to a lesser extent Cu^{2+}, detectable in the dog and the monkey after high doses of EMB is certainly connected with this process. At EMB doses of 400 mg/kg an interaction is evident from the reduced Zn^{2+} and Cu^{2+} concentrations in certain animal organs (BUYSKE et al. 1966; FIGUEROA et al. 1971). Even at therapeutic doses (25 mg of EMB/kg) a fall in the Zn^{2+} concentration in the plasma can still be recorded in man (CAMPBELL and ELMES 1975). Like INH and PAS, EMB readily diffuses into the body fluids and organs. Distribution throughout the body water must be reckoned with. EMB is bound to a small extent to proteins and to a considerable extent to the erythrocytes (Table 3, p. 419), which represent the deep compartment for EMB (PEETS and BUYSKE 1962; PLACE et al. 1966; PUJET and PUJET 1972; AOYAGI 1977; CHEN et al. 1984). The serum concentration correspondingly falls off multiphasically (Tables 1 and 2). The EMB concentration in the sputum corresponds to that in the serum, while the pleural fluid contains 30% to 40% of the serum concentration. Active concentrations are also reached in fibrosclerotic foci. In mice, with the exception of the level in the brain, the EMB concentrations (in the liver, kidney, heart, spleen, lung, and muscle) are more than twice the concentration in the plasma (KELLY et al. 1981).

EMB passes through the placental barrier, therapeutically active concentrations being measured in the foetal blood after the administration of an EMB dose of 15 mg/kg (SHNEERSON and FRANCIS 1979). Only a small quantity of EMB diffuses into the CSF but, like INH, ETH/PTH, and RMP, the drug is still suitable for the treatment of meningitis (Table 7, p. 423).

Table 3. Excretion of ^{14}C-EMB in the urine and the faeces of tuberculosis patients (% of administered dose, PLACE et al. 1966)

Urine portion	Patient A, ♀		Patient B, ♂	Patient C, ♂
	Dose and route of administration			
	10 mg i.v.	25 mg/kg p.o.	25 mg/kg p.o.	25 mg/kg p.o.
0– 24 h	72,6	54,2	54,3	53,5
0– 48 h	81,6	62,7	66,8	59,7
0– 72 h		67,0	70,2	63,4
0– 96 h			71,3	64,9
0–120 h			72,9	66,3
0–144 h			73,9	67,3
Faeces				
0– 24 h	0,2	6,3	12,8	0,1
0– 48 h	0,3	12,1	18,7	12,7
0–72 h				22,2
0–96 h			20,3	
Total excretion	81,9	79,1	94,2	89,5

Table 4. Excretion of EMB and its biotransformation products (% of the administered dose) in the 24-h urine (PLACE et al. 1966)

Patient	Dose and route of administration	EMB	Biotransformation products	Total excretion
A. J.	10 mg, i.v.	65	8	73
A. J.	25 mg/kg, p.o.	39	15	54
B.	25 mg/kg, p.o.	32	8	40
T.	25 mg/kg, p.o.	44	10	54
B. (first dose)	25 mg/kg, p.o.	43	11	54
B. (after 6 months) of treatment)	25 mg/kg, p.o.	54	7	61
D.	50 mg/kg, p.o.	36	8	44
F.	50 mg/kg, p.o.	38	8	46
M.	50 mg/kg, p.o.	40	5	45

Therapy with EMB has in individual cases resulted in serious damage to the optic nerve, a connection being assumed to exist between this damage and a release of Zn^{2+} and Cu^{2+} ions caused by EMB. Studies aimed specifically at the depigmentation of the tapetum lucidum in the dog after the administration of high doses of EMB indicate that this hypothesis is correct (BUYSKE et al. 1966; FIGUEROA et al. 1971). At a dose of 25 mg EMB/kg over a treatment period of 8 weeks, however, only a reduction of the plasma Zn^{2+} content from 82 μg/100 ml to 71 μg/100 ml can be observed in man, the Cu^{2+} content remaining unaffected (CAMPBELL and ELMES 1975). Thus, the release of Zn^{2+} cannot be the sole cause of the EMB-determined damage to the optic nerve. On the basis of animal experiments a modification of the permeability of optic nerve membranes is considered as a possibility (BORCHARD et al. 1975).

EMB undergoes glomerular filtration and tubular secretion, the biotransformation products being subject to glomerular filtration (Table 8, p. 424). In man up to 91% (p.o.) and 94% (i.v.) of the dose is excreted with the urine (Tables 3 and 4); in the dog up to 90% is excreted (PEETS and BUYSKE 1962; BUYSKE et al. 1966), 60%–80% still in biologically active form (PLACE and THOMAS 1963; PEETS et al. 1965; PLACE et al. 1966). Other authors report lower values for the urinary excretion (PUJET and PUJET 1972; HÖFFLER 1981). Between 10% and 20% is excreted with the faeces (PEETS et al. 1965; DUME et al. 1971). A slight impairment of the renal function does not have any far-reaching effects on the excretion of EMB, though its half-life is prolonged if such impairment is considerable (Table 10, p. 426, DUME et al. 1971; ZELLER and RÓKA 1973; KROENING 1974; ZITKOVA and TOUSHEK 1978; HÖFFLER 1981). Further pharmacokinetic parameters are reproduced in Tables 6, 9, and 11, pp. 421, 425 and 433.

References

Aoyagi T (1977) Clinical problems on the binding of protein to antituberculous drugs. Kekkaku 52:459–468

Beggs WH, Auran NE (1972) Uptake and binding of ^{14}C-ethambutol by tubercle bacilli and the relation of binding to growth inhibition. Antimicrob Agents Chemother 2:390–394

Bemski G (1973) PMR study of the interaction of ethambutol with polynucleotides and related compounds. FEBS Letters 30:79–83

Borchard U, Dreistein A, Hamacher J (1975) Influence of ethambutol on resting and action potential of the peripheral nerve. Naunyn-Schmiedebergs Arch Pharmacol 287 Suppl: R 18

Buyske DA, Sterling W, Peets E (1966) Pharmacological and biochemical studies on ethambutol in laboratory animals. Ann NY Acad Sci 135:711–725

Campbell IA, Elmes PC (1975) Ethambutol and the eye; zinc and copper. Lancet II:711

Chen MM, Lee CS, Perrin JH (1984) Absorption and disposition of ethambutol in rabbits. J Pharm Sci 73:1053–1055

Dume T, Wagner C, Wetzels E (1971) Zur Pharmakokinetik von Ethambutol bei Gesunden und Patienten mit terminaler Niereninsuffizienz. Dtsch Med Wochenschr 96:1430–1434

Eule H, Werner E (1970) Ethambutol-Serumspiegel bei unterschiedlicher Dosierung; Vergleich von vier verschiedenen Bestimmungsmethoden. Z Erkr Atmungsorgane 133:443–448

Figueroa R, Weiss H, Smith JC Jr, Hackley BM, McBean LD, Swassing CR, Halsted JA (1971) Effect of ethambutol on the ocular zinc concentration in dogs. Am Rev Respir Dis 104:592–594

Forbes M, Kuck NA, Peets EA (1965) Effect of ethambutol on nucleic acid metabolism in Mycobacterium smegmatis and its reversal by polyamines and divalent cations. J Bacteriol 89:1299–1305
Forbes M, Peets EA, Kuck NA (1966) Effect of ethambutol on mycobacteria. Ann NY Acad Sci 135:726–731
Höffler D (1981) Die Dosierung wichtiger Antibiotika und Tuberkulostatika bei Niereninsuffizienz. Internist (Berlin) 22:601–606
Jenne JW, Beggs WH (1973) Correlation of in vitro and in vivo kinetics with clinical use of isoniazid, ethambutol and rifampin. Am Rev Respir Dis 107:1013–1021
Jungbluth H, Urbanczik R (1974) Ethambutol-Serumspiegel nach oraler und intravenöser Verabreichung. Prax Pneumol 28:499–504
Kanther R (1970) Myambutol: chemistry, pharmacology, and toxicology. Antibiot Chemother 16:203–214
Kelly RG, Kaleita E, Eisner HJ (1981) Tissue distribution of (^{14}C)ethambutol in mice. Am Rev Respir Dis 123:689–690
Kroening U (1974) Die Konzentrationsbestimmung von Ethambutol im Vollblut und ihre Bedeutung für den Nachweis der Kumulation des Medikamentes. Pneumonologie 151:135–146
Kuck UA, Peets EA, Forbes M (1963) Mode of action of ethambutol on Mycobacterium tuberculosis, strain H37Rv. Am Rev Respir Dis 87:905–906
Omer LMO (1978) Tagesprofile und Profilverlaufskontrollen von Ethambutol bei älteren Tuberkulosekranken. Prax Pneumol 32:252–256
Peets EA, Buyske DA (1962) Studies of the metabolism in the dog of ethambutol C^{14}, a drug having antituberculosis activity. Pharmacologist 4:171
Peets EA, Sweeney WM, Place VA, Buyske DA (1965) The absorption, excretion and metabolic fate of ethambutol in man. Am Rev Respir Dis 91:51–58
Place VA, Thomas JP (1963) Clinical pharmacology of ethambutol. Am Rev Respir Dis 87:901–904
Place VA, Peets EA, Buyske DA (1966) Metabolic and special studies of ethambutol in normal volunteers and tuberculosis patients. Ann NY Acad Sci 135:775–795
Pujet J-C, Pujet C (1972) Dosages sanguines et humoraux de l'éthambutol administré par perfusion intraveineuse. Bordeaux Méd:1215–1222
Reutgen H (1975) Wirkungsmodi antituberkulöser Verbindungen: Ethambutol. In: Meissner G, Schmiedel A †, Nelles A † (Hrsg) Infektionskrankheiten und ihre Erreger, Band 4, Teil III. Fischer, Jena, pp 299–318
Reutgen H, Iwainsky H (1970) Zum Wirkungsmechanismus des Ethambutols. Z Erkr Atmungsorgane 133:457–459
Reutgen H, Iwainsky H (1972) Untersuchungen zum endogenen Stoffwechsel von Mykobakterien. 5. Mitt. Über den Einfluß von Ethambutol auf den endogenen Stoffwechsel von *Mycobacterium smegmatis*. Z Naturforschung 27b:1405–1411
Shepherd RG, Baughn C, Cantrall ML, Goodstein B, Thomas JP, Wilkinson RG (1966) Structure-activity studies leading to ethambutol, a new type of antituberculous compound. Ann NY Acad Sci 135:686–710
Shneerson JM, Francis RS (1979) Ethambutol in pregnancy – foetal exposure. Tubercle 60:167–169
Tsukamura M, Mizuno S (1967) Mode of action of ethambutol. Effect of ethambutol on the incorporations of several isotopic compounds into lipids, nucleic acids and protein by M. smegmatis. Kekkaku 42:437–442
Youatt J (1965) Changes in the phosphate content of mycobacteria produced by isoniazid and ethambutol. Aust J Exp Biol Med Sci 43:305–314
Zeller F, Róka L (1973) Ethambutolausscheidung bei Tuberkulosepatienten mit mäßig eingeschränkter Nierenfunktion. Prax Pneumol 27:36–43
Zitkova L, Toushek I (1978) Pharmacokinetics of cycloserin and ethambutol. Probl Tuberk 56 issue 3: 23–25

XIV. RMP

1. Mode of Action

RMP is taken up very rapidly by mycobacteria, to the extent of ~80% of the available quantity within 1 h. Continuation of the incubation to 24 h yields only a slight further increase (Table 1, TOYOHARA 1971). The incorporation of ^{14}C-RMP is largely the same in RMP-sensitive and RMP-resistant mycobacteria. The development of resistance leads to a change in the affinity of RMP for the DNA-dependent RNA polymerase. The enzyme isolated from sensitive microorganisms of *M. phlei* is, for example, 90% inhibited by 1 μg RMP/ml, while that obtained from a resistant population remains unaffected by this dose (WHITE et al. 1971).

A disturbance of the nucleic acid and/or protein synthesis was already suspected from the very first studies on the incorporation of radiolabelled compounds (LEONI and TECCE 1963; TSUKAMURA et al. 1963). Specific studies did not in fact reveal any change in the DNA synthesis but showed a very specific inhibition of DNA-dependent RNA polymerases of bacterial origin by this ansamycin antibiotic. The corresponding mammalian RNA polymerases are only impaired at substantially higher RMP concentrations (Fig. 1, HARTMANN et al. 1967; HONICKEL et al. 1968; WEHRLI and STAEHELIN 1971; KONNO et al. 1973b; BOLT 1975; KONNO et al. 1977). Obviously differences in the polymerase amino acid sequence play a role, only slight alterations leading to a considerable reduction of the RMP activity.

Since the ansa ring of RMP is decisive for the biological effect, reactions taking place within the context of biotransformation in vivo, such as the formation of deacetyl-RMP or demethyl-RMP, do not always result in loss of the antimicrobial activity (POGO 1971; WEHRLI and STAEHELIN 1971).

As a result of the formation of a stable RMP complex with the RNA polymerase, the configuration (largely of the β-subunit) of the enzyme is modified to the extent that RNA synthesis can not begin to start (MICHEL-BRIAND 1978), though any synthesis already in progress is not inhibited (HONICKEL et al. 1968; HANDSCHIN et al. 1976). Thus, RMP has no effect on *E. coli* if it is added 2 min after the start of the experiment (UMEZAWA et al. 1968).

Studies on mycobacteria have confirmed these findings obtained on *E. coli*, *B. subtilis*, and *Staph. aureus*. The polymerases of BCG and *M. smegmatis* are completely inhibited by just 0.1 μg–1 μg RMP/ml (Fig. 2; DICKINSON et al. 1972; KONNO et al. 1972, 1973b; MIŠOŇ and TRNKA 1973; KONNO et al. 1977). In *M. smegmatis* the incorporation of uracil is prevented after 2 min and that of

Table 1. Uptake of ^{14}C-RMP by *M. tuberculosis* (TOYOHARA 1971, Dubos medium, 10 μg RMP/ml, data given in Cpm/g dry weight of bacteria, 2960 KBq/ml = 80 μCi)

Incubation time (h)	1	6	24
M. tuberculosis H37Rv	718	748	887
M. tuberculosis H37Rv, RMP-resistant	699	750	831

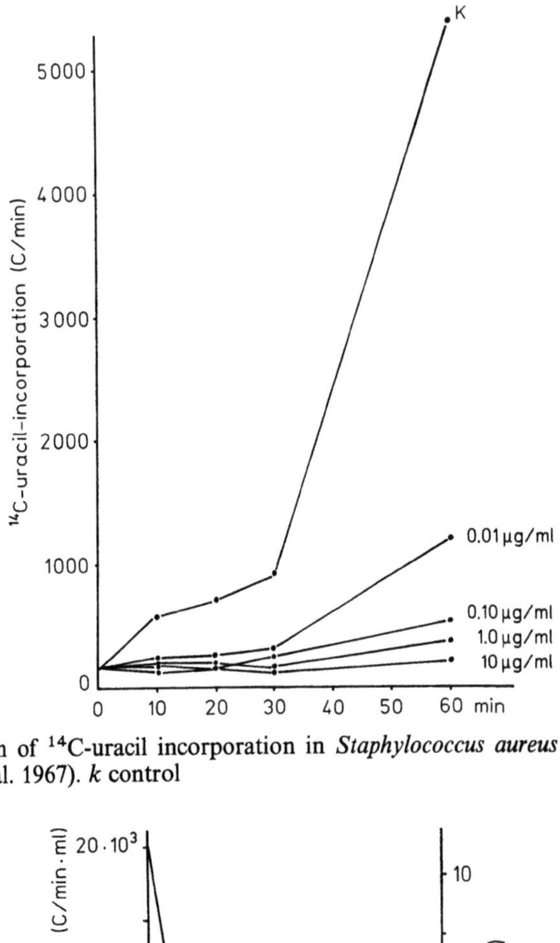

Fig. 1. Inhibition of ^{14}C-uracil incorporation in *Staphylococcus aureus* by rifamycin B (HARTMANN et al. 1967). *k* control

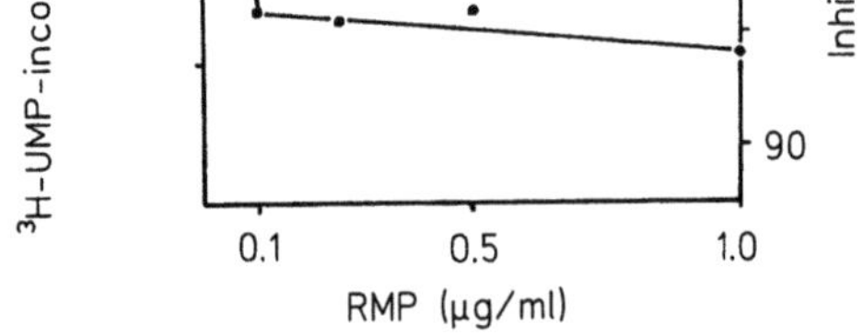

Fig. 2. Inhibition of the polymerase activity of *Mycobacterium bovis* (BCG) by RMP (KONNO et al. 1972)

phenylalanine after 6 min. As long as certain concentrations and exposure times are not exceeded, the inhibition is reversible. Fifteen min after the removal of the RMP, the incorporation of uracil can once again be detected (WHITE et al. 1971). In the event of longer action times, modifications of the cytoplasm and the ribosomes can be established before cell destruction becomes clearly apparent (BLUNDELL and WILD 1971; KONNO et al. 1973a).

2. Biotransformation

a) Biotransformation Pattern in Man and in Animals

The RMP concentrations in the nutrient media used to determine antimycobacterial activity, especially solid nutrient media, fall off rapidly. To make shorter incubation times possible, rapidly proliferating species such as *Sarcina lutea, B. brevis, Staph. aureus,* and others are used for the activity determinations instead of slow-growing mycobacteria.

Microbiological assays of RMP-containing body fluids, however, sometimes display considerable differences when tested with different microorganisms, indicating the presence of biotransformation products of RMP with different action spectra. These biotransformation products can be separated by thin-layer chromatography and identified by their characteristic color (Figs. 3 and 4; KOLOS and EIDUS 1972; SUNAHARA and NAKAGAWA 1972; NAKAGAWA and SUNAHARA 1973; WINSEL et al. 1976).

Considerable differences exist between the individual mammalian species in the fractions of the biotransformation products. In man and in the guinea pig deacetyl-RMP is predominant, while in the rat demethyl-RMP is the main metabolite and in the dog and the mouse the deacetylation and demethylation proceed more or less to the same extent. By contrast, rabbits excrete RMP largely in the unchanged form (TENCONI and BERETTA 1970).

In man, the fraction of deacetyl-RMP is about 80% in the bile and about 30% in the urine, while the fraction of demethyl-RMP is very small. The 3-formyl-RMP SV formed by hydrolytic cleavage constitutes some 10% of the biotransformation products excreted with the urine (MAGGI et al. 1969; RITTER 1973; WINSEL et al. 1976; ACOCELLA 1978). In addition, the formation of a conjugate

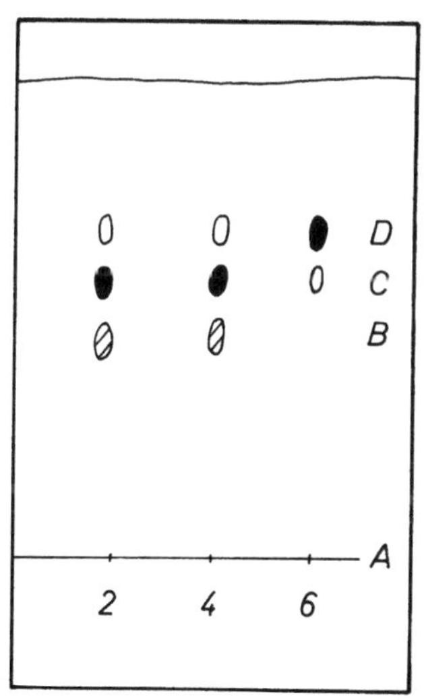

Fig. 3. Biotransformation products of RMP in the urine (NAKAGAWA and SUNAHARA 1973, thin-layer chromatogram, schematic representation, benzene-hexane extract; solvent system: chloroform/methanol 9:1). *A* start; *B* 3-formyl-rifamycin SV; *C* RMP; *D* RMP-quinone; *2, 4, 6:* times of urine sample collection after administration of the drug

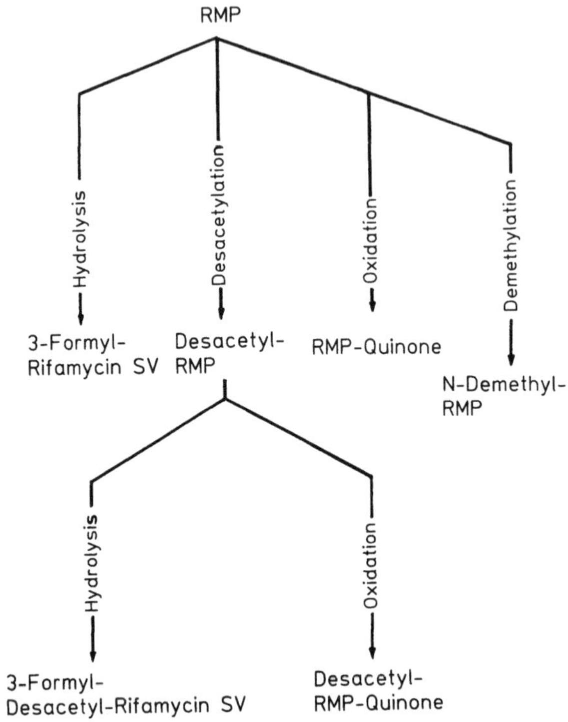

Fig. 4. Biotransformation routes of RMP (detection of biotransformation products in the urine, NAKAGAWA and SUNAHARA 1973)

between deacetyl-RMP and glucuronate has been discussed as a possibility (NAKAGAWA and SUNAHARA 1973; ACOCELLA and CONTI 1980).

The 3-formyl-RMP isolated in man was for a long time overlooked because its R_F-value is similar to that of deacetyl-RMP. The RMP-quinone detected need not be produced as a result of biotransformation. For example, it could be formed by oxidation during the thin-layer-chromatographic resolution itself. In vivo it is probably reduced again by RMP-inductable NADPH-cytochrome C-reductase (KOLOS and EIDUS 1972; SUNAHARA and NAKAGAWA 1972; NAKAGAWA and SUNAHARA 1973; OTANI and REMMER 1975). According to the studies performed so far, all the biotransformation products have practically the same antimycobacterial activity (TOYAHARA 1971).

b) Modification of the Biotransformation Rate of RMP by Auto-Induction (see also General Part, A.II.3–4, p. 409)

RMP belongs to the group of drugs with an induction activity. As a result of the induction of microsomal enzymes in the liver, RMP is increasingly biotransformed to deacetyl-RMP. Accordingly, after repeated administration of RMP the total excretion in the bile is increased with a simultaneous reduction of the excretion with the urine. This induction process is already measurable after a short time in the case of daily or intermittent administration of RMP by a reduced excretion with the urine or shortening of the serum $t_{50\%}$ of the RMP. Significant differences emerge in tests with microorganisms having a lower sensitivity to deacetyl-RMP, while the antimycobacterial activity is affected only slightly by the induction (see Fig. 5, p. 410; CANETTI et al. 1970; GRASSI 1971; IOFFE 1973; IWAINSKY et al. 1976; WINSEL et al. 1976; ACOCELLA 1978; ACOCELLA et al. 1978; HOLDINESS 1984). The experimentally determined differences in the results pertaining to the inductive effect of RMP only became clarified after RMP and deacetyl-RMP had been determined separately in the serum and urine by chemical and microbiological methods, in the last time also with HPLC (HOUIN et al. 1983; LOOS et al. 1985). It was discovered that the excretions of RMP and of deacetyl-RMP are accelerated simultaneously (ACOCELLA 1978; MOUTON et al. 1979). In clinical treatment, the induction phase lasts 4 weeks–8 weeks, depending on the rythm of application (IWAINSKY et al. 1974). After 7 days without the drug, the values return to their initial level.

RMP is apparently a selective inductor of the oxidative biotransformation of drugs (ZILLY et al. 1977). This is indicated by the increases – observed after RMP therapy – of the NADPH-cytochrome C-reductase, cytochrome P 450, and glucuronyl-transferase and by the absence of the induction phase in patients with liver damage (HAKIM et al. 1971; SCHOENE et al. 1972; OTANI and REMMER 1975). Because of the unusual shift of the absorption maximum of the cytochrome P 450-CO-complex in comparison with other inductors (3-methylcholanthrene, hexobarbital) after administration of RMP, the latter is ascribed atypical inductor properties (HEUBEL and NETTER 1979).

3. Pharmacokinetics

Just 5 min after intravenous administrations, the ^{14}C-RMP concentration in mouse tissue is higher than that in the blood. At the same time, beginning renal excretion and elimination via the gastric mucosa are discernible. After 4 h the RMP concentration in the lungs falls again to that in the blood. At this time the liver, myocardium, salivary glands, pancreas, and brown fat tissue all exhibit high concentrations. The RMP is largely excreted after 24 h, being still detectable after 4 days only in the liver and the intestines. In the CNS, on the other hand, no RMP can be detected throughout the entire period (BOMAN 1975). In the rat the RMP concentration is lower than that in the serum in only a few organs, namely the brain, testicles, fat tissue, pleural fluid, sputum, and milk (Fig. 5, MEYER-BRUNOT et al. 1967). The concentration in other organs is 2–3 times as high as that in the serum. As one would expect of a drug that is excreted with the bile, the RMP concentrations in the liver and the gall-bladder are particularly high. According to experiments on guinea pigs, a depot effect must be reckoned with in the lesion (BLASI et al. 1971).

In man RMP is rapidly distributed throughout the body water (ACOCELLA 1967; FURESZ et al. 1967). Seventy-five – 98% is bound to the serum proteins, half of this to albumin (Table 3, p. 419, BEEUWKES et al. 1969; BINDA et al. 1971; BOMAN 1974; BOMAN and RINGBERGER 1974; AOYAGI 1977; ABAI and TOMCHANI 1979). Tables 2 and 3 show the course of the RMP concentration in the serum as a function of the dose after oral administration (FURESZ 1970; KÖHLER and

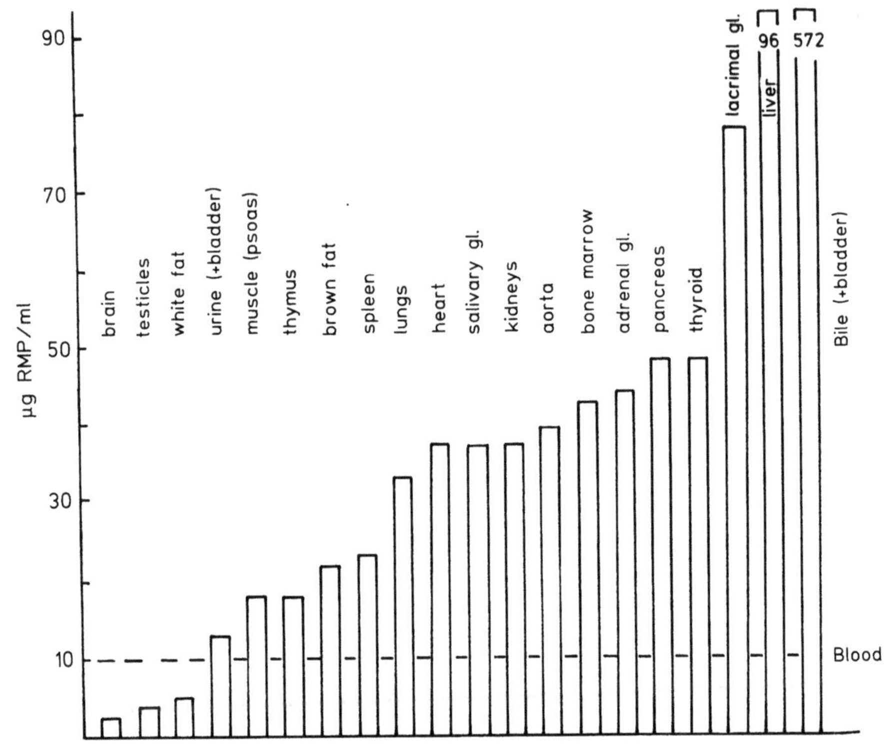

Fig. 5. RMP concentrations in the blood and tissue of rats (MEYER-BRUNOT et al. 1967, 20 mg RMP/kg i.v.)

WINSEL 1982) and Fig. 6 the corresponding course after intravenous infusion (NITTI et al. 1977). The concentrations in the spleen correspond to that in the serum; those in the lungs, the fat tissue, and milk are lower and those in the sputum and pathologically altered lung tissue are substantially lower (~35% of the RMP concentration in the serum). The increase of the RMP concentration in the pleural fluid takes place more slowly, a maximum being reached only after 5 h–11 h. After 12 h the values are again lower than in the plasma (TSUKAMURA 1972; BOMAN 1974; PAWLOWSKA and PNIEWSKI 1975; DOLD and PETERSEN 1978). In view of the biotransformation pattern, the presence of an oxidizing enzyme in the sputum is suspected (BEEUWKES et al. 1969; HUSSELS 1969; DEVINE et al. 1970; SUNAHARA and NAKAGAWA 1972; KISLITSYNA and KOTOVA 1975; KISS et al. 1975; PAWLOWSKA and PNIEWSKI 1975).

Unlike the ototoxic antibiotics, RMP does not accumulate in the perilymph.

RMP quickly passes into the foetal circulation, 10 to 30% of the concentration in the maternal serum being measured. Elimination takes place slowly in the foetus, which should be borne in mind in the event of prolonged daily administration (TERMINE and SANTUARI 1968). The course of the concentration in the CSF is like damped oscillation (Table 7, p. 423). The concentration maxima are lower than in the blood, but RMP concentrations exceeding the MIC can be de-

Table 2. RMP concentration in human serum (μg/ml) in dependence on the dose (FURESZ 1970)

n	Dose (mg) p.o.	Blood sample taken after h					
		2	4	8	12	16	24
6	100	0.9	0.5	0.1	–	–	–
27	150	1.9	1.2	0.4	–	–	–
10	250	3.2	3.0	1.1	0.3	–	–
5	300	5.7	3.5	1.6	0.4	–	–
13	450	7.9	6.8	5.4	2.1	0.6	0.1
12	600	8.8	7.4	–	–	1.2	0.2
10	750	20.9	17.6	10.3	4.9	–	0.4
9	900	27.7	22.5	15.4	8.3	–	1.6

Table 3. RMP concentration in the serum (μg/ml) of tuberculosis patients in dependence on the orally administered dose (KÖHLER and WINSEL 1982)

RMP dose	*n*	RMP concentration (μg/ml)			
		3 h	6 h	9 h	regression
600 mg	82	15.3 ± 5.6	10.7 ± 4.1	7.4 ± 3.6	−0.9999
900 mg	132	25.1 ± 6.3	17.6 ± 4.6	12.7 ± 3.2	−0.9997
1800 mg	132	33.5 ± 8.6	23.1 ± 7.0	17.1 ± 5.7	−0.9981

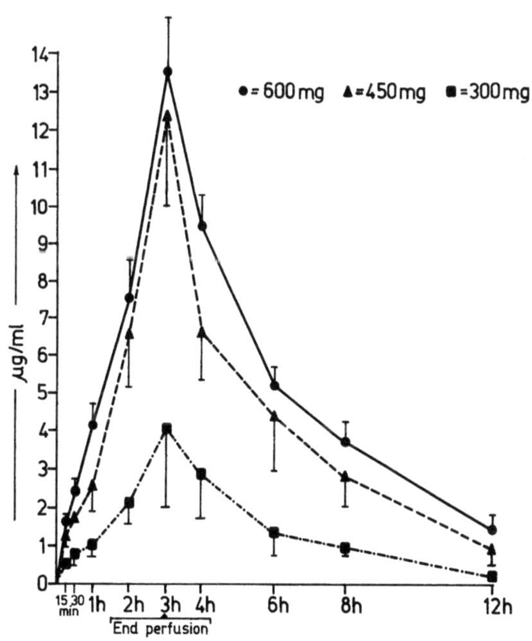

Fig. 6. RMP concentration in serum after intravenous infusion in dependence on the dose (NITTI et al. 1977)

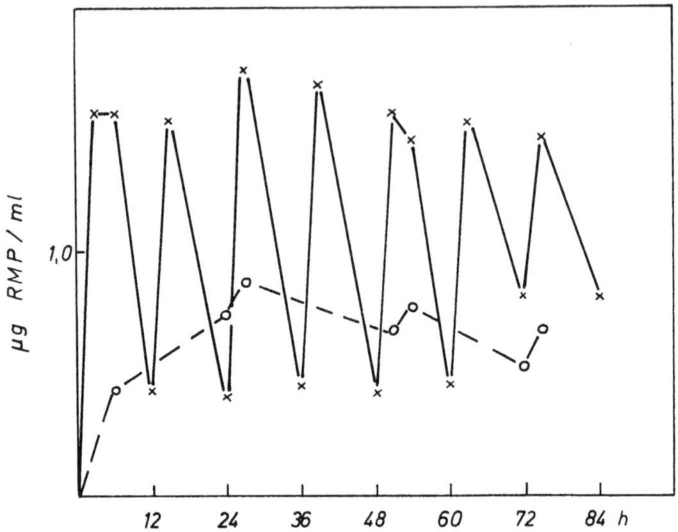

Fig. 7. RMP concentration in the serum and CSF in man (D'OLIVEIRA, 1972). Administration of 300 mg RMP every 12 h, mean values of 10 patients. ×——× serum concentration; o——o CSF concentration.

tected for a longer time. The scatter of the individual values in the CSF is wider than in the serum, probably because of differences in the degree of inflammation (Fig. 7, D'OLIVEIRA 1972). RMP has been proposed for the treatment of meningitis tuberculosa (PILHEU 1975).

The enterohepatic circulation and the biliary excretion are in the foreground in the excretion of RMP. Between 41% and 67% of the administered dose is recovered (FURESZ et al. 1967; ACOCELLA et al. 1972; NAKAGAWA and SUNAHARA 1973). RMP and deacetyl-RMP are excreted predominantly via the liver and bile. Deacetyl-RMP is not reabsorbed (VERBIST and ROLLIER 1971; DECROIX and DJUROVIC 1972; BOMAN 1974). Some 10% to 15% of the administered dose is excreted with the urine (Table 4, KÖHLER and WINSEL 1982), the urinary excretion being higher in women than in men (WINSEL et al. 1985). The fraction of deacetyl-RMP in the urine is lower than that in the bile. The excretion via the kidneys is dose-dependent. There is a direct correlation between the individual RMP clear-

Table 4. Excretion of RMP and its biotransformation products with the urine (mg/24 h) in dependence on the orally administered dose (KÖHLER and WINSEL 1982)

RMP dose	*n*	RMP excretion (mg/24 h)	% of the dose
600 mg	71	62.1 ± 27.9	10.4 ± 4.7
900 mg	108	121.1 ± 53.8	13.5 ± 6.0
1800 mg	134	230.5 ± 97.5	12.8 ± 5.4

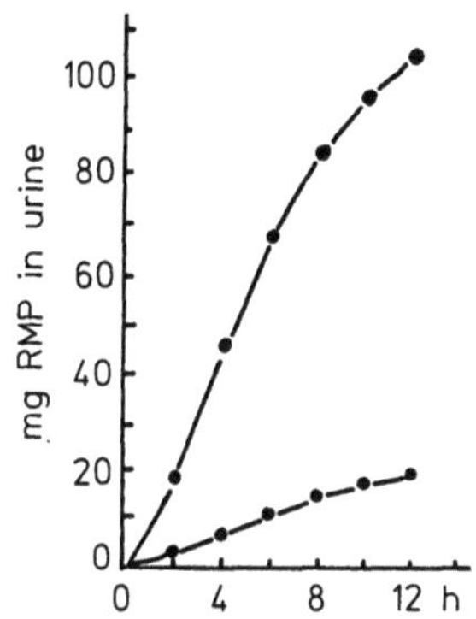

Fig. 8

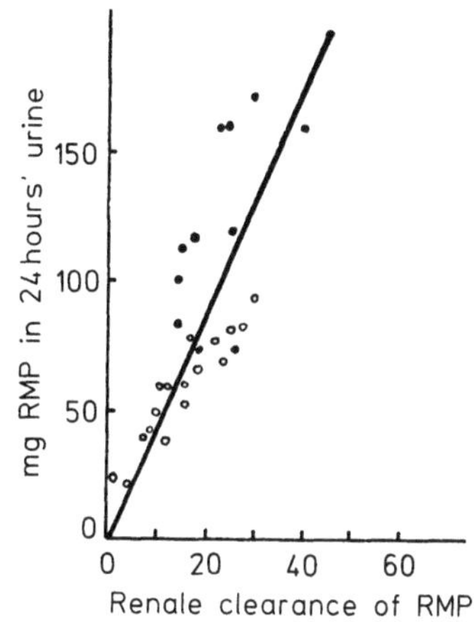

Fig. 9

Fig. 8. Excretion of total RMP (*top*) and deacetyl-RMP (*bottom*) with the urine (NAKAGAWA and SUNAHARA 1973, cumulative curves after 450 mg RMP p.o.)

Fig. 9. Correlations between RMP excretion with the urine and renal RMP clearance (NAKAGAWA and SUNAHARA 1973). ● First dose; ○ administration after 2 and/or 3 months of daily treatment

ance and the quantity of RMP excreted with the urine (Fig. 8 and 9, NAKAGAWA and SUNAHARA 1973; JANISZEWSKI and SZEWCZYK 1975). The maximum RMP concentration in the urine is measured at between 3 h and 6 h after administration of the substance (IOFFE 1973).

During the induction phase, the biliary excretion increases and accordingly the RMP concentration and RMP excretion with the urine decrease (IWAINSKY et al. 1971; SUNAHARA and NAKAGAWA 1972). RMP competitively inhibits the excretion of bilirubin via the liver. After administration of RMP an increased quantity of bilirubin is thus excreted with the urine (VERBIST and ROLLIER 1971).

In order to keep down the costs of the RMP, which is relatively expensive, attempts have been made to reduce its rate of excretion with a simultaneous increase of its serum concentration by prescribing it simultaneously with probenecid. However, the concentrations increases thus obtained do not justify this approach (KENWRIGHT and LEVY 1973; ALLEN et al. 1975; FALLON et al. 1975).

A different utilization of the two routes of excretion has been observed in animal experiments. In mice excretion with the urine is the predominant route, while

Table 5. Renal biliary excretion of RMP in various animal species (% of the dose, TENCONI and BERETTA 1970)

Route of excretion	Mouse	Rat	Guinea pig	Rabbit	Dog
Urinary (24 h)	19%	13%	4%	5%	10%
Biliary (4 h)	7%	37%	17%	16%	1%

it is the route least used in the guinea pig. In the rat excretion with the bile is the most important, while this route is used least in the dog (Table 5, TENCONI and BERETTA 1970).

Further data on pharmacokinetic parameters, and the like are given in Tables 6 and 8, 9, 11 (pp. 421, 424, 425, 433). RMP excretion with urine decreases with progression of renal insufficiency but plasma levels are not influenced (TITARENKO et al. 1983). For more information about dosage to patients with kidney damage see Table 10, p. 426. Information on the induction properties of RMP and on their effects is given in Sections II.3 and II.4 of the General Part (pp. 409 and 410).

References

Abai AM, Tomchani A (1979) Rifampicin binding by the blood serum proteins. Probl Tuberk 57 issue 1: 54–59
Acocella G (1967) A comparative study on the concentration of two antibiotics in the human appendix wall. Chemotherapia 12:36–40
Acocella G (1978) Clinical pharmacokinetics of rifampicin. Clin Pharmacokinet 3:108–127
Acocella G, Conti R (1980) Interaction of rifampicin with other drugs. Tubercle 61:171–177
Acocella G, Mattiussi R, Segre G (1978) Multicompartmental analysis of serum, urine and bile concentrations of rifampicin and desacetyl-rifampicin in subjects treated for one week. Pharmacol Res Commun 10:271–288
Acocella G, Bonollo L, Garimoldi M, Mainhardi M, Tenconi LT, Nicolis FB (1972) Kinetics of rifampicin and isoniazid administered alone and in combination to normal subjects and patients with liver disease. Gut 13:47–53
Allen BW, Ellard GA, Mitchison DA, Hatfield ARW, Kenwright S, Levi AJ (1975) Probenecid and serum-rifampicin. Lancet II:1309
Aoyagi T (1977) Clinical problems on the binding of protein to antituberculous drugs. Kekkaku 52:459–468
Beeuwkes H, Buytendijk HJ, Maesen FPV (1969) Der Wert des Rifampicin bei der Behandlung von Patienten mit bronchopulmonären Affektionen. Arzneimittelforsch 19:1283–1285
Binda G, Domenichini E, Gottardi A, Orlandi B, Ortelli E, Pacini B, Foust G (1971) Rifampicin, a general review. Arzneimittelforsch 21:1907–1977 (M, B, Ph)
Blasi A, Ninni A, Olivieri D, Caputi M (1971) Livelli ematici, livelli tessutali e livelli lesionali della rifamicina nella cavia infettata con micobatteri tubercolari. Giorn Ital Mal Tor 25:283–287
Blundell MR, Wild DC (1971) Altered ribosomes after inhibition of Escherichia coli by rifampicin. Biochem J 121:391–398
Bolt HM (1975) Nebenwirkungen von Rifampicin und ihre biochemischen Grundlagen. Dtsch Med Wochenschr 100:63–65
Boman G (1974) Clinical and experimental studies on rifampicin: distribution, kinetics and drug interactions. Thesis, Stockholm
Boman G (1975) Autoradiographic studies of the distribution of rifampicin. Scand J Respir Dis Suppl 93:3
Boman G, Ringberger V-A (1974) Binding of rifampicin by human plasma proteins. Eur J Clin Pharmacol 7:369–373
Canetti G, Djurovic V, Le Lirzin M, Thibier R, Lepeuple A (1970) Étude comparative de l' évolution des taux sanguins de rifampicine chez l' homme par deux méthodes microbiologiques différentes. Rev Tuberc Pneumol 34:93–106
Decroix G, Djurovic V (1972) Taux sanguin de rifampicine chez les tuberculeux cirrhotiques. Rev Tuberc Pneumol 36:1003–1008

Devine IF, Johnson DP, Hagerman CR, Pierce WE, Rhode SL, Peckinpaugh RO (1970) Rifampin. Levels in serum and saliva and effect on the meningococcal carrier state. JAMA 214:1055–1059

Dickinson JM, Jackett PS, Mitchison DA (1972) The effect of pulsed exposures to rifampicin on the uptake of uridine-^{14}C by *Mycobacterium tuberculosis*. Am Rev Respir Dis 105:519–527

Dold U, Petersen KF (1978) Sputumkonzentrationen von Rifampicin vor und nach Bromhexin-Gabe. Prax Klin Pneumol 32:543–550

Fallon RJ, Allan GW, Lees AW, Smith J, Tyrrell WF (1975) Probenecid and rifampicin serum levels. Lancet II:792–796

Furesz S (1970) Chemical and biological properties of rifampicin. Antibiot Chemother 16:316–351

Furesz S, Scotti R, Pallanza R, Mapelli E (1967) Rifampicin: A new rifamycin. III. Absorption, distribution and elimination in man. Arzneimittelforsch 17:534–537

Grassi GG (1971) Aspetti dell' attività antimicobatterica della rifampicina. Giorn Ital Mal Tor 25:77–88

Hakim J, Feldmann G, Boucherot J, Boivin P, Guibout P, Kreis B (1971) Effect of rifampicin, isoniazid and streptomycin on the human liver: a problem of enzyme induction. Gut 12:761

Handschin J, Wunderli W, Wehrli W (1976) The binding of rifampicin to RNA polymerase at various transcription steps. EXPEAM 32:796

Hartmann G, Honikel KO, Knüsel F, Nüesch J (1967) The specific inhibition of the DNA-directed RNA synthesis by rifamycin. Biochim Biophys Acta 145:843–844

Heubel F, Netter KJ (1979) Atypical inductive properties of rifampicin. Biochem Pharmacol 28:3373–3378

Holdiness MR (1984) Clinical pharmacokinetics of the antituberculosis drugs. Clin Pharmacokin 9:511–544

Honikel K, Sippel A, Hartmann G (1968) Mode of action of antibiotics on DNA-directed polymerase reactions. Hoppe-Seyler's Z Physiol Chem 349:957

Houin G, Beucler A, Richelet S (1983) Pharmacokinetics of rifampicin and desacetylrifampicin in tuberculous patients after different rates of infusion. Ther Drug Monit 5:67–72

Hussels H-J (1969) Zur Methodik der Serum-Konzentrationsbestimmungen des neuen Antibiotikums Rifampicin. Med Lab 22:195–203

Ioffe RA (1973) Rifampicin passage with urine during treatment of tuberculous patients. Probl Tuberk 51 issue 12: 43–46

Iwainsky H, Eule H, Winsel K, Werner E (1971) Pharmakokinetic of high rifampicin-dosages during intermittent controlled chemotherapy. Acta Tuberc Pneumol Belg 62:326–327

Iwainsky H, Winsel K, Werner E, Eule H (1974) On the pharmacokinetics of rifampicin I: Influence of dosage and duration of treatment with intermittent administration. Scand J Respir Dis 55:229–236

Iwainsky H, Winsel K, Werner E, Eule H (1976) On the pharmacokinetics of rifampicin (RMP) during treatment with intermittent administration II. Influence of age and sex of the patients. Scand J Respir Dis 57:5–11

Janiszewski M, Szewczyk I (1975) Assessment of the diagnostic usefulness of a chemical method of determination of rifampicin in the urine. Gruzlica 37:157–162

Kenwright S, Levi AJ (1973) Impairment of hepatic uptake of rifamycin antibiotics by probenecid and its therapeutic implications. Lancet II:1401–1405

Kislitsyna NA, Kotova NI (1975) Rifampicin concentration in pathological formations of resected lungs. Probl Tuberk 53 issue 6: 79–81

Kiss J, Farago E, Juhasz I, Bacsa S, Fabian E (1975) Untersuchung des Rifampicinspiegels im Blutserum und Lungengewebe des Menschen. Tuberkulózis (Budapest) XXVIII:82–86

Köhler H, Winsel K (1982) Klinische und experimentelle Untersuchungen zur Optimierung der Chemotherapie der Lungen- und Nierentuberkulose. Promotion B-Arbeit, Friedrich-Schiller-Universität, Jena

Kolos OT, Eidus LL (1972) A simple thin-layer chromatographic method for the separation and identification of rifampin and its metabolites. J Chromatogr 68:294–295

Konno K, Oizumi K, Hayshi I, Oka S (1972) Action mode of rifampicin on Mycobacterium tuberculosis. Kekkaku 47:255–260

Konno K, Oizumi K, Ariji F, Yamaguchi J, Oka S (1973a) Mode of action of rifampin on mycobacteria. I. Electron microscopic study of the effect of rifampin on *Mycobacterium tuberculosis*. Am Rev Respir Dis 107:1002–1005

Konno K, Oizumi K, Oka S (1973b) Mode of action of rifampin on mycobacteria. II. Biosynthetic studies on the inhibition of ribonucleic acid polymerase of *Mycobacterium bovis* BCG by rifampin and uptake of rifampin-^{14}C by *Mycobacterium phlei*. Am Rev Respir Dis 107:1006–1012

Konno K, Motomiya M, Oizumi K, Ariji F (1977) Mode of action of antituberculosis drugs on tubercle bacilli. Kekkaku 52:661–668

Leoni L, Tecce G (1963) Azione della rifamicina SV sulle reazioni della sintesi proteica in vitro. Chemotherapia 7:194–199

Loos U, Musch E, Jensen JC, Mikus G, Schwabe HK, Eichelbaum M (1985) Pharmacokinetics of oral and intravenous rifampicin during chronic administration. Klin Wochenschr 63:1205–1211

Maggi N, Furesz S, Pallanza R, Pelizza G (1969) Rifampicin desacetylation in the human organism. Arzneimittelforsch 19:651–654

Meyer-Brunot HG, Schmid K, Keberle H (1967) Stoffwechsel und Pharmakokinetik von Rifampicin bei Tier und Mensch. Proc V^th Int Congress Chemotherapy Vienna Vol I/2:763–770

Michel-Briand Y (1978) Mécanismes d'action des antibiotiques, à propos de quelques exemples. CR Soc Biol 172:609–627

Mišoň P, Trnka L (1973) Zum Wirkungsmechanismus von Rifampicin. Mschr Lungenkrankh Tbk-Bekpfg 16:259–264

Mouton RP, Mattie H, Suart K, Kreukniet J, de Wael J (1979) Blood levels of rifampicin, desacetyl-rifampicin and isoniazid during combined therapy. J Antimicrob Chemother 5:447–454

Nakagawa H, Sunahara S (1973) Metabolism of rifampicin in the human body. 1st report. Kekkaku 48:167–176

Nitti V, Virgilio R, Patricolo MR, Juliano A (1977) Pharmacokinetic study of intravenous rifampicin. Chemotherapy 23:1–6

D'Oliveira JJG (1972) Cerebrospinal fluid concentrations of rifampin in meningeal tuberculosis. Am Rev Respir Dis 106:432–437

Otani G, Remmer H (1975) Participation of microsomal NADPH-cytochrome C reductase in the metabolism of rifampicin. Naunyn-Schmiedebergs Arch Pharmacol 287 Suppl: R76

Pawlowska I, Pniewski T (1975) On the methodology of determination of rifampicin (RMP) concentration in sputum. Gruzlica 43:969–975

Pilheu JA (1975) Rifampicin concentrations in cerebrospinal fluid of patients with tuberculous meningitis. Am Rev Respir Dis 111:240

Pogo BGT (1971) Biogenesis of vaccinia: effect of rifampicin on transcription. Virology 44:576–581

Ritter W (1973) Neue Ergebnisse über Biotransformation und Pharmakokinetik von Antituberkulotika. Prax Pneumol 27:139–145 (B, Ph)

Schoene B, Fleischmann RA, Remmer H, Oldershausen HF v (1972) Induction of drug-metabolizing enzymes in human liver. Naunyn-Schmiedebergs Arch Pharmacol 274 Suppl: R 101

Sunahara S, Nakagawa H (1972) Metabolic study and controlled clinical trials of rifampin. Chest 61:526–532

Tenconi LT, Beretta E (1970) Urinary and biliary metabolites of rifampicin in different animal species. In: Baker SBDC, Tripod J, Jacob J (eds) Proc Europ Soc for the Study of Drug Toxicity 11:80–85. Excerpta Media Foundation, Amsterdam

Termine A, Santuari E (1968) Il passaggio trans-placentare delle rifampicina. Dosaggio del farmaco nel siero materno e fetale e nel liquido amniotico. Ann Ist Forlanini 28:431–439

Titarenko OT, Vakhmistrova TI, Perova TL (1983) Rifampicin excretion with urine in patients with renal insufficiency treated with rifampicin alone or in combination with isoniazid. Antibiotiki 28:698–702
Toyohara M (1971) An experimental study on the antituberculous activity of rifampicin. Kekkaku 46:211–216
Tsukamura M (1972) Permeability of tuberculous cavities to antituberculosis drugs. Tubercle 53:47–52
Tsukamura M, Imazu S, Tsukamura S, Mizuno S, Toyama H, Termine A, Rossi P (1963) Studies on the mode of action of rifamycin SV. Chemotherapia 7:478–481
Umezawa H, Mizuno S, Yamazaki H, Nitta K (1968) Inhibition of DNA-dependent RNA synthesis by rifamycins. J Antibiotics 21:234–235
Verbist L, Rollier F (1971) Pharmacological study of rifampicin after repeated high dosage during intermittent combined therapy. II. Bilirubin levels and other biochemical determinations. Respiration 28 Suppl: 17–28
Wehrli W, Staehelin M (1971) Actions of the rifamycins. Bact Rev 35:290–309
White RJ, Lancini GC, Silvestri LG (1971) Mechanism of action of rifampin on *Mycobacterium smegmatis*. J Bacteriol 108:737–741
Winsel K, Iwainsky H, Werner E, Eule H (1976) Trennung, Bestimmung und Pharmakokinetik von Rifampicin und seinen Biotransformationsprodukten. Pharmazie 31:95–99
Winsel K, Eule H, Werner E, Iwainsky H (1985) Zur Pharmakokinetik des Rifampicins (RMP) bei intermittierender Behandlung von Patienten mit Lungentuberkulose. Pharmazie 40:253–256
Zilly W, Breimer DD, Richter E (1977) Stimulation of drug metabolism by rifampicin in patients with cirrhosis or cholestasis measured by increased hexobarbital and tolbutamide clearance. Europ J Clin Pharmacol 11:287–293

Subject Index

Handbook of Experimental Pharmacology

Continuation of "Handbuch der experimentellen Pharmakologie"

Editorial Board
G. V. R. Born, A. Farah,
H. Herken, A. D. Welch

Springer-Verlag
Berlin Heidelberg New York
London Paris Tokyo

Volume 44
Heme and Hemoproteins

Volume 45: Part 1
Drug Addiction I

Part 2
Drug Addiction II

Volume 46
Fibrinolytics and Antifibronolytics

Volume 47
Kinetics of Drug Action

Volume 48
Arthropod Venoms

Volume 49
Ergot Alkaloids and Related Compounds

Volume 50: Part 1
Inflammation

Part 2
Anti-Inflammatory Drugs

Volume 51
Uric Acid

Volume 52
Snake Venoms

Volume 53
Pharmacology of Ganglionic Transmission

Volume 54: Part 1
Adrenergic Activators and Inhibitors I

Part 2
Adrenergic Activators and Inhibitors II

Volume 55
Psychotropic Agents

Part 1
Antipsychotics and Antidepressants

Part 2
Anxiolytics, Gerontopsychopharmacological Agents and Psychomotor Stimulants

Part 3
Alcohol and Psychotomimetics, Psychotropic Effects of Central Acting Drugs

Volume 56, Part 1 + 2
Cardiac Glycosides

Volume 57
Tissue Growth Factors

Volume 58
Cyclic Nucleotides

Part 1
Biochemistry

Part 2
Physiology and Pharmacology

Volume 59
Mediators and Drugs in Gastrointestinal Motility

Part 1
Morphological Basis and Neurophysiological Control

Part 2
Endogenous and Exogenous Agents

Volume 60
Pyretics and Antipyretics

Springer

Handbook of Experimental Pharmacology

Continuation of "Handbuch der experimentellen Pharmakologie"

Editorial Board
G. V. R. Born, A. Farah,
H. Herken, A. D. Welch

Springer-Verlag
Berlin Heidelberg New York
London Paris Tokyo

Volume 61
Chemotherapy of Viral Infections

Volume 62
Aminoglycoside Antibiotics

Volume 63
Allergic Reactions to Drugs

Volume 64
Inhibition of Folate Metabolism in Chemotherapy

Volume 65
Teratogenesis and Reproductive Toxicology

Volume 66
Part 1: **Glucagon I**
Part 2: **Glucagon II**

Volume 67
Part 1
Antibiotics Containing the Beta-Lactam Structure I
Part 2
Antibiotics Containing the Beta-Lactam Structure II

Volume 68, Part 1+2
Antimalarial Drugs

Volume 69
Pharmacology of the Eye

Volume 70
Part 1
Pharmacology of Intestinal Permeation I
Part 2
Pharmacology of Intestinal Permeation II

Volume 71
Interferons and Their Applications

Volume 72
Antitumor Drug Resistance

Volume 73
Radiocontrast Agents

Volume 74
Antieliptic Drugs

Volume 75
Toxicology of Inhaled Materials

Volume 76
Clinical Pharmocology of Antiangial Drugs

Volume 77
Chemotherapy of Gastrointestinal Helminths

Volume 78
The Tetracycline

Volume 79
New Neuromuscular Blocking Agents

Volume 80
Cadmium

Volume 81
Local Anesthetics

Volume 82
Radioimmunoassay in Basic and Clinical Pharmacology

Volume 83
Calcium in Drug Actions

Springer